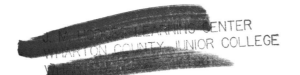

Medical and Health Sources for *Health Care U.S.A.*

The names of the clinics, centers, physicians, and other health professionals listed in this book were provided by the following government health agencies, professional medical and health associations, academic institutions, and voluntary health associations as well as by our own survey of leading medical centers.

Alcohol, Drug Abuse and Mental Health Administration
American Academy of Environmental Medicine
American Association for the Study of Headaches
American Association of Suicidology
American Association of Tissue Banks
American Association of University Affiliated Programs
American Burn Association
American College of Nurse Midwives
American Fertility Society
American Geriatric Society
American Liver Foundation
American Medical Association
American Osteopathic Association
American Speech-Language Association
Association of American Medical Colleges
Association of Sleep Disorders Centers
Children's Cancer Study Group
Children's Hospice International
Commission on Accreditation on Rehabilitation Facilities
Cystic Fibrosis Foundation
Health Care Financing Administration
Huntington's Disease Society
Multiple Sclerosis Society
Muscular Dystrophy Association
National Association of Alcoholism Treatment Programs
National Cancer Institute
National Center for Education in Maternal and Child Health
National Kidney Foundation

National Heart, Lung and Blood Institute
National Institute of Allergy and Infectious Diseases
National Institute of Arthritis and Musculoskeletal and Skin Diseases
National Institute of Child Health and Human Development
National Institute of Diabetes and Digestive and Kidney Diseases
National Institute of General Medical Sciences
National Institute of Handicapped Research
National Institute of Neurological and Communicative Disorders and Stroke
National Institute on Alcohol Abuse and Alcoholism
National Institute on Drug Abuse
National Neurofibromatosis Foundation
National Psoriasis Foundation
National Society for Children and Adults with Autism
National Sudden Infant Death Syndrome Clearinghouse
National Tay-Sachs and Allied Diseases Association
Orton Dyslexia Society
Paget's Disease Foundation
Parkinson's Disease Foundation
Pediatric Oncology Group
Phobia Society of America
Retinitis Pigmentosa Foundation
Spina Bifida Association of America
United Parkinson Foundation
Western Psychiatric Institute, University of Pittsburgh School of Medicine

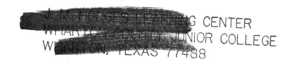

HEALTH CARE
U.S.A.

Jean Carper

74323

PRENTICE HALL PRESS · New York

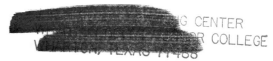

Published by Prentice Hall Press
A Division of Simon & Schuster, Inc.
Gulf +Western Building
One Gulf +Western Plaza
New York, NY 10023

PRENTICE HALL PRESS is a trademark of Simon & Schuster, Inc.

Library of Congress Cataloging-in-Publication Data

Carper, Jean.
Health care U.S.A.

Includes bibliographies.
1. Medical care—Information services—United States—Directories. 2. Diseases—Information services—United States—Directories. 3. Medical centers—United States—Directories. 4. Medicine—Research—United States—Directories. 5. Consumer education—United States—Directories. I. Title.
[DNLM: 1. Health Services—United States—directories. W 22 AA1 C2h]
R118.4.U6C37   1987   362.1'02573   86-25556
ISBN 0-13-609686-7
ISBN 0-13-609694-8 (pbk.)

Manufactured in the United States of America

10 9 8 7 6 5 4 3 2 1

First Edition

*To my mother, Natella Boyer Carper,
for her enduring good spirit and temperament*

Acknowledgments

The idea for this book originated in 1983 and since that time a great number of people have been involved in making it a reality. I especially want to thank Elizabeth Brooks, an indefatigable and meticulous researcher who cheerfully saw this book through four years of information gathering, updating, and verification; Ann Barker, who did important final checking and revisions of the many lists of experts; Sheila Harvill and Laura Gilliam, for typing the long lists onto computer.

I would also like to express my profound gratitude to the dozens of people who read the manuscript and galleys for content, accuracy, and style. Among them, Abigail Trafford, a superb journalist and editor who helped shape the book with her excellent suggestions and editing; Storm Whaley, associate director for communications, the National Institutes of Health, and his staff and other specialists at NIH who both supplied much research material and suggested changes on the manuscript; the numerous executive directors and staffs of the voluntary health associations who spent many hours collecting and providing information and verifying it; the public information staffs of medical colleges who sent information about their physicians and medical facilities; and the many physicians and other health specialists who read the text of the sections for medical accuracy.

Also thanks to my agent, Raphael Sagalyn, for his expanded vision of the book and his faith in its ultimate publication; to my original editor, Victoria Skurnick, who added immeasurably to the scope of the book; and to Paul Aron, my final editor, whose appreciation of the book's intent and potential was mainly responsible for its completion and publication.

Contents

INTRODUCTION

Anyone who is in medical trouble wants to know where to find help, help of all kinds, the broadest, most precise, most compelling help available—help from the experts, help from people in similar trouble, help from those who have triumphed and survived, help from books, help from researchers, help from the government, help from agencies, professional associations, and, most of all, help from the best, most knowledgeable physicians and other health professionals in the country.

That is the reason for this book. It is a national directory of medical information to help you find the resources to cope with the great number of disorders, diseases, and conditions that may strike you, your family or your friends. Most of the medical problems discussed in this book are quite serious—life-threatening or physically or mentally disabling. All of them are chronic or permanent, requiring attention over a period of time. This is not a book of symptoms, of self-diagnosis, of acute or emergency do-it-yourself medical care. This is a book of where to go after you know you have a problem—usually after your primary physician knows you have a problem. It is a book of resources, references and support systems, as well as of physician and health specialists. In many instances it will provide names to contact on your own; in others it is a source for a second opinion or a referral from your primary physician.

As far as we know, this is the first book of its kind: a compendium that puts together a vast and diverse amount of consumer health information in one place (names and phone numbers of specialists, researchers, clinics and centers as well as hotlines, publications, associations and government agencies), making it instantly accessible when you *need* it—not after a crisis has passed.

Also important and unique is that *Health Care U.S.A.*'s list of specialists was not arbitrarily compiled by the author or by a small select group of physicians or other experts. The lists of centers, physicians and other health care professionals included in each chapter came from established, respected medical sources such as physicians' professional associations, medical accreditation bodies, voluntary health associations and government agencies. Thus, *Health Care U.S.A.* represents a *national consensus* of the best sources of medical information according to leading organized bodies of medical expertise. It is a sourcebook that gives you access to the best and most highly acclaimed medical care.

We have tried to make the book broadly based to make it possible for you to find sources close to home, no matter where you live. The sources of the lists of experts are noted within each section.

Generally, *Health Care U.S.A.* is organized to present five points of vital information about each medical problem. First, there is a description of the disease or problem: its prevalence, symptoms, diagnosis, latest types of treatments, including standard "state-of-the-art" treatment, and sometimes experimental treatments. Second, whenever available there is a roster of medical experts on the subject, such as clinics, centers, physician specialists, and hospital-based services. Some examples include pain clinics, sexual dysfunction clinics, government cancer and arthritis centers, government-accredited hospices, drug abuse clinics geared to adolescents, phobia and depression specialists. Third, you will find in each section a list of books, free

1

and for-sale literature, audio- and videotapes and other available materials, and special services to help you learn more and cope better. The fourth component of each section is a list of self-help, voluntary health organizations and federal government health agencies that provide ongoing mutual support and valuable information. Fifth, there is notice of who is doing selected experimental therapy and how you can find them should there be cause to think you could benefit from the research.

As I wrote and compiled this book, I tried to keep in mind one thing: if I were seeking help for a particular medical problem, what would I want to know, what sources would I want to know existed, whom would I need to consult, where could I find reliable information and help? Is there any special new or experimental therapy I would like to know about?

I was constantly amazed and thrilled at the wealth of everyday helpful information that only a few health specialists knew about, and yet was of tremendous benefit. While working on the book, I met the parents of a brain-damaged child who did not have the faintest idea where to find community support and help. Using information from *Health Care U.S.A.*, I could tell them of a center in their area. A friend in Chicago needed a depression expert; I could refer her to one from a list circulated by the National Institute of Mental Health. When a friend of one of my researchers was contemplating back surgery because of extreme pain, we consulted the list of pain clinics and located one near her home in New England.

A prime source of information was that vast reservoir of medical knowledge and research—the National Institutes of Health (NIH). NIH has experts in virtually every field of medicine; publishes innumerable reports, pamphlets, magazines and journals, and funds by far most of the medical research in the nation, some of it through established, specialized centers, such as the comprehensive cancer centers and multipurpose arthritis centers. In addition, we did surveys of more than 100 of the country's voluntary health organizations and 75 of the nation's leading medical schools. We asked the organizations what specific services and materials they offered to the public and, in some cases, for the names of leading specialists in their area of concern. We asked the medical schools for information

about specialized patient services offered at their medical centers.

We contacted numerous professional medical and health associations, health-related accrediting agencies, and health-related government agencies for resources they were associated with or knew about. We also ran computerized library searches to discover the existence of important books we had not learned about from other sources.

Health Care U.S.A. reflects two of the strongest new directions in the health care field: a growing emphasis on cooperative team professional medicine and a new reliance on paraprofessional and mutual self-help support from people who have been through medical difficulties and survived to share their experience and knowledge with others. In other words, help from our neighbors, and an increasing responsibility for the state of one's own health.

Thus, the book's emphasis is on medical *centers* of excellence, which typically include many outstanding individual doctors, rather than just a few specialists. Physicians, even the best ones, are not islands unto themselves. As medicine grows more sophisticated and humanistic, it becomes a more cooperative and complex venture. If you have cancer, for example, you don't necessarily need to find the best surgeon or the best radiologist. What you really want is the best oncology "team." A group of professionals can determine the best overall approach, regardless of each doctor's medical speciality.

Much of the best medical care is increasingly multidisciplinary, dependent on various specialists coordinated by a leader or overseer. That is not to say you should not seek out an expert physician, for the individual still makes the critical difference, but sometimes it is more important to get to the proper center than to simply rely on one physician. Any center of excellence will have not one star, but many. Usually you can expect top-notch treatment at such centers no matter whom you encounter there because the extremely competent and creative physicians or health professionals directing that center attract and demand satellite health professionals of equally high quality. That is why this book emphasizes medical centers, clinics, and teams as the best guides to excellent overall care. In nearly all cases the name of the director or a contact at the center is included.

Not surprisingly, the search for medical specialists sometimes leads to universities and medical schools. In such a setting physicians are encouraged to keep up on the latest research and, in fact, conduct much of it. Thus, in a special section at the back of the book you will find lists of certain specialists who are heads of departments at medical schools and can be contacted for sources of specialized medical care.

It should be stressed that the search for specialists should not be conducted at the exclusion of your family physician but in conjunction with him or her. Primary medical care by general practitioners is still the first line of defense against disease and a major force in getting and staying well. The search for a specialist should be a joint venture—a link between you and your family doctor to find the best care. Many physicians desire second opinions and consultations with specialists and often take the initiative in suggesting them. You should not be reluctant to consult your family doctor about specialists noted in this book.

Included in many sections of this book are references to those doing research on a disease or disorder, almost always under the auspices of the National Institutes of Health. Such research not only gives hope, but, in some cases, it can have immediate application for those who are suffering. It is possible that you may be able to participate in such research studies, or benefit from them less directly, by seeking treatment from the researcher as a private patient although you are not part of the study. Your own primary physician may also tune into the latest research and apply it to your case. Surely in the case of cancer, knowledge of the most current procedures can sometimes make a vital difference. It has been estimated that if every cancer patient in the United States had the most up-to-date "state-of-the-art" treatment, the general survival rate would be increased by 15 percent.

At the same time, American health care is changing significantly to give us a greater awareness of self-responsibility. Health care is no longer relegated to the health professional alone. *Health Care U.S.A.* encourages participation in your medical future. For some, that may mean more emphasis on self-help, mutual support, and wider choices outside traditional medical channels. Sometimes the medical establishment is slow to respond. For example, phobias, once treated by traditional psychotherapy and psychoanalysis, which proved virtually useless, are now successfully managed by phobia-treatment centers that usually include recovered phobics as part of the treatment team. Also, the role of psychological attitude in the cause and progression of numerous diseases is emerging as increasingly important.

This new focus on medical self-determination led us to include information for those who want to know about some unconventional medical choices. There are sources of alternative medical care, such as "clinical ecology" allergists, and advocates of new approaches to treating alcoholism and cancer. The mention of such clinics and therapies does not imply an endorsement of them but an offering of information with which to make informed choices.

Because of the new confidence in the ability of fellow sufferers to help each other, you'll find lists of mutual support organizations, with local chapters and support groups, hotlines, and also therapies dependent on the newfound power of paraprofessionals to heal, as they can with phobias.

You'll also find in each section listings of pamphlets, booklets, books and sometimes audio and videocassettes, to help enlighten you and make your input into your own medical care more powerful and meaningful. We tried to choose books that offer the most up-to-date medical information in fast-moving fields, as well as some classics.

Telephone numbers are included in almost all cases although with the realization that they may change. Therefore, some of the phone numbers are general numbers for medical centers or hospitals that stay the same even though a particular physician may move on. If a phone number is not listed the omission may have been dictated by a physician or organization to encourage contact only by mail or through other physicians. We attempted to verify the phone numbers, addresses, and spellings of names; however, there may be some errors. We apologize for these in advance. As for the selection of centers, clinics, organizations and individuals, we probably missed some that should be in the book, despite the help of many excellent sources. Any medical specialists or resources we missed will be included in future editions of this book if we are made aware of them.

We cannot recommend or endorse the physicians, centers, clinics and other health professionals listed here; that is beyond our expertise and competence. Those listed have credentials respected by their peers, and are presented to help consumers make better, more informed choices. We expect that readers will exercise their own judgment about any individual doctor, center, or health professional.

Health Care U.S.A. contains information on all major, life-threatening, disabling and chronic medical problems on which there is a significant and defined body of medical and self-help resources. The health problems that touch the most people are included, as well as some less prevalent disorders, such as Paget's disease and psoriasis. If certain diseases and disorders are missing it is not because we accidentally overlooked them. They are not included because we could not find sufficient resource information to make their inclusion worthwhile.

Often the availability of such information depends on how much active interest government agencies or citizen's groups take in a particular disease or disorder. Diseases that are intensively investigated by the National Institutes of Health and vigorously promoted by voluntary citizens' groups are bound to generate much more information and sources of help than those diseases that have no organized constituency. Thyroid and similar endocrine diseases jump to mind. We could not find self-help groups or any special clinics organized to provide resources on these diseases. When such information is generated on medical problems not found on these pages, we will include it in updates of this directory.

Health Care U.S.A. was read for accuracy before publication by medical experts, including a number of specialists at the National Institutes of Health. However, there are many controversies in medicine. Often experts in the same field do not agree with each other. Statistics, such as figures on how many people have certain diseases, are almost always estimates and are subject to much disagreement, especially between voluntary health organizations, which some accuse of inflating estimates, and government agencies, which tend to be conservative. Some experts prefer upbeat reporting of medical facts; others complain that "good news" reporting of promising new therapies builds false hopes. This book seeks to tread a fine line between legitimate optimism and undue pessimism, and between the interests of voluntary organizations and academic and government scientists, while recognizing both.

In the final analysis, of course, all material was filtered through the judgment of the author, a medical and consumer writer for 20 years. *Health Care U.S.A.* is a first. Three years were spent compiling the data, and because there can be changes during that time, many of the lists were rechecked as close to publication date as possible. Any changes that occurred during production of the book will be updated in future editions. Since we intend to update *Health Care U.S.A.* every two years, we invite readers to share with us opinions and any special information that might make future editions of the book more helpful.

Health Care U.S.A. can tell you where to look and where to go for medical help. It is a vast source of consumer medical information compiled in one reference book for the first time. I hope it gives you new power to find the medical resources to make your life and the lives of your family and friends longer and better.

—JEAN CARPER

NATIONAL HEALTH HOTLINES AND HELPLINES

ACQUIRED IMMUNE DEFICIENCY SYNDROME (AIDS)
(800) 342-AIDS (general-information recording)
(800) 447-AIDS (specific information)
  —U.S. Public Health Service

(800) 221-7044
  —National Gay/Lesbian Crisisline (3–9 P.M. EST)

ALCOHOLISM
(800) 328-9000
  —Hazelden Foundation

ALZHEIMER'S DISEASE AND SENILE DEMENTIA
(800) 621-0379
(800) 572-6037 (in Illinois)
—Alzheimer's Disease and Related Disorders Association

ASTHMA (AND LUNG DISEASES)
(800) 222-LUNG
—National Jewish Hospital/National Asthma Center

CANCER
(800) 4-CANCER
(800) 638-6070 (Alaska)
(808) 524-1234 in Oahu, HI (call collect on neighboring islands)
—National Cancer Institute

CHILDREN
(800) 237-5055
(800) 282-9161 (in Florida)
—Shriners Hospital Referral Line (for children under 18 years of age, needing burn treatment or orthopedic care)

CYSTIC FIBROSIS
(800) FIGHT-CF
(301) 881-9130 (in Maryland)
—Cystic Fibrosis Foundation

DIABETES
(800) 232-3472
(703) 549-1500 (in Virginia)
—American Diabetes Association

(800) 223-1138
(212) 889-7575 (in New York)
—Juvenile Diabetes Foundation International

DIGESTIVE DISEASES
(301) 652-9293 (Tuesday, 7–9 P.M. EST, toll call)
—American Digestive Disease Society

DOWN SYNDROME
(800) 221-4602
(212) 460-9330 (in New York)
—National Down's Syndrome Society

DRUG ABUSE
(800) 662-HELP
—National Institute on Drug Abuse
(800) 554-KIDS
—National Federation of Parents for Drug-Free Youth
(800) 241-7946
—PRIDE
(800) COCAINE (treatment referrals, no counseling)
—Fair Oaks Hospital, Fair Oaks, NJ

DYSLEXIA
(800) ABC-D123
—The Orton Dyslexia Society

EPILEPSY
(800) 426-0660
(206) 323-8174 (in Washington)
—University of Washington

EYES
(800) 424-8567
(202) 727-2142 (in District of Columbia)
—Library of Congress, National Library Services for the Blind and Physically Handicapped
(800) 424-8666
(202) 393-3666 (in District of Columbia)
—American Council for the Blind

HEALTH INFORMATION
(800) 336-4797 (referrals to other sources of information; answers individual questions on side effects of medications)
—National Health Information Clearinghouse

HEARING
(800) 638-8255 (voice/TDD)
(301) 897-8682 (in Hawaii, Maryland, and Alaska)
—National Association for Hearing and Speech Action
(800) 521-5247 (Hearing Aid Hotline)
—National Hearing Aid Society
(800) 424-8576 (Hearing Helpline)
(703) 642-0580 (in Virginia)
—The Better Hearing Institute

HEART
(800) 241-6993
—Association of Heart Patients

KIDNEY
(800) 638-8299
(800) 492-8361 (in Maryland)
—American Kidney Fund

LEPROSY (HANSEN'S DISEASE)
(800) 543-3131
(201) 794-8650 (in New Jersey and Alaska)
—American Leprosy Missions

LIVER
(800) 223-0179
(201) 857-2626 (in New Jersey)
—American Liver Foundation

LUPUS
(800) 558-0121
—Lupus Foundation of America

MULTIPLE SCLEROSIS
(800) 872-2767
—Action for Research in Multiple Sclerosis

ORGAN DONATIONS
(800) 528-2971
(713) 528-2971 (in Texas)
—The Living Bank
(800) 24-DONOR (for physicians and medical
personnel only)
—North American Transplant Coordinators
Organization

PARKINSON'S DISEASE
(800) 344-7872
(714) 640-0218 (in California)
—Parkinson's Educational Program USA

REHABILITATION
(800) 346-2742 (voice/TDD)
—National Rehabilitation Information
Center

RETINITIS PIGMENTOSA
(800) 638-2300
(301) 225-9400 (in Maryland)
(800) 638-1818 (eye donations)
—Retinitis Pigmentosa Foundation

SCLERODERMA
(800) 722-HOPE
—United Scleroderma Foundation

SICKLE-CELL DISEASE
(800) 421-8453
(213) 936-7205 (in California)
—National Association for Sickle Cell
Disease

SMOKING CESSATION
(800) 253-7077
—Seventh-day Adventists

**SPEECH AND LANGUAGE
PROBLEMS**
(800) 638-TALK
—National Association for Hearing and
Speech Action

SPINA BIFIDA
(800) 621-3141 (outside Illinois)
—Spina Bifida Association of America

SPINAL CORD INJURY
(800) 526-3456
(800) 638-1733 (in Maryland)
—Maryland Institute for Emergency
Medical Services Systems
(800) 328-8253
(800) 862-0179 (in Minnesota)
—Spinal Cord Society
(800) 225-0292
(201) 379-2690 (in New Jersey)
—American Paralysis Association

**SUDDEN INFANT DEATH SYNDROME
(SIDS)**
(800) 221-SIDS
—National Sudden Infant Death Syndrome
Foundation

SURGERY
(800) 638-6833 (Second Opinion)
(800) 492-6603 (in Maryland)
—U.S. Department of Health and Human
Services

FEDERAL HEALTH AGENCIES

Public Health Service
Department of Health and Human Services
200 Independence Ave. S.W., Room 716G
Washington, DC 20201
(202) 245-7694

Centers for Disease Control
Department of Health and Human Services
Public Inquiries
Building 1, Room B63
1600 Clifton Rd., N.E.
Atlanta, GA 30333
(404) 329-3534

Food and Drug Administration
Department of Health and Human Services
5600 Fishers Lane
Rockville, MD 20857
(301) 443-2410

Public inquiries about the use or safety of a drug:

Office of Consumer and Professional Affairs
Food and Drug Administration, HFN17
5600 Fishers Lane
Rockville, MD 20857
(301) 295-8012

Public inquiries about the use or safety of a medical or biologic device:

Consumer Inquiries
Food and Drug Administration, HFE-88
5600 Fishers Lane, Room 1663
Rockville, MD 20857
(301) 443-3170

National Institutes of Health
Public Inquiries
Building 31, Room 2B-10
9000 Rockville Pike
Bethesda, MD 20892
(301) 496-2535

If you have questions about Medicare or Medicaid contact your local Social Security Office, or:

Health Care Financing Administration
Inquiries Staff, BERC
Room 9F1
East Low Rise Building
6325 Security Blvd.
Baltimore, MD 21207
(301) 594-9890

Administration on Developmental Disabilities
Office of Human Development Services
Department of Health and Human Services,
Room 348-F
200 Independence Ave., S.W.
Washington, DC 20201
(202) 245-2890

Alcohol, Drug Abuse, and Mental Health
Administration
Parklawn Building
5600 Fishers Lane
Rockville, MD 20857
(301) 443-4883 (alcohol)
(301) 443-4536 (mental health)
(301) 443-6780 (drug abuse)

HOW TO GET TREATMENT AT THE NATIONAL INSTITUTES OF HEALTH

At the Warren Grant Magnuson Clinical Center, a large modern hospital in the heart of the National Institutes of Health campus in Bethesda, Maryland, NIH investigators carry on experimental treatments for all kinds of diseases, disorders and conditions. Some of these "clinical trials" last for several years; some are changed as time goes on, and new ones are begun. Each month, physician-researchers at the NIH Clinical Center accept a limited number of patients to participate in their studies.

To get into NIH's clinical center, you should be referred by a physician or dentist; your disorder, disease or certain particular aspects of your illness must fit into studies being conducted at the center; you must understand and be willing to participate in the research study. In some cases, you cannot have had extensive medical treatment elsewhere, which would confuse the results of the study. For example, in a study to determine whether radiation is as effective as surgery in the treatment of breast cancer, patients must be admitted before they have had either. In other NIH studies, the disorder may be long-standing, perhaps not responsive to previous treatments.

If you are accepted, there is no charge for the medical, surgical or other hospital services necessary for the research. You usually have to pay your own transportation to and from Bethesda, a suburb of Washington, DC. After the treatment, you return to the care of your referring physician or family. (Some of the procedures are slightly different for those with incapacitating mental disorders.)

Few would dispute that care at the NIH Clinical Center is among the best in the country. The physicians and other scientists conducting the studies are often the cream of the crop and can sometimes come up with remarkable lifesaving diagnoses and treatments that later become standard medical procedures.

On the other hand, the purpose of the treatment at the Center is research, and some of the experimental therapies may not succeed. Also, not everyone who is admitted receives "experimental" treatment; it is usually done on a random selection basis. At any rate, you can be assured of at least receiving the best state-of-the-art treatment and the chance to benefit from a successful *new* treatment. In cases where the illness is poorly controlled by conventional therapy, a person has very little to lose by trying a new treatment.

Some of the major studies being conducted at the NIH Clinical Center are noted throughout this book. Physicians can obtain information about requesting admission for a patient by calling the Patient Referral Service at (301) 496-4891, or by writing:

Office of the Director
The Clinical Center
Building 10, Room 2C-146
National Institutes of Health
Bethesda, MD 20892

SOME LEADING MEDICAL AND HEALTH ORGANIZATIONS FOR CONSUMERS AND HEALTH PROFESSIONALS

Alzheimer's Disease and Related Disorders
  Association
70 E. Lake St., Suite 600
Chicago, IL 60601
(312) 853-3060
(Consumers)

American Academy of Allergy and
  Immunology
611 E. Wells St.
Milwaukee, WI 53202
(414) 272-6071
(Physicians)

American Academy of Dermatology
1567 Maple Ave.
Evanston, IL 60201
(312) 869-3954
(Physicians)

American Academy of Facial Plastic and
  Reconstructive Surgery
1101 Vermont Ave., N.W., Suite 404
Washington, DC 20005
(202) 842-4500
(Physicians)

American Academy of Family Physicians
1740 W. 92nd St.
Kansas City, MO 64114
(816) 333-9700
(Physicians)

American Academy of Neurology
2221 University Ave., S.E., Suite 335
Minneapolis, MN 55414
(612) 623-8115
(Physicians)

American Academy of Ophthalmology
655 Beach St., Suite 300
San Francisco, CA 94109
(415) 561-8500
(Physicians)

American Academy of Pediatrics
141 Northwest Point Blvd.
P.O. Box 927
Elk Grove Village, IL 62009-0927
(312) 869-9327
(Physicians)

American Academy of Physical Medicine and
  Rehabilitation
122 S. Michigan Ave., Suite 1300
Chicago, IL 60603-6107
(312) 922-9366
(Physicians)

American Association of Biofeedback
  Clinicians
2424 Dempster
Des Plaines, IL 60016
(312) 827-0440
(Health professionals)

American Association of Blood Banks
1117 N. 19th St., Suite 600
Arlington, VA 22209
(703) 528-8200
(Health professionals)

American Association of Homes for the Aging
1129 20th St., N.W., Suite 400
Washington, DC 20036
(202) 296-5960
(Health professionals)

American Association on Mental Deficiency
1719 Kalorama Rd., N.W.
Washington, DC 20009
(202) 387-1968
(Health professionals)

American Brittle Bone Society
1256 Merrill Drive
West Chester, PA 19382
(215) 692-6248
(Consumers)

American Cancer Society, Inc.
90 Park Ave.
New York, NY 10016
(212) 599-8200
(Consumers)

American Chiropractic Association
1916 Wilson Blvd.
Arlington, VA 22201
(703) 276-8800
(Health professionals)

American College of Chest Physicians
911 Busse Highway
Park Ridge, IL 60068
(312) 698-2200
(Physicians)

American College of Obstetricians and
  Gynecologists
600 Maryland Ave., S.W., Suite 300 East
Washington, DC 20024
(202) 638-5577
(Physicians)

American Council on Science and Health
1995 Broadway, 18th Floor
New York, NY 10023
(212) 362-7044
(Consumers)

American Diabetes Association, Inc.
1660 Duke St.
Alexandria, VA 22314
(703) 549-1500
(Consumers)

American Digestive Disease Society
7720 Wisconsin Ave., N.W.
Bethesda, MD 20014
(301) 652-9293
(Physicians and consumers)

American Fertility Society
2131 Magnolia Ave., Suite 201
Birmingham, AL 35256
(205) 251-9764
(Physicians)

American Foundation for the Blind, Inc.
15 W. 16th St.
New York, NY 10011
(212) 620-2000
(Consumers)

American Gastroenterological Association
6900 Grove Rd.
Thorofare, NJ 08086
(609) 848-1000
(Physicians)

American Geriatrics Society
770 Lexington Ave., Suite 400
New York, NY 10021
(212) 308-1414
(Physicians)

American Heart Association, Inc.
7320 Greenville Ave.
Dallas, TX 75231
(214) 750-5300
(Consumers)

American Holistic Medical Association
2727 Fairview Ave. East #D
Seattle, WA 98102
(206) 322-6842
(Physicians and health professionals)

American Hospital Association
840 Lakeshore Drive
Chicago, IL 60611
(312) 280-6000
(Hospitals)

American Liver Foundation
998 Compton Ave.
Cedar Grove, NJ 07009
(201) 857-2626
(Consumers)

American Lung Association
1740 Broadway
New York, NY 10019
(212) 315-8700
(Consumers)

American Medical Association
535 N. Dearborn St.
Chicago, IL 60610
(312) 645-5000
(Physicians)

American Osteopathic Association
212 E. Ohio St.
Chicago, IL 60611
(312) 280-5882
(Physicians)

American Psychiatric Association
1400 K St., N.W.
Washington, DC 20005
(202) 682-6000
(Physicians)

American Psychological Association, Inc.
1200 17th St., N.W.
Washington, DC 20036
(202) 955-7600
(Health professionals)

American Rheumatism Association
17 Executive Park Dr., N.E., Suite 480
Atlanta, GA 30329
(404) 633-3777
(Physicians and health professionals)

American Society of Anesthesiologists
515 Busse Highway
Park Ridge, IL 60068
(312) 825-5586
(Physicians)

American Society of Clinical Hypnosis
2250 E. Devon Ave., Suite 336
Des Plaines, IL 60018
(312) 297-3317
(Health professionals)

American Society of Clinical Oncology
435 N. Michigan Ave., Suite 1717
Chicago, IL 60611
(312) 644-0828
(Physicians and health professionals)

American Society of Plastic and Reconstructive
  Surgeons
233 N. Michigan Ave., Suite 1900
Chicago, IL 60601
(312) 856-1818
(Physicians)

American Speech-Language-Hearing
  Association
10801 Rockville Pike
Rockville, MD 20852
(301) 897-5700
(Health professionals)

American Urological Association
1120 N. Charles St.
Baltimore, MD 21201
(301) 727-1100
(Physicians)

Arthritis Foundation
1314 Spring St., N.W.
Atlanta, GA 30309
(404) 872-7100
(Consumers)

Biofeedback Society of America
c/o Francine Butler, Ph.D.
10200 W. 44th Ave., #304
Wheat Ridge, CO 80033
(303) 422-8436
(Health professionals)

Center for Medical Consumers
237 Thompson St.
New York, NY 10012
(212) 674-7105
(Consumers)

Cooley's Anemia Foundation
105 E. 22nd St., Suite 911
New York, NY 10010
(212) 598-0911
(Consumers)

Endocrine Society
9650 Rockville Pike
Bethesda, MD 20814
(301) 530-9660
(Physicians and researchers)

Epilepsy Foundation of America
4351 Garden City Drive
Landover, MD 20785
(301) 459-3700
(Consumers)

Gerontological Society of America
1411 K St., N.W., Suite 300
Washington, DC 20005
(202) 393-1411
(Health professionals)

Health Research Group
2000 P St., N.W., Suite 700
Washington, DC 20036
(202) 872-0320
(Consumers)

March of Dimes Birth Defects Foundation
1275 Mamaroneck Ave.
White Plains, NY 10605
(914) 428-7100
(Consumers)

Muscular Dystrophy Association
810 Seventh Ave., 27th Floor
New York, NY 10019
(212) 586-0808
(Consumers)

National Council on Alcoholism, Inc.
12 W. 21st St., 7th Floor
New York, NY 10010
(212) 206-6770
(Consumers)

National Easter Seal Society
2023 W. Ogden Ave.
Chicago, IL 60612
(312) 243-8400
(Consumers)

National Kidney Foundation
2 Park Ave.
New York, NY 10016
(212) 889-2210
(Consumers)

National Migraine Foundation
5252 N. Western Ave.
Chicago, IL 60625
(312) 878-7715
(Physicians and health professionals)

National Multiple Sclerosis Society
205 E. 42nd St.
New York, NY 10017
(212) 986-3240
(Consumers)

National Women's Health Network
224 7th St., S.E.
Washington, DC 20003
(202) 543-9222
(Consumers)

North American Transplant Coordinators
   Organization (NATCO)
7115 Blanco Rd., Suite 114-126
San Antonio, TX 78216
(Health professionals)

Skin Cancer Foundation
475 Park Ave., S.
New York, NY 10016
(212) 725-5176
(Consumers)

Society of Nuclear Medicine
136 Madison Ave., 8th Floor
New York, NY 10016
(212) 889-0717
(Physicians and health professionals)

Traditional Acupuncture Institute
American City Building, Suite 100
Columbia, MD 21044
(301) 596-6006
(Health professionals and consumers)

United Cerebral Palsy Association
66 E. 34th St.
New York, NY 10016
(212) 481-6300
(Consumers)

ACQUIRED IMMUNE DEFICIENCY SYNDROME (AIDS)

AIDS is a recently discovered viral disease in which the immune system is disabled; it renders victims of the disease vulnerable to a number of infections that inevitably prove fatal. Although researchers believe they have identified the virus responsible, AIDS is incurable to date. As of March 1986, about 16,000 cases of AIDS had been diagnosed, resulting in 8,220 deaths. Reported cases are primarily among so-called "high-risk" groups. Recent figures show that 73 percent of AIDS victims are homosexual or bisexual men; 17 percent are intravenous drug users; and 0.6 percent are hemophiliacs who depend for survival on blood-clotting factor derived from donor blood. Other AIDS victims include recipients of blood transfusions, children of women with AIDS, and heterosexual partners of those carrying the AIDS virus. There is increased concern that the virus is a growing threat to the heterosexual population.

Some experts predict the AIDS epidemic will spread and accelerate: Two to three million Americans may be infected within five to ten years. One million Americans may already be infected with the virus, although most are free of illness. Once infected, a person is believed to carry the AIDS virus for life and be capable of infecting others *without* developing the symptoms. About 10 percent of those individuals exposed to the virus have developed symptoms; however, since the infection is new and the incubation period of the virus is long, experts do not know how many of these people will eventually succumb to AIDS. One estimate is that as many as 40 percent of those infected with the AIDS virus may eventually develop the symptoms and die unless a cure is found. At one time, researchers thought the incubation period for the virus was several years; evidence now indicates that the virus can remain dormant for five or more years before exerting its deadly damage. A number of factors, including genetic susceptibility, nutrition, other infections that "activate" the immune system, or a history of drug abuse, may make a person more vulnerable to the virus.

AIDS is not highly contagious. There is no evidence it is transmitted by casual contact, such as sneezing, coughing, or shaking hands. It is believed that intimate contact in which the virus enters the bloodstream through needles or breaks in the skin is required for transmission. AIDS has been spread primarily by sexual contact among homosexual and bisexual men. About one-fourth of the cases, however, are found among heterosexuals, mainly intravenous drug users.

Cause: AIDS is believed to be caused by an unusual virus known as human T-cell lymphotropic virus, or HTLV-3. The virus specifically assaults the T4 lymphocytes, white blood cells that are important in defending the body against certain potentially lethal infections.

Symptoms: Early symptoms resemble those of less serious illnesses, such as colds or flu, and include swollen lymph glands in the neck, armpits, and groin; fatigue and loss of appetite; fever or night sweats; dry cough; shortness of breath; and persistent diarrhea.

The AIDS virus attacks and weakens the immune system, exposing the person to a number of "opportunistic infections" that the body would ordinarily be able to fight off. In some cases, the virus enters the brain, causing confusion, memory loss, and dementia. Death results after the body succumbs to severe infections, such as *Pneumocystis carinii,* a rare pneumonia, or Kaposi's sarcoma, a type of cancer. The average survival period is about one year after diagnosis of AIDS.

Diagnosis: Alert physicians are now acquainted with the symptoms and are more likely to look for and identify AIDS. However, diagnosis is sometimes difficult because symptoms resemble those of many other infections. Diagnosis is usually made after a thorough physical examination, medical history, and appropriate labora-

tory tests, such as blood tests and a test that spots abnormalities in the functioning of the immune system. A screening test can identify individuals who have been exposed to the virus. The screening test is used primarily to prevent donations of contaminated blood and the spread of AIDS through transfusions. Donating blood does not involve a risk of acquiring AIDS because equipment is sterilized between donors.

Treatment: Researchers are seeking new treatments for AIDS; however, at this writing no therapy has proved successful in reversing the immune deficiency. Treatment is directed at controlling the secondary symptoms, such as deadly infections and cancer. Many experimental drugs are being investigated that may attack the virus directly or help restore functioning of the weakened immune system. Some treatments appear promising. Bone marrow transplants are also being tried. At the present time, prevention, not treatment, is at the forefront of controlling AIDS.

WHERE TO FIND HELP FOR AIDS

Many physicians and other health professionals and agencies have responded to the AIDS crisis by establishing special clinics and programs to help persons who have contracted the disease. Such networks can offer support and can refer persons with AIDS to physicians and centers experienced in treating the disease. The following groups provide information on local resources and treatment.

CALIFORNIA
AIDS Project/Los Angeles
837 N. Cole St., Suite 3
Los Angeles, CA 90038
(213) 871-1284

California Department of Health Services
AIDS Activities
PO Box 160146
Sacramento, CA 95816-0146
(916) 445-0553

San Diego AIDS Project
4304 Third Ave.
PO Box 81082
San Diego, CA 92138
(619) 294-2437

San Francisco AIDS Foundation
333 Valencia St., 4th Floor
San Francisco, CA 94103
(415) 864-4376

COLORADO
Colorado AIDS Project
PO Box 18529
Denver, CO 80218
(303) 837-0166

DISTRICT OF COLUMBIA
AIDS Action Project
Whitman-Walker Clinic
2335 18th St., N.W.
Washington, DC 20009
(202) 332-5295 or 332-AIDS

St. Francis Center
3800 Macomb St., N.W.
Washington, DC 20016
(202) 234-5613

FLORIDA
AIDS Education Project
PO Box 4073
Key West, FL 33041
(305) 294-8302

Health Crisis Network
PO Box 52-1546
Miami, FL 33152
(305) 634-4636

GEORGIA
AID Atlanta (AIDA)
1132 W. Peachtree St., N.W., Suite 112
Atlanta, GA 30309
(404) 872-0600

HAWAII
Life Foundation
320 Ward Ave., Suite 104
Honolulu, HI 96814
(808) 537-2211

ILLINOIS
Howard Brown Memorial Clinic
2676 N. Halsted St.
Chicago, IL 60614
(312) 871-5777 or (800) AID-AIDS

LOUISIANA
Foundation for Health Education
PO Box 51537
New Orleans, LA 70151
(504) 244-6900

MARYLAND
Health Education Resource Center
101 W. Read St., Suite 819
Baltimore, MD 21201
(301) 945-AIDS

MASSACHUSETTS
Fenway Community Health Center
AIDS Action Committee
16 Haviland St.
Boston, MA 02215
(617) 267-7573

MICHIGAN
United Community Services
51 W. Warren Ave.
Detroit, MI 48201
(313) 833-0622

MINNESOTA
Minnesota AIDS Project
PO Box 300122
Minneapolis, MN 55403
(612) 824-1772

NEW YORK
New York City Health Department
Hotline: (718) 485-8111

Gay Men's Health Crisis
PO Box 274
132 W. 24th St.
New York, NY 10011
(212) 807-6655

OHIO
Health Issues Task Force
PO Box 14925 Public Square Station
Cleveland, OH 44114
(216) 651-1448

OREGON
Cascade AIDS Project
408 S.W. Second Ave., Suite 403
Portland, OR 97204
(503) 233-8299

PENNSYLVANIA
Philadelphia Community Health Alternatives
Philadelphia AIDS Task Force
PO Box 7259
Philadelphia, PA 19109
(215) 624-2879

TENNESSEE
Lifestyle Health Services
1729 Church St.
Nashville, TN 37203
(615) 329-1478

TEXAS
KS/AIDS Foundation
3317 Montrose, Box 1155
Houston, TX 77006
(713) 524-2437

VIRGINIA
Richmond AIDS Information Network
Fan Free Clinic
1721 Hanover Ave.
Richmond, VA 23220
(804) 358-6343

WASHINGTON
Northwest AIDS Foundation
PO Box 3449
Seattle, WA 98114
(206) 326-4166

WISCONSIN
Brady East STD Clinic
Milwaukee AIDS Project
1240 E. Brady St.
Milwaukee, WI 53202
(414) 273-2437

SOURCE: *Journal of the American Medical Association.*

NATIONAL HOTLINES AND AGENCIES

National AIDS Hotline
(800) 342-AIDS (general-information
   recording)
(800) 447-AIDS (specific information)
(202) 646-8182—District of Columbia
(202) 245-6867—Alaska and Hawaii (call
   collect)

Operated by the federal government between
8:30 A.M. and 5:30 P.M., EDT. Offers a recorded
message on the most up-to-date information on
AIDS. Questions, including how to find medical
treatment, are answered by employees of the
United States Public Health Service.

National VD Hotline
(800) 227-8922

Answers questions on sexually transmitted diseases, including AIDS. Makes referrals to clinics
and some private physicians specializing in venereal disease treatment throughout the country.
Will send additional information by mail. The
hotline is funded partly by the federal government and partly by private sources.

Centers for Disease Control (CDC)
Office of Public Inquiries
1600 Clifton Rd., N.E.
Atlanta, GA 30333
(404) 329-3534

CDC, part of the U.S. Public Health Service,
is the federal agency most concerned with helping AIDS sufferers and other interested persons
get accurate information about the disease and
find adequate treatment.

AIDS RESEARCH AT THE NATIONAL INSTITUTES OF HEALTH

Experimental treatment aimed at the underlying cause of AIDS as well as rehabilitating the
immune system is under way at the Clinical Center at National Institutes of Health in Bethesda,
Maryland, for a few selected patients referred
by physicians. For more information your physician can contact:

The Clinical Center
Building 10, Room 2C146
National Institutes of Health
Bethesda, MD 20892
(301) 496-4831 (Allergy and Infectious
   Diseases Consultant)

BOOKS

AIDS: The Medical Mystery, **Frederick P.
Siegal, M.D.,** and **Marta Siegal,** New
York: Grove Press, 1984.

The AIDS Epidemic, edited by **Kevin M. Cahill,
M.D.,** New York: St. Martin's Press, 1983.
The AIDS Epidemic: How You Can Protect

Yourself and Your Family—Why You Must,
James I. Slaff, M.D., and **John K.
Brubaker,** New York: Warner Books, 1985.
The AIDS Fact Book, **Ken Mayer, M.D.,** and
Hank Pizer, New York: Bantam Books,
1983.

The Truth About AIDS, **Ann Fettner,** New
York: Holt, Rinehart and Winston, 1984.
Understanding AIDS: A Comprehensive Guide,
edited by **Victor Gone,** New Brunswick,
NJ: Rutgers University Press, 1986.

MATERIALS, FREE AND FOR SALE

Free

Free Facts About AIDS, 8 pages.
What Everybody Should Know About AIDS, 16
pages
*What Gay and Bisexual Men Should Know
About AIDS,* 16 pages.
Why You Should Be Informed About AIDS, 16
pages.

Centers for Disease Control
Office of Public Inquiries
1600 Clifton Rd., N.E.
Atlanta, GA 30333
(404) 329-3534

Answers About AIDS.

American Council on Science and Health
AIDS Report
47 Maple St.
Summit, NJ 07901

Free with self-addressed, stamped envelope

Medical Answers About AIDS, booklet.

Gay Men's Health Crisis
Box 274
142 W. 24th St.
New York, NY 10011

For sale

Directory of AIDS-related Services, lists
services throughout the country, 104 pages.

The United States Conference of Mayors
1620 I St., N.W., 4th Floor
Washington, DC 20006
(202) 293-7330

ALCOHOLISM

Alcoholism is one of our most serious health problems. Approximately ten million Americans, or 10 percent of those who drink, suffer from alcoholism and problems related to it. More than three million teenagers, aged 14 to 17, have the symptoms of developing alcoholism. Alcohol directly or indirectly causes about 95,000 deaths each year. (Some experts put the figure as high as 200,000.) About one-half, or 25,000 of our traffic fatalities every year, are related to alcohol. Young adults who have been drinking account for an estimated 40 to 60 percent of that toll, and drunk driving is the leading cause of death among individuals 15 to 24 years old. Alcohol is also linked to a number of physical disabilities and diseases, including cirrhosis of the liver, that result in about 30,000 deaths each year. Fetal alcohol syndrome is a birth defect causing mental retardation. Alcohol is also heavily involved in suicides and homicides.

Cause: Alcoholism is considered a physical addiction characterized by a tolerance to the drug and a physical reaction when it is withdrawn. There is no single cause of alcoholism: It is generally considered to be a combination of psychological and/or environmental and biological causes.

Persuasive new evidence shows that biological or genetic predisposition to alcoholism may be much more important than previously believed. Research indicates that alcoholics metabolize alcohol abnormally, and that some people are born with a malfunctioning liver enzyme system that could make them more vulnerable to alcohol addiction. The brain waves of alcoholics and their children (even though they have not been exposed to alcohol) often differ from those of nonalcoholics. Although biology is not destiny, a tendency to alcoholism may be inherited and then triggered by psychological and environmental factors.

Symptoms: Reaction to alcohol is entirely individual, but alcoholism is usually defined as loss of control over drinking to the extent that it interferes with family and social life, job performance, and, sometimes, health. A person is said to have a drinking problem if the following signs are present: a decided change in personality or behavior, frequent drunkenness or drunk driving, trouble on the job, family or financial problems because of drinking, early morning drinking, drinking when confronted with stressful situations, arrests for drunkenness, and alcohol-induced blackouts. These are signs, but there is no typical alcoholic.

As the dependence deepens, there is a need to drink more, eventual loss of control over drinking, specific painful psychological and physical withdrawal symptoms (extreme nervousness, anxiety, sweating, nausea, trembling), and, in some cases, delirium tremens (D.T.s), which can be deadly without proper medical care.

Diagnosis: All or some of the above signs may lead the individual, a family member, or a physician or other health professional to apply the label of alcoholic. Recently, a biochemical blood test, developed by researchers, has been able to spot male alcoholics in almost every case. Apparently, the use of alcohol over a long period of time causes subtle changes in the blood chemistry that can be detected by chemical analysis. This test does not prove the person was born with a different blood chemistry, simply that his blood has a chemical profile known to be common in alcoholics, perhaps caused by the consumption of alcohol.

Treatment: The current treatment for alcoholics is rather standard: The alcoholic must stop drinking and not take alcohol again—total, lifelong abstinence. In some cases, the alcoholic must first be detoxified to rid the body of alcohol. Detoxification helps the body adjust to the absence of alcohol and produces a clear mind capable of desiring and helping in recovery. This process may bring about severe withdrawal symptoms and is ideally done under the care of a physician or health-care professional, often in a hospital; in many acute cases, the withdrawal may necessitate medication to help control symptoms, such as seizures. Detoxification is not dangerous or as discomforting, with modern drug treatment. At the same time, the patient is put on a good diet and receives medical treatment for any physical problems resulting from alcohol abuse. This may halt the progression of alcohol-induced disease, and, in some cases, reverse the damage to a degree.

The difficulty, of course, is to prevent the return to alcohol. Some physicians prescribe Antabuse, a drug that produces nausea and other discomforts when mixed in the body with alcohol; however, there can be side effects. Antabuse is not for everyone; nor is it considered adequate treatment when used alone. Psychotherapy is usually an integral part of alcoholism recovery—individual or group psychotherapy, family therapy, or counseling—helping the person to admit

to his or her alcoholism, discover possible psychological reasons for it, and overcome it.

Most health professionals believe that support groups, including Alcoholics Anonymous, are vitally important in helping people stay away from alcohol. Also, the more recent employer assistance programs have proved remarkably effective in helping control alcoholism because of the alcoholic's desire to retain a job.

There are many types of facilities for treating alcoholism—inpatient and outpatient units in hospitals, community mental health centers, local agencies, private clinics, Veterans' Administration hospitals, and a large network of referral services. Many alcoholics do not need to be hospitalized, although hospitalization is indicated for some and may be necessary for those who have serious problems with other drugs, requiring medical attention during withdrawal.

Increasingly, especially among the young, alcoholism is only one part of a pattern of drug dependency. The new generation of addicts are often characterized by ''polyabuse''—a dependence on both alcohol and drugs or a variety of chemicals. Most facilities that treat alcoholism also treat the entire range of drug and chemical dependency.

Experts say there is no single type of facility that has the best record for treating alcoholism. Success depends on many factors, including the patient's personal and social resources. It has been noted that alcoholics with the involvement and support of family, friends, and employers are more apt to succeed in recovering.

WHERE TO FIND TREATMENT FOR ALCOHOLISM

Many hospitals throughout the country, too numerous to list here, have inpatient and outpatient alcoholism treatment programs. The units almost always offer combined alcohol and other chemical dependency treatment. For referrals to hospitals and other facilities in your area contact your state's office of alcohol abuse listed below.

You can also buy a copy of the *National Directory of Drug-Abuse and Alcoholism Treatment and Prevention Programs* (document number S/N 01702401252-1), which lists about 7,500

programs nationwide. Order the directory from the Superintendent of Documents, Government Printing Office, Washington, DC 20402. For alcohol- and drug-treatment programs geared primarily to adolescents, see the chapter on drug abuse, page 199.

Additionally, on page 23, you will find a list of leading alcoholism treatment facilities, including the well-known Betty Ford Center in California.

STATE ALCOHOLISM AND DRUG-ABUSE AGENCIES

You can often get excellent local information about alcohol- and drug-abuse treatment and prevention programs from state offices of alcohol and drug abuse. Some agencies publish comprehensive directories to local facilities.

ALABAMA

Department of Mental Health and Mental
  Retardation
Ken Wallis, Acting Commissioner
200 Interstate Park Drive
PO Box 3710
Montgomery, AL 36193
(205) 271-9209

ALASKA

Department of Health and Social Services
Office of Alcoholism and Drug Abuse
Matthew Felix, Coordinator
Pouch H-05F, 114 Second St.
Juneau, AK 99811
(907) 586-6201

ARIZONA

Arizona Department of Health Services
Alcohol Abuse and Alcoholism Section
Gwen G. Smith, Program Representative
Office of Community Behavioral Health
1740 W. Adams, Room 001
Phoenix, AZ 85007
(602) 255-1152

Arizona Department of Health Services
Drug Abuse
Ed Zborower, Program Representative
Office of Community Behavioral Health
1740 W. Adams
Phoenix, AZ 85007
(602) 255-1152

ARKANSAS

Arkansas Office on Alcohol and Drug Abuse
  Prevention
Paul T. Behnke, Director
1515 W. Seventh Ave., Suite 310
Little Rock, AR 72201
(501) 371-2603

CALIFORNIA

Department of Alcohol and Drug Programs
Chauncey Veatch III, Esq., Director
111 Capitol Mall, Suite 450
Sacramento, CA 95814
(916) 445-0834

COLORADO

Alcohol and Drug Abuse Division
Colorado Department of Health
Robert B. Aukerman, Director
4210 E. 11th Ave.
Denver, CO 80220
(303) 331-8201

CONNECTICUT

Connecticut Alcohol and Drug Abuse
  Commission
Donald J. McConnell, Executive Director
999 Asylum Ave., 3rd Floor
Hartford, CT 06105
(203) 566-4145

DELAWARE

Division of Alcoholism, Drug Abuse, and
  Mental Health
Bureau of Alcoholism and Drug Abuse
Sally Allshouse, Chief
1901 N. Dupont Highway
New Castle, DE 19720
(302) 421-6101

DISTRICT OF COLUMBIA

Office of Health Planning and Development
Simon Holliday, Chief
1875 Connecticut Ave., N.W., Suite 836A
Washington, DC 20009
(202) 673-7481

FLORIDA

Alcohol and Drug Abuse Program
Department of Health and Rehabilitation
  Services
Linda Lewis, Director
1317 Winewood Blvd., Room 157A
Tallahassee, FL 32301
(904) 488-0900

GEORGIA
Division of Mental Health, Mental
  Retardation, and Substance Abuse
Georgia Department of Human Resources
Patricia A. Redmond, Director
878 Peachtree St., N.E., 3rd Floor
Atlanta, GA 30309
(404) 894-6352

HAWAII
Alcohol and Drug Abuse Branch
Mental Health Division
Department of Health
Joyce Ingram-Chinn, Branch Chief
PO Box 3378
Honolulu, HI 96801
(808) 548-4280

IDAHO
Substance Abuse Section
Department of Health & Welfare
Charles E. Burns, Supervisor
450 W. State St., 4th Floor
Boise, ID 83720
(208) 334-4368

ILLINOIS
Department of Alcoholism & Substance Abuse
Edward T. Duffy, Director
State of Illinois Center
100 W. Randolph St., Suite 5-600
Chicago, Il 60610
(312) 917-3840

INDIANA
Division of Addiction Services
Department of Mental Health
Joseph E. Mills III, Director
117 E. Washington St.
Indianapolis, IN 46204
(317) 232-7816

IOWA
Department of Substance Abuse
Mary L. Ellis, Director
507 10th St.
Suite 500, Colony Building
Des Moines, IA 50319
(515) 281-3641

KANSAS
Alcohol and Drug Abuse Services
James A. McHenry, Jr., Ph.D.
Commissioner
2700 W. Sixth St., 2nd Floor
Biddle Building
Topeka, KS 66606
(913) 296-3925

KENTUCKY
Cabinet for Human Resources
Michael Townsend, Director
Division of Substance Abuse
Department for Mental Health and Mental
  Retardation
275 E. Main St.
Frankfort, KY 40621
(502) 564-2880

LOUISIANA
Office of Prevention and Recovery from
  Alcohol and Drug Abuse
Vern Ridgeway, Assistant Secretary
PO Box 53129
2744-B Wooddale Blvd.
Baton Rouge, LA 70892
(504) 922-0728

MAINE
Office of Alcoholism and Drug Abuse
  Prevention
Neill Miner, Director
State House Station #11
Augusta, ME 04333
(207) 289-2781

MARYLAND
Alcoholism Control Administration
John Bland, Director
201 W. Preston St., 4th Floor
Baltimore, MD 21201
(301) 225-6541, 6542

Maryland State Drug Abuse
  Administration
Howard B. Silverman, Acting Director
201 W. Preston St.
Baltimore, MD 21201
(301) 383-3312

MASSACHUSETTS
Division of Alcoholism
Edward Blacker, Ph.D., Director
150 Tremont St.
Boston, MA 02111
(617) 727-1960

Division of Drug Rehabilitation
Thomas P. Salmon, Director
150 Tremont St.
Boston, MA 02111
(617) 727-8614

MICHIGAN
Office of Substance Abuse Services
Robert Brook, Administrator
3500 N. Logan St.
PO Box 30035
Lansing, MI 48909
(517) 373-8603

MINNESOTA
Chemical Dependency Program Division
Cynthia Turnure, Ph.D., Executive Director
Department of Human Services
Space Center
444 Lafayette Rd.
St. Paul, MN 55101
(612) 296-3991

MISSISSIPPI
Division of Alcohol and Drug Abuse
Ann D. Robertson, M.S.W., Director
1102 Robert E. Lee Office Building
Jackson, MS 39201
(601) 359-1297

MISSOURI
Division of Alcohol and Drug Abuse
R.B. Wilson, Director
2002 Missouri Blvd.
PO Box 687
Jefferson City, MO 65101
(314) 751-4942

MONTANA
Alcohol and Drug Abuse Division
State of Montana
Department of Institutions
Robert Anderson, Administrator
1539–11th Ave.
Helena, MT 59620
(406) 444-2827

NEBRASKA
Division on Alcoholism and Drug Abuse
Cecilia Willis, Ph.D., Director
Box 94728
Lincoln, NE 68509
(402) 471-2851, x5583

NEVADA
Bureau of Alcohol and Drug Abuse
Department of Human Resources
Richard Ham, Chief
505 E. King St.
Carson City, NV 89710
(702) 885-4790

NEW HAMPSHIRE
Office of Alcohol and Drug Abuse Prevention
Geraldine Sylvester, Director
Health and Welfare Building
Hazen Drive
Concord, NH 03301
(603) 271-4627, 4630

NEW JERSEY
Division of Alcoholism
New Jersey Department of Health
Riley Regan, Director
129 E. Hanover St.
Trenton, NJ 08608
(609) 292-8949

Division of Narcotic and Drug Abuse Control
New Jersey Department of Health
Richard Russo, M.S.P.H., Director
129 E. Hanover St.
Trenton, NJ 08608
(609) 292-5760

NEW MEXICO
Alcoholism Bureau
Joe Gallegos, Acting Chief
Behavioral Health Services Division
Crown Building
PO Box 968
Santa Fe, NM 87504-0968
(505) 984-0020, x493

Drug Abuse Bureau
Ellen Costilla, Chief
Behavioral Health Services Division
PO Box 968
Santa Fe, NM 87504-0968
(505) 984-0020, x331

NEW YORK
Division of Substance Abuse Services
John S. Gustafson, Deputy Director
Executive Park, Box 8200
Albany, NY 12203
(518) 457-7629

New York State Division of Alcoholism and
   Alcohol Abuse
Robert V. Shear, Director
194 Washington Ave.
Albany, NY 12210
(518) 474-5417

NORTH CAROLINA
Division of Mental Health, Mental
   Retardation, and Substance Abuse Services
Alcohol and Drug Abuse Section
Thomas F. Miriello, Deputy Director
325 N. Salisbury St.
Raleigh, NC 27611
(919) 733-4670

NORTH DAKOTA
State Department of Human Services
Division of Alcoholism and Drug Abuse
Tom R. Hedin, Director
State Capitol
Bismarck, ND 58505
(701) 224-2769

OHIO
Bureau of Drug Abuse
David D. Lippert, Acting Administrator
170 N. High St., 3rd Floor
Columbus, OH 43215
(614) 466-7893

Ohio Department of Health
Bureau of Alcohol Abuse and Alcoholism
   Recovery
Wayne Lindstrom, Chief
170 N. High St., 3rd Floor
Columbus, OH 43215
(614) 466-3445

OKLAHOMA
Programs Division
Thomas Stanitis, M.A., M.H.S., Chief of
   Programs
PO Box 53277, Capitol Station
Oklahoma City, OK 73152
(405) 521-0044

OREGON
Program Office for Alcohol and Drug Abuse
Department of Human Resources
Jeffrey N. Kushner, Assistant Director
301 Public Service Building
Salem, OR 97310
(503) 378-2163

PENNSYLVANIA
Office of Drug and Alcohol Programs
Luceille Fleming, Deputy Secretary for Drug
   and Alcohol Programs
PO Box 90, Department of Health
Health and Welfare Building, 8th Floor
Harrisburg, PA 17108
(717) 787-9857

PUERTO RICO
Puerto Rico Department of Addiction Control
   Services
Alejandrina S. deLugo
Assistant Secretariat of Alcoholism
PO Box 21414, Rio Piedras Station
Rio Piedras, PR 00928
(809) 763-5014, 7575

RHODE ISLAND
Department of Mental Health, Mental
   Retardation, and Hospitals
Division of Substance Abuse
William H. Pimental, Assistance Director
Substance Abuse Administration Building
Cranston, RI 02920
(401) 464-2091

SOUTH CAROLINA
South Carolina Commission on Alcohol and
   Drug Abuse
William J. McCord, Director
3700 Forest Drive, Suite 300
Columbia, SC 29204
(803) 758-2521

SOUTH DAKOTA
Division of Alcohol and Drug Abuse
Lois Olson, Director
Joe Foss Building
523 E. Capitol
Pierre, SD 57501-3182
(605) 773-3123

TENNESSEE
Tennessee Department of Mental Health and
  Mental Retardation
Robert Currie, Assistant Commissioner
Division of Alcohol and Drug Abuse Services
James K. Polk Building
505 Deaderick St., 4th Floor
Nashville, TN 37219
(615) 741-1921

TEXAS
Texas Commission on Alcohol and Drug
  Abuse
Ross Newby, Executive Director
1705 Guadalupe St.
Austin, TX 78701
(512) 475-2577

UTAH
Division of Alcoholism and Drugs
F. Leon PoVey, Director
150 W. North Temple
PO Box 45500
Salt Lake City, UT 84145
(801) 533-6532

VERMONT
Office of Alcohol and Drug Programs
Richard Powell II, Director
103 S. Main St.
Osgood Building
Waterbury, VT 05676
(802) 241-2170

VIRGINIA
Department of Mental Health/Mental
  Retardation
Wayne Thacker, Director
Office of Substance Abuse Services
PO Box 1797
109 Governor St.
Richmond, VA 23214
(804) 786-3906

WASHINGTON
Bureau of Alcoholism & Substance Abuse
Glen Miller, Director
Mailstop, OB-44W
Olympia, WA 98504
(206) 753-5866

WEST VIRGINIA
Division of Alcoholism and Drug Abuse
Office of Behavioral Health Services
Jack Clohan, Jr., Director
State Capitol
1800 Washington St., E.
Charleston, WV 25305
(304) 348-2276

WISCONSIN
Wisconsin Office of Alcohol and Other Drug
  Abuse
Larry W. Monson, Director
1 W. Wilson St., Room 441
PO Box 7851
Madison, WI 53702
(608) 266-3442

WYOMING
Division of Community Programs
Jean DeFratis, Substance Abuse Program
  Manager
Hathaway Building, 3rd Floor
Cheyenne, WY 82002
(307) 777-7115, x7118

SOURCE: *Alcohol, Drug Abuse, and Mental Health Administration.*

SOME ALCOHOLISM TREATMENT PROGRAMS

All of these centers are members of the National Association of Alcoholism Treatment Programs. They include a range of treatment
services—inpatient, outpatient and residential;
about one-half are affiliated with hospitals.

ALABAMA
Alcoholism Recovery Services, Inc.
2701 Jefferson Ave., S.W.
Birmingham, AL 35211
(205) 923-6552

Lloyd Nolan Hospital
701 Ridgeway Rd.
Fairfield, AL 35064
(205) 783-5156

Intercept Program
Livingston-Tombigbee
Highway 11 N., Drawer AA
Livingston, AL 35470
(205) 652-9511

Brookwood/Parkside
Cottage Hill Station
PO Box 91174
Mobile, AL 36691
(205) 633-0906

Humana Hospital E. Montgomery
Family Recovery Program
PO Box 17720
Montgomery, AL 36193
(205) 277-5483

Meadhaven Baptist Medical Center
Alcohol & Drug Treatment Services
2105 E. South Blvd.
Montgomery, AL 36198
(205) 284-1224

Brookwood/Parkside
PO Box 128
Warrior, AL 35180
(205) 647-1945

ARIZONA
West Valley Camelback Hospital
5625 W. Thunderbird Rd.
Glendale, AZ 85306
(602) 588-4700

Care Unit
John C. Lincoln Hospital
9211 N. Second St.
Phoenix, AZ 85020
(602) 870-6356

Phoenix General Hospital
Womans Center for Alcoholism Treatment
1950 W. Indian School Rd.
Phoenix, AZ 85015
(602) 279-4411

St. Luke's Behavioral Health Center
1800 E. Van Buren
Phoenix, AZ 85006
(602) 251-8484

Sedona Villa
PO Box 4245
Sedona, AZ 86340
(602) 282-3583

Sierra Tucson
Box 8307
Tucson, AZ 85738
(602) 624-4000

St. Joseph's Hospital
O'Reilly Care Center
350 N. Wilmot
Tucson, AZ 85732
(602) 296-3211

Tucson General Hospital–Westcenter
3838 N. Campbell Ave.
Tucson, AZ 85719
(602) 327-5431

ARC Meadows
Highway 93 N., Box 97
Wickenburg, AZ 85358
(602) 684-2815

ARKANSAS
Intercept Program
Delta Medical Center
505 S. New York St.
Brinkley, AR 72021
(501) 276-0672

Ouachita Hospital
Chemical Dependence Unit
638 California St.
Camden, AR 71701
(501) 836-1330

Care Unit
Sparks Regional Medical Center
1311 S. I St., 4th Floor W.
Fort Smith, AR 72901
(501) 441-5500

Intercept Program
Gurdon Municipal Hospital
Third & Walnut Sts.
Gurdon, AR 71743
(501) 353-4401

Care Unit
Arkansas Rehabilitation Institute
9601 Interstate 630, Exit 7
Little Rock, AR 72205
(501) 223-7507

Care Unit
St. Michael Hospital
315 E. Fifth St.
Texarkana, AR 75502
(501) 774-CARE

Intercept Program
Central Ozarks
Highway 14 N., Drawer 219
Yellville, AR 72687
(501) 449-6211

CALIFORNIA
Assist Foundation
1156 Oak St., #213
Alameda, CA 94501
(415) 523-5483

Phoenix Recovery Centers, Inc.
1124 Ballena Blvd., 2nd Floor
Alameda, CA 94501
(415) 521-4135

Discover Recovery
Martin Luther Hospital Medical Center
1830 W. Romneya Drive, Box 3304
Anaheim, CA 92803
(714) 491-5661

Care Unit
Western Medical Center/Anaheim
1025 S. Anaheim Blvd.
Anaheim, CA 92805
(714) 533-6220

Care Unit
Bellflower Doctors Hospital
9542 E. Artesia Blvd.
Bellflower, CA 90706
(213) 920-8826

Care Unit
Alta Bates Hospital
3001 Colby Plaza at Ashby
Berkeley, CA 94705
(415) 549-3080

Phoenix Program
St. Joseph Medical Center–CDS
Buena Vista & Alameda Sts.
Burbank, CA 91505
(818) 843-5111

Care Unit
Valley Park Medical Center
7011 Shoup Ave.
Canoga Park, CA 91307
(818) 348-0500

Brightside ACT Center/Carmel
24945 Valley Way
Carmel, CA 93923
(408) 624-4995

Recovery Resources of Memorial Hospital
1905 Memorial Drive
Ceres, CA 95307
(209) 572-7276

Phoenix Program
Mt. Diablo Hospital
2540 East St.
Concord, CA 94520
(415) 674-2200

Coronado Hospital ADRU
250 Prospect Place
Coronado, CA 92118
(619) 435-6251

Care Unit
Costa Mesa Medical Center Hospital
301 Victoria St.
Costa Mesa, CA 92627
(714) 650-1090

Starting Point/Orange County
350 W. Bay St.
Costa Mesa, CA 92627
(714) 642-3505

Selton Medical Center
1900 Sullivan Ave.
Daly City, CA 94015
(415) 992-4000

Fresno Community Hospital–ARU Units
Fresno & R Sts.
Fresno, CA 93715
(209) 442-3940

Glendale Adventist Medical Center
801 S. Chevy Chase Drive
Glendale, CA 91205
(818) 247-9303

Glendale Adventist Research Center
335 Mission Rd.
Glendale, CA 91205
(818) 242-3116

Memorial Hospital of Glendale
1420 S. Central Ave.
Glendale, CA 91204
(818) 502-2361

Starting Point/Hayward Hospital
22455 Maple Court
Hayward, CA 94541
(415) 537-7714

LifeStarts, Centinela Hospital
555 E. Hardy St.
Inglewood, CA 90301
(213) 677-HELP

Comprehensive Care Corporation
18551 Von Karman
Irvine, CA 92714
(714) 253-7233

Intercept Program
Kingsburg General Hospital
1200 Smith St.
Kingsburg, CA 93631
(209) 897-5841

Recovery Centers of America
25301 Cabot Rd., #101
Laguna Hills, CA 92653
(714) 581-1445

McDonalds Center at Scripps Memorial
   Hospital
9888 Genesee Ave.
La Jolla, CA 92038
(619) 458-4300

Intercept Program
Mountains Community Hospital
29101 Hospital Rd.
Lake Arrowhead, CA 92352
(714) 336-2061

Westworld Community Healthcare, Inc.
23072 Lake Center Drive, #200
Lake Forest, CA 92630
(714) 768-2981

Doctors Hospital of Lakewood
5300 N. Clark Ave.
Lakewood, CA 90712
(213) 866-9711

New Beginnings
Lodi Community Hospital
800 S. Lower Sacramento Rd.
Lodi, CA 95240
(209) 334-2770

Memorial Coastview
2801 Atlantic Ave., Box 1428
Long Beach, CA 90801
(213) 426-6619

New Beginnings
Dominguez Medical Center
171 W. Bort St.
Long Beach, CA 90805
(213) 639-2664

Care Unit
Cedars–Sinai Medical Center
8700 Beverly Blvd.
Los Angeles, CA 90048
(213) 855-4766

New Beginnings
Century City Hospital
2070 Century Park E.
Los Angeles, CA 90067
(213) 201-6730

Care Unit
Hospital of Los Angeles
5035 Coliseum St.
Los Angeles, CA 90016
(213) 295-6441

Schick Shadel Hospital
Frawley Corporation
1901 Ave. of the Stars, #1530
Los Angeles, CA 90067
(213) 553-9771

New Beginnings
Community Hospital at Los Gatos
815 Pollard Rd.
Los Gatos, CA 95030
(408) 378-6141

Daniel Freeman Marina Hospital
4650 Lincoln Blvd.
Marina Del Rey, CA 90291
(213) 827-4427

Phoenix Program
Merced Community Medical Center
301 E. 13th St.
Merced, CA 95340
(209) 385-7142

Care Unit
Mission Community Hospital
27700 Medical Center Rd.
Mission Viejo, CA 92691
(714) 582-2900

New Beginnings
Modesto City Hospital
730 17th St.
Modesto, CA 95354
(209) 577-2100

Recovery Center of the Monterey Peninsula
  Hospital
576 Hartnell
Monterey, CA 93940
(408) 373-0924

St. Catherine Hospital
Marine Blvd. & Etheldore St.
Moss Beach, CA 94038
(415) 728-5533

Phoenix Program
El Camino Hospital
2500 Grant Rd.
Mountain View, CA 94040
(415) 940-7250

Coldwater Canyon Hospital
6421 Coldwater Canyon
North Hollywood, CA 91606
(818) 506-4764

Gladman Memorial Hospital
2633 E. 27th St.
Oakland, CA 94601
(415) 536-8111

Merritt Peralta Institute
Chemical Dependence Recovery Hospital
435 Hawthorne Ave.
Oakland, CA 94609
(415) 652-7000

New Beginnings
Ojai Valley Community Hospital
1306 Maricopa Highway
Ojai, CA 93023
(805) 646-5567

New Beginnings
Ontario Community Hospital
550 N. Monterey Ave.
Ontario, CA 91764
(714) 988-3844

Care Unit
Hospital of Orange
401 S. Tustin Ave.
Orange, CA 92666
(714) 633-9582

St. Joseph Hospital
Recovery Services
1100 W. Stewart Drive
Orange, CA 92667
(714) 771-8080

Starting Point/Orangevale
8773 Oak Ave.
Orangevale, CA 95662
(916) 988-5700

Care Unit
Channel Island Community Hospital
2130 N. Ventura Rd.
Oxnard, CA 93030
(805) 487-5358

Care Unit
Palmdale Hospital Medical Center
1212 E. Ave. S
Palmdale, CA 93550
(805) 265-6410

Pasadena Community Hospital
1845 N. Fair Oaks
Pasadena, CA 91103
(818) 348-7811

Intercept Program
Del Puerto Hospital
S. 9th & E Sts.
Patterson, CA 95363
(209) 892-2348

Phoenix Program
Petaluma Valley Hospital
400 N. McDowell
Petaluma, CA 94953
(707) 778-2730

New Beginnings
Doctors Hospital of Pinole
2151 Appian Way
Pinole, CA 94564
(415) 724-1520

New Beginnings
Placentia Linda Community Hospital
1301 Rose Drive
Placentia, CA 92670
(714) 524-4894

Betty Ford Center at Eisenhower
39000 Bob Hope Drive
Rancho Mirage, CA 92270
(619) 340-0033

St. Elizabeth Hospital
Chemical Dependency Service
Sister Mary Columbia Drive
Red Bluff, CA 96080
(916) 527-2112

New Beginnings
Redding Medical Center
1450 Liberty St.
Redding, CA 96001
(916) 243-2933

South Bay Hospital
Chemical Dependency Service
514–N. Prospect Ave.
Redondo Beach, CA 90277
(213) 318-4708

Intercept Program
Parkview Community Hospital
3865 Jackson St.
Riverside, CA 92503
(714) 359-3002

Knollwood Center
Riverside Community Hospital
5900 Brockton Ave.
Riverside, CA 92506
(714) 788-3500

Starting Point/Roseville
333 Sunrise Blvd.
Roseville, CA 95678
(916) 781-1560

Care Unit
Community Hospital of Sacramento
2251 Hawthorne St.
Sacramento, CA 95815
(916) 920-1507

Starting Point/Sacramento
1001 Grand Ave.
Sacramento, CA 95838
(916) 929-5383

Starting Point Outpatient Program
2220 Watt Ave. Suite C13
Sacramento, CA 95825
(916) 489-2999

Alisal Community Hospital
333 N. Sanborn Rd.
Salinas, CA 93905
(408) 424-5663

San Bernardino Community Hospital
1500 W. 17th St.
San Bernardino, CA 92411
(714) 887-8111

Hillside Hospital
1940 El Cajon Blvd.
San Diego, Ca 92104
(619) 692-1215

New Beginnings at San Diego
Physicians & Surgeons Hospital
446 26th St.
San Diego, CA 92102
(619) 239-6026

Care Unit
Marshal Hale Memorial Hospital
3773 Sacramento St.
San Francisco, CA 94118
(415) 666-7781

Starting Point/St. Mary's
450 Stanyan St.
San Francisco, CA 94117
(415) 668-1000

Good Samaritan Hospital
Phoenix Program
2425 Samaritan St.
San Jose, CA 95124
(408) 559-2200

Care Unit
San Jose Hospital
675 E. Santa Clara St.
San Jose, CA 95112
(408) 977-4423

Santa Clara County
Alcoholism Services
976 Lenzen Ave.
San Jose, CA 95126
(408) 299-6498

Alcohol Services
3220 S. Higuera, Suite 201
San Luis Obispo, CA 93401
(805) 544-3307

Phoenix Program
Mills Memorial Hospital
100 S. San Mateo Drive
San Mateo, CA 94401
(415) 579-2100

Recovery Alliance at San Pedro
Pennisula Hospital
1300 W. 7th St.
San Pedro, CA 90732
(213) 514-5300

Phoenix Program
Family Medical Center
9260 Alcosta Blvd., C-21
San Ramon, CA 94583
(415) 829-2492

Care Unit
Goleta Valley Community Hospital
351 S. Patterson
Santa Barbara, CA 93160
(805) 683-5747

Pinecrest Hospital
2415 De La Vina St.
Santa Barbara, CA 93105
(805) 682-2511

Azure Acres CDRC
2264 Green Hill Rd.
Sebastopol, CA 95472
(707) 823-3385

Phoenix Program
St. Joseph Oak Park Hospital
2510 N. California
Stockton, CA 95204
(209) 467-6300

Sierra Memorial Hospital
9449 San Fernando Rd.
Sun Valley, CA 97342
(213) 767-3310

Maynord's Chemical Dependency Recovery
  Center
19325 Cherokee Rd.
Tuolumne, CA 95379
(209) 928-3737

Care Unit
Emanuel Medical Center
825 Delbon Ave.
Turlock, CA 95380
(209) 668-4357

Health Care Medical Center
14662 Newport Ave.
Tustin, CA 92680
(714) 838-9600

Starting Point/Vallejo
525 Oregon St.
Vallejo, CA 94590
(707) 557-8233

Intercept Program
Trinity General Hospital
410 N. Taylor St.
Weaverly, CA 96093
(916) 623-5541

Aero Medical Advisors
8820 S. Sepulveda Blvd.
Westchester, CA 90045
(213) 641-7186

Presbyterian Intercommunity
Hospital–CDC
12401 E. Washington Blvd.
Whittier, CA 90602
(213) 698-0811

Glenn General Hospital
1133 W. Sycamore St.
Willows, CA 95988
(916) 934-2894

St. Jude Hospital–Yorba Linda
16850 E. Bastanchury Rd.
Yorba Linda, CA 92686
(714) 993-3000

COLORADO
Cottonwood Hill, Inc.
13455 W. 58th Ave.
Arvada, CO 80002
(303) 420-1702

Washington House, Inc.
7373 Birch St.
Commerce City, CO 80022
(303) 289-3391

ARU Denver
1834 Gilpan
Denver, CO 80128
(303) 234-5614

Care Unit
Mercy Medical Center
1619 Filmore St.
Denver, CO 80206
(303) 393-3461

Presbyterian–St. Lukes Medical Center/AMI
  Rocky Mountain Health Care Center
601 E. 19th Ave.
Denver, CO 80203
(303) 839-6000

Harmony Foundation, Inc.
PO Box 1989
Estes Park, CO 80517
(303) 586-4491

Parkside Lodge of Florence
521 W. 5th St.
Florence, CO 81226
(303) 784-4806

New Beginnings at Fort Collins
Suite 004, William Stover Building
503 Remington
Fort Collins, CO 80524
(303) 493-3389

ARU Bridge House
436 S. 7th St.
Grand Junction, CO 81501
(303) 245-4213

The Ark
Box 626
Green Mountain Falls, CO 80819
(303) 684-9483

New Beginnings at Denver
1325 Everett Court
Lakewood, CO 80125
(303) 231-9090

Care Unit
Montrose Memorial Hospital
800 Third St.
Montrose, CO 81401
(303) 249-7635

Parkside Lodge of Colorado
8801 Lipan St.
Thornton, CO 80221
(303) 430-0800

CONNECTICUT
Blueridge Center
1095 Blue Hills Ave.
Bloomfield, CT 06002
(203) 243-1331

Guenster Rehabilitation Center, Inc.
276 Union Ave.
Bridgeport, CT 06607
(203) 384-9301

Parkside Lodge of Connecticut
Route 7, Box 668
Canaan, CT 06018
(203) 824-5426

Greenwich Hospital, ARC
Perryridge Rd.
Greenwich, CT 06830
(203) 869-7000

Eagle Hill Treatment Center
28 Alberts Hill Rd.
Sandy Hook, CT 06482
(203) 426-8085

DISTRICT OF COLUMBIA
New Beginnings at Psychiatric Institute of
    Washington, DC
2141 K St., N.W., 9th Floor
Washington, DC 20037
(202) 828-1880

Recovery Centers of America
1010 Wisconsin Ave., N.W., Suite 900
Washington, DC 20007
(202) 298-3230

FLORIDA
Center for Recovery at JFK Memorial Hospital
4800 S. Congress Ave.
Atlantis, FL 33462
(305) 433-3600

Bowling Green Inn
PO Box 337
Bowling Green, FL 33834
(813) 375-2218

Care Unit of Coral Springs
3275 N.W. 99th Way
Coral Springs, FL 33065
(305) 753-5200

Humana Hospital–Daytona Beach
400 N. Clyde Morris Blvd.
Daytona Beach, FL 32020
(904) 258-1030

Palm Beach Institute
The Friary Inc.
Route 2, Box 174
Gulf Breeze, FL 32561
(904) 932-9375

CDU Daytona Beach General Hospital
1340 Ridgewood Ave.
Holly Hill, FL 32017
(904) 677-5100

Care Unit of Jacksonville Beach
1320 Roberts Drive
Jacksonville Beach, FL 32250
(904) 241-5133

Glenbeigh–Marc Inc.
1001 N. U.S. Highway 1, 8th Floor
Jupiter, FL 33458
(305) 747-6565

Brookwood/Parkside
PO Box 2388
Kissimmee, FL 32742-2388
(305) 933-5222

Sun Coast Chemical Dependency Co-
     Dependency Program
1793 Penelope Lane
Largo, FL 33544
(813) 585-9986

Recovery Center
Highland Park General Hospital
1660 N.W. 7th Court
Miami, FL 33136
(305) 325-7008

Humana Hospital–Biscayne
20900 Biscayne Blvd.
Miami, FL 33180
(305) 932-0250

Naples Research & Counseling Center
9001 Tamiami Trail E.
Naples, FL 33962
(813) 775-4500

Care Unit
North Miami General Hospital
1701 N.E. 127th St.
North Miami, FL 33161
(305) 893-4030

Care Unit
Baptist Hospital
1101 W. Moreno St.
Pensacola, FL 32522
(904) 434-4866

Parkside Lodge of Pinellas
Metropolitan General Hospital
7950 66th St. N.
Pinellas Park, FL 33565
(813) 541-7548

Care Unit
St. Anthony's Hospital
601 12th St. N.
St. Petersburg, FL 33705
(813) 825-1200

Care Unit of Tampa at St. Francis
301 E. 7th Ave.
Tampa, FL 33602
(813) 273-9472

St. Francis Parkside Lodge
301 E. 7th Ave.
Tampa, FL 33602
(813) 273-9472

BRC–Town & Country Hospital
6001 Webb Rd.
Tampa, FL 33615
(813) 885-6666

Palm Beach Institute
Family of Programs
1014 N. Olive Ave.
West Palm Beach, FL 33401
(305) 833-7553

GEORGIA
Outpatient Addiction Clinic
4470 Chamblee-Dunwoody Rd., #100
Atlanta, GA 30338
(404) 451-0358

Safe Centers, Inc.
6255 Barfield Rd., #120
Atlanta, GA 30328
(404) 843-3292

University Hospital
1350 Walton Way
Augusta, GA 30910
(404) 722-9022

Gwinnett Treatment Center
55 Morningside Drive
Buford, GA 30518
(404) 945-1057

Brookwood/Parkside
804 Industrial Blvd.
Dublin, GA 31040
(305) 275-0353

IDAHO
St. Benedicts ACT Center
2003 Lincoln Way
Coeur d'Alene, ID 83814
(208) 667-9591

Walker ACT Center
1120 Montana
Godding, ID 83330-0541
(208) 934-8461

Care Unit
Mercy Medical Center
1512 12th Ave. Rd.
Nampa, ID 83651
(208) 466-4531

ILLINOIS
Care Unit
St. Joseph Hospital
915 E. 15th St.
Alton, IL 62002
(618) 463-5600

Care Unit
Copley Memorial Hospital
Lincoln & Weston Aves.
Aurora, IL 60505
(312) 859-0600

Parkside Lodge of Champaign
809A W. Church St.
Champaign, IL 61820
(217) 398-8616

Care Unit
Central Community Hospital
5701 S. Wood St.
Chicago, IL 60636
(312) 737-9171

New Day Center
Hyde Park Community Hospital
5800 Stony Island
Chicago, IL 60637
(312) 643-9200

Care Unit
Jackson Park Hospital & Medical Center
7531 S. Stoney Island Ave.
Chicago, IL 60649
(312) 947-2330

Martha Washington Hospital
2312 W. Irving Park Rd.
Chicago, IL 60618
(312) 583-9000

Care Unit
Mount Sinai Hospital Medical Center
California Ave. at 15th St.
Chicago, IL 60680
(312) 650-6509

New Beginnings
Lincoln West Medical Center
2544 W. Montrose Ave.
Chicago, IL 60618
(312) 722-2273

Care Unit
St. Elizabeth Hospital
1431 N. Claremont Ave.
Chicago, IL 60622
(312) 278-5015

Lutheran Center Countryside
6502 Joliet Rd.
Countryside, IL 60525
(312) 354-9403

Kishwaukee Community Hospital–CDTC
Route 23 & Bethany Rd.
Dekalb, IL 60115
(815) 756-2722

Alexian Brothers Medical Center
Alcoholism Treatment Center
800 W. Biesterfield
Elk Grove Village, IL 60007
(312) 981-3524

Care Unit
Elmhurst Memorial Hospital
200 Berteau Ave.
Elmhurst, IL 60126
(312) 941-4551

Chapman Center
Evanston Hospital
2650 Ridge Ave.
Evanston, IL 60201
(312) 492-6465

Talbot Hall CDU
St. Elizabeth Medical Center
2100 Madison
Granite City, IL 62040
(618) 798-3069

Ingalls Memorial Hospital
One Ingalls Drive
Harvey, IL 60426
(312) 333-2300

Highland Park Hospital CDP
718 Glenview Rd.
Highland Park, IL 60035
(312) 480-3719

New Day Center
Hinsdale Hospital
120 N. Oak St.
Hinsdale, IL 60521
(312) 887-2652

ARC–Chicago
1776 Moon Lake Blvd.
Hoffman Estates, IL 60194
(312) 882-0070

Parkside Lodge South
Resolve Center
411 W. Division
Manteno, IL 60950
(815) 468-3241

Parkside Lodge of Mundelein
24647 N. Highway 21
Mundelein, IL 60060
(312) 634-2020

Lutheran Center for Substance Abuse
1700 Luther Lane
Park Ridge, IL 60068
(312) 696-6050

Parkside Medical Services
205 W. Touhy Rd.
Park Ridge, IL 60068
(312) 696-8200

Parkside Youth Center
1700 N. Western Ave.
Park Ridge, IL 60068
(312) 698-4730

Proctor Community Hospital
5409 N. Knoxville
Peoria, IL 61614
(309) 691-1055

ATEP–Rockford Memorial Hospital
2400 Rockton Ave.
Rockford, IL 61103
(815) 968-6861

Parkside Lodge of Rockford
475 Executive Parkway
Rockford, IL 61108
(815) 229-3030

Care Unit
Swedish American Hospital
1400 Charles St.
Rockford, IL 61108
(815) 966-2273

Care Unit
Skokie Valley Hospital
9600 Gross Point Rd.
Skokie, IL 60076
(312) 677-3910

INDIANA
Anderson Center of St. John's
2210 Jackson St.
Anderson, IN 46014
(317) 646-8444

Care Unit
Our Lady of Mercy Hospital
U.S. Highway 30
Dyer, IN 46311
(219) 322-6716

Renaissance Center for Addiction Treatment
PO Box 1329, 600 East Blvd.
Elkhart, IN 46515
(219) 522-5522

Parkside Lodge at Mulberry Center
500 S.E. Fourth St.
Evansville, IN 47713
(812) 426-8201

Care Unit
Memorial Hospital of Michigan City
5th & Pine Sts.
Michigan City, IN 46360
(219) 872-9134

Pathways Center of Memorial Hospital
615 N. Michigan St.
South Bend, IN 46601
(219) 284-7482

Hamilton Center, Inc.
620 Eighth Ave.
Terre Haute, IN 47804
(812) 231-8226

IOWA
Iowa Methodist Medical Center
1200 Pleasant St.
Des Moines, IA 50308
(515) 283-6431

Mercy Alcohol & Drug Recovery Program
Mercy Medical Plaza #105, 421 Laurel St.
Des Moines, IA 50314
(515) 247-4441

Our Primary Purpose
University at Penn
Des Moines, IA 50316
(515) 263-5582

Mercy Health Center
Mercy Drive
Dubuque, IA 52001
(319) 589-9635

KANSAS
Arkansas City Memorial Hospital
216 W. Birch
Arkansas City, KS 67005
(316) 442-2500

St. John's at Concordia
1100 Highland Drive
Concordia, KS 66901
(913) 243-1234

St. Catherine's Hospital
608 N. 5th
Garden City, KS 67846
(316) 275-6111

St. Anthony Hospital
2220 Canterbury Rd.
Hays, KS 67601
(913) 628-1121

Hoisington Lutheran Hospital
Alcohol & Drug Treatment Center
250 W. 9th St.
Hoisington, KS 67544
(316) 653-2114

Parkside Lodge of Kansas
2100 N. Jackson St.
Hutchinson, KS 67502
(316) 663-4800

Primary Outpatient Treatment Center
1106 St. Mary's Rd.
Junction City, KS 66441
(913) 762-5352

Bethany Medical Center CDP
51 N. 12th St.
Kansas City, KS 66102
(913) 281-8954

St. Joseph Memorial Hospital
923 Carroll Ave.
Larned, KS 67550
(316) 285-3161

St. John's of Greater Kansas City
11111 Nall, Suite 219
Leawood, KS 66211
(913) 491-5440

Labette County Medical Center
Katy Hospital Behavioral Medicine
400 Katy St.
Parsons, KS 67357
(316) 421-0004

Adolescent Treatment Center
1646 N. 9th St.
Salina, KS 67401
(913) 825-7103

St. John's Hospital
139 N. Pennsylvania
Salina, KS 67401
(913) 827-5591

Shawnee Mission Medical Center ARU
9100 W. 74th St.
Shawnee Mission, KS 66201
(913) 676-2540

St. Francis Hospital Medical Center
1700 W. 7th St., 3rd Floor
Topeka, KS 66606
(913) 295-8360

Care Unit
Stormont–Vail Regional Medical Center
1500 S.W. 10th St.
Topeka, KS 66606
(913) 354-6797

St. Luke's Hospital
Chemical Dependency Unit
1323 N. A St.
Wellington, KS 67152
(316) 326-2227

St. John's of Wichita, I
Adolescent Treatment Center
250 N. Rock Rd., Suite 150
Wichita, KS 67206
(316) 688-5124

St. John's of Wichita, II
1919 N. Amidon, Suite 310
Wichita, KS 67203
(316) 832-0820

KENTUCKY
Care Unit
Our Lady of Bellefonte Hospital
St. Christopher Drive
Ashland, KY 41101
(606) 836-3148

Care Unit
Resevoir Hill
800 Park St.
Bowling Green, KY 42101
(502) 843-5100

Care Unit
St. Luke Hospital
512 S. Maple Ave.
Falmouth, KY 41040
(606) 572-3500

LOUISIANA
Baton Rouge Chemical Dependency Units
PO Box 4109
Baton Rouge, LA 70821
(504) 387-7950

Silkworth Center at Parkland Hospital
2414 Bunker Hill Drive
Baton Rouge, LA 70808
(504) 928-6633

CDU of Acadiana
PO Box 91526
Lafayette, LA 70509
(318) 234-5614

St. Patrick Hospital CDTC
524 S. Ryan
Lake Charles, LA 70601
(318) 433-7872

Bowling Green of St. Tammany
701 Florida Ave
Mandeville, LA 70448
(504) 626-5661

Lakewood Hospital
Behavioral Medicine Center
PO Drawer 2267
Morgan City, LA 70381
(504) 631-4515

New Beginnings
F. Edward Hebert Hospital
1 Sanctuary Drive
New Orleans, LA 70114
(504) 363-2580

Humana Hospital–Brentwood
1800 Irving Place
Shreveport, LA 71101
(318) 424-6761

Physicians & Surgeons Hospital
1530 Lime Ave.
Shreveport, LA 71104
(318) 227-3950

MAINE
Care Unit
Jackson Brook Institute
175 Running Hill Rd.
South Portland, ME 04106
(207) 761-2200

MARYLAND
Recovery Associates
5411 Old Frederick Rd., Suite 2
Baltimore, MD 21229
(301) 788-1717

New Beginnings at Hidden Brook
522 Thomas Run Rd.
Bel Air, MD 21014
(301) 879-1919

New Beginnings at Warwick Manor
Warwick Rd. Route 1, Box 178
East New Market, MD 21631
(301) 943-8108

Changing Point
PO Box 167, College Ave.
Ellicott City, MD 21043
(301) 465-9500

Oakview Treatment Center
3100 Health Park Drive
Ellicott City, MD 21043
(301) 461-9922

New Beginnings
Meadows Recovery Center
730 Maryland, Route 3
Gambrills, MD 21054
(301) 923-6022

Melwood Farm
PO Box 182
Olney, MD 20832
(301) 924-5000

Bowling Green Inns/Manor Care
10750 Columbia Pike
Silver Spring, MD 20901
(301) 593-9600

Saint Luke Institute, Inc.
2420 Brooks Drive
Suitland, MD 20746-5294
(301) 967-3700

Sheppard & Enoch Pratt Hospital
6501 N. Charles St.
Towson, MD 21204
(301) 823-8200

New Beginnings at White Oak
PO Box 56
Woolford, MD 21677
(301) 228-7000

MASSACHUSETTS
NCCADAC
183 N. Common St.
Lynn, MA 01905
(617) 596-2224

The Mediplex Group
2101 Washington St.
Newton, MA 02162
(617) 969-0480

New Day Center
Fuller Memorial Hospital
NORCAP Center
111 Dedham St.
Norfolk, MA 02056
(617) 668-0385

Hillcrest Hospital
165 Tor Court
Pittsfield, MA 01201
(413) 443-7414

Addiction Recovery Corp.
411 Waverly Oak Rd.
Waltham, MA 02154
(617) 893-0602

A.I.H.S.
36 Commerce Way
Woburn, MA 01801
(617) 938-8888

Bay Colony Health Services Inc.
200 W. Cummings Park, #40
Woburn, MA 01801
(617) 935-3025

Doctors Hospital of Worcester
107 Lincoln St.
Worcester, MA 01605
(617) 799-9000

MICHIGAN
New Day Center
Battle Creek Adventist Hospital
165 N. Washington Ave.
Battle Creek, MI 49106
(616) 964-7121

Bay Haven at Samaritan Health Center
713 Ninth St.
Bay City, MI 48708
(517) 894-3799

New Horizons Recovery Center
960 Agard, Box 1264
Benton Harbor, MI 49022
(616) 927-5179

Insight at Colombiere
9075 Big Lake Rd.
Clarkson, MI 48016
(313) 625-0400

Samaritan Health Center
5555 Conner Ave.
Detroit, MI 48213
(313) 579-4960

Horizon Center
610 Abbott
East Lansing, MI 48823
(517) 332-1144

New Day Center
Tri-County Community Hospital
1131 E. Howard City/Edmore Rd.
Edmore, MI 48829
(517) 427-5116

Insight at Botsford General Hospital
28050 Grand River
Farmington Hills, MI 48024
(313) 471-8583

Insight
2425 S. Linden Rd., Box 1007
Flint, MI 48504
(313) 733-5981

Insight at Fifth Avenue
420 W. Fifth Ave.
Flint, MI 48503
(313) 234-6040

Insight at Flint Osteopathic Hospital
3921 Beecher Rd.
Flint, MI 48504
(313) 762-4627

Insight at Hurley Medical Center
One Hurley Plaza
Flint, MI 48502
(313) 257-9412

Insight Community Services
Suite 305, Phoenix Building
801 S. Saginaw St.
Flint, MI 48502
(313) 238-2068

Insight Intensive Outpatient Clinic
G-3255 Beecher Rd.
Flint, MI 48504
(313) 733-3988

Insight Outpatient Clinic
The Leemen Centre
G-2241 S. Linden Rd.
Flint, MI 48504
(313) 733-0900

Outpatient Chemical Dependency Clinic
801 S. Saginaw St., Suite 300
Flint, MI 48502
(313) 238-2158

Care Unit of Grand Rapids
1931 Boston, S.E.
Grand Rapids, MI 49503
(616) 243-2273

Lutheran Center for Substance Abuse–
    Michiana
311½ E. Main
Niles, MI 49047
(616) 684-6211

Saginaw Osteopathic Hospital
515 N. Michigan Ave.
Saginaw, MI 48602
(517) 771-5317

New Day Centers, Inc.
2620 S. Cleveland Ave.
St. Joseph, MI 49085
(616) 428-2041

Insight at Riverside
Osteopathic Hospital
150 Traux
Trenton, MI 48183
(313) 676-4200

MINNESOTA
Fountain Lake Treatment Center
408 Fountain St.
Albert Lea, MN 56007
(507) 373-2384

Focus Unit
St. Joseph Medical Center
523 North St.
Brainerd, MN 65401
(218) 829-2861

Care Unit
Buffalo Memorial Hospital
303 Catlin St.
Buffalo, MN 55313
(612) 682-5490

Hazeldon Foundation
Box 11
Center City, MN 55012
(612) 257-4010

ARC West
14400 Martin Drive
Eden Prairie, MN 55344
(612) 934-7555

Care Unit
Golden Valley Health Center
4101 Golden Valley Rd.
Golden Valley, MN 55422
(612) 588-2771

ARC Parkview
3705 Park Center Blvd.
Minneapolis, MN 55416
(612) 929-5531

Hazelden Pioneer House
11505 36th Ave., North
Plymouth, MN 55441
(612) 559-2022

New Connection Program
73 Leech St.
St. Paul, MN 55102
(612) 224-4384

New Beginnings at Waverly
Route 1, Box 86
Waverly, MN 55390
(612) 658-4811

MISSISSIPPI
Brookwood/Parkside
5354 I-55
S. Frontage Rd.
Jackson, MS 39212
(601) 372-9788

MISSOURI
Care Unit
DePaul Health Center
12303 DePaul Drive
Bridgeton, MO 63044
(314) 344-7400

Care Unit
Freeman Hospital
1102 W. 32nd St.
Joplin, MO 63104
(314) 771-0500

Care Unit
Baptist Medical Center
6601 Rockhill Rd.
Kansas City, MO 64131
(816) 276-7856

Care Unit
Grim-Smith Hospital
112 E. Patterson
Kirksville, MO 63501
(816) 665-7222

New Beginnings
Kirksville Osteopathic Medical Center
900 E. LaHarpe
Kirksville, MO 63501
(816) 665-3713

St. Joseph Hospital
Family Recovery Program
525 Couch Ave.
Kirkwood, MO 63122
(314) 966-1633

Care Unit
Hospital of St. Louis
1755 S. Grand Blvd.
St. Louis, MO 63104
(314) 771-0500

Hyland Center
St. Anthony's Medical Center
10010 Kennerly Rd.
St. Louis, MO 63128
(314) 525-7200

New Beginnings
Lutheran Medical Center
2639 Miami St.
St. Louis, MO 63118
(314) 577-5849

Parkside Lodge of St. Louis
4201 McKibbon Rd.
St. Louis, MO 63134
(314) 428-4201

St. John's Mercy Medical Center
The Edgewood Program
615 S. New Ballas
St. Louis, MO 63141
(314) 569-6500

Care Unit
St. Mary's Health Center
6420 Clayton Rd.
St. Louis, MO 63117
(314) 768-8605

Intercept Program
Kelling Hospital
114 W. Kelling Ave.
Waverly, MO 64096
(816) 493-2211

MONTANA
Rimrock Foundation
PO Box 30374, 1231 N. 29th St.
Billings, MT 59101
(406) 248-3175

Care Unit
St. James Hospital East
2500 Continental Drive
Butte, MT 59701
(406) 782-0408

Francis Mahon Deaconess Hospital
Chemical Dependency Center
621 Third St. S.
Glasgow, MT 59230
(406) 228-2776

St. Patrick ACT Center
500 W. Broadway
Missoula, MT 59806
(406) 543-7271

NEBRASKA
Catholic Health Corporation
920 S. 107 Ave., Suite 200
Omaha, NE 68114
(402) 393-7661

Eppley Chemical Dependency Services
3612 Cuming St.
Omaha, NE 68131
(402) 397-3150

NEVADA
Care Unit Hospital of Nevada
5100 W. Sahara
Las Vegas, NV 89102
(702) 362-8404

Care Unit
Community Hospital of North Las Vegas
1409 E. Lake Mead Blvd.
North Las Vegas, NV 89030
(702) 642-6905

NEW HAMPSHIRE
Beech Hill Hospital
PO Box 254
Dublin, NH 03444
(603) 563-8511

Hampstead Hospital
East Rd.
Hampstead, NH 03841
(603) 329-5311

Care Unit
Lake Shore Hospital
200 Zachary Rd.
Manchester, NH 03103
(603) 645-6700

Spofford Hall
Route 9A, Box 225
Spofford, NH 03462
(603) 363-4545

Seminole Point Hospital Corporation
Woodland Rd., Box 1000
Sunapee, NH 03782
(603) 763-2545

NEW JERSEY
New Day Center
Hackettstown Community Hospital
651 Willow Grove St.
Hackettstown, NJ 07840
(201) 852-5100

Sunrise House Foundation
PO Box 600
Lafayette, NJ 07848
(201) 383-6300

New Beginnings at Lakehurst
440 Beckerville Rd.
Lakehurst, NJ 08733
(201) 657-4800

Monmouth CDTC, Inc.
152 Chelsea Ave.
Long Branch, NJ 07740
(201) 222-5190

Parkside Lodge of New Jersey
E. Second & Pancoast Aves.
Moorestown, NJ 08057
(609) 235-7900

The A.R.T.S.
Health Industry of New Jersey
70 Parker Ave., 5th Floor
Passaic, NJ 07055
(201) 472-0364

Seabrook House, Inc.
PO Box 5055, Polk Lane
Seabrook, NJ 08302
(609) 455-7575

Future Health Systems, Inc.
47 Maple Ave.
Summit, NJ 07901
(201) 273-5400

NEW MEXICO
Care Unit
Hospital of Albuquerque
505 High St., N.E.
Albuquerque, NM 87102
(505) 848-8088

Care Unit
Lovelace Medical Center
5400 Gibson Blvd., S.E.
Albuquerque, NM 87108
(505) 262-7252

Lea Regional Hospital Pavilion
Lovington Highway, Box 3000
Hobbs, NM 88240
(505) 392-4566

Care Unit
St. Mary's Regional Health Center
S. Main & Chisum Sts.
Roswell, NM 88201
(505) 623-2273

New Beginnings at Amethyst Hall
6930 Weicker Lane
Velarde, NM 87582
(505) 852-2704

NEW YORK
Arms Acres
Box X
Carmel, NY 10512
(914) 225-3400

Alive & Well
900 Walt Whitman Rd.
Melville, NY 11747
(516) 466-4444

Breakthrough
Gracie Square Hospital
420 E. 76th St.
New York, NY 10021
(212) 988-4400

ICD Alcoholism Program
340 E. 24th St.
New York, NY 10010
(212) 679-0100

Robert Sbriglio, M.D.
77 Fifth Ave., Apt. 3-B
New York, NY 10003
(212) 472-5643

Conifer Park
150 Glenridge Rd
Scotia, NY 12302
(518) 399-6446

ARC Westchester
PO Box 37, Route 118
Yorktown Heights, NY 10598
(914) 962-5000

NORTH CAROLINA
Woodhill Treatment Center
PO Box 5014
Asheville, NC 28813
(704) 253-3681

Care Unit
Alamance County Hospital
327 Graham-Hopedale Rd.
Burlington, NC 27215
(919) 226-4382

Charlotte Treatment Center
1715 Sharon Rd. W., Box 240197
Charlotte, NC 28224
(704) 554-8373

Oakleigh at Durham
309 Crutchfield St.
Durham, NC 27704
(919) 479-3000

New Day Center
Park Ridge Hospital
Howard Gap Rd.
Fletcher, NC 28732
(704) 684-8501

Fellowship Hall
PO Box 6929
Greensboro, NC 27415
(919) 621-3381

Carolinas Hospital
Alcoholism Program Service
PO Box 18871
Raleigh, NC 27619
(919) 872-5358

Care Unit
Rowan Memorial Hospital
612 Mocksville Ave.
Salisbury, NC 28144
(704) 638-1300

NORTH DAKOTA
Heartview Foundation
1406 Second St., N.W.
Mandan, ND 58554
(701) 663-2321

OHIO
Care Unit
Christ Hospital
2139 Auburn Ave.
Cincinnati, OH 45219
(513) 369-1116

Care Unit
Hospital of Cincinnati
3156 Glenmore Ave.
Cincinnati, OH 45211
(513) 481-8822

Glenbeigh Hospital–Cleveland
18120 Puritas Rd.
Cleveland, OH 44135
(216) 953-0177

Brookwood/Parkside
349 Ridenour Rd.
Columbus, OH 43230
(614) 471-2552

Care Unit
Mercy Hospital
1430 S. High St.
Columbus, OH 43207
(614) 445-5200

Care Unit
Miami Valley Hospital
1 Wyoming St.
Dayton, OH 45409
(513) 461-9670

Samaritan Hall
4780 Salem Ave.
Dayton, OH 45416
(513) 276-5031

Serenity Hall
Richland Hospital
1451 Lucas Rd., Box 637
Mansfield, OH 44901
(419) 589-5511

Care Unit
Marietta Memorial Hospital
Matthew & Ferguson Sts.
Marietta, OH 45750
(614) 373-8816

Care Unit
Community Medical Center Hospital
1050 Delaware Ave.
Marion, OH 43302
(614) 387-6408

Care Unit
East Ohio Regional Hospital
90 N. Fourth St.
Martins Ferry, OH 43935
(614) 633-4241

Care Unit
Massillon Community Hospital
875 Eighth St., N.E.
Massillon, OH 44646
(216) 837-6897

Southwest General Hospital
18697 Bagley Rd.
Middleburg Heights, OH 44130
(216) 826-8200

Care Unit
Williams County General Hospital
909 Snyder Ave.
Montpelier, OH 43453
(419) 485-5511

Shepherd Hill
200 Messimer Drive
Newark, OH 43055
(614) 522-8484

Southern Hills Hospital ATS
727 Eighth St.
Portsmouth, OH 45662
(614) 354-2281

Glenbeigh Hospital
Route 45
Rock Creek, OH 44084
(216) 563-3400

Care Unit
Salem Community Hospital
1995 E. State St.
Salem, OH 44460
(216) 332-7348

Community Hospital Recovery Center
2615 E. High St.
Springfield, OH 45505
(513) 325-0531

Flower Hospital Center for Alcoholism
  Treatment
5200 Harroun Rd.
Sylvania, OH 43560
(419) 885-1444

Tennyson Center
St. Vincent Medical Center
2465 Collingwood
Toledo, OH 43620-1195
(419) 255-5665

Toledo Hospital ATC
2142 N. Cove Blvd.
Toledo, OH 43606
(419) 241-3662

Dettmer Hall
3130 N. Dixie Highway
Troy, OH 45373
(513) 335-5624

Serenity Hall Centers
29000 Center Ridge Rd.
Westlake, OH 44145
(216) 835-6059

Glenbeigh Family Center
301 E. 293rd St.
Willowick, OH 44094
(216) 585-2600

Greene Hall
1141 N. Monroe Dr.
Xenia, OH 45385
(513) 372-8011

Alcoholic Clinic of Youngstown
2151 Rush Blvd.
Youngstown, OH 44507
(216) 744-1181

Good Samaritan Medical Center
800 Forest Ave.
Zanesville, OH 43701
(614) 454-5469

OKLAHOMA
Care Unit
Jane Phillips Episcopal Memorial Medical
   Center
3500 E. Frank Phillips Blvd.
Bartlesville, OK 74006
(918) 333-5027

Country View
12300 E. 91st St.
Broken Arrow, OK 74012
(918) 252-2541

Care Unit
Enid Memorial Hospital
402 S. Fourth St.
Enid, OK 73701
(405) 242-7713

Comanche County Memorial Hospital
3401 W. Gore Blvd.
Lawton, OK 73505
(405) 344-8620

Care Unit
St. Anthony Hospital
1000 N. Lee St.
Oklahoma City, OK 73102
(405) 272-6835

St. John's of Oklahoma City
6125 W. Reno, Suite 400
Oklahoma City, OK 73127
(405) 495-3080

Cherokee Nation of Oklahoma
Box 948
Talequah, OK 74464
(918) 456-0671

Brookhaven Hospital
201 S. Garnett
Tulsa, OK 74128
(813) 438-4257

Care Unit
Hillcrest Medical Center
Utica on the Park
Tulsa, OK 74104
(918) 560-5711

OREGON
Sacred Heart General Hospital
675 W. Broadway
Eugene, OR 97402
(503) 686-6888

Serenity Lane Inc.
616 W. 16th St.
Eugene, OR 97401
(503) 687-1110

Mount Hood Medical Center
Box 718
24700 S.E. Stark
Gresham, OR 97030
(503) 661-9204

Care Unit
St. Anthony Hospital
1601 S.E. Court Ave.
Pendleton, OR 97801
(503) 276-3021

Care Unit
Physicians & Surgeons Hospital
1927 N.W. Lovejoy St.
Portland, OR 97209
(503) 225-0031

New Day Center
Portland Adventist Medical Center
6012 S.E. Yamhill
Portland, OR 97215
(503) 231-3995

PENNSYLVANIA
Gateway Rehabilitation Center
Moffett Run Rd.
Aliquippa, PA 15001
(412) 766-8700

Care Unit
Slate Belt Medical Center
701 Slate Belt Blvd., Route 3
Bangor, PA 18013
(315) 588-6011

Livengrin Foundation, Inc.
4833 Hulmeville Rd.
Bensalem, PA 19020
(215) 639-2300

Care Unit
Butler Memorial Hospital
911 E. Brady St.
Butler, PA 16001
(412) 284-4357

UHS/Keystone Center
2001 Providence Rd.
Chester, PA 19013
(215) 876-9000

Mirmont Alcoholism Rehabilitation Center
501 N. Lansdowne Ave.
Drexel Hill, PA 19026
(215) 284-8198

Eagleville Hospital
100 Eagleville Rd.
Eagleville, PA 19408
(215) 539-6000

ARC–The Terraces
1170 S. State St.
Ephrata, PA 17522
(717) 627-0790

Care Unit
Hamot Medical Center
201 State St.
Erie, PA 16550
(814) 870-6133

Susquehanna Valley Center
10th Floor, Brady Hall, S. Front St.
Harrisburg, PA 17101
(717) 782-5310

Bowling Green Inn–Brandywine
495 Neward Rd.
Kennett Square, PA 19348
(215) 268-3588

Clear Brook, Inc.
R.D. No. 10, E. Northhampton St.
Laurel Run, PA 18702
(717) 823-1171

Malvern Institute
940 King Rd.
Malvern, PA 19355
(215) 647-0330

Spencer Hospital
1034 Grove St.
Meadville, PA 16335
(814) 336-4357

South Hills Health System
4129 Brownsville Rd.
Pittsburgh, PA 15227
(412) 881-2255

Roxbury
PO Box L, 601 Roxbury Rd.
Shippensburg, PA 17257
(717) 532-4217

Caron Foundation
Box 277, Galen Hall Rd.
Wernersville, PA 19565
(215) 678-2332

New Beginnings at Cove Forge
PO Box B
Williamsburg, PA 16693
(814) 832-2131

RHODE ISLAND
Edgehill Newport
200 Harrison Ave.
Newport, RI 02840
(401) 849-5700

SOUTH CAROLINA
Baker Hospital
2750 Speissegger Drive
Charleston, SC 29405
(803) 744-2110

New Beginnings at Fenwick Hall
Box 688, 1709 River Rd.
Johns Island, SC 29455
(803) 559-2461

North Greenville Hospital
807 N. Main St.
Travelers Rest, SC 29690
(803) 834-5131

SOUTH DAKOTA
Care Unit
Dakota Midland Hospital
Highway 281 N. & 15th Ave., N.W.
Aberdeen, SD 57401
(605) 622-3425

Keystone Treatment Center, Inc.
1010 E. Second, Box 159
Canton, SD 57013
(605) 987-2751

Intercept Program
Custer Community Hospital
1039 Montgomery St.
Custer, SD 57730
(605) 673-2229

River Park
801 E. Dakota Ave.
Pierre, SD 57501
(605) 224-6177

TENNESSEE
ARC Chattanooga
8614 Harrison Bay Rd.
Harrison, TN 37341
(615) 344-3737

New Beginnings
University Medical Center
1411 Baddour Parkway
Lebanon, TN 37087
(615) 444-8165

Methodist Outreach, Inc.
2009 Lamar Ave.
Memphis, TN 38114
(901) 276-5401

Care Unit
St. Joseph Hospital
220 Overton Ave.
Memphis, TN 38105
(901) 529-2902

Care Unit
Baptist Hospital
2000 Church St.
Nashville, TN 37236
(615) 329-7777

Cumberland Heights
Route 2 River Rd.
Nashville, TN 37209
(615) 352-1757

Meharry–Hubbard Hospital
1005 DB Todd Blvd.
Nashville, TN 37208
(615) 327-5532

Vanderbilt Institute for Treatment of
   Alcoholism
4th Floor, Zerfloss Building, 21st Ave. S.
Nashville, TN 37232
(615) 322-6158

New Beginnings
John W. Harton Regional Medical Center
PO Box 460
Tullahoma, TN 37388
(615) 455-0020

TEXAS
Care Unit
Hendrick Medical Center
1242 N. 19th
Abilene, TX 79601
(915) 677-2287

BRC–Alvin
Alvin Community Hospital
301 Medic Lane
Alvine, TX 77511
(713) 331-6141

St. Anthony's Hospital
200 N.W. Seventh Ave.
Amarillo, TX 79176
(806) 378-6797

Parkside Lodge of Dallas/Ft. Worth
Route #1, Box 223AB
Argyle, TX 76226
(817) 455-2201

The Faulkner Center
1900 Rio Grande
Austin, TX 78705
(512) 482-0075

Shoal Creek Hospital
Renaissance Program for Chemical
   Dependency
3501 Mills Ave.
Austin, TX 78731
(512) 452-0361

Care Unit
Baptist Hospital of Southeast Texas
3510 Stagg Drive
Beaumont, TX 77704
(409) 839-5387

Care Unit
Palo Duro Hospital
2 Hospital Drive
Canyon, TX 79015
(806) 655-7723

Starlite Village Hospital
PO Box 317
Center Point, TX 78013
(512) 634-2212

Chemical Dependency Unit of South Texas
PO Box 81326
Corpus Christi, TX 78412
(512) 993-6100

Care Unit
Corpus Christi Osteopathic Hospital
1502 Tarleton
Corpus Christi, TX 78415
(512) 884-2524

New Beginnings
Southside Community Hospital
4626 Weber Rd.
Corpus Christi, TX 78411
(512) 854-2031

Care Unit
Baylor University Medical Center
3500 Gaston Ave.
Dallas, TX 75246
(214) 820-2300

Deer Park Hospital
4525 Glenwood Ave.
Deer Park, TX 77536
(713) 479-0955

Brookwood/Parkside
4601 Interstate 35 N.
Denton, TX 76201
(817) 565-8100

Harris Hospital H.E.B.
2219 W. Euless Blvd.
Euless, TX 76039
(817) 283-1561

BRC–Fort Worth
6825 Manhattan Blvd., #501
Fort Worth, TX 76112
(817) 496-8833

Care Unit–Dallas/Fort Worth
1066 W. Magnolia
Fort Worth, TX 76104
(817) 336-2828

Schick Shadel Hospital
4101 Frawley Dr.
Fort Worth, TX 76118
(817) 284-9217

Dallas–Fort Worth Medical Center
444 Duncan Perry Rd.
Grand Prairie, TX 75051
(214) 641-5263

Behavioral Health System, Inc.
3838 N. Belt, #230
Houston, TX 77032
(713) 590-4413

Care Unit
Memorial Northwest Hospital
1635 N. Loop W.
Houston, TX 77008
(713) 880-7506

P.A.C.T.
2616 S. Loop W., #225
Houston, TX 77054
(713) 666-9811

La Hacienda Treatment Center
Hospital Services of Texas, Inc.
PO Box 1
Hunt, TX 78024
(512) 238-4222

Brookwood/Parkside
5638 Medical Center Drive
Katy, TX 77450
(713) 392-3456

Brookwood/Parkside
PO Box 168
Liverpool, TX 77577
(713) 439-7474

Intercept Program
Mason Memorial Hospital
203 College St.
Mason, TX 76856
(915) 347-2684

Clearview
PO Box 4757
Midland, TX 79704
(915) 697-5200

Intercept Program
West Plains Medical Center
708 S. First St.
Muleshoe, TX 79347
(806) 272-7561

Care Unit
Memorial Hospital
1204 Mound St.
Nacogdoches, TX 75961
(409) 560-5200

Intercept Program
New Boston General Hospital
520 Hospital Drive
New Boston, TX 75570
(214) 628-5687

Park Place Recovery Center
3050 39th St.
Port Arthur, TX 77642
(409) 983-4951

Brookwood/Parkside
14747 Jones Maltsberger Rd.
San Antonio, TX 78247
(512) 494-1237

New Day Center
Hays Memorial Hospital
1301 Redwood Rd.
San Marcos, TX 78666
(512) 353-8979

Intercept Program
Brazos Valley Hospital
526 Ward St.
Sealy, TX 77474
(409) 885-4952

White River Retreat, Inc.
Star Route 2, Box 123
Spur, TX 79370
(806) 263-4211

Citizens Medical Center
Behavioral Medicine Center
2701 Hospital Drive
Victoria, TX 77901
(512) 572-5179

Campbell Memorial Hospital
Behavioral Medicine Unit
713 E. Andersen
Weatherford, TX 76086
(817) 594-8751

Brookwood/Parkside
Box 98
200 Green Rd.
Willmer, TX 75172
(214) 525-6285

Intercept Program
Wortham Hospital
S. Highway 14, Box 428
Wortham, TX 76693
(817) 765-3363

UTAH
St. Benedict's ACT
3017 Taylor Ave.
Ogden, UT 84403-0908
(801) 627-2150

St. Benedict's ACT Center
3293 Harrison Blvd., #120
Ogden, UT 84403
(801) 627-1780

St. Benedict's ACT Center–Ogden
5475 S. 500 E.
Ogden, UT 84405-6978
(801) 479-2250

Dayspring–Utah Valley Regional Medical
  Center
1034 N. Fifth W.
Provo, UT 84603
(801) 373-7850

Adapt Center
2700 W. 5600 S.
Roy, UT 84067
(801) 773-6870

Highland Ridge Hospital
4578 Highland Drive
Salt Lake City, UT 84119
(801) 272-9851

I.H.C. Hospital, Inc.
Regional Medical Center
36 S. State St., 22nd Floor
Salt Lake City, UT 84111
(801) 533-8282

LDS Hospital–Dayspring
325 Eighth Ave.
Salt Lake City, UT 84143
(801) 321-5580

Mill Creek–Dayspring
772 E. 3300 S., #100
Salt Lake City, UT 84106
(801) 487-9000

St. Benedict's ACT Center
1255 E. 3900 S.
Salt Lake City, UT 84124
(801) 263-1300

VERMONT
Brattleboro Retreat
75 Linden St.
Brattleboro, VT 05301
(802) 257-7785

Founders Hall
Hospital Hall
Hospital Drive
St. Johnsbury, VT 05301
(802) 748-9374

VIRGINIA
Arlington Hospital ATP
1701 N. George Mason Drive
Arlington, VA 22205
(703) 558-6536

New Beginnings at Serenity Lodge
2097 S. Military Highway
Chesapeake, VA 23320
(804) 543-6888

Dominion Hospital–CDP
2960 Sleepy Hollow Rd.
Falls Church, VA 22044
(703) 536-2000

Complete Alcoholism Treatment Services
Fairfax Hospital
3300 Gallows Rd.
Falls Church, VA 22046
(703) 698-1530

Arlington Health Services Corporation
Route 3, Box 52
Harrisonburg, VA 22801
(703) 434-7396

Riverside Hospital ATP
J. Clyde Morris Blvd.
Newport News, VA 23601
(804) 599-2684

St. Johns Hospital
Route 2, Box 389
Richmond, VA 23233
(804) 784-3501

Mt. Regis Center
405 Kimbal Ave.
Salem, VA 24153
(703) 389-4761

WASHINGTON
Care Unit
St. Joseph Hospital
1006 N. H. St.
Aberdeen, WA 98520
(206) 533-8500

Care Unit
Monticello Medical Center
600 Broadway
Longview, WA 98632
(206) 636-7363

Care Unit
Ballard Community Hospital
5409 Barnes Ave., N.W.
Seattle, WA 98107
(206) 789-7209

Care Unit
Riverton General Hospital
12844 Military Rd. S.
Seattle, WA 98168
(206) 242-2260

Schick Shadel Hospital
12101 Ambaum Blvd., S.W.
Seattle, WA 98166
(206) 244-8100

Care Unit
Deaconess Medical Center
W. 800 Fifth Ave.
Spokane, WA 99210
(509) 458-2273

New Beginnings
Lakewood General Hospital
5702 100th St., S.W.
Tacoma, WA 98499
(206) 582-4357

St. Joseph Community Hospital
PO Box 1600
Vancouver, WA 98668
(206) 690-4550

WEST VIRGINIA
Care Unit
Charleston Area Medical Center
Brooks & Washington Sts.
Charleston, WV 25301
(304) 348-6060

WISCONSIN
Parkside Lodge of Wisconsin
2185 Shopiere Rd.
Beloit, WI 53511
(608) 365-2709

Elmbrook Memorial Hospital ATP
19333 W. North Ave.
Brookfield, WI 53005
(414) 785-2233

Parkside Lodge of Wisconsin
313 Stoughton Rd.
Edgerton, WI 53534
(608) 884-3381

DePaul–Pathway
2697 Grand Ave.
Hartford, WI 53027
(414) 673-7950

Parkside Lodge of Wisconsin
320 Lincoln St.
Janesville, WI 53547
(608) 754-2264

St. Catherine's Hospital ATP
3556 Seventh Ave.
Kenosha, WI 53140
(414) 396-4382

St. Francis Medical Center, Inc.
700 West Ave. S
La Crosse, WI 54601
(608) 785-0940

New Start Program
Madison General Hospital
202 S. Park St.
Madison, WI 53715
(608) 267-6291

DePaul–Holy Family Chemical
    Dependency Unit
21st & Western Aves.
Manitowoc, WI 54220
(414) 683-3030

DePaul–Brown Deer
8464 W. Brown Deer Rd.
Milwaukee, WI 53225
(414) 355-7992

DePaul Rehabilitation Hospital
4143 S. 13th St.
Milwaukee, WI 53221
(414) 281-4400

DePaul St. Anthony's
1004 N. 10th St.
Milwaukee, WI 53203
(414) 271-1965

Kettle Moraine Hospital
4839 N. Hewitts Point Rd.
Oconomowoc, WI 53066
(414) 567-0201

DePaul Port Washington
743 N. Montgomery St.
Port Washington, WI 53074
(800) 242-2112

The A-Center of Racine
2000 Domanik Drive
Racine, WI 53404
(414) 632-6141

St. Croix Valley Memorial Hospital–C.D.C.
204 S. Adams St.
St. Croix Falls, WI 54024
(715) 483-3261

DePaul Oakland Clinic
3510 N. Oakland Ave.
Shorewood, WI 53211
(414) 961-1121

Sacred Heart Hospital
Alcohol & Drug Unit
216 N. Seventh St.
Tomahawk, WI 54487
(715) 543-2181

Brady Hall
Route 2, Box 236A
Turtle Lake, WI 54889
(715) 986-4340

Clarence Snyder Hall
Route 2, Box 193
Turtle Lake, WI 54889
(715) 986-4520

Dewey Center
Milwaukee Psychiatric Hospital
1220 Dewey Ave.
Wauwatosa, WI 53213
(414) 258-2600

DePaul Lincoln Clinic
10401 W. Lincoln Ave.
West Allis, WI 53227
(414) 546-8140

SOURCE: *National Association of Alcoholism Treatment Programs.*

CONTROLLED DRINKING: AN ALTERNATIVE TREATMENT AND A MINORITY VIEW

Nearly all treatment for alcoholism in this country is based on total abstinence, the guiding principle behind Alcoholics Anonymous. But there is an alternative alcohol treatment that is increasingly popular in Europe and is gaining some ground here, although it has many critics. It starts with the assumption that many problem drinkers may benefit from learning how to control drinking rather than avoiding alcohol altogether. Advocates of this point of view note that there is little help for millions of Americans who do not consider themselves alcoholics but would like to learn how to handle their drinking better— to moderate their drinking rather than eliminate it.

Some European researchers maintain they have had success in training alcoholics to drink moderately. In this country, one of the leading advocates of controlled drinking is Dr. William R. Miller, director of the Alcohol Research and Treatment Program at the University of New Mexico. Dr. Miller reports that his controlled drinking program has been successful with many people who are not considered hard-core or "addictive" alcoholics. These people seemingly do not have a biological dependence on alcohol and do not have close relatives who are alcoholics. Dr. Miller says he has been successful in teaching about two-thirds of these "nonaddictive" alcoholics how to drink moderately.

Controlled drinking is definitely a minority view, and only a handful of clinics offer this approach to problem drinking. Critics maintain it is dangerous because it tempts alcoholics into falsely believing they can drink. Advocates of the method argue it may save millions who are now only problem drinkers from becoming full-fledged alcoholics, and may offer help to certain alcoholics who want moderation, not abstinence.

GOVERNMENT ALCOHOL RESEARCH CENTERS

The National Institute on Alcohol Abuse and Alcoholism supports several major centers at medical centers to do both basic (animal and laboratory) and patient-oriented research on the effects and mechanisms of alchohol and alcoholic behavior. Each of the centers has a special area of interest. Here are the centers that do research involving people, and their main areas of interest.

Alcohol Research Group
1816 Scenic Avenue
Berkeley, CA 94709
Robin Room, Ph.D. Studies on the epidemiology of alcohol problems.

Pacific Institute for Research
The Prevention Center
2532 Durant Ave.
Berkeley, CA 94704
Lawrence Wallack, D.P.H. Several studies to find innovative approaches to the prevention of alcohol-related problems, including traffic accidents.

Scripps Clinic and Research Foundation
10666 N. Torrey Pines Rd.
La Jolla, CA 92037
Floyd E. Bloom, M.D. Several studies focusing on the effects of alcohol on the central nervous system.

University of Colorado Medical Center
4200 E. Ninth Ave.
Denver, CO 80262
Richard Dietrich, Ph.D. Several studies focusing on the effects of alcohol on the central nervous system, and the genetic factor.

University of Connecticut Health Center
Farmington Ave.
Farmington, CT 06032
Roger E. Meyer, M.D. Studies on causes of alcoholism and response to various treatments.

University of Florida
J. Hills Miller Health Center, J-14
Gainesville, FL 32610
Kenneth F. Finger, Ph.D. Several studies focusing on alcohol abuse among the elderly.

Washington University School of Medicine
Department of Psychiatry
4940 Audubon Ave.
St. Louis, MO 63110
Samuel B. Guze, M.D. Several studies concentrating on the neurobiology, genetics, and family history of alcoholism.

Alcohol Research Center
Veterans Administration Hospital
130 W. Kingsbridge Rd.
Bronx, NY 10468
Charles S. Lieber, M.D. Some studies on depression in alcoholics.

ALCOHOL RESEARCH AT THE NATIONAL INSTITUTES OF HEALTH

Several studies on alcoholic patients are under way at the Clinical Center at the National Institutes of Health in Bethesda, Maryland, including drug treatment for brain dysfunction due to chronic alcoholism, alcohol-withdrawal treatment, research to reduce the craving for alcohol and identification of the biological and genetic factors in alcoholism. Selected patients, referred by physicians, may be accepted. For more information your physician can contact:

Office of the Director
The Clinical Center
Building 10, Room 2C146
National Institutes of Health
Bethesda, MD 20992

ORGANIZATIONS AND AGENCIES

Alcoholics Anonymous
PO Box 459
Grand Central Station
New York, NY 10163

AA is by far the most widely recognized self-help group for alcoholics, with a worldwide membership of more than one million. AA maintains no membership lists, insists on anonymity for its members, and is best known for its mutual support groups that meet periodically. Each group is self-supporting, although no dues or fees are required for membership. Sponsors open meetings for anyone, and closed meetings for alcoholics only. Program is based on a "12-step" guide to recovery. Publishes a book, *Alcoholics Anonymous,* pamphlets, booklets and a monthly periodical, *The AA Grapevine,* containing information, interpretation and inspiration, written by AA members. AA groups meet in hundreds of treatment centers. AA will provide more information upon request.

The Calix Society
7601 Wayzata Blvd.
Minneapolis, MN 55426
(612) 546-0544

A society, dedicated to helping Catholics maintain sobriety through affiliation with and participation in Alcoholics Anonymous. The creed is total abstinence and the promotion of spiritual development of members. Calix is Latin for chalice and reflects the Society's goals of substituting "the cup that sanctifies for the cup that stupefies." Publishes brochures, a newsletter, and a list of local Calix Units. Will provide more information and location of local units upon request.

Hazelden Foundation
PO Box 11
Center City, MN 55012
(612) 257-4010
(800) 328-9000

A nonprofit organization for chemical dependency rehabilitation. Maintains several programs in Minnesota, including the Hazelden Rehabilitation Center, a large private treatment center accommodating about 1,600 people a year. Also a rehabilitation program in West Palm Beach, Florida. Has a half-way house and a live-in 5-day family program. Numerous books, booklets, audiotapes, videotapes, films on alcoholism and drug addiction. Quarterly newsletter. Will provide more information and a catalogue of materials upon request.

National Association for Children of
  Alcoholics
31706 Coast Highway #201
South Laguna, CA 92677
(714) 499-3889

National nonprofit, membership organization for the children of alcoholics serving primarily as an information networking source. Helps individuals find treatment for children. Makes referrals to other self-help organizations. Publishes a quarterly newsletter, and operates a clearinghouse for information on children of alcoholics.

National Association of Alcoholism Treatment
  Programs, Inc.
2082 Michelson Drive
Irvine, CA 92715
(714) 476-8204

A national trade association of both nonprofit and profit-making alcohol treatment centers.

Represents about 450 treatment centers throughout the country. Bimonthly newsletter offers for sale a list of its member-programs throughout the country. Available to the public.

National Clearinghouse for Alcohol
  Information
PO Box 2345
Rockville, MD 20852
(301) 468-2600

An information source sponsored by the federal government. Provides information on all aspects of alcoholism to the public and professionals working in the field of alcoholism. Will answer questions over the phone and send detailed information upon request.

National Council on Alcoholism
12 W. 21st St.
New York, NY 10010
(212) 206-6770

A national voluntary health organization with 200 state and local affiliates dedicated to combating alcoholism. An information source for the public, it makes treatment referrals for alcoholics and their families and provides pamphlets, booklets, audiovisual materials and a bimonthly newsletter, *The Amethyst.*

National Institute on Alcohol Abuse and
  Alcoholism
Parklawn Building
5600 Fishers Lane
Rockville, MD 20852
(301) 443-4883 (public affairs)

The agency within the federal government's Department of Health and Human Services most concerned with the problems of alcoholism. Sponsors research nationwide. Publishes numerous materials, including *Alcohol Health and Research World,* a quarterly magazine of up-to-date information of developments in the alcohol field, which is available by subscription.

Toughlove
PO Box 1069
Doylestown, PA 18901
(215) 348-7090

A national alcohol and drug abuse prevention program geared toward helping parents, families, and friends cope with individuals who are chemically dependent or potentially chemically dependent. Has a listing of about 1,500 local groups for parents and children, and helps parents organize local groups. Provides books, audiocassettes, a bimonthly newsletter, makes referrals to local groups. Will provide more information upon request.

Women for Sobriety
PO Box 618
Quakertown, PA 18951
(215) 536-8026

A national self-help organization for women with drinking problems with local chapters throughout the country. Designed to fill a vacuum for women who may want additional support from other women; supports women through local self-help groups that meet weekly; publishes and sells materials on alcoholism, including pamphlets, books, a newsletter and audiotapes; and conducts workshops. Will provide more information and a list of chapters upon request.

BOOKS

The number of books, pamphlets, booklets and audiovisual materials on alcoholism is vast. Those listed below are among the most outstanding but the list is by no means comprehensive. For a catalogue of publications on all aspects of alcoholism, contact the National Council on Alcoholism, 733 Third Ave., New York, NY 10017; or the Hazelden Foundation, PO Box 11, Center City, MN 55012.

Alcohol Problems and Alcoholism: A Comprehensive Survey, **James E. Royce, Ph.D.,** New York: Macmillan/Free Press, 1981.

Alcoholism: The Facts, **D.W. Goodwin,** New York: Oxford University Press, 1981.

Alcoholism: Treatable Illness, **J. George Strachan,** Hazelden Foundation, Rev. 1982.

Bill W.: Biography of the Founder of AA, **Robert Thomsen,** New York: Harper & Row, 1975.

End of the Rainbow, **Mary Ann Crenshaw,** New York: Macmillan Publishing Co., 1981.

Goodbye Hangovers, Hello Life, **Jean Kirkpatrick, Ph.D.,** New York: Atheneum, 1986.

Having Been There, edited by **Allan Luks,** New York: Charles Scribner's Sons, 1979 (short stories)

Helping your Alcoholic Before He or She Hits Bottom, **Roque Fajardo,** New York: Crown Publishers, 1976.

How To Live With a Problem Drinker and

Survive, **Gary G. Forrest,** New York: Atheneum, 1980.

I'll Quit Tomorrow, **Vernon Johnson,** New York: Harper & Row, 1980.

I'm Black and Sober, **Chaney Allen,** Minneapolis: CompCare Publications, 1978.

Lost Years: Confessions of a Woman Alcoholic, **Megan Moran,** New York: Doubleday, 1985.

The Natural History of Alcoholism: Causes, Patterns and Paths to Recovery, **George E. Vaillant, M.D.,** Cambridge, MA, Harvard University Press, 1983.

No Laughing Matter, **Fr. Joseph C. Martin,** New York: Harper & Row, 1982.

The Quality of Mercy, **Mercedes McCambridge,** New York: Times Books, 1982.

Toughlove, **Phyllis** and **David York,** New York: Doubleday, 1982; Bantam Books, 1983.

Toughlove Solutions, **Phyllis** and **David York,** New York: Doubleday, 1984; Bantam Books, 1985.

Turnabout: Help for a New Life, **Jean Kirkpatrick, Ph.D.,** New York: Doubleday, 1977; (a recovered alcoholic and founder of Women for Sobriety; also available from Women for Sobriety, Inc.).

Twenty-Four Hours a Day: A Handbook, Hazelden Foundation.

Will America Sober Up? **Allan Luks,** Boston: Beacon Press, 1984.

MATERIALS, FREE AND FOR SALE

Free

AA at a Glance, pamphlet.
A Message for Teenagers, pamphlet.
Information on AA, pamphlet.
Problems Other than Alcohol, pamphlet.

Alcoholics Anonymous
PO Box 459
Grand Central Station
New York, NY 10163
(no charge for single copies)

Alcohol and the Unborn Baby, 16 pages.
Is Beer a Four Letter Word?, 60 pages.
Someone Close Drinks Too Much, 15 pages.

National Clearinghouse for Alcohol
   Information
PO Box 2345
Rockville, MD 20852
(301) 468-2600

Guide to Alcohol Programs for Youth, 28 pages.
Treating Alcoholism: The Illness, the Symptoms,
   the Treatment, 16 pages.

National Institute on Alcoholism and Alcohol
   Abuse
Parklawn Building
5600 Fishers Lane
Rockville, MD 20852
(301) 443-4883

For sale

Alcoholism: The Family Disease, 48 pages.
Al-Anon Is for Adult Children of Alcoholics, 12
   pages.
Getting in Touch with Al-Anon.
Lois's Story, 9 pages.

Al-Anon Family Group Headquarters
PO Box 182
Madison Square Station
New York, NY 10159-0182
(212) 683-1771

ABC's of Drinking and Driving, 16 pages.
About Alcohol, 16 pages, also available in Span-
   ish.
About Alcoholism, 16 pages.
About Alcoholism Services, 16 pages.
Alcohol and Drug Coloring Book, Tough Love,
   18 pages.
Alcoholic in the Family?, 16 pages.

What Every Teenager Should Know About Alco-
   hol, 16 pages.

National Council on Alcoholism
733 Third Ave.
New York, NY 10017
(212) 986-4433

Toughlove: A Self-Help Manual for Parents
   Troubled by Teenage Behavior, 98 pages.
Toughlove: A Self-Manual for Kids, 134 pages.

Toughlove
PO Box 1069
Doylestown, PA 18901

The New Life Diary Booklets:
For Women Alcoholics
The Nature of Guilt
Six Essays on Depression
So You Want to Quit
The Woman Who Drinks Too Much

Women for Sobriety, Inc.
PO Box 618
Quakertown, PA 18951

Audiocassette tapes

Alcoholism: A Family Affair. **Dr. Patricia
O'Gorman** on "Children of Alcoholics" and
"The Alcoholic Marriage." With interviews of
couples and individuals.
The Doctor Talks to You About Alcoholism,
Frank A. Seixas, M.D., medical director of
the National Council on Alcoholism.

National Council on Alcoholism
733 Third Ave.
New York, NY 10017
(212) 986-4433

Alcoholics
Combating Depression
The First Year
Guilt Feelings
Happiness and Sobriety
Keys to Recovery
Self-Imaging
So You Want to Quit
Special Needs of Women
The Woman Alcoholic

Women for Sobriety, Inc.
PO Box 618
Quakertown, PA 18951

INFORMATION ABOUT CONTROLLED DRINKING

A self-help manual

How to Control Your Drinking by Dr. William R. Miller is a manual with detailed instructions on how to change drinking habits, to control drinking without abstinence. Dr. Miller has evaluated the self-help manual by following up a number of its users for a two-year period, and says the self-help manual is as effective in teaching the control of drinking as is face-to-face treatment in his center. Available from University of New Mexico Press, Albuquerque, NM 87131 or through bookstores.

Dr. William R. Miller
Director, Alcohol Research and Treatment
    Project
Department of Psychology
The University of New Mexico
Albuquerque, NM 87131
(505) 277-4121

ALZHEIMER'S DISEASE AND DEMENTIA

See also Rehabilitation, page 460.

Mental deterioration in the elderly, popularly known as "senility" or dementia, is by no means an inevitable consequence of aging; nor is it our human destiny or Seventh Age, as Shakespeare called it. Although dementia is a significant problem in an aging population, most people live into their eighties and nineties with no signs of serious mental deterioration. In fact, experts are increasingly convinced that more Americans will remain mentally vigorous and vital as they grow old, and that the primary cause of dementia—Alzheimer's disease—will be conquered. Researchers have discovered that many conditions once blamed on general aging are indeed specific diseases or disorders that may be overcome.

It is critical to remember that severe loss of mental faculties or dementia in the elderly does not happen without cause; that cause should always be sought, and in 95 percent of the cases it can be diagnosed and sometimes treated.

About 5 percent of people over age 65 have mental impairment serious enough to be called dementia. About two million Americans have a form of dementia called Alzheimer's disease. This is a specific, progressive brain disease characterized by a deterioration of memory, intellectual capabilities and personality. Dementia is now recognized as a syndrome in which intellectual deterioration is severe enough to interfere with occupational or social performance.

Causes: Most memory loss and related dementia in old age is increasingly viewed as a disease that somehow is associated with aging, but not caused by aging *per se*. Contrary to popular thinking, severe mental impairment in the aged is not due primarily to "hardening of the arteries," although vascular disease at least partially accounts for 10 to 20 percent of the cases of dementia. Much dementia—perhaps from 10 to 30 percent—is reversible, caused by as many as sixty different factors, including depression, overmedication, malnutrition, brain tumor, heart, liver, and kidney disease and a variety of infections. In about 5 percent of the cases of dementia, no cause is ever determined.

By far the major cause of dementia among the elderly is Alzheimer's disease, accounting for 50 to 60 percent of the cases. The disease is named after the German physician Dr. Alois Alzheimer, who first reported the disease in 1907. Alzheimer's is an organic brain disease, a progressive, as yet incurable degeneration of brain cells. Although the risk of Alzheimer's increases as we age, it is not caused simply by growing older. It is a specific brain disease that strikes only certain victims for a mysterious reason.

New findings show that Alzheimer's initially kills a select group of neurons deep in the brain. The death of these cells, it is believed, produces a chemical deficiency in the brain that short-circuits message transmission. As the disease becomes more severe, the brain literally shrivels and may develop large holes. The brain's cells are also characterized by certain abnormal tangles and plaques.

What destroys the brain cells is unknown. Some scientists speculate that the cells are killed by a virus, perhaps a slow-acting one that infects a person in early life but does not produce symptoms until old age. Other researchers note that the brain cells of Alzheimer's patients have large deposits of aluminum, a known brain poison. Why this happens is unknown. There is no evidence that exposure to aluminum in antacids, antiperspirants, or cookware increases the risk of Alzheimer's. Some researchers theorize that the disease is linked to a decrease in immune functions. Recent studies found that Alzheimer's occurred more frequently in a group of people who had suffered serious head injuries up to 35 years before onset of the disease. There is also evidence that Alzheimer's may be genetically influenced, although factors other than a genetic predisposition determine the onset of the disease. Brain changes similar to those found in Alzheimer's show up eventually (after age 40) in nearly all persons born with Down syndrome.

It was once thought that Alzheimer's was a form of "early senility," but experts now know it is identical to the dementia found in the elderly. Alzheimer's has been diagnosed in a person as young as 28, but it is rare in those under age 60.

Symptoms: It almost always begins with memory loss (especially related to recent events) and confusion that can progress to an inability to carry on a conversation, recognize relatives, or even to speak, as well as irritability, lethargy, inappropriate responses, paranoia and delusions. The final stage of Alzheimer's is invariably coma, resulting in death.

Diagnosis: Because so-called "senility" is so widely accepted as a sign of normal aging, many physicians neglect to search for a cause. You should certainly seek another opinion if a physician dismisses the symptoms as "mere aging" or "hardening of the arteries." A thorough physical examination is in order to rule out any reversible causes when dementia is suspected. Of all disorders, depression is reportedly most often confused with Alzheimer's disease.

Alzheimer's is not easy to diagnose—there is no simple blood or brain test to spot the disease—although according to one expert, with proper clinical and laboratory procedures, it can be identified in nine out of ten cases. Such an assessment, he says, requires mental status tests; standard physical, psychiatric and neurologic examinations; a CT brain scan; a comprehensive biochemical screening; an assessment of the vitamin B_{12} level, and thyroid-function tests. Some authorities believe the newer, more sophisticated magnetic resonance imaging of the brain's functioning may also be useful. However, the final diagnosis of Alzheimer's can be made only at autopsy by examining the configuration of brain cell endings.

Treatment: Nothing can cure Alzheimer's, although some experimental drugs can slightly improve the brain functioning and memory of some Alzheimer's patients for very short periods of time—up to two hours. This gives some hope that drugs eventually may be able to retard or reverse the brain deterioration in Alzheimer's patients. There are experimental treatment programs at some leading institutions that accept some Alzheimer's patients, and some experts believe Alzheimer's will be understood and conquered within a decade.

In the meantime, elderly patients with mental impairment need special management, which may include drugs such as tranquilizers, antipsychotics, or antidepressants to treat the symptoms. A person with irreversible dementia may eventually need full-time long-term care at a nursing home or other facility. More than half of the occupants at most nursing homes are Alzheimer's patients.

Since Alzheimer's can have such a devastating effect on the lives of other family members, it is often said that the disease produces not one but many patients in a family. Families in which Alzheimer's occurs usually need intense emotional support. They may be faced with caring for the steadily declining individual under difficult circumstances for many years. An Alzheimer's victim may live from 10 to 20 years after the onset of the disease.

WHERE TO FIND HELP FOR ALZHEIMER'S AND OTHER AGING-RELATED DISEASES

A growing number of medical centers now have programs of geriatric medicine, staffed with physicians well acquainted with diseases that primarily strike the elderly, including dementia. Here are some of the leading centers of geriatrics medicine. Included are the one full department of geriatrics at Mount Sinai School of Medicine in New York City, medical schools that have grants from the National Institute on Aging to start geriatrics departments and medical schools that have residency or fellowship programs to train physicians who want to specialize in geriatric medicine.

All of these physicians and centers are knowledgeable about diseases that strike the elderly, and should be excellent sources of treatment, information and referral.

SOME LEADING SPECIALISTS AND CENTERS IN GERIATRIC MEDICINE

ALABAMA
Harold W. Schnaper, M.D.
Director, Center for Aging
University of Alabama at Birmingham
933 19th St. S.
Birmingham, AL 35294
(205) 934-4399

Veronica J. Scott, M.D.
Assistant Professor of Medicine
Division of Gerontology and Medical
   Geriatrics
University of Alabama at Birmingham
9–33 South
Veterans Administration Medical Center
Birmingham, AL 35294
(205) 933-8101, x6842

ARKANSAS
William J. Carter, M.D.
Division of Geriatrics
John L. McLellan Memorial VA Medical
   Center
4300 W. 7th St.
Little Rock, AR 72205
(501) 661-1202, x2811

CALIFORNIA
Philip G. Weiler, Jr., M.D.
Professor of Community Health
Department of Community Health, TB 168
University of California School of Medicine
Davis, CA 95616
(916) 752-2793

J. Edward Spar, M.D.
Gary W. Small, M.D.
Lissy F. Jarvik, M.D.
Geriatric Psychiatry
University of California, Los Angeles
760 Westwood Plaza
Los Angeles, CA 90024
(213) 825-0038, 0291, 0545

Robert L. Kane, M.D.
Professor of Medicine
Multicampus Division of Geriatric
   Medicine
UCLA School of Medicine
10833 Le Conte Ave.
Los Angeles, CA 90024
(213) 393-0411, x7696

R. Bruce Sloane, M.D.
Lon S. Schneider, M.D.
Department of Psychiatry and the Behavioral
    Sciences
University of Southern California School of
    Medicine
1934 Hospital Place
Los Angeles, CA 90033
(213) 226-5575

Jerome S. Tobis, M.D.
Department of Physical Medicine and
    Rehabilitation
Route 81
University of California Irvine Medical Center
101 The City Drive
Orange, CA 92668
(714) 634-5626

Robert Marcus, M.D.
Associate Director
Geriatric Research, Educational Clinical Center
    182B
VA Medical Center
3801 Miranda Ave.
Palo Alto, CA 93404
(415) 858-3933

Gerald M. Reaven, M.D.
Geriatric Research Educational Clinical Center
    182B
VA Medical Center
Affiliated with Stanford University School of
    Medicine
3801 Miranda Ave.
Palo Alto, CA 94304
(415) 493-5000, x4510

Lawrence Z. Feigenbaum, M.D.
University of California, San Francisco
Mount Zion Hospital and Medical Center
PO Box 7921
San Francisco, CA 94120
(415) 567-6600, x7261

Howard L. Lichtenstein, M.D.
Assistant Clinical Professor of Medicine
University of California
San Francisco VA Medical Center (117)
4150 Clement St.
San Francisco, CA 94121
(415) 221-4810

CONNECTICUT
Leo M. Cooney, Jr., M.D.
Associate Professor of Medicine
Mary E. Tinetti, M.D.
Ronald Miller, M.D.
Assistant Professors of Medicine
Yale University School of Medicine
333 Cedar St.
PO Box 333
New Haven, CT 06510
(203) 785-2204

DISTRICT OF COLUMBIA
Gregory Pawlson, M.D.
Director, Geriatrics Services
Associate Chairman Department of Health
    Care Sciences
George Washington University
1229 25th St., N.W., Room 322
Washington, DC 20037
(202) 676-4269

FLORIDA
George J. Caranasos, M.D.
Ruth S. Jewett, M.D., Professor of Medicine
    in Geriatrics
Department of Medicine
PO Box J-277
University of Florida
Gainesville, FL 32610
(904) 392-3197

Richard R. Streiff, M.D.
George J. Caranasos, M.D.
University of Florida
Medical Service
Gainesville, FL 32602
(904) 373-6016

William Reefe, M.D.
Chief, Division of Gerontology
Veterans Hospital
University of Miami School of Medicine
1201 N.W. 16th St.
Miami, FL 33125
(305) 324-4455, x3559 or 324-3204

Eric Pfeiffer, M.D.
Director, Suncoast Gerontology Center
University of South Florida
12901 N. 30th St.
Box 50
Tampa, FL 33612
(813) 974-4355

Bruce E. Robinson, M.D.
Director, Division of Geriatric Medicine
Internal Medicine
University of South Florida
12901 N. 30th St.
Tampa, FL 33612
(813) 974-2271

GEORGIA
Paul D. Webster III, M.D.
Chairman, Department of Medicine
Medical College of Georgia (BIW 548)
Augusta, GA 30912
(404) 828-2941

IDAHO
Robert E. Vestal, M.D.
Clinical Pharmacology and Geriatrics Units
 (151)
VA Medical Center
500 W. Fort St.
Boise, ID 83702
(208) 338-7250

ILLINOIS
Ben Gierl, M.D.
Director of Geropsychiatric Program
Illinois State Psychiatric Institute
1601 W. Taylor St., Room 412N
Chicago, IL 60612
(312) 996-1185

Donald F. Pochyly, M.D.
Associate Chief of Staff for Geriatrics and
 Extended Care (181)
Stritch School of Medicine
Loyola University, Chicago
Hines, IL 60141
(312) 343-7200, x3235 or 3236

J. N. Krale, M.D.
Chief, Division of Geriatrics
Department of Family Practice
Southern Illinois University
421 N. 9th St.
Springfield, IL 62702
(217) 782-0215

IOWA
Ian M. Smith, M.D.
Professor of Internal Medicine and Family
 Medicine
University of Iowa Hospitals and Clinics
Iowa City, IA 52242
(319) 356-2727

KANSAS
Frederick F. Holmes, M.D.
Division of General and Geriatric Medicine
University of Kansas Medical Center
Kansas City, KS 66103
(913) 588-6005

KENTUCKY
John Wright, M.D.
Medical Director of Geriatrics
University of Louisville School of Medicine
411 E. Muhammad Ali Blvd.—Senior House,
 Inc.
Louisville, KY 40204
(502) 588-6502

MARYLAND
John R. Burton, M.D.
Deputy Director, Department of Medicine
Director, Division of Geriatric Medicine
Francis Scott Key Medical Center
4940 Eastern Ave.
Baltimore, MD 21224
(301) 955-0520

MASSACHUSETTS
Richard E. Fine, M.D.
Acting Director
Geriatric Research Education Clinical Center
Boston University School of Medicine
200 Springs Rd.
Bedford, MA 01730
(617) 275-7500, x631

R. Knight Steel, M.D.
Chief, Geriatrics Section
Boston University School of Medicine
720 Harrison Ave., Suite 1101
Boston, MA 02118
(617) 638-8383, 8300

John W. Rowe, M.D.
Associate Professor of Medicine
Director, Division on Aging
Harvard Medical School
643 Huntington Ave.
Boston, MA 02215
(617) 732-1840 or 735-4580

Richard W. Besdine, M.D.
Hebrew Rehabilitation Center for Aged
Harvard Medical School
1200 Centre St.
Boston, MA 02131
(617) 325-8000, x291

Roger B. Hickler, M.D.
Director, Division of Geriatric Medicine
Department of Medicine
University of Massachusetts Medical School
55 Lake Avenue, N.
Worcester, MA 01605
(617) 856-3197

MICHIGAN
Jeffrey Halter, M.D.
Director
Turner Geriatric Clinic
1010 Wall St.
Ann Arbor, MI 48109
(313) 764-6831

William Kelley, M.D.
University of Michigan Medical School
University Hospital
1405 E. Ann St.
Ann Arbor, MI 48109
(313) 764-6831

MINNESOTA
Patrick W. Irvine, M.D.
Assistant Professor
Department of Medicine
University of Minnesota
St. Paul—Ramsey Medical Center
640 Jackson St.
St. Paul, MN 55101
(612) 221-3464

MISSOURI
Stan Ingman, Ph.D.
MA306 Medical Sciences Building
University of Missouri Medical Center
Columbia, MO 45212
(314) 882-8030

Rodney M. Coe, Ph.D.
St. Louis University School of Medicine
1402 S. Grand Blvd.
St. Louis, MO 63104
(314) 577-8531

NEBRASKA
J. F. Potter, M.D.
Section of Geriatrics and Gerontology
Department of Internal Medicine
University of Nebraska Medical Center
42nd and Dewey
Omaha, NE 68105
(402) 559-4427

NEW YORK
David Hamerman, M.D.
Department of Medicine
Montefiore Medical Center
Albert Einstein College of Medicine
111 E. 210 St.
Bronx, NY 10467
(212) 920-6721

Evan Calkins, M.D.
Professor of Medicine
Head, Division of Geriatrics and
   Gerontology
State University of New York at Buffalo
VA Medical Center III-T
3495 Bailey Ave.
Buffalo, NY 14215
(716) 831-3176

Conn J. Foley, M.D.
Medical Director
Jewish Institute for Geriatric Care
271-11 76th Ave.
New Hyde Park, NY 11042
(516) 343-2100, x301

Kenneth P. Scileppi, M.D.
Division of Geriatrics and Gerontology
Cornell University Medical Center
525 E. 68th St.
New York, NY 10021
(212) 472-6754

Robert Butler, M.D.
Chairman
Department of Geriatrics and Adult
   Development
Leslie S. Libow, M.D.
Vice Chairman and Clinical Director
Mount Sinai School of Medicine
Annenberg 13-30
1 Gustave L. Levy Place
New York, NY 10029
(212) 650-5561
Dr. Butler sees patients on a consultation basis
   only.

Michael L. Freedman, M.D.
Department of Medicine
New York University School of Medicine
550 First Ave.
New York, NY 10016
(212) 340-6269, x6271

David D. Bonacci, M.D.
Director, Geriatric Psychiatry Program
University of Rochester School of Medicine
  and Dentistry
Department of Psychiatry
300 Crittenden Blvd.
Rochester, NY 14642
(716) 275-3540

Anthony Izzo, M.D.
Medical Director and Head of Geriatric
  Program
Monroe Community Hospital
University of Rochester School of Medicine
  and Dentistry
435 E. Henrietta Rd.
Rochester, NY 14606
(716) 473-4080, x318

Myron Miller, M.D.
Director, Program in Geriatrics
SUNY Health Science Center at Syracuse
Weiskotten Hall, Room 1258
766 Irving Ave.
Syracuse, NY 13210
(315) 473-5167

NORTH CAROLINA
Paul Beck, M.D.
Director, Program on Aging
Professor of Medicine
Department of Medicine
University of North Carolina
141 MacNider 202H
Chapel Hill, NC 27514
(919) 966-5945

Harvey Jay Cohen, M.D.
Director, Division of Geriatric Medicine
Center for the Study of Aging and Human
  Development
Duke University Medical Center, Box 3003
Durham, NC 27710
(919) 684-2248

Lou DeMaria, M.D.
Duke-Watts Family Medicine Center
407 Crutchfield St.
Durham, NC 27704
(919) 471-2571

Harold Kallman, M.D.
Professor, Department of Family Medicine
Director, Division of Geriatric Medicine
East Carolina University School of Medicine
PO Box 1846
Greenville, NC 27835-1846
(919) 757-2597

William R. Hazzard, M.D.
Chairman, Department of Medicine
Bowman Gray School of Medicine
300 S. Hawthorne Rd.
Winston-Salem, NC 27103
(919) 748-4305

NORTH DAKOTA
Robin S. Staebler, M.D.
Chairman, Department of Family Medicine
University of North Dakota School of
  Medicine
221 S. 4th
Grand Forks, ND 58201
(701) 777-4216

OHIO
David Bienenfeld, M.D.
Director, Division of Geriatric Psychiatry
University of Cincinnati College of Medicine
7206 MSB
231 Bethesda Ave.
Cincinnati, OH 45267
(513) 872-5574

J. D. Frengley, M.D.
Director of Geriatric Medicine
Cleveland Metropolitan General–Highland
  View Hospital
Case Western Reserve University School of
  Medicine
3395 Scranton Rd.
Cleveland, OH 44109
(216) 459-3951

John F. McGreevey, Jr., M.D.
Director, Office of Geriatric Medicine/
  Gerontology
Department of Medicine
Medical College of Ohio at Toledo
C.S. 10008
Toledo, OH 43699
(419) 381-3567

OREGON
Richard C. U'Ren, M.D.
Associate Professor
Department of Psychiatry
Outpatient Clinic OP336
Oregon Health Science University
3181 S.W. Sam Jackson Park Rd.
Portland, OR 97201
(503) 225-8613

John R. Walsh, M.D.
Chief, Gerontology Section
VA Medical Center
Oregon Health Sciences University
3710 S.W. U.S. Veterans Hospital Rd.
PO Box 1034
Portland, OR 97207
(503) 222-9221, x2403

PENNSYLVANIA
Jerry Johnson, M.D.
Chief, Geriatrics
VA Medical Center
University & Woodland Ave.
Philadelphia, PA 19104
(215) 382-2400, x5892

RHODE ISLAND
Marsha D. Fretwell, M.D.
Director, Section of Geriatrics
Department of Medicine
Roger Williams General Hospital
Brown University
Providence, RI 02908
(401) 456-2060

TENNESSEE
William B. Applegate, M.D.
Head, Section on Geriatrics and Gerontology
Department of Community Medicine
University of Tennessee Center for the Health
    Sciences
66 N. Pauline
Memphis, TN 38163
(901) 528-5903, x5927

TEXAS
George Niederehe, Ph.D.
Geriatric Psychology
University of Texas Mental Sciences Institute
Texas Medical Center
1300 Moursund
Houston, TX 77030
(713) 791-6633

UTAH
James S. Wood, M.D.
University of Utah Medical Center
50 N. Medical Drive
Salt Lake City, UT 84132
(801) 581-7818

VIRGINIA
Richard W. Lindsay, M.D.
Head, Division of Geriatrics
Department of Internal Medicine
University of Virginia School of Medicine
PO Box 157
University of Virginia Hospital
Charlottesville, VA 22908
(804) 924-5835

David Gardner, M.D.
Acting Chairman
Division of General Medicine and Primary
    Care
Medical College of Virginia
PO Box 102, MCV Station
Richmond, VA 23298
(804) 786-3774

WASHINGTON
Igamar Adress, M.D.
Division of Gerontology & Geriatric
    Medicine
University of Washington
325 Ninth Ave. ZA-87
Seattle, WA 98104
(206) 223-3089

WISCONSIN
Elaine A. Leventhal, M.D., Ph.D.
H6/249 Clinical Sciences Center
Department of Medicine
University of Wisconsin School of Medicine
600 Highland Ave.
Madison, WI 53792
(608) 263-5241

Edmund H. Duthie, Jr., M.D.
Chief, Section of Geriatrics/Gerontology (III P)
Department of Medicine
Medical College of Wisconsin
5000 W. National Ave.
Milwaukee, WI 53295
(414) 384-2000, x2896 or 2897

Albert A. Fisk, M.D.
Director
Mount Sinai Medical Center, Geriatrics
   Institute
University of Wisconsin Medical School
PO Box 342
Milwaukee, WI 53201
(414) 289-8342

SOURCE: *National Institute on Aging and American Geriatrics Society.*

GOVERNMENT-SPONSORED RESEARCH ON ALZHEIMER'S DISEASE

The National Institute on Aging has established 10 research-treatment centers to study Alzheimer's disease and related dementias. These 10 centers are operated by some of the nation's leading authorities on the disease; the centers may accept some patients for treatment and research, and physicians on the staff at the centers may be available for consultations with your physician.

CALIFORNIA
Robert Katzman, M.D.
Department of Neurosciences (M-008)
University of California, San Diego
School of Medicine
La Jolla, CA 92093
(619) 452-4606

Caleb E. Finch, Ph.D.
Andrus Gerontology Center
University Park, MC-0191
University of Southern California
Los Angeles, CA 90089-0191
(213) 743-5168

KENTUCKY
William R. Markesbery, M.D.
Director, Sanders-Brown Research Center on
   Aging
University of Kentucky
Lexington, KY 40536
(606) 233-6040

MARYLAND
Donald L. Price, M.D.
Department of Pathology
The Johns Hopkins Hospital
600 N. Wolfe St.
Baltimore, MD 21205
(301) 955-5632

MASSACHUSETTS
John H. Growdon, M.D.
Department of Neurology Service
ACC 730
Massachusetts General Hospital
Fruit Street
Boston, MA 02114
(617) 726-1728

MISSOURI
Leonard Berg, M.D.
Department of Neurology and Neurological
   Surgery
Washington University
School of Medicine
Suite #16304
Barnes Hospital Plaza
St. Louis, MO 63110
(314) 367-3122

NEW YORK
Kenneth L. Davis, M.D.
Department of Psychiatry
Mount Sinai School of Medicine
Fifth Ave. and 100th St.
New York, NY 10029
(212) 579-1633

NORTH CAROLINA
Allen D. Roses, M.D.
Division of Neurology
PO Box 2900
Duke University Medical Center
Durham, NC 27710
(919) 684-6274

PENNSYLVANIA
Francois Boller, M.D., Ph.D
Departments of Neurology and Psychiatry
Western Psychiatric Institute and Clinic
3811 O'Hara St.
Pittsburgh, PA 15213
(412) 624-1557

WASHINGTON
George M. Martin, M.D.
Department of Pathology SM-30
University of Washington
Seattle, WA 98195
(206) 543-5088

SOURCE: *National Institute on Aging.*

RESEARCH AT THE NATIONAL INSTITUTES OF HEALTH

The federal government has experimental treatment programs at the Clinical Center in Bethesda, Maryland, in which selected patients with Alzheimer's or other types of old-age dementia can participate. Participation is by physician referral only. For more information your physician can contact:

Office of the Director
The Clinical Center
Building 10, Room 2C-146
National Institutes of Health
Bethesda, MD 20205
(301) 496-4891

ORGANIZATIONS

Alzheimer's Disease and Related Disorders
   Association, Inc.
360 N. Michigan Ave.
Chicago, IL 60601
(312) 853-3060

This nonprofit national membership organization offers information and advocacy for those with Alzheimer's and related diseases and their families. More than 140 local chapters located around the country. Answer questions and offer pamphlets, articles, and a quarterly newsletter. Will provide more information and a list of local chapters upon request.

National Institute on Aging
9000 Rockville Pike
Building 31, Room 5C35
Bethesda, MD 20892
(301) 496-1752

The agency within the National Institutes of Health most concerned with Alzheimer's disease and other health problems of the aging. Supports research on aging-related diseases, and is a source of information to the public and health professionals.

BOOKS

A Guide to Alzheimer's Disease: For Families, Spouses and Friends, **Barry Reisberg, M.D.,** New York: Free Press, 1981.

Another Name for Madness, **Marion Roach,** New York: Houghton Mifflin Co., 1985.

Brain Failure: An Introduction to Current Concepts of Senility, **Barry Reisberg, M.D.,** New York: Free Press, 1981.

Day Care for Dementia, **John Panella,** White Plains, NY: Burke Rehabilitation Center, 1983. Director of Alzheimer's and Day Care Program, Burke Rehabilitation Center, 785 Mamaroneck Ave. White Plains, NY 10605.

Dementia: A Practical Guide to Alzheimer's Disease and Related Illness, **Leonard L. Heston, M.D.,** and **June A. White,** New York: W. H. Freeman and Company, 1984.

Loss of Self, **Carl Eisdorfer, M.D.,** New York: Norton, 1986.

The End of Senility, **Dr. Arthur S. Freese,** New York: Arbor House, 1978.

The Myth of Senility: Misconceptions About the Brain and Aging, **Robin Marantz Henig,** Garden City, NY: Anchor Press/Doubleday, 1981.

The 36-Hour Day: A Family Guide to Caring for Persons with Alzheimer's Disease, Related Dementing Illnesses, and Memory Loss in Later Life, **Nancy L. Mace** and **Peter V. Rabins, M.D.,** Baltimore: The Johns Hopkins University Press, 1981.

The Truth About Senility and How to Avoid It, **Laurence Galton,** New York: Crowell, 1979.

Your Brain is Younger Than You Think: A Guide to Mental Aging, **Richard M. Torack,** Chicago: Nelson Hall, 1981.

FREE MATERIALS

Alzheimer's Disease: Q and A, 12 pages.

The Dementias: Hope Through Research, 32 pages.

Progress Report on Alzheimer's Disease, Volume II, 28 pages, 1984.

Senility: Myth or Madness. Fact sheet.

National Institute on Aging
Information Center
2209 Distribution Circle
Silver Spring, MD 20910

ANOREXIA NERVOSA
AND BULIMIA

ANOREXIA NERVOSA

Anorexia nervosa is an eating disorder of self-starvation that can be psychologically and physically devastating. The sufferer, usually an adolescent girl, refuses to eat, insisting that she is too fat or gets full on only subsistent amounts of food. The body's hormonal and chemical balance is upset, and death may result if the starvation is sustained.

The number of Americans with this disease is rising. Once considered rare in women over age 20, anorexia now reportedly is spreading to affect women over age 25. The disease has occurred in children as young as 11 and women as old as 60. Also, although it is still primarily a disorder of the middle and upper classes, there is evidence it can occur in all socio-economic groups. According to some reports, the incidence of anorexia has doubled in the past 10 years. According to conservative estimates, one-half of 1 percent of the population, or 1 out of 200 American girls between the ages of 12 and 18 will become anorexic. Some believe the figure is 1 out of every 100 young women. Boys, too, can develop anorexia; in fact, about 5 percent of the victims are adolescent boys.

Cause: Unknown. The common theory has been that anorexia is a psychological disturbance resulting from a striving for perfection and approval, and a family that is seemingly loving but has underlying problems of dependency. Researchers also believe there may be biochemical reasons, perhaps preceding the attack of anorexia. The biochemical link is unknown and is a subject of intense research. Many authorities believe the cause to be a combination of psychological and physiological factors.

Symptoms: The most striking symptom is weight loss; it may start with a diet, but then progresses to an obsession with losing weight. Anorexics with severe disorders can weigh as little as 60 or 70 pounds and still believe they are too fat. They usually deny they are hungry, exercise to the point of fatigue and weakness, have a distorted body image, and are compulsive and withdrawn. Anorexia may also cause hormonal changes, lowered blood pressure, lack of sexual interest, amenorrhea (cessation of menstruation), and reduced functioning of the thyroid gland. In less than 5 percent of the cases sudden death occurs, usually from heart failure.

Diagnosis: It's important to detect anorexia nervosa early. The disease is characterized by emaciation, as if a person were starving to death, which is literally true. There are no specific laboratory tests, although the above-mentioned hormonal changes may be noted.

Treatment: Most treatment involves trying to get the patient to gain weight. This is usually done with a combination of nutritional therapy, individual psychotherapy, and family counseling. In some cases, the patient must be hospitalized until the condition is stabilized. Drugs are sometimes used to relieve depression, but antidepressants have had only limited success in treating the disease itself. Anorexia is an exceedingly difficult condition to overcome and may require long-term treatment. At one large treatment center the average length of hospitalization for anorexia nervosa patients is five to six months. Also, a return to normal weight may be temporary. Some experts say it takes from three to five years before the disease can be considered cured.

BULIMIA

A related disorder, bulimia, is characterized by binging and then purging by vomiting or using diuretics or laxatives. Bulimia is often called the "sister" to anorexia. Bulimia has different characteristics. Individuals with bulimia, unlike those with anorexia, do not have a distorted body image and do not focus on excessive thinness; they may be normal weight or 15 pounds under or over. They do not avoid food, but overeat, and then are seized with an irresistible urge to get rid of it. Unlike people with anorexia, those with bulimia are often aware of their abnormal eating patterns and hunger.

Bulimia typically remains hidden because there are no noticeable weight changes. However, physical changes may occur, such as dehydration, low levels of potassium, which can lead to kidney or cardiovascular failure, and menstrual irregularities. Typical sufferers are in their late teens, twenties and early thirties. Treatment techniques are similar to those for anorexia and may include dietary education, group therapy, psychotherapy, even relaxation techniques and biofeedback. Recently bulimia has been successfully treated with antidepressants, and apparently these drugs are highly successful in some persons.

WHERE TO FIND TREATMENT FOR EATING DISORDERS

In the past few years, numerous eating disorder clinics and individual therapists treating eating disorders have appeared. You can locate such centers and therapists in your area by contacting one of the three self-help national organizations on anorexia and bulimia listed below. Many of the clinics and centers are connected with leading hospitals, universities, and medical schools. Though such centers are not the only excellent clinics, they are among the best and offer the latest treatment techniques available. Some are also doing research on eating disorders. Some eating disorder programs affiliated with leading medical centers are listed below.

SOME LEADING EATING DISORDERS CLINICS

ALABAMA
University of Alabama at Birmingham
Weight Reduction and Eating Disorders Center
Department of Nutrition Sciences
WEBB 212
University Station
Birmingham, AL 35294
Director: Roland L. Weinsier, M.D., D.P.H.
(205) 934-5112

ARIZONA
University of Arizona Health Sciences Center
Eating Disorders Program
Tucson, AZ 85724
Director: Catherine M. Shisslak, Ph.D.
(602) 626-6509

ARKANSAS
University of Arkansas for Medical Sciences
Department of Psychiatry
4301 W. Markham St. Slot 589
Little Rock, AR 72205
Director: William G. Reese, M.D.
(501) 661-5483

CALIFORNIA
University of California, Irvine
California College of Medicine
Eating Disorders Program
Irvine, CA 92717
Director: Barton Blinder, M.D.
(714) 831-6631

University of California, Los Angeles
Eating Disorders Clinic
Neuropsychiatric Institute
Los Angeles, CA 90024
Joel Yager, M.D. (adult outpatients)
Michael Strober, M.D. (adolescent in- and
  outpatients)
Lew Baxter, M.D. (adult inpatients)
(213) 825-0173

University of California
Davis Medical Center
Eating Disorders Clinic
Sacramento, CA 95817
Director: Kay Blacker, M.D.
(916) 453-3574

Stanford University Medical Center
Behavioral Medicine Clinic
Stanford, CA 94305
Clinic Chief: W. Stewart Agras, M.D.
Department Chairman: Thomas Gonda, M.D.
(415) 723-7107

COLORADO
University of Colorado Health Sciences Center
Adolescent Clinic
Denver, CO 80202
Director: Henry Cooper, M.D.
(303) 394-8461

CONNECTICUT
Yale University School of Medicine
Yale Behavioral Medicine Clinic
New Haven, CT 06510
Director: Hoyle Leigh, M.D.
(203) 785-2617, 2122

DISTRICT OF COLUMBIA
George Washington University Medical Center
Eating Disorders Clinic
2150 Pennsylvania Ave., N.W.
Washington, DC 20037
Codirectors: Joan Barber, M.D., and Robert
  Hendren, D.O.
(202) 676-3457, 8298

Georgetown University
Diet Management Clinic
Washington, DC 20007
Director: Aaron Altschul, Ph.D.
(202) 625-3674

Washington Hospital Center
Eating Disorders Unit
110 Irving St., N.W.
Washington, DC 20010
Director: Sue Bailey, M.D.
(202) 829-2026

FLORIDA
University of Florida Clinic
Eating Disorders Clinic
Department of Psychiatry
PO Box J-256
Gainesville, FL 32610
Director: Jon Hodgin, M.D.
(904) 392-0214

University of Miami School of Medicine
Anorexia Nervosa Clinic
Jackson Memorial Hospital
1611 N.W. 12th Ave.
Miami, FL 33136
Director: Guido Diaz, M.D.
(305) 549-7087

University of South Florida
College of Medicine
Eating Disorders Clinic
12901 N. 30th St., Box 14
Tampa, FL 33612
Director: Pauline S. Powers, M.D.
(813) 974-4242

GEORGIA
Eating Disorders Clinic
Emory University Woodruff Health Sciences
  Center
Parkwood Hospital
Atlanta, GA 30322
Director: Donald E. Manning, M.D.
(404) 321-0111, x3297

ILLINOIS
Northwestern University
Northwestern Memorial Hospital
Eating Disorder Clinic
Chicago, IL 60611
Directors: Craig Johnson, M.D., and Steven
  Stern, M.D.
(312) 908-8100

University of Chicago Medical Center
Center for Behavioral Medicine and Health
  Promotion
Department of Psychiatry
5841 S. Maryland Ave.
Chicago, IL 60637
Codirectors: Paul Camic, Ph.D., and Joan
  Falk, Ph.D.
(312) 947-1000

IOWA
University of Iowa Hospitals and Clinics
Eating Disorders Clinic
University of Iowa Psychiatric Hospital
Iowa City, IA 52242
Director: George Winokur, M.D.
(319) 353-3719

KENTUCKY
Eating Disorders Recognition and Intervention
  Program
Norton Psychiatric Clinic
PO Box 35070
Louisville, KY 40232
Director: Barbara A. Fitzgerald, M.D.
(502) 562-8853

LOUISIANA
Ochsner Clinic
Psychiatry Department
1514 Jefferson Highway
New Orleans, LA 70121
Director: Rudolph H. Ehrensing
(504) 838-4000
(adolescent and young women only)

Tulane University Hospital
Eating Disorders Program
New Orleans, LA 70112
Director: Susan G. Willard, M.S.W.,
  B.C.S.W.
(504) 588-5405

MARYLAND
Johns Hopkins University
Eating and Weight Disorder Clinic
Baltimore, MD 21205
Director: Arnold Andersen, M.D.
(301) 955-5514

MASSACHUSETTS
Cambridge Hospital
Eating Disorders Program
Cambridge, MA 02139
Director: Donald Meyer, M.D.
(617) 498-1150

Children's Hospital
Anorexia Nervosa and Related Disorders Clinic
Boston, MA 02115
Director: Eugene Piazza, M.D.
(617) 735-6728

Frances Stern Nutrition Center
Tufts University School of Medicine
New England Medical Center
171 Harrison Ave.
Boston, MA 02111
Director: Johanna Dwyer, R.D., D.Sc.
(617) 956-5273

Massachusetts General Hospital
Eating Disorder Clinic
Boston, MA 02114
Director: David Herzog, M.D.
(617) 726-3588

Mount Auburn Hospital
Outpatient Psychiatry Center
Cambridge, MA 02138
Director: Lloyd Sederer, M.D.
(617) 492-3400, x1443

University of Massachusetts Medical Center
Bulimia Group
Worcester, MA 01605
Director: Terry Rumpf, Ph.D.
(617) 856-3260
(group therapy)

MICHIGAN
University of Michigan Medical Center
Eating Disorders Clinic
Ann Arbor, MI 48109
Director: Kenneth R. Castagna, M.S.W.
(313) 764-0210

MINNESOTA
Mayo Clinic
Rochester, MN 55905
Director: Alexander Lucas, M.D.
(507) 284-3758

University of Minnesota Hospital and Clinic
Anorexia Nervosa and Bulimia Treatment
    Program
Box 393 UMHC
Minneapolis, MN 55455
Director: Elke Eckert, M.D.
(612) 626-6188

MISSISSIPPI
University of Mississippi Medical Center
Eating Disorders Program
Jackson, MS 39216
Director: Will Johnson, Ph.D.
(601) 984-5805

NEBRASKA
University of Nebraska Hospital and Clinic
Eating Disorders Program
Omaha, NE 68105
Director: Paul Pearson, M.D.
(402) 559-5524

NEW YORK
Anorexia Nervosa Treatment Program
Albert Einstein College of Medicine/
    Montefiore Medical Center
Bronx, NY 10467
Director: Preston Zucker, M.D.
(212) 920-6605

Eating Disorders Clinic
Albert Einstein College of Medicine/
    Montefiore Medical Center
Bronx, NY 10467
Director: Marjorie Boeck, M.D.
(212) 920-6613

Anorexia Nervosa Service
Columbia Presbyterian Medical Center
622 W. 168th St.
New York, NY 10032
Director: Dr. Joseph Silverman
(212) 694-5514

Eating Disorders Institute
The New York Hospital–Cornell Medical
    Center
Westchester Division
21 Bloomingdale Rd.
White Plains, NY 10605
Director: Gerard P. Smith, M.D.
(914) 682-9100

NORTH CAROLINA
Duke University Medical Center
Clinical Specialty Unit
Durham, NC 27706
Director: Kenneth Rockwell, M.D.
(919) 684-3992

East Carolina University School of Medicine
Eating Disorders
Psychiatric Medicine
Greenville, NC 27834
Director: James L. Mathis, M.D.
(919) 757-2666

OHIO
Case Western Reserve University School of
    Medicine
Behavior Therapy Clinic
University Hospitals of Cleveland
2074 Abington Rd.
Cleveland, OH 44106
Director: Elizabeth A. Klonoff, Ph.D.
(216) 844-8550

Ohio State University Hospitals
Eating Disorders Clinic
256-A Upham Hall
473 W. 12th Ave.
Columbus, OH 43210
Director: Katherine Dixon, M.D.
(614) 421-8232

University of Cincinnati Medical Center
Eating Disorders Center
231 Bethesda Ave.
Cincinnati, OH 45267-0559
Director: Susan Wooley, Ph.D.
(513) 872-5118

PENNSYLVANIA
Behavioral Medicine Clinic
The Milton S. Hershey Medical Center
The Pennsylvania State University
Hershey, PA 17033
Coordinator: John Hon
(717) 531-8521

Bulimia Center
Jefferson Medical College of Thomas Jefferson
    University
11th & Walnut Sts.
Philadelphia, PA 19107
Director: Harvey J. Schwartz, M.D.
(215) 928-6104

Eating Disorder Service
Center for Behavioral Medicine
Hospital of the University of Pennsylvania
36th and Spruce Sts.
Philadelphia, PA 19104
Director: John Paul Brady, M.D.
(215) 662-3503

Temple University Health Services Center
Eating Disorders Service
Philadelphia, PA 19140
Director: Ira Steisel, Ph.D.
(215) 221-3106

Outpatient Eating Disorders Program
Western Psychiatric Institute and Clinic
University of Pittsburgh
School of Medicine
3811 O'Hara St.
Pittsburgh, PA 15213
Director: L. K. George Hsu, M.D.
(412) 624-1000

TENNESSEE
University of Tennessee, Memphis
College of Medicine
Nutritional Support Services and Consultation
   Program for Nutritional Disorders and
   Surgery
956 Court Ave., E222
Memphis, TN 38105
Director: George S. M. Cowan, Jr., M.D.
(901) 528-6635

TEXAS
University of Texas Health Science Center
Eating Disorders Clinic
5323 Harry Hines Blvd.
Dallas, TX 75235
Directors: David Waller, M.D., and Bettie
   Hardy, M.D.
(214) 688-2218

UTAH
University of Utah School of Medicine
Eating Disorders Clinic
50 N. Medical Drive
Salt Lake City, UT 84132
Director: Arthur Elster, M.D.
(801) 581-8989

VIRGINIA
Medical College of Virginia
Eating Disorders Program
MCV Station, Box 710
Richmond, VA 23298
Directors: Prakash Ettigi, M.D., and Joel
   Silverman, M.D.
(804) 786-9157, 0762

WISCONSIN
Medical College of Wisconsin
Eating Disorders Program
8700 W. Wisconsin Ave.
Milwaukee, WI 53226
Director: Harold Harsch, M.D.
(414) 257-5373

University of Wisconsin Hospital and Clinics
Eating Disorders Program
Madison, WI 53706
Director: John Stephenson, M.D.
(608) 263-6406

SOURCE: *Author's survey of medical schools.*

ORGANIZATIONS

American Anorexia Bulimia Association
133 Cedar Lane
Teaneck, NJ 07666
(201) 836-1800

A national self-help membership organization for
anyone involved with eating disorders. Support
group affiliates in many parts of the country,
led by a recovered anorexic and a mental health
professional. Provides information to the public,
counseling and referrals to medical help. Sponsors conferences and meetings. Produces fact
sheets, reprints, and a newsletter five times annually. Special services: a network to enable an-

orexics to correspond with or talk to recovered anorexics. Will provide more information and name of local group upon request.

National Anorexic Aid Society
5796 Karl Rd.
Columbus, OH 43229
(614) 436-1112

A national self-help organization for those with anorexia and their families. Maintains three local mutual support groups and keeps a roster of other support groups around the country. Makes referrals to counselors and physicians and publishes a bimonthly newsletter. Special services: affiliated with The Center for the Treatment of Eating

Disorders, an outpatient counseling and multi-disciplinary treatment facility. Will provide more information upon request.

National Association of Anorexia Nervosa and
    Associated Disorders
PO Box 271
Highland Park, IL 60035
(312) 831-3438

A national membership organization for anorexics, their families, other interested persons. Offers information, fact sheets and a bi-monthly newsletter. Provides a list of therapists in your area. Will provide more information upon request.

BOOKS

The Anorexia Nervosa Reference Book,
    Roger Slade, New York: Harper and Row,
    1984.
The Art of Starvation: A Story of Anorexia and
    Survival, **Sheila MacLeod,** New York:
    Schocken Books, 1982.
The Best Little Girl in the World, **Steven**
    Levenkron, Ph.D., Chicago: Contemporary
    Books, 1978.
Bulimarexia: The Binge/Purge Cycle, **Marlene**
    B. White and **William White,** New York:
    Norton, 1983.
Bulimia, **Janice M. Cauwels,** Garden City,
    NY: Doubleday, 1983.
Fat Is a Feminist Issue, **Susie Orbach,** New
    York: Berkley Publishers, 1979.
The Golden Cage: The Enigma of Anorexia
    Nervosa, **Hilde Bruch, M.D.,** Boston:
    Harvard University Press, 1977.
The Hunger Scream, **Ivy Ruckman,**

New York: Walker and Company,
    1983.
Obsession: Reflections On the Tyranny of
    Slenderness, **Kim Chernin,** New York:
    Harper and Row, 1982.
The Slender Balance, **Susan Squire,** New
    York: Putnam, 1983.
Solitaire, **Aimee Liu,** New York: Harper &
    Row, 1979.
Starving for Attention, **Cherry Boone O'Neill,**
    New York: Continuum, 1982.
Treating and Overcoming Anorexia Nervosa,
    Steven Levenkron, Ph.D., New York:
    Charles Scribner's Sons, 1982.
When Will We Laugh Again? Dealing with
    Anorexia Nervosa and Bulimia, **Barbara**
    Kinoy, Ph.D., and officials of the
    American Anorexia/Bulimia Association,
    New York: Columbia University Press,
    1984.

FREE MATERIALS

Adolescent Eating Disorders: Anorexia and
    Bulimia, 8 pages, Publication # 352-004.

Virginia Cooperative Extension Service
Virginia Polytechnic Institute and State
    University
Blacksburg, VA 24061

Facts About Anorexia Nervosa, 8 pages.

National Institute of Child Heath and Human
    Development, Room 2A32, Building 31
9000 Rockville Pike
Bethesda, MD 20892

ARTHRITIS, RHEUMATIC DISEASES, AND BONE DISEASES

See also Rehabilitation for special devices and resources for the physically handicapped, page 475, and Pain Clinics, page 429.

Arthritis, which literally means "joint inflammation," is a catch-all term describing not one disease but a family of more than 100 separate rheumatic diseases and disorders. It is one of our most prevalent afflictions: About one in seven or as many as 40 million Americans suffer from some form of arthritis—including some 250,000 children. It can affect not only the joints, but also the connective tissues (the muscles, tendons, and ligaments) and the protective coverings of some internal organs.

Although most people associate arthritis with general aches and pains, it comes in numerous forms, each with unique causes, symptoms, and patterns. Most of it is progressive and chronic. In a minority of cases it is serious and crippling.

An estimated 1 out of 10 arthritis sufferers—more than three million—are affected seriously enough to curtail their normal activities. Technically, there is no cure for most forms of arthritis. The causes are still mysterious and some types are thought to be autoimmune diseases in which certain tissues are attacked by the body's own malfunctioning immune system. Because arthritis is so varied and complex, treatment is individualized as much as possible. Most forms of arthritis can be treated, some very successfully, with exercise, drugs, and, in severe instances, surgery.

Specialists called rheumatologists treat arthritis (for a list of where to find some leading rheumatologists, *see* page 569) often with the help of orthopedic surgeons. (*See* page 630 for a list of some leading orthopedic surgeons.)

OSTEOARTHRITIS

This is the most common type of arthritis, which virtually all humans get if they live long enough. Although osteoarthritis can show up in people of all ages, it is far more common in the elderly and progresses with age. X-rays reveal that almost everyone over age 60 has it to some degree. It is what gives the joints of many elderly people their characteristic knobby look, especially in the hands.

Osteoarthritis in most individuals is the least serious of the arthritic disorders. Unlike rheumatoid arthritis, it is neither an inflammatory nor a systemic disease. It usually comes from a deterioration of cartilage and general mechanical

73

wear and tear on the joints. The cartilage of the joints breaks down, and a bony overgrowth often appears at the edges of the joint. It can affect the hips, knees, spine and the end joints of the fingers. Pain is generally mild to moderate and localized. The disease seldom interferes greatly with normal activities: Its effects are confined to the joints; it doesn't "spread" to other parts of the body, and there is little inflammation. It is still not known why some people are targets for the disease and others are not, or why some get it earlier in life and with more severity, while it troubles others little or not at all. Heredity plays a part in osteoarthritis of the fingers.

Cause: Doctors do not understand precisely how and why osteoarthritis develops. Some researchers believe it may result from repeated minor injuries to the joints or more serious impact injuries. People who are overweight are especially vulnerable to osteoarthritis in the hip and knee joints. There is also some evidence that osteoarthritis may be related to a genetic defect. Crippling can occur when severe osteoarthritis affects the hips or knees.

Symptoms: Pain, stiffness, and loss of normal motion are usually present; affected joints may become tender and swollen.

Diagnosis: Diagnosis is usually not difficult and is usually made by X-rays, physical examinations, and a history of symptoms.

Treatment: Special exercise to keep joints mobile and reduce pain, sometimes drugs and sometimes surgery, if necessary, to replace such joints as the hip.

RHEUMATOID ARTHRITIS

Rheumatoid arthritis is what most people think of as "arthritis." It is far more serious than osteoarthritis and can result in severe crippling; however, only one-sixth of those diagnosed with rheumatoid arthritis suffer serious crippling or deformity. Many doctors think much of this can be avoided by early treatment. The disease can strike from infancy to old age. Most commonly, it appears between the ages of 40 and 50. For an unknown reason, it is three times more likely to strike women than men.

Rheumatoid arthritis attacks the synovium, the joints' membrane lining, that produces lubricant and nutrition for the joint. These linings of the joints—both large and small—become inflamed, causing swelling, heat, and pain. Enzymes in the inflamed cells can, over time, digest the cartilage and bone of the joint, destroying it, and causing crippling. Rheumatoid arthritis often involves the rest of the body, causing weakness, fatigue, loss of appetite, and stiffness. It may attack other parts of the body, such as skin, blood vessels, eyes, lungs, and nerves. The disease comes on gradually and usually follows an irregular course. One-third of the sufferers may go into long periods of remission; for most, it is progressive and persistent.

Cause: Multiple and unknown. Researchers suspect it is due to an autoimmune reaction, possibly triggered by a virus or bacteria.

Studies show that victims of arthritis often have increased levels of antibodies to the same virus that causes mononucleosis, indicating that the two diseases may be related, and adding evidence to the theory that rheumatoid arthritis may be triggered by a virus in genetically susceptible individuals. Doctors also observe that symptoms of rheumatoid arthritis either appear or seem to worsen during periods of emotional stress.

Symptoms: Typically, the joints are hot, stiff, and painful. Joints most often affected are those at the base and middle of the fingers, base of the toes, wrists, and knees. Joints of the shoulders, hips, elbows, and ankles may also be involved. Since the disease may strike the connective tissue and organs throughout the body, other common symptoms are fatigue, fever, weakness, and weight loss.

Diagnosis: It is diagnosed by a history of symptoms, physical examination, blood tests (sometimes to detect what is called "rheumatoid factor"), and tissue analysis.

Treatment: Physical therapy, anti-inflammatory drugs (usually high doses of aspirin), prescription drugs, or surgical joint replacement when the joints are severely damaged.

Drugs: The most widely used for both rheumatoid arthritis and osteoarthritis are the nonsteroidal anti-inflammatory drugs (NSAID) of which aspirin is the prototype. Aspirin is both a painkiller and an anti-inflammatory drug. Although a couple of aspirin are enough to relieve headaches, much higher doses, generally 12 to 24 five-grain aspirin tablets a day, are necessary to counteract inflammation and reduce swelling and damage from arthritis. Such a high dosage can cause severe side effects, including gastrointestinal bleeding and hearing problems.

Other potent drugs, including gold injections, the less toxic oral gold compounds, and penicillamine may produce remission and prevent joint damage. Many rheumatologists also use immunosuppressant drugs with good results.

When all else fails and rheumatoid arthritis cannot be controlled by state-of-the-art drug treatment, some doctors have tried high doses of radiation of the lymphoid system to suppress the immune system. Such radiotherapy has, in preliminary studies, successfully reduced joint swelling, stiffness, and tenderness and increased mobility and activity. However, because serious infections have occurred in people undergoing this therapy, its long-term use is doubtful.

Surgery: It is sometimes necessary to surgically remove the diseased synovium, the joint lining. If the joint function has been destroyed, an artificial joint may be necessary. Doctors consider artificial joint replacement to be one of the most dramatic advances in the treatment of arthritis and other kinds of bone diseases. Total hip replacement, introduced some 15 years ago, has proved notably successful in alleviating pain and restoring function. From 75,000 to 100,000 operations to totally replace hips are done every year. The short-term failure rate for this surgery is reported to be only 1 or 2 percent, but infections can result and, in some cases, the artificial joint must be removed. New techniques are rapidly improving hip replacement, as well as artificial joint replacements of the knee, finger, elbow, ankle and shoulder.

It is especially important to choose a surgeon who does numerous operations. A surgeon who does many procedures is apt to be more skilled than one who does only two or three such operations a year. Such surgery, of course, is only a last resort. It can be expensive, painful, and usually entails a long recovery period. In rare cases it can be detrimental, leaving the joint worse than before. Some experts say a candidate for joint replacement surgery should get a second opinion, and perhaps even a third.

Many orthopedic surgeons now do joint replacement surgery. For a list of some outstanding orthopedic surgeons and centers, *see* page 630. The following two hospitals have done a large number of artificial joint replacement procedures.

Brigham and Women's Hospital
75 Francis St.
Arthritis Center
Boston, MA 02115
Dr. Clement B. Sledge, M.D.

Dr. Sledge has a special interest in joint replacement in children with arthritis.

Hospital for Special Surgery
535 E. 70th St.
New York, NY 10021

The Hospital for Special Surgery is a preeminent center for joint replacement. Orthopedic surgeons at the hospital perform 1,200 joint replacement surgeries a year, on hips, knees, elbows, wrists, and fingers. About one-fifth of the surgeries involve artificial joints custom-designed with the aid of a computer. Surgery is performed for a variety of joint and bone diseases.

Exercise: Exercise is increasingly regarded as excellent therapy for the relief of symptoms and the prevention of crippling arthritis of all types. Most people with rheumatoid arthritis need a prescribed program of routine exercise to preserve the function and the range of motion of the joints. Regular daily exercise helps strengthen muscles, connective tissues, tendons, and ligaments and maintains the health of cartilage. Without exercise, joints may become stiffer and more inflexible, and muscles and cartilage may deteriorate. Proper exercise can produce dramatic results in maintaining mobility. Generally, swimming and walking are considered most beneficial, but the types of exercise depend on which joints are affected and to what extent. For best results, exercise programs should be individually tailored. A physical therapist or physiatrist (a physician specializing in physical medicine) can design such a program, and many local Arthritis Foundation chapters sponsor exercise programs.

JUVENILE ARTHRITIS

Arthritis in children, like arthritis in adults, is not one but a class of several diseases that differ according to the joints involved, severity, age of onset, and complications. Some of the arthritic conditions are not found in adults. Most common and most destructive is juvenile rheumatoid arthritis. Juvenile arthritis can retard growth, cause crippling, and, in 10 percent of sufferers lead to an inflammation of the iris of the eye (iritis) that can lead to blindness. These complications can usually be prevented by early detection and treatment.

Cause: Although the causes are unknown, there is evidence of an inherited predisposition to chronic juvenile arthritis.

Symptoms: The disease mimics the symptoms of other diseases, such as infections, and varies greatly among individuals.

Diagnosis: There is no definitive biological test, and diagnosis is usually made by medical history, physical examination, tissue and blood tests, and X-rays of the joints.

Treatment: Similar to that of adults, therapy depends on the type of arthritis and its symptoms. It usually includes medication, rest, and exercise. Surgery has been limited in children because of their continuing growth and the short-term durability of some joint replacements. However, severely crippled children have successfully been given total artificial hip and knee replacements, allowing them to walk. Newer surgical techniques may make severely crippled children better candidates for surgery. Drug regimens for children may differ from those for adults, but usually include aspirin, a few nonsteroidal anti-inflammatory drugs, and, as a last resort, disease-modifying antirheumatic drugs and gold compounds. Corticosteroids are sometimes used in children but may soften the bones and retard growth.

GOUT

Gout or gouty arthritis is a centuries-old disease that until recently was only partly controllable, excruciatingly painful, and potentially debilitating. Now, researchers hail the conquest of gout as one of the major victories of modern medicine. Experts say there is no reason for anyone to suffer the pain and complications of gout since its underlying mechanisms are now understood and its symptoms can be controlled by modern drugs.

Gout is generally an inherited metabolic disease in which excessive amounts of uric acid in the body are deposited in the tissues and spaces of the joints. Crystals from the uric acid accumulate in the joints, causing inflammation and severe pain. Gout is surprisingly widespread, striking more than one-and-a-half million Americans, 90 percent of them men, usually in middle age. Its female sufferers are usually postmenopausal. Gout can strike the knee, ankle, instep of the foot, joints of the shoulder, wrist and elbow, but almost always shows up in the big toe. Usually it occurs in just one joint at a time.

Cause: Generally, a predisposition for gout is inherited. The high levels of uric acid may occur because the body makes too much and the normally functioning kidneys cannot excrete it fast enough. Or more commonly, the body may produce only a normal amount of uric acid, but kidneys function too slowly to get rid of it. Gout can also result from taking drugs that raise uric acid levels—the worst culprit is diuretics.

Symptoms: Throbbing pain in one joint that sometimes comes on suddenly in the night or after an injury. The joint becomes swollen and tender and may turn dark red or purple. Gout is sometimes accompanied by fevers, chills and a rapid heartbeat.

Diagnosis: Gout can be accurately diagnosed by extracting joint fluid and examining it under a microscope for the presence of crystals of sodium urate.

Treatment: Even with no treatment, acute attacks of gout will subside within a couple of weeks; however, with treatment relief comes in a few hours. If untreated, gout can lead to permanent crippling or damage to the joints and kidneys from the buildup of kidney stones or deposits.

Drugs are the treatment of choice for gout. Drugs such as colchicine and indomethacin will stop the acute attack in the joints; newer drugs, such as allopurinol and andprobenecid (taken to prevent the attacks), either decrease the production of uric acid or increase the kidneys' ability to excrete it, thus lowering concentrations of uric acid to the point where crystals no longer form in the joints. Drugs are sometimes combined, and it may take some experimenting to determine which drugs are most effective in each individual. Such drugs have virtually erased the problem of gout as a major debilitating form of arthritis for those who take daily medication.

OTHER FORMS OF ARTHRITIS AND BONE DISEASES

Spinal arthritis (ankylosing spondylitis, also called Marie-Strümpell disease) causes back pain and stiffness and loss of spinal mobility and can lead to fusion and rigidity of the vertebrae. It is an inflammatory disease of the joints of the spine. Although the complete cause of the disorder is unknown, it has a strong hereditary component. Ten to twenty percent of those with the disease have other family members with it. It is usually diagnosed during a person's twenties and thirties. Diagnosis can be made by X-rays, symptom history, and a back examination. It was once thought to strike men almost exclusively, but now experts say it strikes women as well, but usually in a milder form.

The disease is generally not severe, although an estimated 1 percent of those stricken end up with serious disability. Treatment: drugs and stretching and mobility exercise.

Scleroderma (progressive systemic sclerosis) is a disorder of the connective tissue marked by abnormalities of the fine blood vessels. Scleroderma causes thickening and hardening of the skin and can also afflict the gastrointestinal system, heart, lungs and kidneys.

Brittle bone disease (osteogenesis imperfecta) is a serious genetic connective tissue disease that may affect bones, eyes, the inner ear, teeth and skin. Typically the bones are fragile, which may lead to frequent bone fractures and severe deformities. It strikes one out of every 50,000 infants born each year and about 30,000 children are afflicted with it.

Osteoporosis affects about 15 to 20 million Americans and is the most common bone disease among the elderly, notably women after menopause. About eight times as many women as men have osteoporosis. Osteoporosis is a gradual loss of bone mass, usually tied to the lack of estrogen in later years, and is the underlying cause of many bone fractures among the elderly, including many of the nearly 200,000 broken hips suffered each year. Bones, weakened by osteoporosis, may fracture and collapse (for example, in the spine or hip), spontaneously or after only minor injuries. About 1.3 million fractures due to osteoporosis occur every year in people age 45 and over. Osteoporosis can also cause back pain and humped back.

Severe bone loss is not reversible; thus prevention is the only effective way to avoid osteoporosis. Estrogen replacement therapy is successful in preventing osteoporosis in certain women if it is begun soon after menopause. Another preventive may be adequate calcium intake. Normal vitamin D intake is necessary for calcium absorption. Moderate exercise, including walking, is also recommended to prevent bone loss.

LUPUS (SYSTEMIC LUPUS ERYTHEMATOSUS)

Although lupus is rarely thought of by the public as a form of arthritis, it is medically categorized with rheumatic disorders, such as rheumatoid arthritis, osteoarthritis and juvenile arthritis, and is treated by the same specialists (rheumatologists).

Lupus is a potentially fatal disease of the immune system and connective tissue that strikes primarily women during adolescence or young adult life. About 90 percent of those with lupus are young women, although it has been diagnosed in babies as young as two and in adults as old as 97. Nobody knows how many people have lupus because it is frequently mistaken for other diseases. It is believed to be much more common than thought 20 years ago. Some estimate that half a million Americans may have lupus, making it more common than muscular dystrophy, multiple sclerosis and even leukemia. Some say current studies show that about 130,000 Americans have the systemic or serious form of the disease.

Lupus is often relatively mild, but can be life-threatening if it attacks the whole body, injuring the connective tissue in the kidneys, heart and other vital organs. Twenty years ago such attacks of lupus were considered highly fatal, but today they are treatable and death is unusual. It can produce symptoms of arthritis, such as joint inflammation, but it is rarely crippling. Although it can be a serious disease, many experts believe the danger has been overdramatized and is exaggerated in the public's mind.

Cause: Unknown. Lupus is an autoimmune disease in which large numbers of antibodies attack the body's own tissues. Since the disease is so prevalent in women, it is theorized that sex hormones may somehow interfere with the immune system. The possibility that a virus may trigger the disease has also been raised.

Symptoms: A bright red skin rash, weakness, chronic fatigue, joint pain, decreased appetite, frequent infections, low-grade fever of unknown cause, a striking sensitivity to the sun. Also pain and soreness in the joints, usually in the wrists, knuckles, fingers and knees. Like rheumatoid arthritis, the disease causes an inflammation of the membranes around the joints but rarely causes serious joint damage. In serious cases, the disease can damage the organs, notably the kidneys, leading to kidney failure. There may be hair loss and easy bruising. The disease may strike the nervous system and brain, resembling epilepsy or producing various forms of psychoses.

Diagnosis: Lupus is often misdiagnosed because of its wide range of symptoms and recurring remissions. There is no single test for lupus. It is diagnosed by laboratory tests, including some specialized ones for immune status, and a medical history.

Treatment: Usually highly individual, since the course of the disease varies greatly. Drugs, mainly corticosteroids, are used, as well as aspirin and other pain and anti-inflammatory medications. Also, patients must avoid the sun or use sun screens. Surgery is sometimes required to correct deformities as the tendons and ligaments around the joints loosen. Hip replacement is necessary in rare cases. Some lupus patients have had successful kidney transplants and others have responded to a newer technique—plasmapheresis—in which the blood is cleansed of plasma carrying the antibodies. Most people with lupus can lead nearly normal lives, engaging in exercise and other physical activities. Early treatment may also reduce the chance of permanent organ damage. More than 80 percent of patients can expect to live normal life spans.

GOVERNMENT ARTHRITIS CENTERS

The National Institute of Arthritis and Musculoskeletal and Skin Diseases supports Multipurpose Arthritis Centers around the country. These centers were set up to generate new knowledge about the causes and treatment of arthritis and related musculoskeletal diseases and to help insure that new treatments are applied. The centers are associated with major teaching hospitals and are staffed by leading specialists. The centers conduct research on arthritis and put out numerous booklets, pamphlets, videotapes, and bibliographies on the disease. They are also a source of information about services in the community of interest to those with arthritis. Following are the Multipurpose Arthritis Centers and their respective directors.

ALABAMA
Dr. William J. Koopman
Professor
Department of Medicine
University of Alabama
University Station
Birmingham, AL 35294
(205) 934-5304

CALIFORNIA
Dr. Ira Goldstein
Rheumatology Division
Department of Medicine
San Francisco General Hospital
1001 Potrero Ave., Room 330
San Francisco, CA 94110
(415) 821-8189

Dr. Halsted R. Holman
Stanford University Medical Center
701 Welch Rd., Suite 3301
Stanford, CA 94304
(415) 497-5907

CONNECTICUT
Dr. Naomi F. Rothfield
Professor of Medicine
Chief, Division of Rheumatic Diseases
University of Connecticut
School of Medicine
Farmington, CT 06032
(203) 674-2160

ILLINOIS
Dr. Frank R. Schmid
Professor of Medicine
Northwestern University
McGraw Medical School
303 E. Chicago Ave.
Chicago, IL 60611
(312) 649-8197

INDIANA
Dr. Kenneth D. Brandt
Division of Rheumatology
Indiana University
School of Medicine
541 Clinical Drive
Indianapolis, IN 46223
(317) 264-4225

MASSACHUSETTS
Dr. Alan S. Cohen
Chief of Medicine
Boston University
School of Medicine
818 Harrison St.
Boston, MA 02118
(617) 424-5154

Dr. Matthew H. Liang
Brigham and Women's Hospital
75 Frances St.
Boston, MA 02120
(617) 732-5356

MICHIGAN
Dr. Giles G. Bole
Professor of Internal Medicine
R4633 Kresge Medical Research Building
University of Michigan Medical School
Ann Arbor, MI 48109
(313) 764-1205

MISSOURI
Dr. Gordon C. Sharp
Professor and Director
Immunology and Rheumatology
University of Missouri Health Sciences Center
Department of Medicine
Columbia, MO 65201
(314) 882-8738
Comprehensive model care unit for children
with arthritis.

NORTH CAROLINA
Dr. John B. Winfield
Professor and Chief
Division of Rheumatology
932 FLOB, 231H
University of North Carolina
Chapel Hill, NC 27514
(919) 966-4191

OHIO
Dr. Roland W. Moskowitz
Professor of Medicine
Director, Rheumatic Disease Unit
Case Western Reserve University
2073 Abington Rd.
Cleveland, OH 44106
(216) 444-3168

TEXAS
Dr. Norman Talal
Professor of Medicine
Division of Clinical Immunology
University of Texas
Health Science Center
7703 Floyd Curl Drive
San Antonio, TX 78284
(512) 691-6341

SOURCE: *National Institute of Arthritis and Musculoskeletal and Skin Diseases.*

ARTHRITIS AND BONE DISEASE RESEARCH AT THE NATIONAL INSTITUTES OF HEALTH

Several research studies on rheumatoid arthritis and lupus are being performed at the Clinical Center at the National Institutes of Health in Bethesda, Maryland. Participation in such research and treatment programs are usually by physician referral only. For more information, your physician can contact:

Office of the Director
The Clinical Center
Building 10, Room 2C-146
National Institutes of Health
Bethesda, Maryland 20892
Patient Referral Service
(301) 496-4891

ORGANIZATIONS AND AGENCIES

The Arthritis Foundation
1314 Spring St., N.W.
Atlanta, GA 30309
(404) 872-7100

A national voluntary health association with about 75 local chapters throughout the country. Works to find causes, prevention, and cures for arthritis. Provides information on arthritis, patient services, and professional education and training. Publishes numerous booklets, pamphlets, a quarterly newspaper, and develops self-help programs usually carried out by the network of local chapters. A general all around source of information for those with arthritis. In addition, local Arthritis Foundation chapters keep lists of clinics and private physicians in your community who specialize in the treatment of rheumatology. The physicians must meet stringent criteria: They must be board certified in rheumatology, or board certified in internal medicine, and exhibit a special interest in rheumatology as proved by the fact that at least 50 percent of their patients have rheumatological problems. The physicians complete at least 14 hours of postgraduate education in rheumatology every year in a continuing education program. You can find such a physician in your area by calling your local Arthritis Foundation chapter.

Arthritis Information Clearinghouse
PO Box 9782
Arlington, VA 22209
(703) 558-8250

A government-operated clearinghouse for information on arthritis, set up to serve mostly professionals, such as physicians, educators and librarians. Keeps bibliographies on books, journals, film strips, videotapes, other audiovisual materials, posters, exhibits and displays. Responds to requests from the public and will send out free booklets on arthritis, but generally refers requests for additional help to other organizations, such as the Arthritis Foundation.

The National Institute of Arthritis and
    Musculoskeletal and Skin Diseases
9000 Rockville Pike
Building 31, Room 9A04
Bethesda, MD 20892
(301) 496-3583

As one of the federal government's National Institutes of Health, this Institute has primary responsibility for supporting research on the various types of arthritis as well as musculoskeletal and skin diseases. Publishes materials for the public and professionals. Will provide more information upon request.

The American Lupus Society
23751 Madison St.
Torrance, CA 90505
(213) 373-1335

Voluntary health organization for patients and families with about 35 local chapters. A source of information and self-help. Sponsors mutual support meetings. Quarterly newsletter. Helps patients find physician specialists. Will provide more information upon request.

The Lupus Foundation of America
1717 Massachusetts Ave., N.W.
Washington, D.C. 20036
(202) 328-4550
(800) 558-0121

A national association of concerned patients, their families, and physicians, dedicated to developing and supporting research on lupus, raising understanding of the social and human costs of lupus among the public, helping lupus patients understand their disease and improve their welfare, and generating the exchange of scientific information. More than 90 chapters throughout the country hold public meetings on lupus, distribute literature, provide person to person contact among patients with lupus, and answer questions from the public. Will provide more information upon request.

United Scleroderma Foundation
PO Box 350
Watsonville, CA 95077
(408) 728-2202
(800) 722-HOPE

This national nonprofit organization is dedicated to educating and informing patients and the public about scleroderma. It promotes medical research to find a cause and cure; about 30 local chapters offer mutual support. Workshops are held; brochures and a quarterly newsletter are published. Provides physician referrals. Will provide more information upon request.

SOME SPECIAL SERVICES

Self-help course

This course of six two-hour sessions teaches those with arthritis how to take care of themselves. It is conducted by most local chapters of the Arthritis Foundation throughout the country and includes sessions on stretching and range of motion exercises, relaxation to deal with pain, energy conservation, joint protection, and the role of medication and nutrition in fighting arthritis. It is based on the successful program at Stanford University's Arthritis Center. Call your local Arthritis Foundation chapter for details.

Exercise program

This program of warm water exercises is a joint venture of the YMCA and the Arthritis Foundation. Conducted under the supervision of teachers knowledgeable about arthritis exercises, the program is designed to increase joint motion and flexibility. Call your local YMCA or local Arthritis Foundation chapter.

Support groups

Many local Arthritis Foundation chapters also have clubs or support groups where people get together to discuss their common problems, share experiences, and learn how to better cope with their disease. Also, chapters make referrals to other basic services in the community that may be helpful to those with arthritis, such as vocational training, counseling, and so forth.

BOOKS

Arthritis: A Comprehensive Guide, **Dr. James R. Fries,** Boston: Addison Wesley, 1979.
The Arthritis Exercise Book, **Semyon** and **Ann Edgar,** New York: Cornerstone Library/ Simon & Schuster, 1981.

Arthritis Help Book: What You Can Do for Your Arthritis, **Dr. James Fries** and **Dr. Kate Lorig,** Boston: Addison Wesley, 1980.
Arthritis: Relief Beyond Drugs, New York: Harper & Row, 1981.

Buster Crabbe's Arthritis Exercise Book,
Buster Crabbe with **Raphael Cilento,** New
York: Simon & Schuster, 1980.

Coping with Lupus, **Robert H. Phillips,**
Ph.D., Wayne, NJ: Avery Publishing
Group, 1984.

Help for Your Arthritic Hand, **Semyon**
Krewer, New York: Simon & Schuster,
1982.

Lupus: The Body Against Itself, **Dr. Sheldon**
Paul and **Dodi Schultz,** New York:
Doubleday, 1977.

A Manual for Arthritis Self-Management: A
Joint Venture, **Dr. Frank Dudley Hart,**
New York: Arco, 1981, 93-page manual.

Overcoming Arthritis: A Guide to Coping with
Stiff or Aching Joints, **Dr. Frank Dudley**
Hart, New York: Arco, 1981.

The Sun Is My Enemy, **Henrietta Aldjem,**
Boston: Beacon Press, 1976. First person
account by a lupus patient.

Understanding Arthritis, **Arthritis**
Foundation, edited by Irving Kusher,
M.D., Ann Forer, and **Ann B. McGuire,**
New York: Scribner's, 1984.

We Are Not Alone: Learning to Live with
Chronic Illness, **Sefra Pitzele,** Minneapolis,
MN: Thompson and Company, 1985.

Wellness: An Arthritis Reality, **Beth Ziebell,**
Dubuque: Kendall/Hunt, 1981.

MATERIALS, FREE AND FOR SALE

Free (single copy, no charge)

Arthritis Basic Facts, 36 pages.
Arthritis: Diet and Nutrition, 16 pages.
Arthritis Quackery, 10 pages.
Arthritis Surgery, 16 pages.
Aspirin and Related Medications, 14 pages.
Osteoarthritis, 16 pages.
Rheumatoid Arthritis, 20 pages.
Systemic Lupus Erythematosus, 16 pages.

Arthritis Foundation (and local chapters)
PO Box 19000
Atlanta, GA 30326

How to Cope with Arthritis, 19 pages.
Arthritis, Medicine for the Layman, 25 pages.
Osteoporosis: Cause, Treatment, Prevention,
12 pages.

National Institute for Arthritis and
Musculoskeletal and Skin Diseases
9000 Rockville Pike
Building 31, Room 9A04
Bethesda, MD 20892
(301) 496-3583

The Butterfly Mask, writings by lupus patients,
44 pages.
Lupus Erythematosus, 8 page leaflet (also in
Spanish).
Lupus Erythematosus, 14 page booklet (also in
Spanish).

The American Lupus Society
23751 Madison St.
Torrance, CA 90505
(213) 373-1335

Lupus Erythematosus: A Handbook for
Physicians, Patients and their Families, 40
pages.

Lupus Foundation of America
1717 Massachusetts Ave., N.W.
Washington, DC 20036

Audiovisual materials for sale

Jacobson's Progressive Relaxation, **Selma**
Cole. Exercise audiocassette tape. Exercises
for the arthritic to work through all the
different muscle groups in the body.
Stress Management for Arthritis. Audiocassette tape.

Stanford University Multipurpose Arthritis
Center
101 Welch Rd., Suite 3301
Stanford, CA 94304
(415) 497-5900

For children with arthritis

Arty's Arthritis Antics. A workbook for elementary school age children, contains fairy tales,

nursery rhymes, puzzles, and pictures for coloring—all designed to teach children about arthritis.

University of Alabama Multipurpose Arthritis
  Center
University Station
Birmingham, AL 35294

You Have Arthritis Coloring Book, 30 pages. Teaches children who have arthritis about aspirin, exercising, eye exams, etc.

Dr. Gordon C. Sharp
University of Missouri Medical Center
Columbia, MO 65212

ASTHMA AND ALLERGIES

Allergies and asthma are a widespread source of misery, affecting about 35 million Americans. About 9 million Americans have asthma, 15 million have hay fever, and 12 million have some kind of allergic reaction, such as skin rash, hives, swelling, or other reactions to food, medications, airborne particles, or insect stings. Although death is rare from allergies, a surprising number of people still die from asthma—several thousand a year. In fact, asthma deaths are rising, especially among the elderly.

Both allergies and asthma, in the classic definition, involve some peculiar inherited sensitivity of the immune system, and the two conditions are often lumped together, studied together, and treated by the same specialists. Asthma, however, generally causes more discomfort and needs more intensive care. Often, though not always, asthma is tied to allergic reactions.

A true allergy has to do with the immune system; somehow the immune system is hypersensitive to common substances, called allergens. When these allergens enter the bloodstream, they stimulate white blood cells to produce what are called "allergic antibodies" that, in turn, cause inflammation and irritation, usually of the respiratory system. In rare cases of extreme sensitivity, a drug, an insect sting, or a certain food or chemical can send a person into potentially fatal "anaphylactic shock." Generally, however, allergic reactions come on gradually after periods of exposure, usually becoming apparent in childhood.

Common allergies from pollen, molds, and grasses can be easily diagnosed by skin tests and family history. In some cases, drugs or allergy shots are given to prevent the allergic episodes, and sensitive individuals are advised to avoid the allergens when possible. Such allergies can usually be controlled.

ASTHMA

Asthma is a chronic physical condition in which air cannot easily get in and out of the lungs, resulting in episodes of coughing, wheezing and gasping for breath. Contrary to some popular thinking, asthma is *not* psychological and *is* a serious condition. It can be disabling, both to youngsters and adults. Asthma, notably that with an allergic basis, almost always shows up during childhood. About 5 percent of all children under age 15 suffer from asthma. When asthma develops in adults after age 40, it is thought to be caused by unknown nonallergic factors. Males are more likely than females to be asthmatic. About half of all asthmatic youngsters are free of asthma by age 16. In many cases, symptoms begin to subside by age 6.

Cause: Although episodes can be emotionally aggravated, asthma has a physical cause. Asthmatics have extrasensitive bronchial tubes—the network of air passageways throughout the lungs. During an asthmatic state or episode, air cannot get through because the air tubes are narrowed. That happens when the muscles in the airways constrict or go into spasms, when the membranes that line the small respiratory passages called bronchioles swell up, or when the bronchial tubes become clogged with excessive mucus.

Certain events trigger the asthmatic reaction in the lung tissues. Most often asthma is triggered by a so-called allergenic factor, such as pollen, house dust, tobacco smoke or pet dander. Children with hay fever frequently develop asthma. The trigger also can be cold air, vigorous exercise, an infection of the nose or throat, certain foods, chemicals, drugs, including aspirin, or emotional stress. Both asthma and allergies run in families and have a genetic basis that is not completely understood.

Symptoms: Attacks may be mild or severe: they may last minutes or weeks, come on suddenly or develop slowly, be sporadic or occur so regularly as to be a constant wheezing. In severe attacks, asthmatics may feel they are suffocating—able to breathe in, but not to expel air. The victim may panic, begin to perspire and turn blue around the lips and fingernail beds. Usually early warning signs foretell an oncoming attack. Although each sufferer has individual patterns, the most common warning signals are: coughing in the absence of a cold, clearing throat frequently, irregular or noisy, difficult breathing, unusual sweating and flared nostrils.

Diagnosis: It is easy to diagnose asthma, although many cases are not diagnosed and consequently the victim never learns to cope with the disease. Generally, a medical history, especially a strong family history of asthma or allergies, and a physical examination are enough to confirm asthma. Blood tests and lung function tests are often done.

Treatment: Only a decade ago, asthma was difficult to treat. And many children with asthma were overprotected and prevented from engaging in exercise. Now, children with asthma lead nearly normal lives, and sometimes go on to become champion athletes. New drugs make it easier to live with asthma. Some youngsters take these drugs when they feel an episode coming on to help open up the constricted airways. Others take regular doses—say, four times a day— as a preventive. There are also drug inhalers that children can use to ward off a serious episode, or to prevent symptoms from appearing. Some children may need simple physical therapy procedures, three or four times a day, to loosen mucus and drain the lungs. Certain types of exercise, especially swimming, also help open up the airways. Some asthma sufferers do deep-breathing exercises and biofeedback to relax the muscles that control breathing. Experimental hypnosis has been used with some success to control asthma.

In cases in which the asthma is triggered by allergens, avoiding the allergy-inducing agent is a major part of the treatment. This may call for allergy tests to detect the offender, and perhaps allergy shots; however, experts recommend that such allergy shots be used selectively, only when medication and avoidance of the irritants and allergens don't work.

Most cases of asthma can be treated by a family physician or pediatrician, but difficult cases may need special expertise, and, in rare cases, hospitalization.

SOME TREATMENT CENTERS FOR SEVERE ASTHMA

The following centers are well-established, nationally recognized treatment facilities for severe cases of asthma.

Asthmatic Children's Foundation of New York
PO Box 568
Spring Valley Rd.
Ossining, NY 10562
(914) 762-2110

A philanthropic organization that operates a long-term residential treatment and rehabilitation center for severely ill asthmatic children. Also

operates a phone service of referrals around the country and answers other questions about asthma.

National Foundation for Asthma/Tucson
  Medical Center
PO Box 42195
Tucson, AZ 85733
(602) 323-6046

An agency that provides medical care and social rehabilitation for persons of all ages with chronic asthma. Operates outpatient clinic; requires a physician's written referral. Supports research, publishes information for the public.

National Jewish Hospital/National Asthma
    Center
3800 E. Colfax Ave.
Denver, CO 80206
(303) 398-1565

A preeminent national treatment, diagnostic, research and education center that specializes in difficult cases of chronic respiratory diseases and immunological disorders, including asthma. Accepts patients on referral by physicians or public and private health agencies. Provides extensive services on both an inpatient and outpatient basis. Adult as well as pediatric programs. Also publishes information for the public on respiratory diseases. Publications include a newsletter. Has auxiliary chapters and parents' support groups.

GOVERNMENT-SPONSORED ASTHMA, ALLERGIC, AND IMMUNOLOGIC DISEASES RESEARCH CENTERS

The National Institute of Allergy and Infectious Diseases supports major centers around the country that treat patients and do research. All of the centers can be expected to have well-informed clinicians who may be available for treatment or consultations. Following is a list of the centers and their directors.

CALIFORNIA
Eng Tan, M.D.
Scripps Clinic and Research Foundation
10666 N. Torrey Pines Rd.
La Jolla, CA 92037
(619) 455-8925

John L. Fahey, M.D.
University of California at Los Angeles
Center for Health Sciences Building
Los Angeles, CA 90024
(213) 825-6568

Irma Gigli, M.D.
University of California at San Diego Medical
    Center
225 Dickinson St.
San Diego, CA 92103
(619) 294-5580

William L. Epstein, M.D.
Department of Medicine
University of California at San Francisco
400 Parnassus Ave.
San Francisco, CA 94143
(415) 666-2545

DISTRICT OF COLUMBIA
Joseph A. Bellanti, M.D.
Georgetown University School of Medicine
3900 Reservoir Rd., N.W.
Washington, DC 20007
(202) 625-7440

ILLINOIS
Roy Patterson, M.D.
Northwestern University Medical School
303 E. Chicago Ave.
Chicago, IL 60611
(312) 649-8172

IOWA
Hal Richerson, M.D.
Division of Allergy and Immunology
Department of Internal Medicine
University of Iowa Hospitals and Clinics
Iowa City, IA 52242
(319) 356-2117

MARYLAND
Philip S. Norman, M.D.
Johns Hopkins University School of Medicine
Good Samaritan Hospital
5601 Lock Raven Blvd.
Baltimore, MD 21239
(301) 323-2200

Michael A. Kaliner, M.D.
NIAID, Building 10, Room 11C205
National Institutes of Health
Bethesda, MD 20892
(301) 496-9314

MASSACHUSETTS
K. Frank Austen, M.D.
Brigham and Women's Hospital
75 Francis St.
Boston, MA 02115
(617) 732-1995

Ross E. Rocklin, M.D.
Tufts University
School of Medicine
136 Harrison Ave.
Boston, MA 02111
(617) 956-5333

Fred S. Rosen, M.D.
Children's Hospital Medical Center
300 Longwood Ave.
Boston, MA 02115
(617) 735-7601

MINNESOTA
Gerald J. Gleich, M.D.
Mayo Clinic and Foundation
200 First St., S.W.
Rochester, MN 55905
(507) 282-2511

MISSOURI
Charles W. Parker, M.D.
Washington University School of Medicine
660 S. Euclid Ave.
St. Louis, MO 63110
(314) 454-2501

NEW YORK
Nicholas Chiorazzi, M.D.
The Rockefeller University
1230 York Ave.
New York, NY 10021
(212) 570-8329

Greg Siskind, M.D.
Cornell University
1300 York Ave.
New York, NY 10021
(212) 472-8250

Allen P. Kaplan, M.D.
Health Sciences Center
State University of New York at Stony Brook
Stony Brook, NY 11794
(516) 246-2262

NORTH CAROLINA
Rebecca H. Buckley, M.D.
Duke University
Box 2898
Durham, NC 27710
(919) 684-2922

TEXAS
Paul Bergstresser, M.D.
University of Texas at Dallas
Health Science Center
5223 Harry Hines Blvd.
Dallas, TX 75235
(214) 688-2145

WISCONSIN
Jordan N. Fink, M.D.
Medical College of Wisconsin
8700 W. Wisconsin Ave.
Box 122
Milwaukee, WI 53226
(414) 257-8296

Richard Hong, M.D.
University of Wisconsin Medical School
600 Highland Ave.
Madison, WI 53792
(608) 263-6201

SOURCE: *National Institute of Allergy and Infectious Diseases.*

ORGANIZATIONS

American Lung Association
National Headquarters
1740 Broadway
New York, NY 10019
(212) 315-8700

A national voluntary health organization concerned with lung diseases, including asthma. Maintains state and local affiliates, basically educational. A major source of information on lung diseases. Pamphlets, booklets, and audiovisual

materials. Numerous services, depending on local affiliate. Local affiliates will provide more
information upon request.

Asthma and Allergy Foundation of America
1835 K St. N.W.
Suite P-900
Washington, D.C. 20006
(202) 293-2950

A voluntary national health organization with
local chapters throughout the country. Information and self-help source for those with allergies
and asthma, physicians, health professionals and
other interested persons. Supports research, offers pamphlets, booklets, books and a bimonthly
newsletter, *The Asthma and Allergy Advance.*
Will answer questions from the public and send
more information and the name of local chapters
upon request.

Asthma Care Association of America
PO Box 568
Spring Valley Rd.
Ossining, NY 10362
(914) 762-2110

A nonprofit corporation dedicated to financially
supporting the care, treatment and rehabilitation
of persons with asthma and other allergies. Supports research and publishes *Journal of Asthma.*
Makes medical referrals. Will provide more information upon request.

National Institute of Allergy and Infectious
    Diseases NIAID/NIH
9000 Rockville Pike
Building 31, Room 7A32
Bethesda, MD 20892
(301) 496-5717

One of the National Institutes of Health that conducts and directs nationwide research program
on the causes, diagnosis, treatment and prevention of allergic and infectious diseases, including
asthma.

BOOKS

The Allergy Encyclopedia, **edited by The
    Asthma & Allergy Foundation of America**
    and **Craig T. Norback,** New York: New
    American Library, 1981.
*Asthma: The Complete Guide to Self-
    Management,* **Allan M. Weinstein, M.D.,**
    New York: McGraw-Hill, 1987.
Asthma and Allergies: An Optimistic Future,
    Patrick Young, Washington: U.S.
    Department of Health and Human Services,
    1980, 179 pages. NIH Publication No. 80-
    388. Based on the report of the Task Force
    on Asthma and Other Allergic Diseases. For
    sale by the Superintendent of Documents,
    U.S. Government Printing Office,
    Washington, DC 20402.
Asthma and Hay Fever, **Alan Knight,** New
    York: Arco Publishing, 1981.
Asthma: The Facts, **Donald J. Lane** and

Anthony Storr, New York: Oxford
    University Press, 1979.
Asthma: Stop Suffering, Start Living, **M. Eric
    Gershwin** and **E.L. Klingelhofer,** Reading,
    MA: Addison-Wesley, 1986.
*Breathe Easy: An Asthmatic's Guide to Clean
    Air,* **Stanley Reichman,** New York: Thomas
    Y. Crowell, Co., 1977.
Breathing Exercises for Asthma, **Karen R.
    Butts,** Springfield, IL: Charles C. Thomas,
    1980. For professionals and parents of
    asthmatic children.
Children With Asthma: A Manual for Parents,
    Dr. Thomas F. Plaut, Amherst, MA:
    PediPress, 1983. Mail order from PediPress,
    125 Red Gate Lane, Amherst, MA 01002.
Living With Your Allergies and Asthma,
    Theodore Berland, New York: St. Martin's
    Press, 1983.

Speaking of Asthma, **Dr. Dietrich Nolte,** New York: Delair, 1980.

Teaching Myself About Asthma, **Guy Parcel,** Galveston, TX: University of Texas Medical

Branch. For children from 7 to 12 years old. Mail order from Division of Health Education, University of Texas Medical Branch, Galveston, TX 77550.

MATERIALS, FREE AND FOR SALE

Free (single copies are free)

Information on the following topics:

About Asthma: What Everyone Should Know.
Asthma Facts.
Controlling Asthma.
Hay Fever Facts.
Hints for Control of the Home Environment for the Allergic Person.
What Happens When a Child Has Asthma.

Local American Lung Associations, listed in the white pages of your telephone directory.

Your Child and Asthma, 27 pages. Includes detailed description of drugs and their side effects.

National Jewish Hospital/National Asthma Center
3800 E. Colfax Ave.
Denver, CO 80206
(303) 388-4461

Asthma Fact and Fiction, 16 pages.
Dust 'n Stuff. Directions for allergy proofing your home.

National Foundation for Asthma/Tucson Medical Center
PO Box 42195
Tucson, AZ 85733
(602)-323-6046

Allergies: Medicine for the Layman, 25 pages.
Asthma, 16 pages.
Drug Allergy, 16 pages.
Dust Allergy, 16 pages.
Insect Allergy, 16 pages.
Poison Ivy Allergy, 16 pages.
Pollen Allergy, 16 pages.
Understanding the Immune System, 22 pages.

National Institute of Allergies and Infectious Diseases
9000 Rockville Pike
Building 31, Room 7A32
Bethesda, MD 20892

For sale

Allergy in Children, 14 pages.
Asthma, 11 pages.
Drug Allergy, 14 pages.
Exercise and Asthma, 16 pages.
Food Allergy, 14 pages.
Hay Fever, 22 pages.
The Immune System, 14 pages.
Insect Stings, 14 pages.
Mold Allergy, 14 pages.
Poison Ivy Allergy, 14 pages.
The Potential for Quackery and Questionable Treatment, 11 pages.
Skin Allergy, 14 pages.

Asthma and Allergy Foundation of America
1835 K St. N.W.
Suite P-900
Washington, D.C. 20006
(202) 293-2950

Asthma: Episodes and Treatment, 20 pages.
Asthma: How To Live With It, 20 pages.
What We Know About Allergies.

Public Affairs Pamphlets
381 Park Ave., S.
New York, NY 10016

SUPERSTUFF—Asthma self-help package

Superstuff is an 86-page full-color book of activities (riddles, rhymes, T-shirt iron-ons, a door sign, puzzles, stories, paper dolls, a board game, a record with a relaxation song) designed to help youngsters and their parents learn how to better understand and cope with asthma. The educational self-help package comes with a news-magazine for parents and instructional booklet. It is designed for the elementary school–age child who has asthma and is receiving medical care, and whose ailment is severe enough to disrupt his or her life-style. It may also be of interest to junior high school–age youngsters. The activity kit is not intended for youngsters whose asthma is well controlled or who have only one or two mild episodes a year. The kit is available from local American Lung Association affiliates listed in the white pages of local telephone directories. A donation is requested to help defray printing costs.

ASTHMA HOTLINE

(800) 222-LUNG
(303) 398-1477—Colorado

A specially trained nurse is available Monday through Friday from 8:30 A.M. to 5:00 P.M., Rocky Mountain Time, to answer questions about asthma, as well as about other lung diseases. In addition, the caller can receive information about the National Jewish Hospital/National Asthma Center (which operates the hotline) or can obtain the names of physicians trained at the Center or who are recommended by the staff, and practice in the caller's area.

ALTERNATIVE ALLERGY TREATMENT: CLINICAL ECOLOGY

In the past few years, a medical field called "clinical ecology" or "environmental medicine" has sprung up to challenge the orthodox view of allergies. In traditional medicine, allergies are viewed as emanating from complex changes in the immune system, as determined by certain prescribed tests. But some physicians who practice what is called "clinical ecology" say that defining an allergy by linking it to the immunological mechanism is too narrow and ignores numerous allergies to environmental factors—such as chemical pollutants in the air and food—that have no underlying immunological basis. Food allergies, for example, have been alleged to trigger behavioral changes, such as hyperactivity in children. Some proponents of clinical ecology believe that about two-thirds of all allergies are not linked to the immune system but are hidden intolerances to certain chemicals, and thus are overlooked or dismissed by conventional allergists, leaving people to suffer needlessly.

The clinical ecologists believe that the onset of allergic reactions may be delayed, leading to chronic diseases. They also contend that these allergies can be controlled by changing the environment—by eliminating certain foods from the diet, for example. Some experts believe that many conditions can be relieved this way, including insomnia, fatigue, anxiety, headaches, depression, alcoholism, arthritis and pain. Clinical ecology is scoffed at by many establishment allergists and immunologists who say it is without scientific theory or proof. Nevertheless, clinical ecology advocates insist that they have much evidence—case histories of success—and sound tests and theories to prove their point of view.

SOME SPECIALISTS IN CLINICAL ECOLOGY

Here are some physicians who practice in "clinical ecology" either in a family practice or other specialty. They are all members or fellows of the American Academy of Environmental Medicine, PO Box 16106, Denver, CO 80216.

ALABAMA
James H. Walker, Sr., M.D.*
1501 15th Ave., S.
Birmingham, AL 35233
(205) 934-9770

Andrew M. Brown, M.D.*
515 S. Third St.
Gadsden, AL 35901
(205) 547-4971

Joseph B. Miller, M.D.*
5901 Airport Blvd.
Mobile, AL 36608
(205) 342-8540

ARIZONA
Kenneth M. Hatfield, D.O.
220 N. Stapley Dr., 2
Mesa, AZ 85203
(602) 833-5383

Talmage W. Shill, M.D.
2520 N. Mesa Dr.
Mesa, AZ 85201
(602) 898-0698

Ralph F. Herro, M.D.*
5115 N. Central Ave.
Phoenix, AZ 85012
(602) 266-2374

James A. Smidt, M.D.
5115 N. Central Ave., #C
Phoenix, AZ 85012
(602) 252-9731

Gene D. Schmutzer, D.O.
2425 North Alvernon Way
Tucson, AZ 85712-2501
(602) 795-0292

ARKANSAS
Robert Collier, M.D.*
601 N. Main
Brinkley, AR 72021
(501) 734-4847

Rheeta M. Stecker, M.D.
1315 Central Ave.
Hot Springs, AR 71901
(501) 624-5206

Harold H. Hedges, M.D.
424 N. University
Little Rock, AR 72205
(501) 664-4810

Aubrey M. Worrell, Jr., M.D.*
3900 Hickory St.
Pine Bluff, AR 71603
(501) 535-8200

Howard G. Kimball, M.D.
1919 W. Main St.
Russellville, AR 72801
(501) 968-3611

CALIFORNIA
Robert T. Pottenger, Jr., M.D.*
166 E. Foothill Blvd.
Arcadia, CA 91106-2507
(818) 796-2048

P. L. Saifer, M.D., M.P.H.*
3031 Telegraph Ave., #215
Berkeley, CA 94705
(415) 849-3346

Cathie Ann Lippman, M.D.
292 S. LaCienega Blvd., #202-20
Beverly Hills, CA 90211
(213) 659-9187

George R. Borrell, M.D.
22030 Sherman Way, #305
Canoga Park, CA 91303
(818) 347-3900

John P. Toth, M.D.
2299 Bacon St.
Concord, CA 94520
(415) 682-5660

Daniel A. Calabrese, M.D.
1660 S. El Camino Real #G-208
Encinitas, CA 92024

Erhardt Zinke, M.D.*
300 N. Main, #12
Fallbrook, CA 92028
(619) 728-4901

Edward L. Binkley, M.D.*
c/o FHP Inc-9930 Talbert Ave.
Fountain Valley, CA 92728

Charles G. Gabelman, M.D.*
24953 Paseo de Valencia, #16C
Laguna Hills, CA 92653
(714) 859-9851

Charles A. Moss, M.D.
8950 Villa La Jolla Drive
La Jolla, CA 92037
(619) 457-1314

Geraldine P. Donaldson, M.D.
1398 Concannon Blvd.
Livermore, CA 94550
(415) 443-8282

Jeffry L. Anderson, M.D.
232 E. Blithedale Ave.
Mill Valley, CA 94941
(415) 383-1262

Michael E. Rosenbaum, M.D.
232 E. Blithedale Ave.
Mill Valley, CA 94941
(415) 383-1262

Dorothy V. Calabrese, M.D.
26111 Marguerite Pkwy
Mission Viejo, CA 92692
(714) 582-2161

Joseph J. McGovern, M.D.
389 30th St.
Oakland, CA 94609
(415) 444-5721

John D. Michael, M.D.
6536 Telegraph Ave., #A201
Oakland, CA 94609
(415) 547-8111

William J. Sayer, M.D.*
145 N. California Ave.
Palo Alto, CA 94301-3911
(415) 321-3361

Ruth G. McGill, M.D.
PO Box 55
Potrero, CA 92063
(817) 481-5347

Sunil P. Perera, M.D.
404 Sunrise Ave.
Roseville, CA 95678
(916) 782-7758

George R. Fricke, M.D.
1355 Florin Rd.
Sacramento, CA 95822
(916) 427-8988

Zane R. Gard, M.D.
6386 Alvarado Court, #5326
San Diego, CA 92120
(619) 583-5863

Darrell Hunsaker, M.D.
Naval Hospital
San Diego, CA 92134
(509) 575-0212

Iris R. Bell, M.D.
1902 Webster St.
San Francisco, CA 94115
(415) 563-9384

Ronald R. Chappler, M.D.
909 Hyde St., #401
San Francisco, CA 94109
(415) 885-4433

Don L. Jewett, M.D., Ph.D.
Room U-471, University of California
San Francisco, CA 94143
(415) 666-5132

Alan S. Levin, M.D.
450 Sutter St., Suite #1138
San Francisco, CA 94108
(415) 922-1444

Frederick T. Guilford, M.D.
101 S. San Mateo Drive, Suite 303
San Mateo, CA 94401
(415) 342-7459

Ronald R. Wempen, M.D.
3620 South Bristol St. Suite 306
Santa Ana, CA 92704
(714) 546-4325

Donald E. Reiner, M.D.
1414 S. Miller, Suite D
Santa Maria, CA 93454
(805) 925-0961

Laszlo I. Belenyessy, M.D.
2901 Wilshire Blvd., Suite 435
Santa Monica, CA 90403
(213) 828-4480

James D. Schuler, M.D.
19755 Balfoor, Box 427
Strathmore, CA 93267
(209) 568-1116

John C. Wakefield, M.D.*
970 W. El Camino Real, Suite 1
Sunnyvale, CA 94087
(408) 732-3037

Melvyn R. Werbach, M.D.
18411 Clark St., #207
Tarzana, CA 91356
(818) 996-6110

Richard A. Hendricks, M.D.
1050 Las Tablas Rd.
Templeton, CA 93465
(805) 434-1836

Phillip H. Taylor, M.D.
325 S. Moorpark Rd.
Thousand Oaks, CA 91361
(805) 497-3839

Cecil A. Bradley, M.D.
33800 Alvarado Niles Rd.
Union City, CA 94587
(415) 348-8110

COLORADO
Harold C. Whitcomb, Jr., M.D.
100 E. Main St.
Aspen, CO 81611
(303) 925-5440

Kendall A. Gerdes, M.D.*
1617 Vine St.
Denver, CO 80206
(303) 377-8837

Vincent A. Lagerborg, M.D., Ph.D.
29 Crestmoor Drive
Denver, CO 80220
(303) 482-6001

Del Stigler, M.D.*
2005 Franklin St., #490
Denver, CO 80205
(303) 831-7335

Mechteld Van Hardenbroek, M.C., M.D.
PO Box 298
Dillon, CO 80435
(303) 468-2478

Nicholas G. Nonas, M.D.
601 E. Hampden
Englewood, CO 80110
(303) 781-9416

Lawrence D. Dickey, M.D.
109 West Olive St.
Fort Collins, CO 80524
(303) 482-6001

S. Crawford Duhon, M.D.*
373 W. Drake Rd.
Fort Collins, CO 80526
(303) 223-3970

Robert B. Richards, M.D.*
419 E. Ninth Ave.
Fort Morgan, CO 80701
(303) 867-2437

John W. Jones, M.D.
405 W. 15th St.
Pueblo, CO 81003
(303) 543-7850

V. Michael Barkett, M.D.
577 E. First St.
Salida, CO 81201
(303) 539-4920

CONNECTICUT
Sidney M. Baker, M.D.*
310 Prospect St.
New Haven, CT 06511
(203) 789-1911

Marshall Mandell, M.D.*
Three Brush St.
Norwalk, CT 06850
(203) 838-4706

Jerrold N. Finnie, M.D.
1185 New Litchfield St.
Torrington, CT 06790
(203) 489-8977

DISTRICT OF COLUMBIA
George H. Mitchell, M.D.
2112 F St., N.W., Suite #404
Washington, DC 20037-2712
(202) 429-9456

FLORIDA
Neil C. Henderson, M.D.*
30 S.E. Seventh St.
Boca Raton, FL 33432
(305) 368-2915

Albert F. Robbins, D.O.
51 S.E. Third St.
Boca Raton, FL 33432
(305) 395-3282

W. W. Mittlestadt, D.O.
4001 N. Ocean Dr., #305
Fort Lauderdale, FL 33308-5928
(305) 491-4656

Randall A. Langston, M.D.
1005 Mar Walt Drive
Fort Walton Beach, FL 32548
(904) 863-4121

Martin Brody, M.D., D.D.S.
7100 W. 20th Ave.
Hialeah, FL 33016
(305) 822-9035

Glen Wagner, M.D.
121 Sixth Ave.
Indialantic, FL 32903
(305) 723-5915

Jeffrey Marcus, M.D., F.A.C.S.
3733 E. Gulf-to-Lake Highway
Inverness, FL 32650
(904) 726-3131

Ronald Z. Surowitz, D.O.
411 W. Indian Town Rd.
Jupiter, FL 33458
(305) 746-7826

Morris Beck, M.D.
7400 N. Kendall Drive, #507
Miami, FL 33156
(305) 271-4711

Stanley J. Cannon, M.D.*
9085 S.W. 87th Ave.
Miami, FL 33176
(305) 279-3020

Douglas Sandberg, M.D.
1500 N.W. 12th Ave., #1208
Miami, FL 33136
(305) 547-6511

Alan J. Serrins, M.D.*
7400 N. Kendall Drive
Miami, FL 33156
(305) 595-1597

Sydney D. Wruble, M.D.
7400 N. Kendall Drive
Miami, FL 33156
(305) 595-1597

Hobart T. Feldman, M.D.*
16800 N.W. Second Ave., #301
North Miami Beach, FL 33169
(305) 652-1062

Robert M. Stroud, M.D.*
32 Iroquois Trail
Ormond Beach, FL 32074
(904) 677-5271

Kenneth N. Krischer, M.D., Ph.D.*
910 S.W. 40th Ave.
Plantation, FL 33317
(305) 584-6655

Herbert I. Moselle, M.D.
201 N.W. 82 Ave., #103
Plantation, FL 33324-1809
(305) 584-5040

William H. Philpott, M.D.*
6101 Central Ave.
St. Petersburg, FL 33710
(813) 381-4673

Ray C. Wunderlich, Jr., M.D.
666 Sixth St., S.
St. Petersburg, FL 33701
(813) 822-3612

GEORGIA

D. Morton Boyette, M.D.*
804 Fourteenth Ave.
Albany, GA 31708
(912) 435-7161

Milton Fried, M.D.
4426 Tilly Mill Rd.
Atlanta, GA 30360
(404) 451-4857

Young S. Shin, M.D.
1135 Hudson Bridge Rd., #7
Stockbridge, GA 30281
(404) 474-3666

J.R.B. Hutchinson, M.D.
1462 Montreal Rd.
Tucker, GA 30084
(404) 939-1090

Ann A. Bailey, M.D.
PO Box 8
Warm Springs, GA 31830
(404) 655-3331

IDAHO

Jack A. Seeley, M.D.
10798 W. Overland
Boise, ID 83709
(208) 377-3368

Charles T. McGee, M.D.*
1717 Lincoln Way, #108
Coeur d'Alene, ID 83814-2537
(208) 664-1478

ILLINOIS

Allan B. Aven, M.D.
1120 E. Central Rd.
Arlington Heights, IL 60005
(312) 253-1070

Theron G. Randolph, M.D.*
505 N. Lakeshore Drive, #6506
Chicago, IL 60611
(312) 828-9480

Gary R. Oberg, M.D.*
4911 Route 31, Suite F
Crystal Lake, IL 60014
(815) 455-1990

Michael E. Rubin, M.D.
1585 Ellinwood
Des Plaines, IL 60016
(312) 297-5500

Peter G. Gilbert, M.D.
415 S. Second
Geneva, IL 60134
(312) 232-7761

Richard E. Hrdlicka, M.D.
123 South St.
Geneva, IL 60134
(312) 232-1900

George E. Shambaugh, Jr., M.D.
40 S. Clay St.
Hinsdale, IL 60521
(312) 887-1130

Tipu Sultan, M.D.*
1050 N. Center St.
Maryville, IL 62062
(618) 344-7234

Guy O. Pfeiffer, M.D.*
1710 Wabash Ave.
Mattoon, IL 61938
(217) 235-3822

Robert C. Filice, M.D.
24 W. 500 Maple Ave., #216
Naperville, IL 60540
(312) 369-1220

Paul J. Dunn, M.D.
715 Lake St.
Oak Park, IL 60301
(312) 383-3800

Thomas E. Benson, M.D.*
1200 N. East St.
Olney, IL 62450
(618) 395-5222

Ralph H. Roeper, D.O.
121 N. Northwest Highway
Palatine, IL 60067
(312) 358-2257

Thomas L. Stone, M.D.
1811 Hicks Rd.
Rolling Meadows, IL 60008
(312) 934-1100

Robert W. Boxer, M.D.*
64 Old Orchard Rd.
Skokie, IL 60077
(312) 677-0260

Mohammad T.K. Ghani, M.D.
10301 Roosevelt Rd.
Westchester, IL 60153
(312) 344-3550

Norene B. Hess, M.D.
700 Oak
Winnetka, IL 60093
(312) 446-1923

Robert T. Marshall, M.D., Ph.D.*
700 Oak
Winnetka, IL 60093
(312) 446-1923

INDIANA
John F. O'Brian, M.D.*
3217 Lake Ave.
Fort Wayne, IN 46805
(219) 422-9471

David A. Darbro, M.D.
2124 E. Hanna
Indianapolis, IN 46227
(317) 787-7221

James K. Hill, M.D.
8803 N. Meridian St., Suite 340
Indianapolis, IN 46260
(317) 846-7341

Frederick H. Simmons, M.D.
1009 N. Baldwin, PO Box 866
Marion, IN 46952
(317) 662-6950

Thomas G. Goodwin, M.D.
343 Merrillville Center
Merrillville, IN 46410
(219) 980-6117

Joseph P. Ornelas, M.D.*
6111 Harrison St.
Merrillville, IN 46410
(219) 980-6180

IOWA
Robert W. Soll, M.D., Ph.D.
105 N. Main St.
Denison, IA 51442
(712) 263-6166

Rafael Tarnopolsky, M.D.
3200 Grand Ave.
Des Moines, IA 50312
(515) 271-1400

KANSAS
Michael E. Aronoff, M.D.
407 S. Clairborne
Olathe, KS 66062
(913) 782-3953

Charles T. Hinshaw, Jr., M.D.
1133 E. Second
Wichita, KS 67214
(316)'262-0951

LOUISIANA
Jacob Tasher, M.D.
Highland Park Plaza, Suite 201
Covington, LA 70433
(504) 892-4677

James Moore Foster, M.D.
1927 Hickory Ave.
Harahan, LA 70183
(504) 738-5375

MARYLAND
Barbara A. Solomon, M.D.
8109 Harford Rd.
Baltimore, MD 21234
(301) 668-5611

William J. Cates, M.D.
17515 Redland Rd.
Derwood, MD 20855
(301) 921-0350

MASSACHUSETTS
Robert E. Rechtschaffen, M.D.
21 Everett Ave.
Belchertown, MA 01007
(413) 323-7212

James A. O'Shea, M.D.*
50 Prospect St.
Lawrence, MA 01841
(617) 683-2632

Donald R. Lombard, M.D.
335 South St.
North Hampton, MA 01060
(413) 584-5959

W. Kenneth Holbrook, D.O.
276 Woburn St.
Reading, MA 01867
(617) 944-2288

J. Aaron Herschfus, M.D.*
62 South Main St.
PO Box 336
Sharon, MA 02067
(617) 784-2084

Sheldon S. Goldberg, M.D.*
120 Maple St.
Springfield, MA 01103
(413) 732-7426

Joseph Patrick Keenan, M.D.
75 Springfield Rd.
Westfield, MA 01085
(413) 568-2304

Richard B. Yules, M.D.
475 Pleasant St.
Worcester, MA 01609
(617) 791-6305

MICHIGAN
John J. Kelly, M.D.
14726 Champaign
Allen Park, MI 48101
(313) 386-5500

Paula G. Davey, M.D.*
425 E. Washington
Ann Arbor, MI 48104
(313) 662-3384

Jerry A. Walker, D.O.
5681 S. Beech Daly Rd.
Dearborn Heights, MI 48125
(313) 292-5620

Richard E. Tapert, D.O.
15850 E. Warren
Detroit, MI 48224
(313) 885-5405

Jack W. De Long, M.D.
111 W. 24th St.
Holland, MI 49423
(616) 396-2325 or 394-4042

Vahagn Agbabian, D.O.
28 N. Saginaw St., #1105
Pontiac, MI 48058
(313) 334-2424

Harry R. Butler, M.D.
1821 King Rd.
Trenton, MI 48183
(313) 676-2800

Cornelius F. Derrick, M.D.
1821 King Rd.
Trenton, MI 48183
(313) 675-0678

MINNESOTA
Mark A. Muesing, M.D.
303 Kingwood
Brainerd, MN 56401
(218) 829-9270

MISSISSIPPI
Thomas S. Glasgow, M.D.
2161 S. Lamar
Oxford, MS 38655
(601) 234-2921

MISSOURI
Weldon L. Sportsman, M.D.*
7504 N. Oak St.
Kansas City, MO 64118
(816) 436-7100

James W. Willoughby, M.D.*
PO Box 271
Liberty, MO 64068-0271
(816) 781-0902

Clarence C. Cohrs, M.D.*
423 E. Logan St.
Moberly, MO 65270
(816) 263-1747

William R. Lamb, M.D.
Route 2, Box 61-23
Nixa, MO 65714-9802
(417) 725-4385

Jeannette S. Schoonmaker, M.D.
Route 2, Box 61-23
Nixa, MO 65714-9802
(417) 869-4833

William Louis Traxel, M.D.
666 Lester St.
Poplar Bluff, MO 63901
(314) 686-2411

Howard J. Aylward, Sr., M.D.*
6651 Chippewa
St. Louis, MO 63109
(314) 647-8895

MONTANA
Catherine H. Steele, M.D.
2509-7th Ave., S.
Great Falls, MT 59405
(406) 727-3655

Charles H. Steele, M.D.*
2509-7th Ave., S.
Great Falls, MT 59405
(406) 727-3655

Ralph K. Campbell, M.D.
Finley Point Route
Polson, MT 59860
(406) 883-2232

NEVADA
Reed W. Hyde, M.D.
600 Shadow Lane
Las Vegas, NV 89106
(702) 382-8928

F. Fuller Royal, M.D.
6105 W. Tropicana Ave.
Las Vegas, NV 89103
(702) 871-2700

Joseph F. Tangredi, M.D.
650 Shadow Lane
Las Vegas, NV 89106
(702) 382-3421

I. Marshall Postman, M.D.
1101 West Moana Lane
Reno, NV 89509
(702) 826-4900

NEW JERSEY
Richard N. Podell, M.D.
29 South St.
New Providence, NJ 07974
(201) 464-3800

Charles Harris, M.D.
20 Hospital Drive
Toms River, NJ 08753
(201) 244-3050

Faina Munits, M.D.
15 Rosemont Terrace
West Orange, NJ 07052
(201) 736-3743

NEW MEXICO
Jacqueline Krohn, M.D.
5 Kiowa Lane
Los Alamos, NM 87544
(505) 662-9620

NEW YORK
Bernard S. Puglisi, M.D.*
57 Munger St.
Bergen, NY 14416
(716) 494-1331

James M. Miller, M.D.
40 Front St.
Binghamton, NY 13905
(607) 722-0957

I-Tsu Chao, M.D.
1641 E. 18th St.
Brooklyn, NY 11229
(718) 998-3331

Martin Feldman, M.D.
1695 E. 21st St.
Brooklyn, NY 11210
(718) 744-4413

Doris J. Rapp, M.D.*
1421 Colvin Blvd.
Buffalo, NY 14223
(716) 877-8475

Juan Wilson, M.D.*
1900 Hempstead Turnpike
East Meadow, NY 11554
(516) 794-0404

Alfred V. Zamm, M.D.*
111 Malden Lane
Kingston, NY 12401
(914) 338-7766

Robert M. Giller, M.D.
960 Park Ave.
New York, NY 10028
(212) 472-2002

Jesse M. Hilsen, M.D.
1449 Lexington Ave.
New York, NY 10128
(212) 861-1979

Karl E. Humiston, M.D.*
104 E. 40th St., #906
New York, NY 10016
(212) 986-9385

Warren M. Levin, M.D.*
444 Park Ave., S., 12th Floor
New York, NY 10016
(212) 839-0950

Harold H. Markus, M.D.
161 Ave. of the Americas, 14th Floor
New York, NY 10013
(212) 675-2550

H. L. Newbold, M.D.*
115 E. 34th St., #20K
New York, NY 10016-4631
(212) 679-8207

Joseph S. Rechtschaffen, M.D.
11 E. 68th St.
New York, NY 10021
(212) 737-3136

Morton M. Teich, M.D.*
930 Park Ave.
New York, NY 10028
(212) 988-1821

Wellington S. Tichenor, M.D.
30 Central Park S.
New York, NY 10019
(212) 371-8510

Michael B. Schachter, M.D.
Mountainview Medical Building
Mountainview Ave.
Nyack, NY 10960
(914) 358-6800

A. Stephen Rechtschaffen, M.D.
108 Montgomery St.
Rhinebeck, NY 12572
(914) 876-7082

Sherry A. Rogers, M.D.
2800 W. Genessee St.
Syracuse, NY 13219
(315) 488-2856

Miklos L. Boczko, M.D.
12 Greenridge Ave.
White Plains, NY 10605
(914) 949-8817

Marvin Boris, M.D.
800 Woodbury Rd.
Woodbury, NY 11797
(516) 921-9000

Stanley Weindorf, M.D.
800 Woodbury Rd.
Woodbury, NY 11797
(516) 921-9000

Joseph S. Wojcik, M.D.
525 Bronxville Rd.
Yonkers, NY 10708
(914) 793-6161

NORTH CAROLINA
R. Edward Huffman, M.D.
146 Victoria Rd
Asheville, NC 28801
(704) 253-3695

Thurman M. Bullock, M.D.
104 E. Seventh Ave.
Chadbourn, NC 28431
(919) 654-3143

Francis M. Carroll, M.D.*
104 E. Seventh Ave.
Chadbourn, NC 28431
(919) 654-3143

F. Keels Dickson, M.D.
485 N. Wendover Rd.
Charlotte, NC 28211
(704) 366-0249

Bhaskar D. Power, M.D.
PO Box 1132
Roanoke Rapids, NC 27870
(919) 535-1411

Walter A. Ward, M.D.
PO Box 24039
Winston-Salem, NC 27114-4039
(919) 760-0240

OHIO
Raymond S. Rosedale, Jr., M.D.
4150 Belden Village St. N.W.
Canton, OH 44718
(216) 492-2844

John H. Boyles, Jr., M.D.*
7076 Corporate Way
Centerville, OH 45459
(513) 223-8872

Heather Morgan, M.D.
138 S. Main St.
Centerville, OH 45459
(513) 439-1797

Richard H. Stahl, M.D.*
822 Portage Trail
Cuyahoga Falls, OH 44221
(216) 928-9412

Francis J. Waickman, M.D.*
1625 W. Portage Trail
Cuyahoga Falls, OH 44223
(216) 923-4879

Richard F. Bahr, M.D.
999 Brubaker Drive
Dayton, OH 45429
(513) 298-8661

David D. Brown, M.D.
830 Fidelity Building
Dayton, OH 45402
(513) 223-3691

William D. Welton, M.D.*
830 Fidelity Building
Dayton, OH 45402
(513) 223-3691

James P. Dambrogio, D.O.
212 N. Main St.
Hubbard, OH 44425
(216) 534-9737

Charles S. Resseger, D.O.
853 S. Norwalk Rd.
Norwalk, OH 44857
(419) 668-9615

Donald D. Khym, M.D.
140 Jackson St.
Sandusky, OH 44870
(419) 625-0654

John W. Rechsteiner, M.D.
1116 S. Limestone St.
Springfield, OH 45505
(513) 325-0223

Jose E. Sanchez, M.D.*
2615 Sunset Blvd.
Steubenville, OH 43952
(614) 264-1692

Alston M. Quillin, M.D.
67 E. Wilson Bridge Rd.
Worthington, OH 43085
(614) 436-7188

OKLAHOMA
John F. Russell, D.O.*
PO Box 188
Bixby, OK 74008-0188
(918) 366-8229

Robert Kenneth Goodloe, D.O.
500 Park Place
Mustang, OK 73064
(405) 376-2419

Clifton R. Brooks, Sr., M.D.
2114 Martingale Dr.
Norman, OK 73072
(405) 329-8437

Howard E. Hagglund, M.D.
2227 W. Lindsey, #1401
Norman, OK 73069
(405) 329-4458

John Lee Davis, III, M.D.
3330 N.W. 56th, Suite #602
Oklahoma City, OK 73112
(405) 843-6619

Richard B. Dawson, M.D.
1117 N. Shartel, Suite 402
Oklahoma City, OK 73103
(405) 235-4421

Donald M. Dushay, D.O.
4444 S. Harvard Ave., #100
Tulsa, OK 74135
(918) 744-0228

Harriet H. Shaw, D.O.
4444 S. Harvard Ave., #100
Tulsa, OK 74135
(918) 744-0228

OREGON
Joseph T. Morgan, M.D.*
1750 Thompson Rd.
Coos Bay, OR 97420
(503) 269-0333

John E. Gambee, M.D.
66 Club Rd.
Eugene, OR 97401
(503) 686-2536

James W. Fitzsimmons, Jr., M.D.
591 Hidden Valley Rd.
Grants Pass, OR 97527
(503) 474-2166

John A. Green, III, M.D.
3674 Pacific Highway
Hubbard, OR 97032
(503) 981-1175

Donald C. Mettler, M.D.*
2525 N.W. Lovejoy, #205
Portland, OR 97210
(503) 228-9497

PENNSYLVANIA
Donald E. Goehring, M.D.*
503 Union Bank Building
Butler, PA 16001
(412) 287-4241

Chin Y. Chung, M.D.
210 E. Second St.
Erie, PA 16507
(915) 455-4429

Roy E. Kerry, M.D.
17 Sixth Ave.
Greenville, PA 16125
(412) 588-2600

Leland J. Green, M.D.
PO Box 508
Lansdale, PA 19446
(215) 855-9501

George C. Miller, II, M.D.
Three Hospital Drive
Lewisburg, PA 17837
(717) 524-4405

Kenneth B. Skolnick, M.D.
1789 Pinehollow Rd.
McKees Rocks, PA 15136
(412) 531-1207

Conrad G. Maulfair, Jr., D.O.
R.R. #2, Box 71 Main St.
Mertztown, PA 19539
(215) 682-2104

Helen Fox Krause, M.D.
9104 Babcock Blvd.
Pittsburgh, PA 15237
(412) 366-1661

Bernard Leff, M.D.
239-4th Ave., 2nd Floor
Pittsburgh, PA 15222
(412) 281-8351

Harold E. Buttram, M.D.
R.D. #3, Clymer Rd.
Quakertown, PA 18951
(215) 536-1890

PUERTO RICO
Jose R. Zaragoza, M.D.*
PO Box 1028
Arecibo, PR 00613
(809) 878-3830

Ramon Casanova-Roig, M.D.*
513 Hostos Ave.
Hato Rey, PR 00918
(809) 764-5715

SOUTH CAROLINA
Allan D. Lieberman, M.D.*
7510 Northforest Drive
North Charleston, SC 29418
(803) 572-1600

SOUTH DAKOTA
John W. Argabrite, M.D.*
Three E. Kemp, PO Box 1596
Watertown, SD 57201
(605) 886-3144

TENNESSEE
William G. Crook, M.D., P.C.*
681 Skyline Drive
Jackson, TN 38301
(901) 423-5100

Fred M. Furr, M.D.
9217 Park W. Blvd., Building E
Knoxville, TN 37923
(615) 693-1502

Cecil E. Pitard, M.D.
403 Newland Professional Building
Knoxville, TN 37916
(615) 522-7714

Peter L. Ballenger, M.D.
1325 Eastmoreland, Suite 205
Memphis, TN 38104
(901) 725-6853

Richard G. Wanderman, M.D.
6584 Poplar Ave., #420
Memphis, TN 38138
(901) 683-2777

Robert C. Owen, M.D.
210-25th. Ave. N., #1016
Nashville, TN 37203
(615) 327-3291

TEXAS
Charles R. Chung, M.D.
1850 Central Drive
Bedford, TX 76021
(817) 267-1521

Floyd H. Brigham, M.D.
700 Faltin St.
Comfort, TX 78013
(512) 995-3882

Richard Allan Berlando, M.D.
6757 Arapaho, Suite 757
Dallas, TX 75248
(214) 458-9944

Alfred R. Johnson, D.O.
8345 Walnut Hill Lane, #205
Dallas, TX 75231
(214) 368-4132

Armando Lopez de Victoria, M.D.
8345 Walnut Hill Lane, Suite 2
Dallas, TX 75231
(214) 368-4132

Glenn R. Monte, D.O.
9709 Bruton Rd.
Dallas, TX 75217-2704
(214) 398-8471

R. W. Noble, M.D.
6757 Arapaho Rd., #757
Dallas, TX 75248-4040
(214) 458-9944

William J. Rea, M.D.*
8345 Walnut Hill Lane, Suite #205
Dallas, TX 75231
(214) 368-4132

Ralph E. Smiley, M.D.*
3209 Rolling Knoll Drive
Dallas, TX 75234
(214) 241-0404

Donald E. Sprague, M.D.*
8345 Walnut Hill Lane, Suite #205
Dallas, TX 75231
(214) 368-4132

William H. Munyon, M.D.
4800 Alberta
El Paso, TX 79905
(915) 533-3020

Gary H. Campbell, D.O.
7421 Meadowbrook Drive
Fort Worth, TX 76112
(817) 457-8992

Charles R. Hamel, M.D.*
3801 Hulen
Fort Worth, TX 76107
(817) 731-9531

George J. Jeutersonke, D.O.
Camp Bowie at Montgomery
Fort Worth, TX 76107
(817) 735-2000

Charles A. Rush, Jr., M.D.*
7601 Glenview Drive
Fort Worth, TX 76118
(817) 284-9251

James C. Whittington, M.D.*
1021 Seventh Ave.
Fort Worth, TX 76104
(817) 332-4585

Dor W. Brown, Jr., M.D.*
109 S. Adams St.
Fredericksburg, TX 78624
(512) 997-2115

Thomas P. Buckley, M.D.
626 Apache Drive
Garland, TX 75043
(214) 271-4912

George B. Marsh, Jr., M.D.*
PO Drawer H
Grand Saline, TX 75140
(214) 962-4247

Kenneth C. Sherman, Sr., M.D.*
445 Woodland Drive
Harlingen, TX 78550
(512) 428-4500

Vickey C. Halloran, M.D.
5629 FM 1960 W., #225
Houston, TX 77069-4215
(713) 370-6351

Jacob Siegel, M.D., P.A.*
8300 Waterbury, #305
Houston, TX 77055-3450
(713) 682-2553

John Parks Trowbridge, M.D.
9816 Memorial Blvd., Suite 205
Humble, TX 77338
(713) 540-2329

Michael E. Truman, D.O.
1709 Precinct Line Rd.
Hurst, TX 76053
(817) 281-0402

William F. Andrew, M.D.*
3716-21st St., Suite 202
Lubbock, TX 79410
(806) 797-3331

Joe A. Izen, M.D.*
3912 Brookhaven
Pasadena, TX 77504
(713) 941-2444

Lee R. Byrd, Jr., M.D.
4700 Lewis Drive
Port Arthur, TX 77640
(409) 982-3131

Harris Hosen, M.D.*
2649 Proctor St.
Port Arthur, TX 77640
(409) 985-5585

Don Mannerberg, M.D.
375 Municipal Drive
Richardson, TX 75080
(214) 669-8707

Albert H. Cobb, Jr., M.D.
PO Box 913
San Marcos, TX 78667
(512) 396-2125

Malcolm C. Maley, M.D.*
808 Olive St., Suite C
Texarkana, TX 75501
(214) 793-1816

Martha B. Strickland, M.D.
1020 Leona Rd.
Uvalde, TX 78801
(512) 278-3220

Charles R. Mabray, M.D.*
4204 N. Laurent St.
Victoria, TX 77901
(512) 578-5233

William E. Wagnon, Jr., M.D.
3500 Hillcrest Dr.
Waco, TX 76708
(817) 754-0375

UTAH
Dennis W. Remington, M.D.
3707 N. Canyon Rd., Suite 8C
Provo, UT 84604
(801) 224-9000

VIRGINIA
Roger D. Neal, M.D.
176 W. Valley St.
Abingdon, VA 24210
(703) 628-9547

Jack H. Eberhart, M.D.
435 Commonwealth Blvd.
Martinsville, VA 24112
(703) 638-3473

John W. Selman, M.D.
435 Commonwealth Blvd.
Martinsville, VA 24112
(703) 638-3743

Henry J. Palacios, M.D.
8005 Algarve St.
McLean, VA 22101
(703) 356-2244

WASHINGTON
George H. Drumheller, Jr., M.D.*
1515 Pacific Ave.
Everett, WA 98201
(206) 258-4361

Allan Magaziner, D.O.
24030—132nd Ave., S.E.
Kent, WA 98042
(206) 631-8920

David Buscher, M.D.*
121 Third Ave.
Kirkland, WA 98033
(206) 827-2151

Albert G. Corrado, M.D.*
750 Swift, Suite 22
Richland, WA 99352
(509) 946-4631

Greg Sinding Johnson, D.O.
8523—15th Ave., N.E.
Seattle, WA 98115
(206) 546-4344

Daniel Pletsch, M.D.
11012 N.E. Fourth Plain Rd.
Vancouver, WA 98662
(206) 256-4118

Murray L. Black, D.O.*
609 S. 48th Ave.
Yakima, WA 98908-3614
(509) 966-1780

Randall E. Wilkinson, M.D.
302 S. 12th Ave.
Yakima, WA 98902-3176
(509) 453-5506

Richard S. Wilkinson, M.D.
302 S. 12th Ave.
Yakima, WA 98902-3176
(509) 453-5506

WEST VIRGINIA
Edwin M. Shepherd, M.D.
3100 MacCorkle Ave., S.E., #606
Charleston, WV 25304
(304) 344-8039

WISCONSIN
Eleazar M. Kadile, M.D.
1901 S. Webster, #3
Green Bay, WI 54301
(414) 432-2204

George F. Kroker, M.D.*
2532 Edgewood Place
La Crosse, WI 54601
(608) 782-2027

David L. Morris, M.D.*
615 S. 10th St.
La Crosse, WI 54601
(608) 782-2027

Melvin G. Apell, M.D.
555 S. Washburn
Oshkosh, WI 54901
(414) 231-5313

Wayne H. Konetzki, M.D.
403 N. Grand Ave.
Waukesha, WI 53186
(414) 547-3055

WYOMING
Gerald L. Smith, M.D.
5320 Education Drive
Cheyenne, WY 82009
(307) 632-5589

SOURCE: *American Academy of Environmental Medicine.*

*Fellow.

BOOKS ON CLINICAL ECOLOGY

Allergies and the Hyperactive Child, **Doris J. Rapp,** New York: Sovereign, 1979.

An Alternative Approach to Allergies, **Theron G. Randolph, M.D.,** and **Ralph W. Moss, Ph.D.,** New York: Harper & Row, 1980; Bantam Books, 1981.

Eating Dangerously: The Hazards of Hidden Allergies, **Richard Mackarness,** New York and London: Harcourt Brace Jovanovich, 1976.

Feingold Cookbook for Hyperactive Children, **Benjamin Feingold, M.D.,** New York: Random House, 1979.

How to Control Your Allergies, **Robert Forman,** New York: Larchmont Books, 1979.

Introduction to Clinical Allergy, **Benjamin Feingold, M.D.,** Springfield, IL: Charles C. Thomas, 1973.

Why Your Child Is Hyperactive, **Benjamin Feingold, M.D.,** New York: Random House, 1975.

The Yeast Connection: A Medical Breakthrough, **William G. Crook, M.D.,** Jackson, TN: Professional Books, 1984.

ORGANIZATIONS OF ALTERNATIVE THERAPIES

American Academy of Environmental
  Medicine
PO Box 16106
Denver, CO 80216

Professional association of physicians, scientists, other health professionals. Investigates inhalant, chemical, and food sensitivities. Quarterly newsletter, journal, a national directory of clinical ecologists. The directory is free with a self-addressed stamped envelope. Will provide more information upon request.

Feingold Association of the United States
Drawer AG
Holtsville, NY 11742
(516) 543-4658

National membership self-help organization based on the Feingold diet for hyperactive children with 150 chapters throughout the country. Dedicated to helping families with hyperactive children through diet. Makes medical referrals. Monthly newsletter with up-to-date nutritional information, food lists, handbooks, teaching manuals, professional packets, and cookbooks. Sponsors workshops. Will provide more information upon request with a self-addressed stamped envelope.

ASTHMA AND ALLERGIES RESEARCH AT THE NATIONAL INSTITUTES OF HEALTH

Researchers at the NIH Clinical Center in Bethesda, Maryland, are treating and studying persons with allergies and asthma. Some areas of interest: patients with recurring anaphylactic shock reactions with the aim of improving the therapy for that problem, selected patients with bronchial asthma and other allergic diseases, notably seasonable allergic asthmatics and aspirin-sensitive patients; patients with food allergies, including those with anaphylactic reactions and delayed onset reactions.

You can usually enter the NIH Clinical Center for treatment and participation in this research only by physician referral. Your physician can contact:

The Clinical Center
Building 10, Room 2C-146
National Institutes of Health
Bethesda, MD 20892
(301) 496-4831

AUTISM

See also Mental Retardation, Developmental and Learning Disabilities, page 355, for centers that specialize in the rehabilitation and care of those with autism and similar disorders.

Autism is a lifelong brain disorder that shows up during the first two-and-a-half years of life. Experts believed until recently that autism was essentially psychological in origin: a form of mental retardation, a kind of schizophrenia, or an emotional withdrawal due to uncaring or unresponsive parents. It was often treated with family counseling or electroshock therapy. But recent research has proved that autism is not psychologically induced. It is a subtle, physically-based brain abnormality that occurs before, during, or soon after birth. Thus, parents need no longer blame themselves for this condition and should avoid physicians or counselors who attribute autism to emotional causes or ''bad parenting.''

Autism is rare. It appears in 5 out of every 10,000 births and is three times more likely to affect males. However, one expert estimates that about half the cases of autism have not been detected or have been misdiagnosed.

Cause: Researchers are not sure what causes autism, but they speculate that it may be caused by unidentified viruses, birth injuries, immune deficiencies, genetic abnormalities, or exposure to toxic chemicals or to certain infections, such as rubella (German measles), during pregnancy.

Symptoms: Autistic infants initially appear quite normal at birth but soon exhibit extremely bizarre behavior. The major characteristics are aloofness, failure to communicate, and peculiar body movements. The child may appear to be deaf; about half are mute. Early signs are toneless or repetitive babbling, aversion to touch, lack of eye contact, and self-destructive behav-ior. Severely disturbed children often bang their heads, jab at their eyes, rock compulsively on their toes, flap their hands, and are exceedingly hyperactive and aggressive.

Although some autistic children—perhaps as many as 10 percent—show signs of extraordinary abilities (artistic or musical talent or astounding feats of memory, such as multiplying large numbers), most are mentally retarded. According to one extensive study, about 60 percent of autistic children had IQs below 50, 20 percent between 50 and 70, and 20 percent over 70.

Autistic children will probably never be completely normal, but many do grow up to work and live independently. A few have even completed college and earned Ph.D.'s. New medical treatments growing out of recent research may significantly improve the outlook for the autistic child.

Diagnosis: There are no medical tests for autism; experts diagnose it by observing the child's behavior and taking history of the child's early behavior. However, there are neurologic and metabolic tests a child should have before the diagnosis is final. Experts recommend that the diagnosis be confirmed at a center where there are specialists in the treatment or care of autistic children—for example, a developmental evaluation center, a mental health center, or a health service. Without the thorough examination offered in such centers, the child could be misdiagnosed. Experts emphasize it is essential to get an early diagnosis of autism so that the child can receive special attention and education.

Treatment: Unquestionably, autism is a serious condition, and children do not ''outgrow'' it, although some children do respond to certain treatments and improve with proper education and management. Because there are many causes for the damage leading to the condition, there is no universal treatment. Some children seem to respond to certain drugs. For example, recent research has shown some improvement in managing some autistic children with a drug called fenfluramine. Investigators theorize that the drug may help correct a biochemical deficiency that interferes with the chemical messengers in the brains of autistic children, producing the bizarre behavior. Amphetamines help control some youngsters who are both hyperactive and autistic; special diets help some autistic children with metabolic defects or problems absorbing their food.

Autistic individuals have a normal life span, and there is some evidence that the symptoms change. Autistic individuals should be reevaluated periodically.

Most important, autistic children need special education. They seem to do best in a highly structured environment and often respond to behavioral modification techniques.

In some cases, as the child ages, institutionalization may be necessary, but usually the child can remain at home, or in residential group homes, sheltered workshops, special vocational settings, supervised farm communities, special summer camps or recreation programs.

SOME LEADING SPECIALISTS AND RESEARCHERS IN AUTISM

The following are some leading specialists in the research and treatment of autism.

CALIFORNIA
Robert Koegel, Jr., Ph.D.
Director
Autism Project
SOC Process Research Institute
University of California
Santa Barbara, CA 93106
(805) 961-2311

Gary LaVigna, Ph.D.
Director
Behavior Therapy, Family Counseling Center
1840 W. Imperial Highway
Los Angeles, CA 90047
(818) 781-9922

O. Ivar Lovaas, Ph.D.
Professor
Department of Psychology
UCLA
Los Angeles, CA 90024
(213) 825-2319

Bernard Rimland, Ph.D.
Director
Institute for Child Behavior Research
4182 Adams Ave.
San Diego, CA 92116
(714) 281-7165

Edward Ritvo, M.D.
Department of Psychiatry
UCLA School of Medicine
Center for the Health Sciences
Los Angeles, CA 90024
(213) 825-0220

Adriana L. Schuler, Ph.D.
Department of Special Education
University of California
Santa Barbara, CA 93106
(805) 961-3477

CONNECTICUT
Donald J. Cohen, M.D.
Professor of Pediatrics, Psychiatry, and
    Psychology
Yale Child Study Center
230 S. Frontage Rd.
New Haven, CT 06510
(203) 785-2511

Amy Lettick, L.H.D.
Director
Benhaven
Maple St.
East Haven, CT 06512
(203) 469-9819

DISTRICT OF COLUMBIA
Mary Coleman, M.D.
Director
Children's Brain Research Institute
2525 Belmont Road, N.W.
Washington, DC 20008
(202) 483-0444

Frederick C. Green, M.D.
Children's Hospital National Medical Center
111 Michigan Ave. N.W.
Washington, DC 20010
(202) 745-5000

FLORIDA
Ralph G. Maurer, M.D.
Associate Professor
Children's Mental Health Unit
Box J-234, JHMC
University of Florida
Gainesville, FL 32610
(904) 392-3611

GEORGIA
Teodoro Ayllon, Ph.D.
Psychology Department
Georgia State University
Atlanta, GA 30303
(404) 658-2283

KANSAS
Ogden R. Lindsley, Ph.D.
Professor of Education
University of Kansas
Lawrence, KS 66045
(913) 864-4432

MICHIGAN
Andrew D. Maltz, Ph.D.
Psychiatry/Psychology Department
Children's Hospital
3901 Beaubien Blvd.
Detroit, MI 48201
(313) 494-5301

MISSISSIPPI
Doris P. Bradley, Ph.D.
Chair
Department of Speech and Hearing
University of Southern Mississippi
Hattiesburg, MS 39401
(601) 266-7221

MISSOURI
Phillip R. Dodge, M.D.
Professor
Pediatrics and Neurology
Medical Center
500 S. Kings Highway
St. Louis, MO 65110
(314) 454-6005

NEW YORK
Richard Masland, M.D.
Neurological Institute
710 W. 168th St.
New York, NY 10032
(212) 305-2500

NORTH CAROLINA
Eric Schopler, Ph.D.
Director
Gary B. Mesibov, Ph.D.
Associate Director
Division TEACCH
310 Medical School, E222-H
University of North Carolina
Chapel Hill, NC 27514
(919) 966-2174

UTAH
William R. Jenson, Ph.D.
Graduate School of Education
327 Milton Bennion Hall
Salt Lake City, UT 84112
(801) 581-7148

WASHINGTON
Robert J. Reichler, M.D.
Director
Harborview Medical Center 2A99
325 9th Ave.
Seattle, WA 98104
(206) 223-8700

WISCONSIN
Anne Donnellan, Ph.D.
Wisconsin Center for Education Research
University of Wisconsin
1025 W. Jackson
Madison, WI 53706
(608) 263-4272

SOURCE: *National Society for Children and Adults with Autism.*

ORGANIZATION

The National Society for Children and Adults
  with Autism
1234 Massachusetts Ave., N.W.
Washington, DC 20005
(202) 783-0125

Voluntary, nonprofit, membership organization
that acts as a clearinghouse for information on
autism, including treatments, education, federal
programs, and specialized facilities such as
camps and group homes. It has 176 chapters
nationwide that make medical referrals. Offers
advice to parents on how to organize in communities to get better services and to protect an
autistic child's rights in the school and health-
care systems. Has a library and bookstore and
publishes a wide range of materials on autism,
including a newsletter.

BOOKS

Autism, Nightmare Without End, **Dorothy
  Johnson Beavers,** Port Washington, NY:
  Ashley Books, 1982.
*Autism: A Practical Guide for Parents and
  Professionals,* **Maria J. Paluszny,** New
  York: Syracuse University Press, 1979.
*The Autistic Child: Language Development
  Through Behavior Modification,* **Ivar
  Lovaas,** New York: Halsted Press, 1977.
*Autistic Children: A Guide for Parents and
  Professionals,* **Lorna Wing,** New York:
  Brunner/Mazel, 1972.

A Child Called Noah, **J. Greenfield,** New
  York: Holt, Rinehart, & Winston, 1970.
Children With Emerald Eyes, **Mira
  Rothenberg,** New York: Dial Press, 1977.
A Miracle to Believe In, **Barry Neil
  Kauffmann,** Garden City, NY: Doubleday,
  1981.
Nadia, **Lorna Selfe,** New York: Harcourt,
  Brace, Jovanovich, 1979.
A Place for Noah, **J. Greenfield,** New York:
  Holt, Rinehart, & Winston, 1978.
The Siege, **Clara Park,** New York: Harcourt,
  Brace, and World, 1982.

BURNS

About two million Americans every year are burned badly enough to see physicians. Seventy-five thousand are hospitalized and about 12,000 die, making burns the third-leading cause of accidental death. Approximately one-third of burn victims are children under age 15. Burn injuries are painful and can cause disfigurement, deformities or loss of function. Sometimes months, even years, of hospitalization are required for lifesaving procedures, reconstruction and rehabilitation.

The chances of survival and recovery without disfigurement are greater if the victim is cared for at a specialized burn center. The establishment of burn centers has given the severely burned a 30 to 50 percent greater chance of surviving. Disfigurement and hospital stays are reduced as a result of new experimental treatments, such as artificial skin and better control of infections and metabolic balance.

Usually a burn victim is rushed to the nearest hospital's emergency room. However, after initial treatment for trauma, the victim should be transferred to a special burn facility if the burns are severe or complex, that is, if the hands, feet, or face are involved or if there are third-degree burns over 15 percent of the body. Fortunately, nearly every American is within reach of hospitals with physicians who have expertise in burn treatment.

WHERE TO FIND TREATMENT FOR SEVERE BURNS

The following hospitals provide specialized burn care. Asterisks indicate those hospitals that reportedly have the capability for managing severe burns even though they have not formally established a burn unit. All others have special burn units. Some hospitals, such as the highly respected Shriner's Hospitals and those designated as children's hospitals, accept only children as patients. Generally, the larger burn units (those with the most beds) and those affiliated with university medical centers are considered the most outstanding burn centers.

HOSPITAL-BASED BURN CENTERS

ALABAMA
Children's Hospital
1600 Seventh Ave., S.
Birmingham, AL 35233
Dr. Marshall Pits
(205) 939-9100
16 beds

University of Alabama Hospitals
619 S. 19th St.
Birmingham, AL 35233
Dr. Alan R. Dimick
(205) 934-3411
13 beds

University of Southern Alabama Medical
  Center Hospital
2451 Fillingim St.
Mobile, AL 36617
Dr. Arnold Luterman
(205) 471-7000
7 beds

ALASKA
Providence Hospital
3200 Providence Drive
Anchorage, AK 99504
Dr. Frederick Hood
(907) 562-2211
10 beds

Fairbanks Memorial Hospital
1650 Cowles St.
Fairbanks, AK 99701
Dr. William Wennen
(907) 452-8181
*5 beds

ARIZONA
Maricopa Medical Center
2601 E. Roosevelt St.
Phoenix, AZ 85008
Dr. John M. Stein
(602) 267-5700
20 beds

St. Mary's Hospital
1601 W. St. Mary's Rd.
Tucson, AZ 85745
Dr. Philip Fleishman
(602) 795-8700
9 beds

ARKANSAS
Arkansas Children's Hospital
804 Wolfe St.
Little Rock, AR 72202
Dr. Fred T. Caldwell
(501) 370-1323
14 beds

University Hospital
University of Arkansas Medical Science
  Campus
4301 W. Markham St.
Little Rock, AR 72205
Dr. Fred T. Caldwell
(501) 661-5000
*6 beds

CALIFORNIA
Terrace Plaza Medical Center
14148 Francisquito Ave.
Baldwin Park, CA 91706
Dr. William T. Choctaw
(818) 338-1101 x260
*9 beds

Alta Bates Hospital
3001 Colby St. at Ashby
Berkeley, CA 94705
Dr. Jerold Z. Kaplan
(415) 540-1573
6 beds

Eden Hospital
20103 Lake Chabot Rd.
Castro Valley, CA 94546
Dr. Ronald Iverson
(415) 537-1234
6 beds

Chico Community Hospital
560 Cohasset Rd.
Chico, CA 95926
Dr. Donald J. Mangus
(916) 345-2411
6 beds

Brotman Medical Center
3828 Delmas Terrace
PO Box 2459
Culver City, CA 90230
Dr. Arthur M. Kahn
(213) 836-BURN
23 beds

Rancho Los Amigos Hospital
7601 E. Imperial Highway
Downey, CA 90242
Dr. G. Brody
(213) 922-7454
*24 beds (reconstructive only)

Valley Medical Center of Fresno
445 S. Cedar Ave.
Fresno, CA 93702
Dr. Val Selivanov
(209) 453-4220
6 beds

Los Angeles County/University of Southern
  California Medical Center
1200 N. State St.
Los Angeles, CA 90033
Dr. Bruce E. Zawacki
(213) 226-7991
37 beds

University of California, Irvine Medical Center
101 The City Drive
Orange, CA 92668
Dr. Bruce M. Achauer
(714) 634-5304
8 beds

University of California, Davis Medical Center
2315 Stockton Blvd.
Sacramento, CA 95817
Dr. F. William Blaisdell
(916) 453-3636
8 beds

San Bernardino County Medical Center
780 E. Gilbert St.
San Bernardino, CA 92404
Dr. Appannagari Gnanavez
(714) 383-3142
9 beds

University Hospital/University of California
  Medical Center
225 Dickinson St.
San Diego, CA 92103
Dr. John Hansbrough
(619) 294-6502
14 beds

St. Francis Memorial Hospital
900 Hyde St.
San Francisco, CA 94120
Dr. Edward Falees
(415) 775-4321
10 beds

San Francisco General Hospital Medical Center
1001 Potrero Ave.
San Francisco, CA 94110
Dr. Donald D. Trunkey
(415) 821-8197
6 beds

Santa Clara Valley Medical Center
751 S. Bascom Ave.
San Jose, CA 95128
Dr. Ronald M. Sato
(408) 279-5242
6 beds

Brookside Hospital
2000 Vale Rd.
San Pablo, CA 94806
Dr. Robert L. Shapiro
(415) 235-7000
6 beds

Sherman Oaks Community Hospital
4929 Van Nuys Blvd.
Sherman Oaks, CA 91403
Dr. A. Richard Grossman
(213) 981-7111
30 beds

Dameron Hospital
525 W. Acacia St.
Stockton, CA 95203
Dr. Genest de L'Arbre
(209) 944-5550
7 beds

Torrance Memorial Hospital Medical Center
3330 Lomita Blvd.
Torrance, CA 90505
Dr. William D. Davies
(213) 325-9110
10 beds

COLORADO
Penrose Hospital
2215 N. Cascade Ave.
Colorado Springs, CO 80903
Dr. Ian G. Walker
(303) 630-5770
8 beds

Children's Hospital
1056 E. 19th Ave.
Denver, CO 80218
Dr. William Carl Bailey
(303) 861-8888
*8 beds

University Medical Center
4200 E. Ninth Ave.
Denver, CO 80262
Dr. Edward Bartle
(303) 394-8052
5 beds

St. Mary's Hospital
10th St. & Grand Ave.
Grand Junction, CO 81501
Dr. William Merkel
(303) 242-9127
*2 beds

Northern Colorado Medical Center
1801 16th St.
Greeley, CO 80631
Dr. James R. Wheeler
(303) 352-4121
*4 beds

CONNECTICUT
Bridgeport Hospital
267 Grant St.
PO Box 5000
Bridgeport, CT 06610
Dr. Michael L. D'Aiuto
(203) 384-3728
22 beds

Hartford Hospital
80 Seymour St.
Hartford, CT 06115
Dr. Philip E. Trowbridge
(203) 542-2515
*5 beds

Yale—New Haven Hospital
20 York St.
New Haven, CT 06504
Dr. Stephen Ariyan
(203) 785-2573
*4 beds

DISTRICT OF COLUMBIA
Children's Hospital National Medical Center
111 Michigan Ave., N.W.
Washington, DC 20010
Dr. Judson G. Randolph
(202) 745-5116, 5152
12 beds

Washington Hospital Center
110 Irving St., N.W.
Washington, DC 20010
Dr. Marion Jordon
(202) 541-7241, 6662
23 beds

FLORIDA
Shands Hospital
University of Florida
Gainesville, FL 32610
Dr. Hal G. Bingham
(904) 392-3054, 3055
6 beds

James M. Jackson Memorial Hospital
1611 N.W. 12th Ave.
Miami, FL 33136
Dr. C. Gillon Ward
(305) 325-7085
8 beds

Orlando Regional Medical Center
1414 S. Kuhl Ave.
Orlando, FL 32806
Dr. Paul Geary
(305) 841-5176
*5 beds

Tampa General Hospital
Davis Islands
Tampa, FL 33606
Dr. C. Wayne Cruse
(813) 253-0711
17 beds

GEORGIA
Grady Memorial Hospital
80 Butler St., S.E.
Atlanta, GA 30335
Dr. Roger Sherman
(404) 588-4307
30 beds

Eugene Talmadge Memorial Hospital—
    Medical College of Georgia
1120 15th St.
Augusta, GA 30912
Dr. Richard C. Treat
(404) 828-3893
6 beds

Humana Hospital
3651 Wheeler Rd.
Augusta, GA 30910
Dr. Joseph Still
(404) 863-3232
10 beds

Medical Center
710 Center St.
Columbus, GA 31901
Dr. Robert K. Worman
(404) 571-1336
*6 beds

HAWAII
Straub Clinic & Hospital
888 S. King St.
Honolulu, HI 96813
Dr. James H. Penoff
(808) 523-2311
*3 beds

ILLINOIS
Children's Memorial Hospital
2300 Children's Plaza
Chicago, IL 60614
Dr. Desmond Kernahan
(312) 880-4094
6 beds

Cook County Hospital
1825 W. Harrison St.
Chicago, IL 60612
Dr. Takayoshi Matsuda
(312) 633-6564, 6570
30 beds

Edgewater Hospital
5700 N. Ashland Ave.
Chicago, IL 60660
Dr. Ramesh Kharwadkar
(312) 878-6000
*4 beds

University of Chicago Hospitals
950 E. 59th St.
Chicago, IL 60637
Dr. Thomas Krizek
(312) 962-6736
20 beds

Foster G. McGaw Hospital, Loyola University
  of Chicago
2160 S. First Ave.
Maywood, IL 60153
Dr. Raymond Warpeha
(312) 531-3988
14 beds

Franciscan Medical Center
2701 17th St.
Rock Island, IL 61201
Dr. Frank E. Miller
(309) 793-3173
14 beds

St. Anthony's Hospital Medical Center
5666 E. State St.
Rockford, IL 61101
Dr. Raymond Hoffman
(815) 226-2000
8 beds

Memorial Medical Center
800 N. Rutledge St.
Springfield, IL 62781
Dr. Elof Erickson
(217) 788-3325
10 beds

INDIANA
St. Joseph's Hospital
700 Broadway
Fort Wayne, IN 46802
Dr. Robert J. Voorhees
(219) 425-3431
7 beds

J. W. Riley Hospital
1100 W. Michigan St.
Indianapolis, IN 46223
Dr. A. Michael Sadove
(317) 264-3927
8 beds (children)

Methodist Hospital of Indiana
1701 N. Senate Blvd.
Indianapolis, IN 46202
Dr. Wally Zollman
(317) 929-8056
*10 beds

W. N. Wishard Memorial Hospital
1001 W. 10th St.
Indianapolis, IN 46202
Dr. Marjorie L. Bush
(317) 630-6471
8 beds (adults)

IOWA
University of Iowa Hospitals & Clinics
650 Newton Rd.
Iowa City, IA 52242
Dr. Albert E. Cram
(319) 356-2496
13 beds

St. Luke's Regional Medical Center
2720 Stone Park Blvd.
Sioux City, IA 51104
Dr. Larry D. Foster
(712) 279-3440
12 beds

KANSAS
University of Kansas Medical Center
39th St. & Rainbow Blvd.
Kansas City, KS 66103
Dr. Mani M. Mani
(913) 588-6540
10 beds

St. Francis Regional Medical Center
929 N. St. Francis Ave.
Wichita, KS 67201
Dr. Thomas E. Kendall
(316) 268-5388
11 beds

KENTUCKY
University Hospital
800 Rose St.
Lexington, KY 40536
Dr. Edward Luce
(606) 233-5260
4 beds

Humana Hospital Suburban
4001 Dutchman's Lane
Louisville, KY 40207
Dr. John M. Weeter
(502) 895-5466
*4 beds

Humana Hospital University
530 S. Jackson
Louisville, KY 40217
Dr. Hiram C. Polk, Jr.
(502) 562-3000
5 beds

Kosair-Children's Hospital
200 E. Chestnut
Louisville, KY 40202
Dr. John M. Weeter
(502) 562-6300
6 beds

LOUISIANA
Baton Rouge General Hospital
3600 Florida St.
PO Box 2511
Baton Rouge, LA 70821
Dr. D. V. Cacioppo
(504) 387-7716
12 beds

West Jefferson Hospital
4500 11th St.
Marrero, LA 70072
Dr. Frank C. DiVincenti
(504) 347-5511
14 beds

Louisiana State University Medical Center
    Hospital
1541 Kings Highway
PO Box 33932
Shreveport, LA 71130
Dr. Edwin Deitch
(318) 674-6133
16 beds

MAINE
Eastern Maine Medical Center
489 State St.
Bangor, ME 04401
Dr. Charles Dixon
(207) 947-3711

Maine Medical Center
22 Bramhall St.
Portland, ME 04102
Dr. David Clark
(207) 871-2991
4 beds

MARYLAND
Francis Scott Key Medical Center
4940 Eastern Ave.
Baltimore, MD 21224
Dr. Andrew Munster
(301) 955-0886
28 beds

MASSACHUSETTS
Boston City Hospital
818 Harrison Ave.
Boston, MA 02118
Dr. Erwin Hirsch
(617) 424-5204
*2 beds

Brigham & Women's Hospital
75 Francis St.
Boston, MA 02115
Dr. Robert H. Demling
(617) 732-7712
10 beds

Massachusetts General Hospital
32 Fruit St.
Boston, MA 02114
Dr. John F. Burke
(617) 726-3354
10 beds

Shriners Burns Institute
51 Blossom St.
Boston, MA 02114
Dr. John P. Remensnyder
(617) 722-3000
30 beds

Worcester City Hospital
26 Queen St.
Worcester, MA 01610
Dr. Margaret S. Skiles
Dr. Felix Catalod
(617) 799-8110
11 beds

MICHIGAN
Michigan Burn Center
University of Michigan Hospitals
Chelsea Community Hospital
1405 E. Ann
Ann Arbor, MI 48109
Dr. Irving Feller
(313) 995-BURN
29 beds

Children's Hospital of Michigan
3901 Beaubien
Detroit, MI 48201
Dr. James R. Lloyd
(313) 494-5678
15 beds

Detroit Receiving Hospital & University
  Health Center
4201 St. Antoine
Detroit, MI 48201
Dr. Martin C. Robson
(313) 494-3216
18 beds

Hurley Medical Center
One Hurley Plaza
Flint, MI 48502
Dr. Musa S. Haffajee
(313) 257-9188
13 beds

Blodgett Memorial Medical Center
1840 Wealthy St., S.E.
Grand Rapids, MI 49506
Dr. David Vander Wall
(616) 774-7670
8 beds

Bronson Methodist Hospital
252 E. Lovell St.
Kalamazoo, MI 49007
Dr. Frank J. Newman
(616) 383-6485 or (800) 632-3430
12 beds

Edward R. Sparrow Hospital
1215 E. Michigan Ave.
Lansing, MI 48909
Dr. Errikos Constant
(517) 483-2677
6 beds

St. Mary's Hospital
830 S. Jefferson Ave.
Saginaw, MI 48601
Dr. Syed Akhtar
(517) 790-5055
6 beds

MINNESOTA
Miller-Dwan Hospital and Medical Center
502 E. Second St.
Duluth, MN 55805
Dr. John W. Wolfe
(218) 727-8762
16 beds

Hennepin County Medical Center
701 Park Ave.
Minneapolis, MN 55415
Dr. John Twomey
(612) 347-2915
12 beds

St. Mary's Hospital
1216 Second St., S.W.
Rochester, MN 55901
Dr. George B. Irons (adults)
(507) 285-5123, 5591
Dr. Robert Telander (children)
(507) 285-6691
*6 beds

St. Paul–Ramsey Medical Center
640 Jackson St.
St. Paul, MN 55101
Dr. Lynn D. Solem
(612) 221-3351
24 beds

MISSISSIPPI
Delta Medical Center
1400 E. Union St.
PO Box 5247
Greenville, MS 38701
Dr. Robert Love
(601) 378-3783
16 beds

MISSOURI
University of Missouri Health Sciences Center
One Hospital Drive
Columbia, MO 65212
Dr. Boyd E. Terry
(314) 882-7994
7 beds

Children's Mercy Hospital
24th at Gillham Rd.
Kansas City, MO 64108
Dr. Ronald J. Sharp
(816) 234-3520
6 beds

St. John's Regional Health Center
1235 E. Cherokee St.
Springfield, MO 65802
Dr. Mark Wittmer
(417) 885-2876
9 beds

Barnes Hospital
Barnes Hospital Plaza
St. Louis, MO 63110
Dr. William H. Monafo
(314) 362-4060
6 beds

St. John's Mercy Medical Center
615 S. New Ballas Rd.
St. Louis, MO 63141
Dr. Vatche H. Ayvazian
(314) 569-6055
9 beds

MONTANA
St. Vincent Hospital
1233 N. 30th St.
Billings, MT 59101
Dr. David F. Sloan
(406) 245-2458
*4 beds

NEBRASKA
St. Elizabeth Community Health Center
555 S. 70th St.
Lincoln, NE 68510
Dr. Robert W. Gillespie
(402) 489-7181
10 beds

NEVADA
Southern Nevada Memorial Hospital
1800 W. Charleston Blvd.
Las Vegas, NV 89102
Dr. Charles A. Buerk
(702) 383-2268
12 beds

NEW JERSEY
Hackensack Medical Center
30 Prospect Ave.
Hackensack, NJ 07601
Dr. Anthony Barbara
(201) 441-2020
*9 beds

St. Barnabas Medical Center
Old Short Hills Rd.
Livingston, NJ 07039
Dr. Frederick Fuller
(210) 533-5920
12 beds

NEW MEXICO
St. Joseph's Hospital
715 Grand, N.E., #308
Albuquerque, NM 87102
Dr. John L. Coon
(505) 247-2449 or (800) 221-3664

University of New Mexico Hospital
2211 Lomas Blvd., N.E.
Albuquerque, NM 87106
Dr. John O. Kucan
(505) 843-2111
10 beds

NEW YORK
Albany Medical Center Hospital
New Scotland Ave.
Albany, NY 12208
Dr. John B. Fortune
(518) 445-3010
8 beds

Bronx Municipal Health Center
Pelham Parkway S. & Eastchester Rd.
Bronx, NY 10461
Dr. Stanley Levenson
(212) 430-8065
*11 beds

Kings County Hospital
451 Clarkson Ave.
Brooklyn, NY 11203
Dr. Winston Mitchell
(718) 735-3131
5 beds

Children's Hospital
219 Bryant St.
Buffalo, NY 14222
Dr. Melvyn Karp
Dr. Theodore Jewett
(716) 878-7435

Sheehan Emergency Hospital
425 Michigan Ave.
Buffalo, NY 14203
Dr. Louis C. Cloutier
(716) 842-2200
10 beds

Nassau County Medical Center
2201 Hempstead Turnpike
East Meadow, NY 11554
Dr. Roger L. Simpson
(516) 542-3207
10 beds

St. Joseph's Hospital
555 E. Market St.
Elmira, NY 14902
Dr. James Marshall
(607) 733-6541
*4 beds

Harlem Hospital Center
506 Lenox Ave.
New York, NY 10037
Dr. James E. C. Norris
(212) 491-1335
5 beds

New York Hospital–Cornell Medical Center
525 E. 68th St.
New York, NY 10021
Dr. Cleon Goodwin
(212) 472-5132
24 beds

St. Vincent's Hospital
153 W. 11th St.
New York, NY 10011
Dr. Ronald N. Ollstein
(212) 790-8941, 8940
6 beds

Strong Memorial Hospital
601 Elmwood Ave.
Rochester, NY 14642
Dr. R. Christie Wray, Jr.
(716) 275-5475
9 beds

University Hospital
Stony Brook, NY 11794
Dr. Harry Soroff
(516) 444-2701
6 beds

Upstate Medical Center
750 E. Adams St.
Syracuse, NY 13210
Dr. William Clark
(315) 473-6083
6 beds

Westchester County Medical Center
Grasslands Reservation
Valhalla, NY 10595
Dr. Roger E. Salisbury
(914) 347-4909
10 beds

Good Samaritan Hospital
1000 Montauk Highway
West Islip, NY 11795
Dr. Richard A. Giery
(516) 957-4000

NORTH CAROLINA
North Carolina Memorial Hospital
Manning Drive
Chapel Hill, NC 27514
Dr. Hugh D. Peterson
(919) 966-4131
23 beds

Charlotte Memorial Medical Center
1000 Blythe Blvd.
Charlotte, NC 28203
Dr. Harold F. Hamit
(704) 331-2525
4 beds

Duke University Hospital
Duke University
Durham, NC 27710
Dr. Gregory Georgiade
(919) 681-2404
7 beds

Pitt County Memorial Hospital
2577 Stantonsburg Rd.
Greenville, NC 27834
Dr. Howard G. Dawkins, Jr.
(919) 752-1406 or (800) 672-7828
4 beds

North Carolina Baptist Hospital
300 S. Hawthorne Rd.
Winston-Salem, NC 27103
Dr. Jesse H. Meredith
(919) 748-7766
6 beds

NORTH DAKOTA
St. Luke's General Hospital
Fifth St. N. & Mills Ave.
Fargo, ND 58122
Dr. David W. Todd
(701) 280-5504
*4 beds

OHIO
Children's Hospital Medical Center–Akron
   Regional Burn Center
281 Locust St.
Akron, OH 44308
Dr. C. R. Boeckmann
(216) 379-8224
12 beds (admits adult burns)

Shriners Burns Institute
202 Goodman St.
Cincinnati, OH 45219
Dr. Bruce G. MacMillan
(513) 751-3900
30 beds

University of Cincinnati Hospital
234 Goodman St.
Cincinnati, OH 45267
Dr. Robert P. Hummel
(513) 872-3100
10 beds

Cleveland Metro General Hospital
3395 Scranton Rd.
Cleveland, OH 44109
Dr. Richard Fratianne
(216) 459-5627
16 beds

Children's Hospital
700 Children's Drive
Columbus, OH 43205
Dr. E. Thomas Boles
(614) 461-2000
14 beds

Ohio State University Hospital
410 W. 10th Ave.
Columbus, OH 43210
Dr. Robert Ruberg
(614) 421-8744
6 beds

Children's Medical Center
One Children's Plaza
Dayton, OH 45404
Dr. Charles D. Goodwin
(513) 226-8300
6 beds

Miami Valley Hospital
One Wyoming St.
Dayton, OH 45409
Dr. R. K. Finley
(513) 223-6192
8 beds

St. Vincent's Medical Center
2213 Cherry St.
Toledo, OH 43608
Dr. Michael Yanik
(419) 259-4734
12 beds

OKLAHOMA
Baptist Medical Center
3300 N.W. Expressway
Oklahoma City, OK 73112
Dr. Paul Silverstein
(405) 949-3345, 3311
32 bcds

Oklahoma Children's Memorial Hospital
940 N.E. 13th St.
Oklahoma City, OK 73104
Dr. William P. Tunell
(405) 271-4733
12 beds

Hillcrest Medical Center
1120 S. Utica Ave.
Tulsa, OK 74104
Dr. Bernard Swartz
(918) 584-1351
20 beds

OREGON
Oregon Burn Center (at Emanuel Hospital)
2801 N. Gantenbein Ave.
Portland, OR 97227
Dr. Philip Parshley
(503) 280-4233
12 beds

PENNSYLVANIA
Lehigh Valley Hospital Center
1200 S. Cedar Crest Blvd.
PO Box 689
Allentown, PA 18105
Dr. Walter J. Okunski
(215) 776-8734
6 beds

Crozer–Chester Medical Center
15th St. & Upland Ave.
Chester, PA 19013
Dr. Charles E. Hartford
(215) 876-0356
19 beds

Geisinger Medical Center
N. Academy Ave.
Danville, PA 17822
Dr. Philip C. Breen
(717) 271-6591
*6 beds

Hamot Medical Center
201 State St.
Erie, PA 16550
Dr. Charles R. Bales
(814) 459-0344
8 beds

Hershey Medical Center
500 University Drive
PO Box 850
Hershey, PA 17033
Dr. William P. Graham
(717) 534-8521

Saint Agnes Medical Center
1900 S. Broad St.
Philadelphia, PA 19145
Dr. Frederick A. DeClement
(215) 339-4339
11 beds

St. Christopher's Hospital for Children
Fifth St. & Lehigh Ave.
Philadelphia, PA 19133
Dr. Stuart J. Hulnick
(215) 427-5000
4 beds

Mercy Hospital
1400 Locust St.
Pittsburgh, PA 15219
Dr. Charles Copeland
(412) 232-8225
7 beds

Western Pennsylvania Hospital
4800 Friendship Ave.
Pittsburgh, PA 15224
Dr. Harvey Slater
(412) 363-2876
18 beds

York Hospital
1001 S. George St.
York, PA 17405
Dr. Robert Davis
(717) 771-2345
*6 beds

RHODE ISLAND
Rhode Island Hospital
593 Eddy St.
Providence, RI 02902
Dr. Lawrence Bowen
(401) 277-4000
*4 beds

SOUTH CAROLINA
Medical University Hospital
171 Ashley Ave.
Charleston, SC 29425
Dr. Dabney R. Yarborough (adults)
(803) 792-3681
Dr. H. Biemann Othersen, Jr. (children)
(803) 792-3851
12 beds

TENNESSEE
Baroness Erlanger Hospital
975 E. Third St.
Chattanooga, TN 37403
Dr. Phil D. Craft
(615) 778-7881
6 beds

Regional Medical Center
842 Jefferson Ave.
Memphis, TN 38103
Dr. William Hickerson
(901) 528-5500
6 beds

Vanderbilt University Hospital
1161 21st Ave.
Nashville, TN 37232
Dr. John B. Lynch
(615) 322-7311
20 beds

TEXAS
St. David's Hospital
800 E. 30th, Suite 309
Austin, TX 78705
Dr. Robert A. Ersek
(512) 479-6805

Baptist Hospital of Southeast Texas
College & 11th Sts.
Beaumont, TX 77704
Dr. Duane Larson
(409) 835-3781

Memorial Medical Center
2606 Hospital Blvd.
PO Box 5280
Corpus Christi, TX 78405
Dr. Robert H. Balme
(512) 881-4360
9 beds

Parkland Memorial Hospital
5201 Harry Hines Blvd.
Dallas, TX 75235
Dr. John Hunt
(214) 637-8546
30 beds

Sun Towers Hospital
1801 N. Oregon St.
El Paso, TX 79902
Dr. Charles Lyon
(915) 532-6281
12 beds

Brooke Army Medical Center
Fort Sam Houston, TX 78234
Dr. Basil A. Pruitt, Jr.
(512) 221-4604, 2943
40 beds

John Peter Smith Hospital
1500 S. Main St.
Fort Worth, TX 76104
Dr. Charles Crenshaw
(817) 921-3431

Shriners Burns Institute
610 Texas Ave.
Galveston, TX 77550
Dr. David N. Herndon
(409) 761-2516
30 beds

University of Texas Medical Branch Hospitals
8th & Mechanic Sts.
Galveston, TX 77550
Dr. Sally Abston
(713) 761-2023
16 beds

Ben Taub General Hospital
1502 Taub Loop
Houston, TX 77030
Dr. Frank Gerow
(713) 791-7000
*8 beds

Hermann Hospital
1203 Ross Sterling Ave.
Houston, TX 77030
Dr. Donald H. Parks
(713) 797-4350
15 beds

Lubbock General Hospital
602 Indiana Ave.
Lubbock, TX 79417
Dr. Richard Baker
(806) 743-3406
*6 beds

Humana Hospital Southmore
906 E. Southmore
Pasadena, TX 77502
Dr. David Katrana
(713) 477-0411
12 beds

Medical Center Hospital
4502 Medical Drive
San Antonio, TX 78284
Dr. A. B. Cruz, Jr.
(512) 696-3030

UTAH
University of Utah Hospital
50 N. Medical Drive
Salt Lake City, UT 84132
Dr. Glenn Warden
(801) 581-2700
12 beds

VERMONT
Medical Center Hospital of Vermont
Colchester Ave.
Burlington, VT 05401
Dr. John Davis
(802) 656-4545
*6 beds

VIRGINIA
University of Virginia Medical Center
Jefferson Park Ave.
Charlottesville, VA 22908
Dr. Richard Edlich
(804) 924-5520
10 beds

Norfolk General Hospital
600 Gresham Drive
Norfolk, VA 23507
Dr. Wendy Marshall
(804) 628-3117
8 beds

Medical College of Virginia Hospital
1200 E. Broad St.
Box 510 MCV Station
Richmond, VA 23298
Dr. Boyd W. Haynes
(804) 786-9240
12 beds

WASHINGTON
St. Joseph's Hospital
3201 Ellis St.
Bellingham, WA 98225
Dr. James Hines
(206) 734-5400, x2501
*2 beds

Children's Orthopedic Hospital
4800 Sand Point Way N.E.
Seattle, WA 98105
Dr. Robert T. Schaller
(206) 526-2042
*8 beds

Harborview Medical Center
325 Ninth Ave.
Seattle, WA 98104
Dr. David Heimbach
(206) 223-3127
40 beds

Sacred Heart Medical Center
W. 101 Eighth Ave.
Spokane, WA 99220
Dr. Charles Miller
(509) 455-3344
*4 beds

St. Joseph's Hospital
1718 S. I St.
Tacoma, WA 98401
Dr. Martin Schaeferle
(206) 591-6677
10 beds

WEST VIRGINIA
Cabell-Huntington Hospital
1340 Hal Greer Blvd.
Huntington, WV 25701
Dr. James A. Coil, Jr.
(304) 526-2390
4 beds

WISCONSIN
University of Wisconsin Hospital and Clinics
600 Highland Ave.
Madison, WI 53792
Dr. Richard Helgerson
(608) 263-1490, 1378
7 beds

St. Mary's Hospital
2323 N. Lake Drive
Box 503
Milwaukee, WI 53211
Dr. George Collentine
(414) 225-8000
20 beds

SOURCE: *American Burn Association.*

GOVERNMENT BURN RESEARCH AND TREATMENT CENTERS

The following centers and physicians are doing or have done clinical and basic research on burn injuries under grants from the National Institutes of Health (National Institute of General Medical Sciences). Such centers are working on the frontiers of burn care and are staffed with physicians considered to be among the most knowledgeable in the country on the latest burn treatments.

CALIFORNIA
Dr. Thomas K. Hunt
University of California, San Francisco School
   of Medicine
Department of Surgery
San Francisco, CA 94143
(415) 666-1865

LOUISIANA
Dr. John J. Spitzer
Louisiana State University Medical Center
1901 Perdido St.
New Orleans, LA 70112
(504) 568-6172

MASSACHUSETTS
Dr. John F. Burke
Massachusetts General Hospital
White Building, Room 403
Boston, MA 02114
(617) 726-2809
Dr. Burke is one of the creators of "artificial skin" for burn victims, and one of the preeminent burn-care authorities in the country.

Dr. Douglas W. Wilmore
Peter Bent Brigham Hospital
75 Francis St.
Boston, MA 02115
(617) 732-7025

NEW YORK
Dr. Dhiraj M. Shah
Albany Medical Center
Department of Surgery
Albany, NY 12208
(518) 445-5672

Dr. G. Thomas Shires
New York Hospital–Cornell University
   Medical Center
525 E. 68th St.
New York, NY 10021
(212) 472-5640

TEXAS
Dr. Charles R. Baxter
University of Texas Health Science Center
Department of Surgery
Dallas, TX 75235
(214) 688-3523

WASHINGTON
Dr. C. James Carrico
Dr. Russell Ross
University of Washington School of Medicine
Seattle, WA 98195
(206) 543-3300

SOURCE: *National Institute of General Medical Sciences.*

ORGANIZATIONS

National Burn Victim Foundation
308 Main St.
Orange, NJ 07050
(201) 731-3112

A nonprofit organization dedicated to serving as the burn victim's advocate. Services include professional counseling for burn victims, a self-help support group, educational programs, and a burned child consultation service. Active mostly in New Jersey.

Phoenix Society
11 Rust Hill Rd.
Levittown, PA 19056
(215) 946-4788

Self-help, voluntary membership service organization for burn victims and their families. Sixty local chapters, with coordinators who are burn victims. Provide mutual support and information about burns and disfigurement prevention. A yearly conference for burn survivors. Newsletter, *Icarus File*, audiovisual materials. Will send more information and name of chapter in your area upon request.

BOOKS

The Burned Child Book, **John Davis, Jr. (age 7),** North Carolina Memorial Hospital, Chapel Hill, NC 27514, 1980 (no charge).

The Fatal Fire, **Dennis Smith, E.P.,** New York: Dutton, 1979.

The Fire That Will Not Die, **Michele McBride,** Palm Springs, CA: ETC Publications, 1979.

The Flames Shall Not Consume You, **Mary Ellen Ton,** Elgin, IL: David C. Cook Publishing Co., 1982.

Life Instead, **Diane Bringold,** Waco, TX: Word Books, 1979.

Manual of Burn Care, **edited by Joan Nicosia**
and **Jane Petro, M.D.,** New York: Raven Press, 1982.

A Matter of Degree: Heat, Life, and Death, **Lucy Kavaler,** New York: Harper and Row, 1981.

Race for Life: The Joel Sonnenberg Story, **Janet Sonnenberg,** Grand Rapids, MI: The Zondervan Corporation, 1983.

Tested by Fire, **Virginia** and **Merrill Womach,** Old Tappan, NJ: Fleming H. Revell Co., 1978.

The Time of My Death, **Alan Jeffy Breslau, E.P.,** New York: Dutton, 1977.

CANCER

Cancer is a complex disease that can attack all organs and parts of the body. It is characterized by uncontrolled growth and spread of abnormal cells. Cancer of all types is the second largest cause of death, killing more than 450,000 persons a year, about one every 70 seconds. In 1986, there were an estimated 930,000 newly diagnosed cases of cancer. About one in four Americans can expect to have cancer at some time in their lives. It strikes people of any age, but occurs more frequently as people get older. It is rare in children, but is still the leading cause of death among children ages 3 to 14.

Cause: Nobody understands precisely how cancer develops, what triggers some cells to become cancerous, or why cancer strikes a certain individual. Scientists believe that the causes are multiple, involving perhaps genetic susceptibility and exposure to cancer-causing agents, such as carcinogenic chemicals and cigarette smoke. Recent studies show that diet—notably low-fat, high-fiber foods—may help protect against the development of certain cancers. Scientists know that the disease often takes a long time to appear as a tumor, and in fact is often a process of 20- to 30-years' duration. Studies show that cancer occurs in two stages. It is first "initiated" or turned on by some agent, and then through the years is stimulated to grow by "promoters" to the stage where the cells start reproducing abnormally. The abnormal cells may form a tumor, which then metastasizes, or spreads from the original site, forming new tumors in other organs. If unchecked, the abnormal growths crowd out normal cells and may cause death.

Symptoms: They vary, depending on which part of the body the cancer attacks. Externally, cancer may appear as a growth or thickening on or under the skin, which increases in size. Internally, it may become noticeable by abnormal bleeding, for example, from the rectum or mouth. Other symptoms are a change in bowel and bladder habits, a sore that does not heal, indigestion and difficulty swallowing, obvious change in a mole or wart, nagging cough or hoarseness. Cancers of the blood, lymphatic tissue and bone may give rise to fatigue, tendency to bruise and bleed easily, increased susceptibility to infections, enlarged lymph nodes and bone pain.

Diagnosis: This also depends on the type and location of cancer and may include physical examination, X-rays, CAT scans, blood tests and ultrasound (high-frequency sound waves). Once a possible cancer is located, the final diagnosis is made through a biopsy, excision of a small amount of the suspicious tissue and examination under a microscope to determine if cancer cells are present. Because cancer almost always gets worse and spreads, it is important to detect the cancer at an early stage. Such early detection will not guarantee a cure, for by the time some cancers are detected, it is too late for effective therapy, but in general the chances of survival are increased by early diagnosis.

Treatment: Fortunately, the diagnosis of cancer is no longer a death knell. As scientists learn more about the nature and progress of the disease, physicians develop more sophisticated ways of combating it. The three mainstays of cancer therapy are surgery, radiation and chemotherapy (drug therapy). Physicians increasingly recognize that cancer is not merely a localized disease; but in many patients it is a whole body, or systemic disease in which cancer cells are circulating throughout the body. If the patient is to survive, these "wandering cells" must also be destroyed or controlled, usually by drugs or radiation. The pattern of cancer varies in individuals, and there is a trend to individualize treatment, often using not just one type of treatment, but several—whatever seems to be best for the individual patient. At the same time, surgery is becoming less mutilating for some kinds of cancer, for example, breast cancer, and much more aggressive for other types.

Another important trend in cancer management is the multidisciplinary or "team" approach. No longer does cancer treatment reside solely with a surgeon, radiologist or chemotherapist; it may involve these experts and also include an immunologist, a pain-control expert, nurses, psychologists, social workers, dietitians, and physical and speech therapists. The management of systemic cancer is increasingly directed or coordinated by a cancer specialist called an oncologist, who helps coordinate and choose the proper treatment for the individual, based on the latest research in *all* specialties, including surgery, radiation, chemotherapy, immunology, hyperthermia (heat), etc.

Consequently, although the overall national death rate from cancer is rising slightly, mainly due to increased lung cancer, death rates are decreasing for certain types of cancer. As a result, certain cancer patients now have a much greater chance of being cured. "Cured" is generally defined as living without cancer symptoms for at least five years. About 85 percent of those people (excluding patients with breast, prostate, and kidney cancers) who do survive five years are expected to live relatively free of the disease. Breast, prostate, and kidney cancers are more likely to recur after five years than other types of cancer.

SPECIFIC CANCERS

There are a growing range of treatments and resources for most kinds of cancers.

Here are the prevalence and five-year survival rates of the major cancers and the state-of-the-art or latest proven treatments for each, according to experts at the National Cancer Institute.

Lung: 144,000 new cases each year. The primary causes are cigarette smoking and exposure to environmental and occupational chemicals. Traditionally, victims have been men, but because of increased cigarette smoking, women are now becoming extremely vulnerable to lung cancer; lung cancer has overtaken breast cancer as the number-one cause of cancer deaths among women.

Survival outlook for lung cancer is poor; only 13 percent survive for five years after diagnosis, and there has been little progress in fighting lung cancer in recent years. One type of cancer, called oat-cell cancer, is becoming slightly more curable; this cancer was previously fatal within six months; now 10 to 20 percent of the victims are living longer. Usual treatment for lung cancer is surgery and radiation. About 90 percent of this type of cancer could be prevented by quitting smoking.

Colon-rectum: 138,000 new cases a year. Both of these cancers are curable in about 50 percent of the cases, usually with surgery. However, early detection of colon cancer is critical. Preliminary studies show that survival rates are dramatically increased when the cancer is discovered early or even when premalignant growths in the colon called polyps are detected and removed. New types of treatment are available for rectal cancer, including surgery, radiation and possibly chemotherapy.

Breast: 120,000 new cases a year. The type of treatment for breast cancer has changed dramatically in recent years. Previously, standard treatment was radical mastectomy to remove the entire breast and the underlying muscles and lymph nodes. Surgery was performed on the spot, immediately following a confirming biopsy. Now, the biopsy and surgery (if necessary) are commonly done in two steps, providing time for the woman and her physician to discuss and decide on treatment. Also, in a number of cases (when the lump is less than one inch in diameter), only the tumor is removed. This procedure, called a lumpectomy, is usually followed by several weeks of high-energy radiation to kill remaining cancer cells. Studies have shown that this limited treatment in many cases of early-stage breast cancer is as effective as the more extensive mastectomy in prolonging life. Chemotherapy is given if the lymph nodes are cancerous.

When mastectomies are performed, they are usually much less mutilating and debilitating than in previous years. Also, reconstruction of the breast, at the time of the mastectomy or later, is increasingly becoming an option, although not all women are candidates. About 74 percent of the women with breast cancer can expect to live at least five years.

Prostate: 86,000 new cases a year. About 71 percent of those treated for prostate cancer survive as long as five years. The most common treatment is surgery, which in the past has left 90 percent of the patients impotent. Recently, a new surgical technique has been developed that does not produce impotence. Furthermore, radiation is sometimes used as an alternative to surgery; it has proved as effective as surgery in many cases and does not produce impotence. Radiation should at least be investigated as an alternative to surgery.

Urinary, including bladder and kidney: 60,000 new cases each year. Kidney cancer is treated by surgery, which may be effective if the cancer has not metastasized, or spread. Drugs are being investigated to control kidney cancer, but none so far is effective. Survival rate for five years is 48 percent. Survival outlook for bladder cancer is improving. About 76 percent can expect to live for five years or more. Treatment consists of surgery, radiation and chemotherapy.

Uterus: 52,000 new cases each year. Death from uterine cancer, which includes cancer of the cervix and the endometrium (or body of the uterus), has been decreasing steadily, mainly due to earlier detection and treatment. Cervical cancer is so treatable that no one should die from it. The cure rate for endometrial cancer is about 84 percent. Standard treatment for cervical cancer is surgery, radiation, or both. Sometimes chemotherapy, in addition to surgery and radiotherapy, is used for endometrial cancer.

Oral: 27,000 new cases each year. This category includes cancer of the lip, tongue, salivary gland, mouth, throat and pharnyx. Oral cancers are twice as likely to occur in males, usually after age 40. Probable causes are heavy smoking and alcohol drinking and chewing tobacco. Five-year survival rate for cancer of the larynx is 67 percent, for nasopharynx, 38 percent among whites. Standard treatment is surgery and radiation. In advanced oral cancers, chemotherapy is advised.

Pancreas: 25,000 new cases a year. Pancreatic cancer is the most difficult of all cancers to treat. Only 2 percent of those stricken survive as long as five years. The disease has almost always spread by the time it is detected. New types of drugs and radiotherapy are being tried. Surgery is sometimes performed to relieve pain and remove the tumor to try to prevent further metastasis.

Leukemia: 49,000 new cases a year. Many kinds of childhood leukemia are curable more than 80 percent of the time, and treatment is steadily improving. The primary treatment is a combination of drugs and radiation that attempts to keep the cancer from attacking the central nervous system. Leukemia in adults is much more difficult to treat, and although 60 percent of the adults with leukemia go into remission, most have a relapse. Adult leukemia is considered about 10 to 20 percent curable.

Ovary: 18,000 new cases a year. Ovarian cancer traditionally is a very difficult cancer to treat, and the five-year survival rate during the past few years has been 38 percent. Recently, however, a major advance—directing radiation over a previously ignored area of the ovary—pioneered at the National Institutes of Health Clinical Center has been found to be much more effective and is for the first time reducing the fatality rate for advanced ovarian cancer. The therapy is complicated and experimental and is available only at cancer research centers.

Skin (melanoma): 22,000 new cases a year. There are about 400,000 new cases annually of non-melanoma skin cancer, which is readily curable. Malignant melanoma is cured in about 80 percent of the cases by surgery. If the melanoma is discovered early, the cure rate is almost 100 percent. It is important to diagnose melanoma early because the effectiveness of treatment depends on the thickness of the melanoma itself. New diagnostic tests for a hereditary type of melanoma have been developed, which will save more lives and probably result in more diagnoses of the cancer.

SURVIVAL RATES

Type	5-Year survival rate	Type	5-Year survival rate
Thyroid	93	Rectum	50
Endometrium	84	Non-Hodgkins lymphoma	48
Testis	88	Ovary	38
Melanoma	80	Leukemia	33
Breast	74	Brain	23
Bladder	76	Stomach	16
Hodgkins	73	Lung	13
Cervix/uterine	66	Esophagus	6
Prostate	71	Pancreas	2
Colon	53		
Kidney	48		

SOURCE: *National Cancer Institute.*

INFORMATION SERVICES

It is essential that a person diagnosed with cancer get the most up-to-date treatment available. In some cases, experimental treatment may be desirable, especially for cancers that are difficult to treat by current therapies. Unfortunately, cancer patients often have to protect themselves from outdated or poor cancer treatment. Some surgeons, for example, continue to perform one-step radical mastectomies even though this procedure is considered outdated.

As a guide, the more difficult the cancer is to treat by standard methods, the more you will want to be sure you are getting top-notch expert care and possibly experimental treatments. As Dr. Vincent DeVita, director of the National Cancer Institute notes, you will probably not need a cancer specialist for cancer of the cervix, for example, which can be competently treated by many gynecologists. On the other hand, if you have ovarian cancer, he says, you will want cancer specialists familiar with the most current and aggressive treatments. Similarly, children with cancer should receive the care of pediatric cancer specialists.

Cancer Information Line

(800) 4-CANCER

(800) 638-6070—Alaska

(202) 636-5700—District of Columbia, Maryland, and Virginia suburbs

(808) 524-1234—Hawaii, Number 6. Oahu, neighboring islands call collect.

These cancer information services are operated by the National Cancer Institute and by organizations under contract to the Institute. You can call them for information on all aspects of cancer, including where to find treatment.

PDQ Information System

The National Cancer Institute has set up a new computer service for physicians throughout the country called PDQ (Physicians Data Query). This system has a directory of physicians in all areas of the country who specialize in treating cancers of various kinds. Your physician can easily find a doctor near you who is a specialist in your kind of cancer. Also, the system describes the current state-of-the-art treatment for each type of cancer and exactly how a physician should proceed in treating it.

The PDQ also notes who is doing current research on new treatments in specific kinds of cancer. Your physician can find out who is doing research on your particular kind of cancer in your locality, and contact the researcher to see whether you might be a candidate for experimental treatment. The system is updated constantly by the National Cancer Institute and can be plugged into computers nationwide, including computers in doctors' offices. The PDQ system was set up to help physicians throughout the country keep up on the latest cancer treatments and research, so that everyone can get the most advanced care. Experts estimate that if everyone got the best cancer treatment currently available, the general cancer survival rates would rise by about 15 percent.

Second Opinion Hotline

(800) 638-6833
Before treatment, and especially before surgery, you may want a second opinion on whether the treatment is necessary or is the best available. Your local medical society, listed in your yellow pages, can suggest a physician for a second opinion. Or call the cancer information line or the national second opinion hotline, both operated by the federal government. You will be referred by the second opinion hotline to an agency, association or insurance company in your area which can tell you how to get a second opinion. Most insurance plans pay for a second opinion for surgery.

GOVERNMENT-SPONSORED CANCER CENTERS

The federal government has attempted to blanket the country with a network of cancer specialists, all adhering to the same general treatment procedures. There are three types: comprehensive cancer centers, clinical cancer centers and community clinical oncology program centers (CCOP). The comprehensive cancer centers are some of the most established cancer centers in the country; they do basic research as well as clinical or patient research. The clinical centers deal only with patients and are spread around to other regions of the country.

The more recently organized CCOPS reach out even further to make latest research findings available to cancer patients through community hospitals, clinics, centers, and physician groups, usually in smaller cities or in areas of cities not covered by other federal cancer centers. Physicians involved in the CCOPS program adhere to treatment and research protocols sponsored by the National Cancer Institute, so the program offers the latest cancer treatment to communities without major cancer centers, and at the same time helps gather research information on a much larger number of cancer patients throughout the country.

You may be able to receive treatment at one of these centers. If you are enrolled in a research program, you will get at the very least the most up-to-date standard cancer treatment, and in addition may receive new experimental treatments that might be more lifesaving than current standard ones.

COMPREHENSIVE AND CLINICAL CANCER CENTERS

ALABAMA
Comprehensive Cancer Center
University of Alabama in Birmingham
University Station
1824 Sixth Ave., S., Room 214
Birmingham, AL 35294
Albert F. LoBuglio, M.D., Director
(205) 934-5077

ARIZONA
University of Arizona Cancer Center
College of Medicine
1501 N. Campbell Ave., Room 7925
Tucson, AZ 85724
Sydney E. Salmon, M.D., Director
(602) 602-6044, 7925

CALIFORNIA

Cancer Research Center
Beckman Research Institute
City of Hope
1450 East Duarte Rd.
Duarte, CA 91010
Charles Mittman, M.D., Director
(818) 357-9711, x2705

UCSD Cancer Center
University of California at San Diego
School of Medicine
La Jolla, CA 92093
Mark R. Green, M.D., Acting Director
(619) 294-6930

Cancer Research Institute
University of Southern California
Comprehensive Cancer Center
PO Box 33804
1441 Eastlake Ave.
Los Angeles, CA 90033-0804
Brian E. Henderson, M.D., Director
Kenneth Norris, Jr.
(213) 224-6416

Jonsson Comprehensive Cancer Center
UCLA Medical Center, Room 10/247
Louis Factor Health Sciences Building
10833 Le Conte Ave.
Los Angeles, CA 90024
Richard J. Steckel, Director
(213) 825-1532

Northern California Cancer Program
1801 Page Mill Rd.
Building B, Suite 200
PO Box 10144
Palo Alto, CA 94303
Saul A. Rosenberg, M.D., Director
(415) 497-7431

CONNECTICUT

Yale University Comprehensive Cancer Center
333 Cedar St., Room WWW 205
New Haven, CT 06510
Alan C. Sartorelli, M.D., Director
(203) 785-4095

DISTRICT OF COLUMBIA

Cancer Research Center
Howard University Hospital
2041 Georgia Ave., N.W.
Washington, DC 20060
Jack E. White, Director
(202) 636-7697

Vincent T. Lombardi Cancer Research Center
Georgetown University Medical Center
3800 Reservoir Rd., N.W.
Washington, DC 20007
John F. Potter, M.D., Director
(202) 625-2042

FLORIDA

Papanicolaou Comprehensive Cancer Center
University of Miami Medical School
1475 N.W. 12th Ave.
PO Box 01690 (D8–4)
Miami, FL 33101
C. Gordon Zubrod, M.D., Director
(305) 548-4810

HAWAII

Cancer Research Center of Hawaii
University of Hawaii at Manoa
1236 Lauhala St.
Honolulu, HI 96813
Dr. Laurence N. Kolonel, Acting Director
(808) 548-8415

ILLINOIS

Illinois Cancer Council
36 S. Wabash Ave., Suite 700
Chicago, IL 60603
Shirley B. Lansky, Director
(312) 346-9813

Northwestern University Cancer Center
Health Sciences Building
303 E. Chicago Ave.
Chicago, IL 60611
Nathaniel I. Berlin, Director
(312) 908-5250, 5251, 5400

University of Chicago Cancer Research Center
5841 S. Maryland Ave.
Box 444
Chicago, IL 60637
John E. Ultmann, M.D., Director
(312) 962-6180

MARYLAND
Johns Hopkins Oncology Center
600 N. Wolfe St., Room 157
Baltimore, MD 21205
Albert H. Owens, Jr., M.D. Center Director,
  Professor of Oncology and Medicine
(301) 955-8822

MASSACHUSETTS
Dana-Farber Cancer Institute
44 Binney St.
Boston, MA 02115
Dr. Baruj Benacerraf, President
(617) 732-3636

MICHIGAN
Meyer L. Prentis Comprehensive Cancer
  Center of Metropolitan Detroit
110 East Warren St.
Detroit, MI 48201
Michael J. Brennan, M.D., Director
(313) 833-1088

MINNESOTA
Mayo Comprehensive Cancer Center
200 First St., S.W.
Rochester, MN 55905
Charles G. Moertel, M.D., Director
(507) 284-2511

NEW HAMPSHIRE
Norris Cotton Cancer Center
Dartmouth-Hitchcock Medical Center
Hanover, NH 03755
O. Ross McIntyre, M.D., Director
(603) 646-5505

NEW YORK
Cancer Research Center
Albert Einstein College of Medicine
Chanin Building, Room 330
1300 Morris Park Ave.
Bronx, NY 10461
Harry Eagle, M.D., Director
(212) 430-2302 or 792-2233

Roswell Park Memorial Institute
666 Elm St.
Buffalo, NY 14263
Gerald P. Murphy, M.D., Director
(716) 845-5570

Columbia University Cancer Center
College of Physicians & Surgeons
701 W. 168th St., Room 1601
New York, NY 10032
I. Bernard Weinstein, M.D., Director
(212) 305-6904

Memorial Sloan-Kettering Cancer Center
1275 York Ave.
New York, NY 10021
Paul Marks, M.D., President
(212) 794-6561

Department of Neoplastic Diseases
Mt. Sinai School of Medicine
Fifth Ave. at 100th St.
New York, NY 10029
James F. Holland, Chairman
(212) 650-6361

Cancer Center
New York University Medical Center
550 First Ave.
New York, NY 10016
Vittorio Defendi, M.D., Director
(212) 340-5349

University of Rochester Cancer Center
601 Elmwood Ave. Box 704
Rochester, NY 14642
Robert A. Cooper, Jr., M.D., Director
(716) 275-4865

NORTH CAROLINA
Lineberger Cancer Research Center
University of North Carolina
School of Medicine (237H)
Chapel Hill, NC 27514
Joseph S. Pagano, M.D., Director
(919) 966-3036

Comprehensive Cancer Center
Duke University Medical Center
227 Jones Building, Research Drive
PO Box 3814
Durham, NC 27710
William W. Shingleton, M.D., Director
(919) 684-2282

Oncology Research Center
Bowman Gray School of Medicine
300 S. Hawthorne Rd.
Winston-Salem, NC 27103
Robert L. Capizzi, M.D., Director
(919) 748-4464

OHIO

Ohio State University Comprehensive Cancer
  Center
410 W. 12th Ave., Suite 302
Columbus, OH 43210
David S. Yohn, M.D., Director
(614) 422-5022

PENNSYLVANIA

Fox Chase Cancer Center
7701 Burholme Ave.
Philadelphia, PA 19111
John R. Durant, M.D., President
(215) 728-2781

RHODE ISLAND

Roger Williams General Hospital
825 Chalkstone Ave.
Providence, RI 02908
Paul Calabresi, M.D., Director
(401) 456-2070

TENNESSEE

St. Jude Children's Research Hospital
332 N. Lauderdale
Memphis, TN 38101
Joseph V. Simone, M.D., Director
(901) 522-0301

TEXAS

UTMB Cancer Center
University of Texas Medical Branch
11th at Mechanic
Microbiology Building
Room 9.104, Route J20
Galveston, TX 77550
John J. Costanzi, M.D., Director
(409) 761-2981, 1862

University of Texas System Cancer Center
M.D. Anderson Hospital & Tumor Institute
6723 Bertner Ave.
Houston, TX 77030
Charles A. LeMaistre, M.D., President
(713) 792-6000

VERMONT

Vermont Regional Cancer Center
University of Vermont
1 S. Prospect St.
Burlington, VT 05401
Roger S. Foster, Jr., M.D., Director
(802) 656-4414

VIRGINIA

Massey Cancer Center
Medical College of Virginia
Virginia Commonwealth University
MCV Station, Box 37
Richmond, VA 23298
Walter Lawrence, Jr., M.D., Director
(804) 786-9322, 9323, 0448

WASHINGTON

Fred Hutchinson Cancer Research Center
1124 Columbia St.
Seattle, WA 98104
Robert W. Day, M.D., Director
(206) 467-4302

WISCONSIN

University of Wisconsin Clinical Cancer
  Center
600 Highland Ave.
Madison, WI 53792
Paul P. Carbone, M.D., Director
(608) 263-8610

COMMUNITY CLINICAL ONCOLOGY PROGRAMS (CCOPs)

ARIZONA
Greater Phoenix CCOP
Internists, Oncologists, Ltd.
1010 E. McDowell, Suite 201
Phoenix, AZ 85006
David K. King, M.D.
(602) 239-2413

ARKANSAS
Arkansas Oncology Clinic CCOP
500 S. University, Suite 401
Little Rock, AR 72205
Billy L. Tranum, M.D.
(501) 664-3008

CALIFORNIA
San Joaquin Valley CCOP
PO Box 1232
Fresno, CA 93715
Phyllis Ager Mowry, M.D., Director
(209) 442-6429

Central Los Angeles CCOP
PO Box 57992
Los Angeles, CA 90057
Armand Bouzaglou, M.D.
(213) 484-7086

Greater Los Angeles CCOP
616 S. Witmer St.
Los Angeles, CA 90017
Jim S. Bonorris, M.D.
(213) 977-2427

San Gabriel Valley CCOP
100 Congress St.
PO Box 7013
Pasadena, CA 91105-7013
Michael P. Kadin, M.D.
(818) 440-5186

Kaiser Foundation Research Institute
Department of Pediatrics, Station D
2025 Morse Ave.
Sacramento, CA 95825
Scott S. Johnson, M.D.
(916) 486-6679

COLORADO
Colorado Cancer Research Program
1719 E. 19th Ave.
Denver, CO 80218
Robert F. Berris, M.D.
(303) 839-7788

CONNECTICUT
Greater Hartford CCOP
114 Woodland St.
Hartford, CT 06105
Dominick N. Pasquale, M.D.
(203) 548-5474

Hospital of St. Raphael CCOP
Main 238
1450 Chapel St.
New Haven, CT 06511
Leonard R. Farber, M.D.
(203) 789-4347

FLORIDA
Halifax Hospital Medical Center
PO Box 1990
Daytona Beach, FL 32015
Herbert D. Kerman, M.D.
(904) 254-4211, x3913

Florida Pediatric CCOP
PO Box 13372, University Station
Gainesville, FL 32604
James L. Talbert, M.D.
(904) 375-6848

GEORGIA
University Hospital CCOP
1350 Walton Way
Augusta, GA 30910
Stephen M. Shlaer, M.D.
(404) 722-9011

HAWAII
Hawaii CCOP
320 Ward Ave., Suite 203
Honolulu, HI 96814
Reginald C. S. Ho, M.D.
(808) 536-7702, x57

ILLINOIS
Saint Mary of Nazareth Hospital Center
2233 W. Division St.
Chicago, IL 60622
Korathu Thomas, M.D.
(312) 770-3205

Evanston Hospital
2650 Ridge Ave.
Evanston, IL 60201
Janardan D. Khandekar, M.D.
(312) 492-3989

Methodist Medical Center of Illinois
222 N.E. Glen Oak Ave.
Peoria, IL 61630
Stephen A. Cullinan, M.D.
(309) 672-5521

Carle Cancer Center CCOP
602 W. University Ave.
Urbana, IL 61801
Alan Kramer Hatfield, M.D.
(217) 337-3010

IOWA
Iowa Oncology Research Association
c/o Kathy Osborn
1048 4th Ave.
Des Moines, IA 50314
Roscoe Morton, M.D.
(515) 244-7586

KANSAS
Wichita CCOP
929 N. St. Francis
Box 1358
Wichita, KS 67201
Henry E. Hynes, M.D.
(316) 268-5784

LOUISIANA
Ochsner Clinic
1514 Jefferson Highway
New Orleans, LA 70121
Carl G. Kardinal, M.D.
(504) 838-3758

MAINE
Eastern Maine Medical Center
489 State St.
Bangor, ME 04401
Alan W. Boone, M.D.
(207) 945-7481

Southern Maine CCOP
22 Bramhall St.
Portland, ME 04102
Ronald J. Carroll, M.D.
(207) 871-2213

MASSACHUSETTS
New England Collaborative CCOP
185 Pilgrim Rd.
Boston, MA 02215
Jacob J. Lokich, M.D.
(617) 732-9237

MICHIGAN
Grand Rapids CCOP
100 Michigan N.E.
Grand Rapids, MI 49503
Edward L. Moorhead, II, M.D.
(616) 774-1230

Kalamazoo CCOP
1521 Gull Rd.
Kalamazoo, MI 49001
Phillip Stott, M.D.
(616) 383-7007

MINNESOTA
400 E. Third St.
Duluth, MN 55805
James E. Krook, M.D.
(218) 722-8364

W. Metro-Minneapolis CCOP
5000 W. 39th St.
St. Louis Park, MN 55416
Joseph M. Ryan, M.D.
(612) 927-3491

MISSISSIPPI
North Mississippi CCOP
806 Garfield
Tupelo, MS 38801
Julian B. Hill, M.D.
(601) 844-9166

MISSOURI
Kansas City CCOP
6601 Rockhill Rd.
Kansas City, MO 64131
Robert J. Belt, M.D.
(816) 361-3500

St. Luke's Hospital
Wornall Rd. at Forty-fourth
Kansas City, MO 64111
Karl H. Hanson, Jr., M.D.
(816) 932-2085

St. Louis CCOP
Mercy Doctors Building
621 S. New Ballas Rd., Suite 3018
St. Louis, MO 63141
Patrick H. Henry, M.D.
(314) 569-6573

MONTANA
Billings Interhospital Oncology Project
1145 N. 29th St., Suite 1B
Billings, MT 59101
Neel Hammond, M.D.
(406) 259-2452

NEVADA
Southern Nevada Research Foundation
2040 W. Charleston Blvd., Suite 204
Las Vegas, NV 89102
John A. Ellerton, M.D.
(702) 384-0013

NEW JERSEY
Bergen-Passaic CCOP
30 Prospect Ave.
Hackensack, NJ 07601
Richard Rosenbluth, M.D.
(201) 441-2363

Essex County Cancer Consortium
Old Short Hills Rd.
Livingston, NJ 07039
Rodger J. Winn, M.D.
(201) 533-5917

Medical Center CCOP Consortium
201 Lyons Ave.
Newark, NJ 07112
Frederick B. Cohen, M.D.
(201) 926-7230

Northern New Jersey CCOP
193 Morris Ave.
Summit, NJ 07901
Abraham Risk, M.D.
(201) 522-2043

NEW YORK
Twin Tiers CCOP
169 Riverside Drive
Binghamton, NY 13905
Robert E. Enck, M.D.
(607) 798-5431

Lutheran Medical Center
150 55th St.
Brooklyn, NY 11220
Hosny Selim, M.D.
(718) 630-7065

Mary Imogene Bassett Hospital CCOP
Atwell Rd.
Cooperstown, NY 13326
Richard J. Horner, M.D.
(607) 547-3339

North Shore University Hospital
300 Community Drive
Manhasset, NY 11030
Vincent P. Vinciguerra, M.D.
(516) 562-4161

Nassau Regional Cancer Program
222 Station Plaza North, Room 300
Mineola NY 11501
Larry Nathanson, M.D.
(516) 663-2310

St. Mary's Hospital CCOP
89 Genesee St.
Rochester, NY 14611
Kishan J. Pandya, M.D.
(716) 464-3521

CCOP of Central New York
101 Union Ave., Suite 817
Syracuse, NY 13203
Kenneth E. Gale, M.D.
(315) 424-1188

NORTH DAKOTA
St. Luke's Hospitals CCOP
5th St. N. at Mills Ave.
Fargo, ND 58122
Lloyd Everson, M.D.
(701) 237-2446

OHIO
Columbus CCOP
111 S. Grant Ave.
Columbus, OH 43215
Jerry T. Guy, M.D.
(614) 461-3049

Dayton CCOP
3525 Southern Blvd.
Kettering, OH 45429
James S. Ungerleider, M.D.
(513) 299-7204, x322

Toledo CCOP
5200 Harroum Rd.
Sylvania, OH 43560
Charles D. Coubau, M.D.
(419) 885-1444, x2003

PENNSYLVANIA
Geisinger Clinic CCOP
N. Academy Ave.
Danville, PA 17822
Albert M. Bernath, M.D.
(717) 271-6413

Allegheny CCOP
320 E. North Ave.
Pittsburgh, PA 15212
Reginald P. Pugh, M.D.
(412) 359-4054

SOUTH CAROLINA
Spartanburg CCOP
101 E. Wood St.
Spartanburg, S.C. 29303
John H. McCulloch, M.D.
(803) 573-6921

SOUTH DAKOTA
Sioux Falls Commmunity Cancer Consortium
1301 S. 9th Ave., Suite 501
Sioux Falls, SD 57105
Robert F. Marschke, Jr., M.D.
(605) 331-3160

TEXAS
Fort Worth/Arlington CCOP
1401 S. Main
Fort Worth, Texas 76104
John L. E. Nugent, M.D.
(817) 336-9371, x7273

VERMONT
Green Mountain Oncology Group
The Rutland Medical Center
Rutland, VT 05701
H. James Wallace, M.D.
(802) 775-7111 x184

VIRGINIA
CCOP of Roanoke
PO Box 13367
Roanoke, VA 24033
Stephen H. Rosenoff, M.D.
(703) 981-7009

WASHINGTON
Virginia Mason Medical Center CCOP
1100 Ninth Ave.
Seattle, WA 98111
Albert B. Einstein, Jr., M.D.
(206) 223-6742

Southwest Washington CCOP
314 S. K St., Suite 108
Tacoma, WA 98405
J. Gale Katterhagen, M.D.
(206) 597-7461

WEST VIRGINIA
West Virginia Cooperative CCOP
3200 MacCorkle Ave., S.E.
Charleston, WV 25304
Steven J. Jubelirer, M.D.
(304) 348-9541

WISCONSIN
Marshfield CCOP
1000 N. Oak Ave.
Marshfield, WI 54449
Tarit K. Banerjee, M.D.
(715) 387-5241

SOURCE: *National Cancer Institute.*

CHILDREN'S CANCER SPECIALISTS

Cancer in children is a special crisis that requires specialized care. About 6,000 youngsters every year develop cancer. About half of the cases are leukemia; most of the rest are cancers of the bone, nervous system, lymph nodes, eye, or kidney (Wilm's Tumor). Survival rates vary according to the type of cancer and the treatment.

Since childhood cancer is rare, many physicians are not experienced in treating it and may not be aware of the latest therapies.

Studies have shown that survival is increased by treatment at a pediatric cancer center and by participating in specially designed studies on the treatment of pediatric cancer. The National

Cancer Institute's designated centers generally have pediatric cancer specialists. NCI's new PDQ system also has the names of childhood cancer specialists in your area. In addition, there are some leading childhood cancer specialists who are part of the National Cancer Institute's Children's Cancer Study Group or its Pediatric Oncology Group. These two groups develop and test new treatments for childhood cancer. The groups' members are among the country's leading authorities on all kinds of pediatric cancer.

Children's Cancer Study Group

CALIFORNIA
Children's Hospital of Los Angeles
PO Box 54700
Terminal Annex
Los Angeles, CA 90054
Jorge Ortega, M.D.
(213) 669-2163

UCLA School of Medicine
Building MDCC, Room A2410
Los Angeles, CA 90024
Stephen Feig, M.D.
(213) 825-5050

USC Cancer Center
1721 N. Griffin Ave.
Phinney Hall, Room 110
Los Angeles, CA 90031
Denman Hammond, M.D., Chair
John Weiner, Ph.D., Admin. Dir.
(213) 223-1373

UCSF/School of Medicine
505 Parnassus St., M665
San Francisco, CA 94143
Arthur Ablin, M.D.
(415) 476-3831

Harbor-UCLA Medical Center
1124 W. Carson St., E-6 Annex
Torrance, CA 90509
Jerry Finkelstein, M.D.
(213) 533-3843

COLORADO
Denver Childrens Hospital
1056 E. 19th Ave.
Denver, CO 80218
David G. Tubergen, M.D.
(303) 861-6750

DISTRICT OF COLUMBIA
Childrens Hospital National Medical Center
111 Michigan Ave., N.W.
Washington, DC 20010
Sanford Leikin, M.D.
(202) 745-2140

ILLINOIS
Children's Memorial Hospital
2300 Childrens Plaza, Room 648
Chicago, IL 60614
Edward Baum, M.D.
(312) 880-4564

INDIANA
Indiana University, Riley Hospital
1100 W. Michigan St., P-132
Indianapolis, IN 46223
Robert M. Weetman, M.D.
(317) 264-8784

IOWA
Iowa University Hospitals & Clinic
2528 HCP
Iowa City, IA 52242
Raymond Tannous, M.D.
(319) 356-3422

MICHIGAN
Mott Childrens Hospital
1405 E. Ann Arbor
Ann Arbor, MI 48109
Ruth Heyn, M.D.
(313) 764-7126

MINNESOTA
University of Minnesota
420 Delaware St, Box 484
Mayo Building
Minneapolis, MN 55455
Mark E. Nesbit, M.D.
(612) 373-4318

Mayo Clinic
200 First St., S.W.
Rochester, MN 55905
Gerald Gilchrist, M.D.
(507) 284-2511

NEW YORK
Babies Hospital
3959 Broadway Building, S. Baulding
New York, NY 10032
Sergio Piomelli, M.D.
(212) 694-5882

Memorial Sloane-Kettering Cancer Center
1275 York Ave.
New York, NY 10021
Peter G. Steinherz, M.D.
(212) 794-7951

Strong Memorial Hospital
260 Crittenden Blvd.
Rochester, NY 14642
Harvey Cohen, M.D.
(716) 275-2981

NORTH CAROLINA
University of North Carolina
509 Burnett-Womack Building, 229H
Chapel Hill, NC 27514
Herbert A. Cooper, M.D.
(919) 966-1178

OHIO
Childrens Hospital Medical Center
Elland Ave. and Bethesda
Cincinnati, OH 45229
Beatrice Lampkin, M.D.
(513) 559-4266

Rainbow Babies & Children Hospital
2101 Adelbert Rd.
Cleveland, OH 44106
Peter Coccia, M.D.
(216) 844-3345

Childrens Hospital of Columbus
700 Childrens Drive
Columbus, OH 43205
Frederick Ruymann, M.D.
(614) 461-2678

OREGON
Doernbecher Childrens Memorial Hospital
3181 S.W. Sam Jackson Park Rd.
Portland, OR 97201
Robert C. Neerhout, M.D.
(503) 225-8194

PENNSYLVANIA
Childrens Hospital of Philadelphia
34th and Civic Center Blvd.
Philadelphia, PA 19104
Anna Meadows, M.D.
(215) 596-9644

Childrens Hospital of Pittsburgh
125 DeSoto St.
Pittsburgh, PA 15213
Vincent Albo, M.D.
(412) 647-5055

TENNESSEE
Department of Pediatrics, Room DD2205
Nashville, TN 37232
John Lukens M.D.
(615) 322-7475

TEXAS
University of Texas at San Antonio
7703 Floyd Curl Drive
San Antonio, TX 78284
Paul Zeltzer, M.D.
(512) 691-6197

UTAH
University of Utah Medical Center
50 N. Medical Drive
Salt Lake City, UT 84132
Richard O'Brien, M.D.
(801) 521-1250

WASHINGTON
Children's Orthopedic Hospital & Medical
    Center
4800 Sand Point Way, N.E., C5371
Seattle, WA 98105
Ronald L. Chard, M.D.
(206) 526-2107

WISCONSIN
University of Wisconsin Medical Center
600 Highland Ave.
Madison, WI 53706
Nasrollah Shahidi, M.D.
(608) 263-6202

The above physicians are the principal investigators of the National Cancer Institute's Children's Cancer Study Group, a government-supported nationwide research and treatment network specializing in children's cancers.

Pediatric Oncology Group

ALABAMA
University of Alabama
Children's Hospital
Division of Hematology/Oncology
1600 Seventh Ave. S.
Birmingham, AL 35233-1711
Robert Castleberry, M.D.
(205) 939-9100

University of South Alabama
2451 Fillingim St.
Mobile, AL 36617
Vipal Mankad, M.D.
(205) 471-7000

ARKANSAS
University of Arkansas
Children's Hospital
Department of Pediatric Hematology/Oncology
804 Wolfe St.
Little Rock, AR 72201
D.H. Berry, M.D.
(501) 372-5622

CALIFORNIA
City of Hope National Medical Center
Department of Pediatric Oncology
1500 E. Duarte Rd.
Duarte, CA 91010
Robert Krance, M.D.
(818) 359-8111

Children's Hospital at Stanford
Department of Pediatric Hematology/Oncology
520 Willow Rd.
Palo Alto, CA 94304
Bertil Glader, M.D.
(415) 327-4800, x225

Stanford University Medical Center
520 Willow Rd.
Palo Alto, CA 94304
Michael P. Link, M.D.
(415) 327-4800

Children's Hospital and Health Center (UCSD)
Hematology Office
8001 Frost St.
San Diego, CA 92123
Gary A. Hartman, M.D.
(619) 576-5811

Naval Regional Medical Center
Pediatric Hematology/Oncology
Box 307, Park Blvd.
San Diego, CA 92134
William J. Thomas, M.D.
(619) 294-6727

University of California
San Diego Medical Center
225 Dickinson St.
San Diego, CA 92103
Faith Kung, M.D.
(619) 294-6737

COLORADO
Fitzsimons Army Medical Center
Pediatric Clinic—Building 507
Colfax and Peoria
Aurora, CO 80045
Askold D. Mosijczuk, M.D.
(303) 361-3837

CONNECTICUT
Yale University School of Medicine
Department of Pediatrics
Room 4087-LMP
333 Cedar St.
New Haven, CT 06510
Diane M. Komp, M.D.
(203) 785-4640

DISTRICT OF COLUMBIA
Walter Reed Army Hospital
Department of the Army
Department of Pediatric Oncology
Section 1 K, Georgia Ave., N.W.
Washington, DC 20307
David A. Maybee, M.D.
(202) 576-1546

FLORIDA
University of Florida
Shands Hospital
JHM Health Center
Gainesville, FL 32610
Samuel Gross, M.D.
(904) 392-5633

Jacksonville Wolfson Children's Hospital
800 Prudential Drive
Jacksonville, FL 32207
Charles Dellinger, M.D.
(904) 393-2889 or 2000, x1111

University of Miami School of Medicine
Jackson Memorial Hospital
1611 N.W. 12th Ave.
Miami, FL 33136
Stuart Toledano, M.D.
(305) 549-7320

Orlando Regional Medical Center
1414 S. Kuhl Ave.
Orlando, FL 32806
Vincent F. Giusti, M.D.
(305) 841-5111

Sacred Heart Children's Hospital
5151 N. Ninth Ave.
Pensacola, FL 32504
Thomas Jenkins, M.D.
(904) 478-1100

All Children's Hospital
801 Sixth St. S.
St. Petersburg, FL 33701
Jerry L. Barbosa, M.D.
(813) 898-7451

University of South Florida Medical Center
12901 N. 30th St.
Tampa, FL 33612
Eva Hvizdala, M.D.
(813) 974-4111

GEORGIA
Emory University School of Medicine
Department of Pediatric Oncology
1365 Clifton Rd. N.E.
Atlanta, GA 30322
Abdel H. Ragab, M.D.
(404) 321-0111

HAWAII
Cancer Center of Hawaii
1236 Lauhala St., Room 509
Honolulu, HI 96813
Robert Wilkinson, M.D.
(808) 548-8530

Tripler Army Medical Center
HST-PE Box 585
Tripler AMC (Oahu), HI 96859
Stephen R. Stephenson, M.D.
(808) 433-6474

KANSAS
University of Kansas Medical Center
Department of Pediatric Oncology
39th & Rainbow Blvd.
Kansas City, KS 66103
Tribhawan Vats, M.D.
(913) 588-6340

St. Francis Regional Medical Center
929 N. St. Francis St.
Wichita, KS 67214
David Rosen, M.D.
(316) 265-3774

LOUISIANA
Louisiana State University
1542 Tulane Ave., 2
New Orleans, LA 70112
Rafael Ducos, M.D.
(504) 568-4564

MARYLAND
Pediatric Oncology, CMSC 801
Johns Hopkins Oncology Center
600 N. Wolfe St.
Baltimore, MD 21205
Brigid G. Leventhal, M.D.
(301) 955-5000

MASSACHUSETTS
Dana-Farber Cancer Institute
Children's Hospital & Joint Cancer for
  Radiation Therapy
44 Binney St.
Boston, MA 02115
Stephen E. Sallan, M.D.
(617) 732-3316

Massachusetts General Hospital
15 Parkman St.
Boston, MA 92114
John Truman, M.D.
(617) 726-2737

MICHIGAN
Children's Hospital of Michigan
Wayne State University
3901 Beaubien Blvd.
Detroit, MI 48201
Y. Ravindranath, M.D.
(313) 494-5516

MISSISSIPPI
University of Mississippi Medical Center
2500 N. State St.
Jackson, MS 39216
Jeanette Pulle, M.D.
(601) 362-4411

Keesler Air Force Base Hospital
Pediatric Division
Keesler Air Force Base, MS 39534
Michael Hensley, M.D.
(601) 377-6631

MISSOURI
University of Missouri Health Sciences Center
Department of Child Health
1 Hospital Drive
Columbia, MO 65201
Nasrollah Hakami, M.D.
(314) 882-4932

St. Luke's Hospital
Wornall Rd. at 44th St.
Kansas City, MO 64111
Anthony Pecoraro, M.D.
(816) 932-2000

Washington University School of Medicine
St. Louis Children's Hospital
400 S. Kingshighway Blvd.
PO Box 14871
St. Louis, MO 63178
Vita J. Land, M.D.
(314) 454-6209

NEW HAMPSHIRE
Dartmouth-Hitchcock Medical Center
Norris Cotton Cancer Center
2 Maynard St.
Hanover, NH 03756
Neil Cornell, M.D.
(603) 646-5527

NEW MEXICO
University of New Mexico School of Medicine
Department of Pediatrics
Surgery Building
2701 Frontier, N.E.
Albuquerque, NM 87131
T. John Gribble, M.D.
(505) 277-4461

NEW YORK
Roswell Park Memorial Institute
666 Elm St.
Buffalo, NY 14263
Arnold Freeman, M.D.
Chief, Department of Pediatrics
(716) 845-2333

Mt. Sinai School of Medicine
One Gustave L. Levy Place
New York, NY 10029
Michael B. Harris, M.D.
Chief, Pediatric Oncology
(212) 650-6031

Pediatric Hematology Center
S.U.N.Y. Upstate Medical Center
750 E. Adams St.
Syracuse, NY 13210
Ronald Dubowy, M.D.
(315) 473-5800

NORTH CAROLINA
Charlotte Memorial Hospital
1000 Blythe Blvd.
Charlotte, NC 28203
Barry L. Golembe, M.D.
(704) 332-2121

Duke University Medical Center
Department of Pediatric Hematology/Oncology
Erwin Rd.
PO Box 2916
Durham, NC 27710
John M. Falletta, M.D.
(919) 684-3401

East Carolina University School of Medicine
Department of Pediatrics
Section on Hematology/Oncology
P.C.M.H.-288W
200 Stantonsburg Rd.
Greenville, NC 27834
Tate Holbrook, M.D.
(919) 757-4676

Bowman Gray School of Medicine
Department of Pediatric Oncology
300 S. Hawthorne Rd.
Winston-Salem, NC 27103
Richard B. Patterson, M.D.
(919) 748-4085

OHIO

Cleveland Clinic Foundation
Department of Pediatric Oncology
9500 Euclid Ave.
Cleveland, OH 44106
Donald Norris, M.D.
(216) 444-2374

OKLAHOMA

Oklahoma Children's Memorial Hospital
Department of Pediatric Hematology/Oncology
PO Box 26307
Oklahoma City, OK 73126
Ruprecht Nitschke, M.D.
(405) 271-5311

PENNSYLVANIA

The Milton S. Hershey Medical Center
Pennsylvania State University
500 University Drive, Box 850
Hershey, PA 17033
James F. Balsley, M.D.
Director, Pediatric Hematology/Oncology
(717) 534-6012

St. Christopher's Hospital for Children
Temple University School of Medicine
5th and Lehigh Ave.
Philadelphia, PA 19133
Donald Pinkel, M.D.
(215) 427-5586

RHODE ISLAND

Rhode Island Hospital
Pediatric Oncology, MPB-1
593 Eddy St.
Providence, RI 02902
Edwin Forman, M.D.
(401) 277-5171

SOUTH CAROLINA

Medical University of South Carolina
Department of Pediatric Oncology
171 Ashley Ave.
Charleston, SC 29425
H. Biemann Othersen, M.D.
(803) 792-3851

TENNESSEE

St. Jude Children's Research Hospital
Department of Pediatric Hematology/Oncology
322 North Lauderdale
PO Box 318
Memphis, TN 38101
Anne Hayes, M.D.
(901) 522-0300

TEXAS

Southwestern Medical School–Dallas
Children's Medical Center
Hematology Clinic
1935 Amelia
Dallas, TX 75232
George R. Buchanan, M.D.
(214) 920-2382

Brooke Army Medical Center
Fort Sam Houston, TX 78234
Terry Pick, M.D.
(512) 221-4932

Cook Children's Hospital
1212 W. Lancaster Ave.
Fort Worth, TX 76102
Paul Bowman, M.D.
(817) 336-5581

University of Texas: Galveston
Division of Hematology/Oncology–Department
    of Pediatrics
Market and 9th Sts.
Galveston, TX 77550
Mary Ellen Haggard, M.D.
(409) 761-2341

Baylor College of Medicine
Department of Pediatric Oncology
6621 Fannin St.
Houston, TX 77030
Donald J. Fernback, M.D.
(713) 791-4122

University of Texas Cancer Center
M.D. Anderson Hospital and Tumor Institute
6723 Bertner Drive
Houston, TX 77030
Jan van Eys, M.D.
(713) 792-2121

VERMONT
University of Vermont College of Medicine
Given Medical Building, Pediatric Division
Colchester Ave.
Burlington, VT 05405
Joseph Dickerman, M.D.
(802) 656-2296

VIRGINIA
University of Virginia School of Medicine
PO Box 386
Charlottesville, VA 22908
Hernan Sabio, M.D.
(804) 924-0211

Fairfax Hospital
3330 Gallows Rd.
Falls Church, VA 22031
Richard Binder, M.D.
(703) 698-1110

Medical College of Virginia
Virginia Commonwealth University
Department of Pediatric Oncology
1200 E. Broad St.
PO Box 646
Richmond, VA 23298
Harold M. Maurer, M.D.
(804) 786-9602

WEST VIRGINIA
West Virginia University Medical Center
Department of Pediatrics
3110 MacCorkle Ave., S.E.
Charleston, WV 25304
Kenneth A. Starling, M.D.
(304) 347-1341, 1342

West Virginia University School of Medicine
Department of Pediatric Oncology
Morgantown, WV 26506
Barbara Jones, M.D.
(304) 293-4451

WISCONSIN
Midwest Children's Cancer Center
Department of Pediatric Oncology
1700 W. Wisconsin
Milwaukee, WI 53233
Bruce Camitta, M.D.
(414) 933-4199

The above physicians are the principal investigators of the National Cancer Institute's Pediatric Oncology Group, a government-supported nationwide research and treatment network specializing in children's cancers.

PSYCHOLOGICAL CANCER THERAPY

There is some evidence that cancer as well as some other chronic illnesses may be influenced by emotional factors including a mind-brain link to the immune system. Therefore, some physicians, psychologists, and counselors try to help control such diseases through psychological techniques, often including purposeful visualization and group therapy or support.

There are numerous individual cases where people seem to do better after such therapy, but there are no long-term, scientifically controlled studies proving it. Therefore, the field is quite controversial.

Here are sources of information about psychological therapy and where to find cancer counselors nationwide, in addition to regular medical therapy.

International Association of Cancer Counselors
Janus Associates
1800 Augusta St., Suite 150
Houston, TX 77057
(713) 780-1057

Cancer Counseling and Research Center
PO Box 1055
Azle, TX 76020
(817) 444-4073

Simonton Cancer Center
875 Via de la Paz
Pacific Palisades, CA 90272
Dr. Carl Simonton
(213) 459-4434

CANCER TREATMENT AT THE NATIONAL INSTITUTES OF HEALTH

The Clinical Center at the federal government's National Institutes of Health in Bethesda, Maryland, is conducting numerous patient-research programs concerning various kinds of cancer, for which you *may* be a candidate. Referral should come from a physician.

Here are a few of the cancer studies, by type of cancer, that were being conducted in 1986.

Several types of recurrent cancers: Tests of interferon and antitumor monoclonal antibodies on patients who do not respond to standard treatments.

Malignant melanoma: Immunology studies of patients between the ages of 15 and 70.

Hodgkin's or non-Hodgkin's lymphoma: Experimental treatment of patients who have received no previous treatment.

Ovarian cancer: Experimental treatment of patients not previously treated with chemotherapy or radiation.

Breast cancer: Experimental drug-therapy and a study comparing the effectiveness of lumpectomy and breast irradiation with modified radical mastectomy.

Selected cancers: Studies of patients between ages 1 and 25.

Oat cell cancer of the lung.

Gastric and pancreatic cancer: "Intraoperative radiation" and radical surgery research on patients without distant metastases.

Bone and soft-tissue cancers: Experimental radiation-drug therapy.

Patients at high risk for recurrent colon or rectal cancer after standard surgery: Experimental therapy.

Stomach cancer: Experimental combination therapy for patients with recurrent stomach cancer.

Prostate cancer: Experimental studies to treat prostate cancer with drugs, radiation and/or endocrinologic treatment.

AIDS/Kaposi's sarcoma: Experimental therapy.

For more information your physician can contact:

Office of the Director
The Clinical Center
Building 10, Room 2C146
National Institutes of Health
Bethesda, MD 20892
(301) 496-4891

ORGANIZATIONS

American Cancer Society
90 Park Ave.
New York, NY 10016
(212) 599-8200

A national voluntary organization dedicated to the control and eradication of cancer through programs of research, education, and service to cancer patients and their families. A major information and self-help source. Pamphlets, brochures, reports, a quarterly magazine, audiovisual materials, and a journal for physicians. Special services: quit-smoking programs, other specialized mutual support and rehabilitation groups for those with various kinds of cancer. Will provide more information upon request.

Association for Brain Tumor
  Research
Suite 200
6232 North Pulaski Road
Chicago, IL 60646
(312) 286-5571

A national voluntary organization supporting research and self-help groups for patients with brain tumors, their families and other interested persons. Booklets, pamphlets, bibliographies. Can tell you how to set up a Brain Tumor Self-Help Group, and will provide a list of institutions and physicians around the country doing experimental brain tumor research and therapy. Will provide more information upon request.

The Candlelighters Foundation
2025 Eye Street, N.W.
Washington, DC 20006
(202) 659-5136

An international organization for the parents of children with cancer and health professionals who treat them. Two hundred fifty self-help groups throughout the country. A major source of information on childhood cancer. Several publications, including quarterly newsletters, bibliography and resource guide. Will provide more information upon request.

Cansurmount
90 Park Ave.
New York, NY 10016
(212) 599-8200

An American Cancer Society program where those who have successfully coped with cancer of all types visit cancer patients undergoing the same kind of treatment. Visitors and patients are matched by age, personality, background.

DES Action
2845 24th Street
San Francisco, CA 94110
(415) 826-5060

A national self-help and information organization for parents and their offspring concerned about the consequences of diethylstilbestrol (DES), a drug taken by over six million women, ostensibly to prevent miscarriages, between 1941 and 1971. The drug is known to cause a rare vaginal cancer and other reproductive birth defects in some of the daughters of the women who took it, and is suspected of causing cancer of the testes and other birth defects in the sons of women who took it during pregnancy. Sponsors DES Cancer Network, a support group of and for DES daughters. Publishes pamphlets and quarterly newsletters. Will provide more information and answer questions from the public upon request.

I Can Cope
American Cancer Society
90 Park Ave.
New York, NY 10016
(212) 599-8200

An American Cancer Society patient education program about living with cancer. An eight-week series of two-hour classes conducted by doctors and other health professionals explains the facts about coping with cancer and answers questions about human anatomy, cancer development, treatment side effects, emotional and sexual issues, self-esteem and community resources. No charge. The program is usually conducted in cooperation with local hospitals or health agencies.

International Association of Laryngectomees
American Cancer Society
90 Park Ave.
New York, NY 10016
(212) 599-8200

A rehabilitation program sponsored by the American Cancer Society in which those who have learned new ways of speaking after removal of their larynx (voice box) because of cancer assist those who are newly recovering from the surgery.

The National Cancer Institute
The National Institutes of Health
9000 Rockville Pike, Building 31, 10A18
Bethesda, MD 20892
(301) 496-5583 (cancer communications office)
(800) 4-CANCER (to order publications and
    get regionally specialized information)

The National Cancer Institute is one of the federal government's National Institutes of Health and is concerned with all aspects of cancer. It funds research; helps make cancer policy; and disseminates information to the general public, physicians, and health professionals on all facets of cancer. NCI puts out numerous publications, answers public inquiries, and can refer you to other sources of information on cancer.

National Leukemia Association
Roosevelt Field, Lower Concourse
Garden City, NY 11530
(516) 741-1190

Reach to Recovery
90 Park Ave.
New York, NY 10016
(212) 599-8200

A national nonmembership organization that funds research and makes financial aid available to those with leukemia who are in need of X-rays or drugs. To be considered for aid, patient must make application and supply a letter from a physician that includes diagnosis. Will provide more information upon request.

An American Cancer Society program where those who have had mastectomies and coped with them visit those who are recovering from recent breast surgery.

BOOKS

Alternatives, **Rose Kushner,** Kensington, MD: Kensington Press, 1984.

The American Cancer Society Cancer Book, New York: Doubleday & Co., 1986.

Brainstorm: A Personal Story, **Karen Osney Brownstein,** New York: Avon Books, 1981.

Cancer: A Patient's Guide, **Chris and Sue Williams,** New York: Wiley, 1986.

Children With Cancer: A Reference Guide for Parents, **Jeanne Munn Bracken,** New York: Oxford University Press, 1986.

A Child's Fight Against Leukemia, **Jonathan B. Tucker,** New York: Holt, Rinehart and Winston, 1982.

Choices: Realistic Alternatives in Cancer Treatment, **Marion Morra** and **Eve Potts,** New York: Avon Books, 1980.

Death Be Not Proud, **John Gunther,** New York: Perennial Library, 1949.

Foods That Fight Cancer, **Patricia Hausman,** New York: Rawson Associates, 1983.

Getting Well Again: A Step-by-Step, Self-Help Guide to Overcoming Cancer for Patients and Their Families, **O. C. Simonton** and **S. Matthews Simonton,** New York: St. Martin's Press, 1978.

The Healing Family: The Simonton Approach for Families Facing Illness, **Stephanie Matthews Simonton,** New York: Bantam Books, 1984.

I Am Whole Again: The Case for Breast Reconstruction After Mastectomy, **Jean Zalon** with **Jean Libman,** New York: Random House, 1978.

In the Company of Others, **Jory Graham,** New York: Harcourt Brace Jovanovich, 1982.

Living With Cancer, **Ernest Rosenbaum,** New York: New American Library, 1982.

Marvella: A Personal Journey, **Marvella Bayh** and **Mary Lynn Katz,** New York: Harcourt Brace Jovanovich, 1979.

We the Victors: Inspiring Stories of People Who Conquered Cancer and How They Did It, **Curtis Bill Pepper,** New York: Doubleday, 1984.

Why Me?, **Rose Kushner,** Philadelphia: E. B. Saunders Co., revised 1982. (breast cancer)

You Can Fight Cancer and Win, **Jane Brody** and **Arthur I. Holleb, M.D.,** New York: Times Books, 1977.

MATERIALS, FREE AND FOR SALE

Free (single copies)

The American Cancer Society also has numerous publications, including a full set of booklets on various types of cancers, including:
Facts on Bladder Cancer, 12 pages.

Facts on Bone Cancer, 12 pages.
Facts on Breast Cancer, 16 pages.
Facts on Cancer of the Brain, 14 pages.
Facts on Cancer of the Larynx, 12 pages.
Facts on Cancer Treatment, 18 pages.
Facts on Colorectal Cancer, 14 pages.

Facts on Leukemia, 14 pages.
Facts on Lung Cancer, 14 pages.
Facts on Ovarian Cancer, 8 pages.
Facts on Prostate Cancer, 10 pages.
Facts on Skin Cancer, 10 pages.
Facts on Stomach and Esophageal Cancers, 14
   pages.

American Cancer Society
90 Park Ave.
New York, NY 10016

*About Glioblastoma Multiforme and Malignant
   Astrocytoma*
About Medulloblastoma
About Meningiomas
About Shunts
Living With a Brain Tumor
A Primer of Brain Tumors, 40 pages,
   illustrated.
Radiation Therapy of Brain Tumors
Treatment of Brain Tumors, 50 pages,
   illustrated.
When Your Child is Ready to Return To School

Association for Brain Tumor Research
6232 N. Pulaski Rd., Suite 200
Chicago, IL 60646

*Fertility and Pregnancy Guide for DES
   Daughters and Sons*

DES Action
2845 24th St.
San Francisco, CA 94110

*Chemotherapy and You: A Guide to Self-Help
   During Treatment*, 30 pages.
*Decade of Discovery: Advances in Cancer
   Research, 1971–1981*, 74 pages.
*Diet and Nutrition: A Resource for Parents of
   Children With Cancer*, 58 pages.
*Eating Hints: Recipes and Tips for Better
   Nutrition During Cancer Treatment*, 86
   pages.
Hospital Days, Treatment Ways, coloring
   book.
*Questions and Answers About DES Exposure
   During Pregnancy and Before Birth*, 20
   pages.
*Radiation Therapy and You: A Guide to Self-
   Help During Treatment*, 24 pages.
Research Reports—a series of booklets:
   Bone Cancer and Other Sarcomas
   Bone Marrow Transplantation

Cancer of the Bladder
Cancer of the Colon and Rectum
Cancer of the Kidney
Cancer of the Lung
Cancer of the Prostate
Cancer of the Uterus
*Hodgkin's Disease and the Non-Hodgkin's
   Lymphomas*
Leukemia
Mesothelioma
Progress in Treatment of Testicular Cancer
*Taking Time: Support for People with Cancer
   and the People Who Care About Them*, 58
   pages.
*Were You or Your Daughter or Son Born After
   1940?* 20 pages, (DES) booklet.
What You Need to Know About Cancer
What You Need to Know About—a series of
   20-page booklets:
   Adult Leukemia
   Cancer of the Bladder
   Cancer of the Brain and Spinal Cord
   Cancer of the Breast
   Cancer of the Colon and Rectum
   Cancer of the Esophagus
   Cancer of the Kidney
   Cancer of the Larynx
   Cancer of the Lung
   Cancer of the Mouth
   Cancer of the Ovary
   Cancer of the Pancreas
   *Cancer of the Prostate and Other Male Geni-
      tourinary Organs*
   Cancer of the Skin
   Cancer of the Stomach
   Cancer of the Testis
   Cancer of the Uterus
   Cancers of the Bone
   Childhood Leukemia
   *Dysplasia, Very Early Cancer and Invasive
      Cancer of the Cervix*
   Hodgkin's Disease
   Melanoma
   Multiple Myeloma
   Non-Hodgkin's Lymphoma

National Cancer Institute
Office of Cancer Communications
Building 31, Room 10A18
Bethesda, Maryland 20892
(301) 496-5583 or (800) 638-6694

For sale

Candlelighters Foundation Bibliography and Resource Guide
Candlelighters Childhood Cancer Foundation Progress Reports:
Bone Marrow Transplantation in Childhood Cancer
When Your Child Has a Life-Threatening Illness

Candlelighters Childhood Cancer Foundation
2025 Eye St., N.W.
Washington, DC 20006

Audiocassette tapes

Also available from the National Cancer Institute:

Conversation After Mastectomy: 35 minutes. Roundtable discussion with four patients who have undergone mastectomies.

Help Yourself: Tips for Teenagers with Cancer: 40 minutes. Four radio-style stories designed to provide information and support for adolescents with cancer.

CEREBRAL PALSY

See also Mental Retardation, Learning and Developmental Disabilities, page 355 and Rehabilitation, page 460.

Cerebral palsy is the common name given to a cluster of disabling conditions caused by damage to the areas of the developing brain that control movement—the motor system. Often, the damage that affects motor coordination also affects other brain functions, sometimes causing seizures, loss of hearing or sight, or mental deficiencies.

Cerebral palsy ranges from damage so mild that a child is merely "awkward" to severe physical handicaps and mental retardation. Cerebral means brain; palsy means paralysis or lack of muscle control. An estimated 5,000 infants develop cerebral palsy every year, and there are approximately 750,000 Americans with cerebral palsy, one-third of them under age 21.

Cerebral palsy usually results from prenatal damage—often something that deprives the developing fetal brain of oxygen, but it can also be caused during or after birth, usually from head injuries. The incidence of some kinds of cerebral palsy has decreased in the past 25 years, partly because of development of a rubella (German measles) vaccine and the prevention of congenital brain dysfunction carried by RH blood factors. However, the increased ability to save premature and low-birth-weight babies is resulting in the survival of more preterm infants with damage to the central nervous system and cerebral palsy.

Cause: An undetermined percentage of the cases of cerebral palsy are caused by damage to the brain of the fetus during pregnancy, usually around the time of birth. The damage can result from infections, oxygen deprivation to the brain, RH blood factor, premature birth, or, very rarely, from a genetic defect such as Lesch-Nyhan syndrome. Cerebral palsy can also develop early in life (the first months or years) from accidental injury, physical child abuse, lead poisoning, or illness, for example, meningitis.

Symptoms: Cerebral palsy is often not detected at birth, but becomes evident as the child develops abnormally. Signs are poor muscle control, difficulty sucking, poor coordination, vision and hearing problems, and muscle spasms. There are three major types of cerebral palsy, depending on the limbs affected and type of motor disturbance. Spastic cerebral palsy, with stiff and difficult movement and a characteristic "scissors" gait, is the most common. A second type, athetoid cerebral palsy, is characterized by involuntary writhing movements, and jerky motions of the body; a third type, called ataxia, is characterized by loss of balance and coordination. There may also be problems with speaking, chewing, swallowing and hand tremors. Some youngsters have symptoms of more than one type. Cerebral palsy is not progressive.

Diagnosis: Parents often spot the signs of central nervous system malfunction and physical examinations by neurologists can confirm cerebral palsy. Special screening tests are used to detect developmental delay and to pinpoint newborn babies, especially the premature, who are at high risk for neurological disabilities like cerebral palsy.

Treatment: There is no cure for cerebral palsy, but it is important to diagnose it early, so the child can get the best care to lessen physical and emotional problems. Such early attention can help prevent changes in muscles, joints, and bones that could lead to serious complications, such as hip dislocation or curvature of the spine. It is especially important to detect hearing problems early so the child can develop normal speech. A child with cerebral palsy may need special surgery to help correct eye, ear and gait problems, and physical therapy and exercise programs; a cerebral palsied child with seizures may need anticonvulsive medication.

The person with cerebral palsy and the family may also need information on mechanical aids—such as special eyeglasses, hearing aids, walkers, and other helps for the disabled, as well as continuing data on special education programs, recreational facilities and vocational training. Some therapists have had remarkable successes with helping cerebral palsied youngsters gain control over their bodies through biofeedback training. Although children with cerebral palsy are atypical, most grow up able to walk and to speak understandably.

Much research is directed at ways to prevent and cure cerebral palsy, as well as at new bioengineering ways to improve the functioning of people who have it.

WHERE TO FIND TREATMENT FOR CEREBRAL PALSY

Neurologists are specialists who deal with cerebral palsy. For a list of leading neurologists who can help you find the proper medical facilities in your area, *see* page 621. *See also* Rehabilitation Centers that Specialize in Infant and Early Childhood Developmental Programs, page 357. Some of these facilities are operated by local Easter Seal Societies and United Cerebral Palsy affiliates.

For expert evaluation and assessment of a person with cerebral palsy, United Cerebral Palsy also recommends a network of centers, called University Affiliated Facilities (UAFs) or University Affiliated Programs (UAPs). (*See* page 366 for listing of centers.) These are federally supported centers located in major universities or medical schools. Some of the centers have specific areas of interest, but they also have multidisciplinary teams that can deal with the full scope of problems, including physical, medical, nutritional, speech, hearing, visual, educational, psychological, social, dental and vocational. They deal with children who have many different types of developmental problems, including cerebral palsy.

You can contact these centers directly, although they usually receive their clients through physician or health professional referral. To find out what special research or emphasis certain centers have you can contact:

American Association of University Affiliated
   Programs for Persons with Developmental
   Disabilities (AAUAP)
8605 Cameron St., Suite 406
Silver Spring, MD 20910
(301) 588-8252

ORGANIZATIONS

National Easter Seal Society, Inc.
2023 W. Ogden Ave.
Chicago, IL 60612
(312)-243-8400/voice
(312)-243-8880/TDD

A national organization with state and local societies formed to give services to people with disabilities from whatever cause, including epilepsy, cerebral palsy, stroke, speech and hearing disorders, geriatric problems, fractures, arthritis, learning and developmental disorders, heart disease, spina bifida, accidents, and multiple sclerosis. About 200 rehabilitation centers nationwide, with various services, depending upon the local unit. A major source of information and self-help. Pamphlets and booklets. Referrals to services are made through local Easter Seal affiliates listed in local phone directories. More information and the location of Easter Seal affiliates near you upon request.

United Cerebral Palsy
60 E. 34th St.
New York, NY 10016
(212) 481-6300, 6343

A nationwide voluntary health organization made up of state and local affiliates with a wide range of services for those with cerebral palsy and other handicaps. A major source of information for the public on cerebral palsy and handicaps. The extent of the services offered depends on the local affiliate, but often includes medical treatment, detection, care, education, psychological counseling, job training, recreational opportunities (camps, hobby groups, sports programs), residential facilities for independent living for older persons, home services, and respite care facilities to relieve parents of the constant care often demanded by the disabled. Pamphlets, booklets, bibliographies, newsletters, manuals. Supports research. Will provide more information and the name of an affiliate near you upon request.

Cerebral Palsy Sports

National Association of Sports for Cerebral
    Palsy, Inc.
66 E. 34th St.
New York, NY 10016
(212) 481-6359

National Association of Sports for Cerebral Palsy (NASCP), affiliated with the United Cerebral Palsy Association, sponsors sports events for all degrees of disabilities, from class I athletes (those with multiple disabilities who may be in wheelchairs), to class VIII, those with minimal handicaps who are ambulatory. The NASCP sends athletes with cerebral palsy to international sports competitions. Sports included: track and field, swimming, weight-lifting, archery, soccer, wheelchair soccer, boccia, riflery, bowling, and cycling. Publishes monthly magazine, *Sportsline,* and various sports manuals and training guides.

BOOKS

About Handicaps (cerebral palsy), **Sara Bonnet Stein,** New York: Walker and Co., 1974.

Care of the Neurologically Handicapped Child, **A. L. Prensky,** New York: Oxford University Press, 1982.

Coping with Cerebral Palsy: Answers to Questions Parents Often Ask, **Jay Schleichkorn, Ph.D.,** Baltimore: University Park Press, 1983.

Functional Aids for the Multiple Handicapped, **Isabel P. Robinault,** New York: United Cerebral Palsy Association, 1973.

Handling the Young Cerebral Palsied Child at Home, **Nancie R. Finnie,** New York: Dutton & Co., 1975.

Holistic Health Care for Children With Developmental Disabilities, **Una Haynes,** Baltimore: University Park Press, 1983.

Howie Helps Himself, 1975; a child with cerebral palsy achieves victory in a wheelchair. Pediatric Projects, Inc., PO Box 2175, Santa Monica, CA 90406.

Non-Vocal Communication Resource Book, **edited by Gregg C. Vanderheiden,** New York: United Cerebral Palsy Foundation, 1978; an inventory of devices, updated by subscription annually.

Program Guide for Infants and Toddlers with Neuromotor and Other Developmental Disabilities, **edited by Frances Connor, Gordon Williamson,** and **John M. Siepp,** New York: Teacher's College Press, c/o Harper & Row Publishers, 1978.

Training Guide to Cerebral Palsy Sports, New York: United Cerebral Palsy Association, 1984, (176-page paperback).

MATERIALS, FREE AND FOR SALE

Free (single copies)

Cerebral Palsy—Facts and Figures, fact sheet
"Four Letter Words" in the Dictionary of the Disabled

Life Can be Beautiful for People with Cerebral Palsy
What Everyone Should Know About Cerebral Palsy, 16 pages.

United Cerebral Palsy Association
66 E. 34th St.
New York, NY 10016
(212) 481-6300

Cerebral Palsy: Hope Through Research, 25
pages.

National Institute of Neurological and
Communicative Disorders and Stroke
9000 Rockville Pike
Bethesda, MD 20892

For sale

*The Doctor Talks to You About Cerebral
Palsy,* **Leon Sternfeld, M.D.** A 60-minute
audiocassette. Soundwords, Inc., 56-11
217th St., Bayside, NY 11364.

CYSTIC FIBROSIS

Cystic fibrosis is an inherited fatal disease affecting approximately 20,000 to 30,000 Americans. It shows up in one out of 2,000 newborns. It can be treated but not cured. Because of better diagnosis and management, the survival time of cystic fibrosis children has been significantly increased in recent years. In 1966, the average lifespan of a cystic fibrosis child was 11 years. Today about half of all cystic fibrosis infants will live to be age 21. It occurs in males and females equally.

Cystic fibrosis stems from an inborn error in metabolism that causes abnormalities in gland secretions—mucus, sweat and saliva—that in turn affect the functioning of the lungs, pancreas and sweat glands. The disease's main characteristic is the production of abnormally thick, sticky mucus that clogs and blocks the bodily channels, interfering with breathing and eventually destroying lung tissue.

Death almost always results from pulmonary complications, including drug-resistant infections, to which cystic fibrosis children are particularly susceptible. The mucus also blocks movement of digestive enzymes in the pancreas, interfering with digestion of fats and proteins. It is said that the condition both strangles and starves its victims.

Cause: Unknown at this time. In late 1985, investigators reported the chromosomal location of the gene that causes cystic fibrosis' metabolic defect, but the specific gene has not yet been identified. Until the specific cystic fibrosis gene is identified, there is no way to correct the error through genetic manipulation or other means.

Researchers do know that the disorder is transmitted by healthy people, called carriers, who do not exhibit symptoms of the illness themselves. About 10 million Americans carry the defective gene. If one parent is a carrier, a child will not inherit the disease, but half of the children will be carriers. When both parents are carriers, a child has a 25 percent chance of inheriting cystic fibrosis. There is no reliable method of detecting carriers in the general population; thus, genetic counseling cannot prevent cystic fibrosis.

Symptoms: The severity of the disorder varies greatly; some youngsters have such a mild form that it is not detected until long after birth. Symptoms generally include a chronic cough, difficulty breathing, susceptibility to serious respiratory problems, malnutrition, salty tasting skin (a sure clue), failure to grow and rounded ends of fingers and toes (clubbing). The illness has no effect on intelligence, motor skills, speech, or learning ability. The symptoms often appear at birth or within the first few months. Sometimes symptoms do not develop until adolescence.

Diagnosis: Most cases are diagnosed early, and this is important if the child is to get the best care to forestall lung damage. However, because the disorder mimics the symptoms of other diseases it is often misdiagnosed or undiagnosed; it can be mistaken for asthma, bronchitis, pneumonia, whooping cough or other respiratory diseases. The digestive malfunctions may be confused with those from celiac disease, a food malabsorption syndrome. The most telltale diagnostic sign of cystic fibrosis is an abnormally high amount of salt in the sweat. Parents often notice this, but it must be confirmed by a specific laboratory test. When cystic fibrosis is diagnosed, brothers, sisters and first cousins should also be screened with the sweat test. X-rays can detect lung damage, and an enzyme test can detect digestive blockage.

Treatment: Proper treatment will prolong a child's life and improve the quality of life. Many children do lead relatively normal, happy lives. Therapy is individualized, but is usually aimed at controlling respiratory infections, excessive salt loss and the pancreatic deficiencies that cause digestive dysfunction. Treatment calls for combating nutritional and digestive problems with dietary supplements, including vitamins and digestive enzymes to help break down foods. This can mean 40 to 60 pills daily. It is necessary to clear the lungs of mucus in order to prevent respiratory infections. This is done by chest physical therapy (postural drainage) several times a day, inhalation of aerosol medications and doses of antibiotics.

CYSTIC FIBROSIS CENTERS

The best place to get treatment and diagnosis is at one of the nation's cystic fibrosis centers. They are associated with leading hospitals and medical centers and offer a team of specialists—physicians, nurses, respiratory therapists, genetic counselors, nutritionists, and social workers—who work together to care for both the physical and the psychological aspects of this terminal disease. Families find other youngsters and families who face similar problems at these centers. This mutual support can prove invaluable, especially since youngsters may require hospitalization for a couple of weeks at a time.

ALABAMA
The Children's Hospital
University of Alabama, Birmingham
1600 Seventh Ave., S.
Birmingham, AL 35233
(205) 939-9583
Center Director: Ralph E. Tiller, M.D.

University of South Alabama Cystic Fibrosis
    Center
USA Children's Specialty Center
Health Services Building
307 University Blvd., Room 101-D
Mobile, AL 36689
(205) 460-7100
Center Director: Robert O. Harris, III, M.D.

ARIZONA
Cystic Fibrosis Center
Phoenix Children's Hospital
909 E. Brill St.
Phoenix, AZ 85006
(602) 239-4350
Center Director: Lucy S. Hernried, M.D.

Tucson Cystic Fibrosis Center
St. Luke's Chest Clinic
Arizona Health Sciences Center
Tucson, AZ 85724
(602) 626-7450
Center Director: Richard J. Lemen, M.D.

ARKANSAS
Arkansas Cystic Fibrosis Center
Arkansas Children's Hospital
804 Wolfe St.
Little Rock, AR 72202
(501) 370-1018
Center Director: Robert H. Warren, M.D.

CALIFORNIA
Cedars-Sinai Medical Center
Cystic Fibrosis Center
8700 Beverly Blvd.
Los Angeles, CA 90048
(213) 855-4421
Center Director: Benjamin M. Kagan, M.D.

Cystic Fibrosis Care, Teaching and Resource
    Center
Children's Hospital of Los Angeles
University of Southern California Medical
    School
4650 Sunset Blvd.
Los Angeles, CA 90027
(213) 669-2287
Center Director: Chun-I Wang, M.D.

Department of Pediatrics
UCLA School of Medicine
The Center for Health Sciences
10833 Le Conte Ave.
Los Angeles, CA 90024
(213) 825-6777
Center Director: E. Richard Stiehm, M.D.

Pediatric Pulmonary Center
Children's Hospital Medical Center
747 52nd St.
Oakland, CA 94609
(415) 428-3305
Center Director: Herman W. Lipow, M.D.

Cystic Fibrosis and Pediatric Pulmonary Care,
    Teaching, and Resource Center
Childrens Hospital of Orange County
455 S. Main St.
Orange, CA 92668
(714) 532-8624
Center Director: Ralph W. Rucker, M.D.

Pediatric Pulmonary Disease Center
Children's Hospital at Stanford
520 Sand Hill Rd.
Palo Alto, CA 94304
(415) 327-4800, x292
Center Director: Norman J. Lewiston, M.D.

Cystic Fibrosis and Pediatric Respiratory
    Diseases Center
University of California at Davis School of
    Medicine
Department of Pediatrics
4301 X St.
Sacramento, CA 95817
(916) 453-3189
Center Director: Geoffrey Kurland, M.D.

Brian Wesley Ray CF Center
San Bernardino County Medical Center
780 E. Gilbert St.
San Bernardino, CA 92415-0935
(714) 383-1654, 3216
Center Director: Richard R. Dooley, M.D.

San Diego Cystic Fibrosis and Pediatric
    Pulmonary Disease Center
University Hospital
225 W. Dickinson St.
San Diego, CA 92103
(619) 294-6810
Center Director: Ivan R. Harwood, M.D.

Cystic Fibrosis Center
Kaiser Permanente Medical Group
2200 O'Farrell St.
San Francisco, CA 94115
(415) 929-5030
Center Director: Avghi M. Thunstrom, M.D.

Cystic Fibrosis Center
University of California at San Francisco
Room M687
Third and Parnassus Ave.
San Francisco, CA 94143
(415) 666-2072
Center Director: Brian Davis, M.D.

COLORADO
University of Colorado
Health Science Center
4200 E. Ninth Ave., C220
Denver, CO 80262
(303) 394-7518
Center Director: Ernest K. Cotton, M.D.

CONNECTICUT
Cystic Fibrosis Center
St. Francis Hospital and Medical Center
114 Woodland St.
Hartford, CT 06105
(203) 548-4355
Center Director: Michelle M. Cloutier, M.D.

Cystic Fibrosis Center
Yale University School of Medicine
333 Cedar St.
New Haven, CT 06510
(203) 785-2480
Center Director: Thomas F. Dolan, Jr., M.D.

DELAWARE
Wilmington Medical Center
501 W. 14th St. (P.O. Box 1668)
Wilmington, DE 19899
(302) 428-2662
Center Director: Elizabeth M. Craven, M.D.

DISTRICT OF COLUMBIA
Metropolitan D.C. Cystic Fibrosis Center for
    Care, Training and Research
Children's Hospital National Medical Center
111 Michigan Ave., N.W.
Washington, DC 20010
(202) 745-2128, 2129
Center Director: Robert J. Fink, M.D.

Georgetown University Pediatric Pulmonary
    and Cystic Fibrosis Center
Georgetown University Hospital
3800 Reservoir Rd., N.W.
Washington, DC 20007
(202) 625-7727, 7015
Center Director: Lucas L. Kulczycki, M.D.

FLORIDA

Cystic Fibrosis and Pediatric Pulmonary
  Disease Center
University of Florida
Shands Teaching Hospital
Box J-296, Hillis Miller Health Center
Gainesville, FL 32610
(904) 392-4458
Center Director: Sarah E. Chesrown, M.D.

Pediatric Pulmonary and Cystic Fibrosis Center
Baptist Medical Center
800 Prudential Drive
Jacksonville, FL 32207
(904) 393-2829
Center Director: Walter C. Kelly, M.D.

Cystic Fibrosis Center
Department of Pediatrics
School of Medicine
PO Box 016820 D820
Miami, FL 33101
(305) 547-6641
Center Director: Robert M. McKey, Jr., M.D.

Cystic Fibrosis Center
Orlando Regional Medical Center
1404 S. Kuhl Ave.
Orlando, FL 32806
(305) 841-5111, x5628
Center Director: Norman A. Helfrich, Jr.,
  M.D.

Cystic Fibrosis Center
Children's Health Center
800 Sixth St., S.
St. Petersburg, FL 33701
(813) 893-2775
Center Director: Jorge S. Vidal, M.D.

GEORGIA

Cystic Fibrosis Care, Teaching and Research
  Center
Emory University School of Medicine
69 Butler St., S.E.
Atlanta, GA 30303
(404) 589-4380
Center Director: Daniel B. Caplan, M.D.

Department of Pediatrics
Section of Pulmonology
Medical College of Georgia
Augusta, GA 30912
(404) 838-4723
Center Director: Karl H. Karlson, Jr., M.D.

IDAHO

Mercy Medical Center
Cystic Fibrosis Center
1512 12th Avenue Rd.
Nampa, ID 83651
(208) 467-1171, x163
Center Director: Eugene M. Brown, M.D.

ILLINOIS

Cystic Fibrosis Center
Children's Memorial Hospital
Northwestern University
2300 Children's Plaza
Chicago, IL 60614
(312) 880-4354
Center Director: John D. Lloyd-Still, M.D.

Pediatric Pulmonary Center
Rush Medical School
Rush–Presbyterian–St. Luke's Medical School
1753 W. Congress Parkway
Chicago, IL 60612
(312) 942-3060
Center Director: Lewis E. Gibson, M.D.

Wyler Children's Hospital
Department of Pediatrics
University of Chicago School of Medicine
Box 133
5841 S. Maryland Ave.
Chicago, IL 60637
(312) 962-6178
Center Director: Lucille A. Lester, M.D.

Cystic Fibrosis Center
Saint Francis Medical Center
Specialty Center
530 N.B. Glen Oak Ave.
Peoria, IL 61603
(309) 672-2745
Center Director: Umesh C. Chatrath, M.D.

INDIANA

Cystic Fibrosis & Chronic Pulmonary Disease
  Clinic
Elkhart General Hospital
PO Box 201
Elkhart, IN 46515
(219) 293-7731
Center Director: Orest Dubynsky, M.D.

Cystic Fibrosis and Pediatric Pulmonary
  Disease Center
Deaconess Hospital
600 Mary St.
Evansville, IN 47747
(812) 426-3455
Center Director: Daniel E. Michel, M.D.

Cystic Fibrosis and Chronic Pulmonary
  Disease Center
Riley Hospital for Children
Indiana University Medical Center
702 Barnhill Drive, Room 293
Indianapolis, IN 46223
(317) 264-7208
Center Director: Howard Eigen, M.D.

Cystic Fibrosis Center
Children's Hospital
Methodist Hospital of Indiana, Inc.
1604 N. Capitol Ave.
Indianapolis, IN 46202
(317) 929-3633
Center Director: Gabriel J. Rosenberg, M.D.

Cystic Fibrosis and Chronic Pulmonary
  Disease Clinic
St. Joseph's Medical Center
811 E. Madison
South Bend, IN 46634
(219) 234-9555
Center Director: Edward A. Gergesha, M.D.

IOWA
Cystic Fibrosis Clinic
Iowa Methodist Medical Center
1200 Pleasant St.
Des Moines, IA 50309
(515) 283-6152
Clinic Director: Veljko Zivkovich, M.D.

Cystic Fibrosis Center
Pediatric Allergy and Pulmonary Division
Department of Pediatrics
University of Iowa Hospitals and Clinics
Iowa City, IA 52242
(319) 356-3485
Center Director: Miles Weinberger, M.D.

KANSAS
Cystic Fibrosis Center
University of Kansas Medical Center
39th St. at Rainbow Blvd.
Kansas City, KS 66103
(913) 588-6377
Center Director: Joseph Kanarek, M.D.

Cystic Fibrosis Care and Teaching Center
St. Joseph Medical Center
3600 E. Harry
Wichita, KS 67218
(316) 689-4707
Center Director: Leonard L. Sullivan, M.D.

KENTUCKY
Cystic Fibrosis Center
Department of Pediatrics
Room C-410, C-415
University of Kentucky Medical Center
800 Rose Street
Lexington, KY 40536-0843
(606) 233-8023
Center Director: Jamshed F. Kanga, M.D.

Louisville Children's Chest Center
University of Louisville
Kosair Children's Hospital
200 E. Chestnut St.
Louisville, KY 40202
(502) 562-8830
Center Director: Garrett Adams, M.D.,
  M.P.H.

LOUISIANA
New Orleans Pediatric Pulmonary Center
Department of Pediatrics
Tulane University School of Medicine
1430 Tulane Ave.
New Orleans, LA 70112
(504) 588-5601
Center Director: William W. Waring, M.D.

Cystic Fibrosis Pediatric Pulmonary Center
Louisiana State University Medical Center
School of Medicine in Shreveport
1501 King's Highway
PO Box 33932
Shreveport, LA 71130-3932
(318) 674-6094
Center Director: Bettina C. Hilman, M.D.

MAINE
Cystic Fibrosis Clinical Center
Eastern Maine Medical Center
489 State St.
Bangor, ME 04401
(207) 947-8311
Center Director: Erlinda A. Polvorosa, M.D.

Central Maine Cystic Fibrosis Center
Central Maine Medical Center
300 Main St.
Lewiston, ME 04240
(207) 795-2830
Center Director: Gilbert R. Grimes, M.D.

Cystic Fibrosis Center
Maine Medical Center
22 Bramhall St.
Portland, ME 04102
(207) 871-2763
Center Director: Martin A. Barron, Jr., M.D.

MARYLAND
The John Hopkins Hospital
CMSC-149
600 N. Wolfe St.
Baltimore, MD 21205
(301) 955-2795
Center Director: Beryl J. Rosenstein, M.D.

Cystic Fibrosis Center
National Institute of Diabetes, Digestive and
  Kidney Diseases
National Institutes of Health
Building 10, Room 9048
Bethesda, MD 20892
(301) 496-3434
Center Director: Milica S. Chernick, M.D.

MASSACHUSETTS
Cystic Fibrosis Center
Children's Hospital Medical Center
300 Longwood Ave.
Boston, MA 02115
(617) 735-6051
Center Director: Harvey R. Colten, M.D.

Cystic Fibrosis Center
Massachusetts General Hospital
ACC 609
15 Parkman St.
Boston, MA 02114
(617) 726-8707, 8708
Center Director: Allen Lapey, M.D.

Cystic Fibrosis Center
Tufts New England Medical Center Hospitals,
  Inc.
Box 343
171 Harrison Avenue
Boston, MA 02111
(617) 956-5085
Center Director: Henry L. Dorkin, M.D.

Baystate Medical Center
Wesson Memorial Unit
140 High St.
Springfield, MA 01105
(413) 787-2515
Center Director: Robert S. Gerstle, M.D.

MICHIGAN
University of Michigan
Cystic Fibrosis Center
Mott Hospital
F2826, Box 66
Ann Arbor, MI 48109-0010
(313) 763-2567
Center Director: William F. Howatt, M.D.

Cystic Fibrosis Center
Harper-Grace Hospitals
3990 John R. St.
Detroit, MI 48201
(313) 494-6673
Director: Patricia Lynne-Davies, M.D.

Cystic Fibrosis Center
Henry Ford Hospital
2799 W. Grand Blvd.
Detroit, MI 48202
(313) 876-2439
Director: Paul A. Kvale, M.D.

Cystic Fibrosis Center
Sinai Hospital of Detroit
6767 W. Outer Drive
Detroit, MI 48235-2899
(313) 493-6824
Director: Alvaro Skupin, M.D.

Cystic Fibrosis Care, Teaching and Resource
  Center
Children's Hospital of Michigan
Wayne State University Medical School
3901 Beaubien Blvd.
Detroit, MI 48201
(313) 494-5541
Center Director: Robert Wilmott, M.D.

CF Center
Mott Children's Health Center
806 Tuuri Place
Flint, MI 48503
(313) 767-5750, x303
Center Director: Frederick S. Lim, M.D.

Cystic Fibrosis Center
Butterworth Hospital
100 Michigan Street, N.E.
Grand Rapids, MI 49503
(616) 774-1898
Center Director: Lawrence E. Kurlandsky,
  M.D.

Greater Lansing Cystic Fibrosis Center
Ingham Medical Center
401 W. Greenlawn
Lansing, MI 48910
(517) 355-4726
Center Director: Richard E. Honicky, M.D.

MINNESOTA
University of Minnesota
Minneapolis, MN 55455
(612) 373-8886
Center Director: Warren J. Warwick, M.D.

Cystic Fibrosis Center
Mayo Foundation
200 First St., S.W.
Rochester, MN 55905
(507) 284-2091
Center Director: Edward J. O'Connell, M.D.

MISSISSIPPI
University of Mississippi Medical Center
2500 N. State St.
Jackson, MS 39216-4505
(601) 984-5205
Center Director: Suzanne T. Miller, M.D.

MISSOURI
Columbia Cystic Fibrosis, Pediatric Pulmonary
  and Gastrointestinal Center
University of Missouri Medical Center
Department of Child Health
One Hospital Drive
Columbia, MO 65212
(314) 882-6921
Center Director: Calvin Woodruff, M.D.

The Children's Mercy Hospital
University of Missouri, Kansas City of School
  of Medicine
24th and Gillham Rd.
Kansas City, MO 64108
(816) 234-3015
Center Director: V. F. Burry, M.D.

Cystic Fibrosis, Pediatric Pulmonary and
  Pediatric Gastrointestinal Center
Cardinal Glennon Memorial Hospital for
  Children
St. Louis University School of Medicine
1465 S. Grand Blvd.
St. Louis, MO 63104
(314) 865-4002
Center Director: Anthony J. Rejent, M.D.

St. Louis Children's Hospital
Washington University School of Medicine
400 S. Kingshighway
St. Louis, MO 63178
(314) 454-6173
Center Director: Robert J. Rothbaum, M.D.

NEBRASKA
Omaha Center for Cystic Fibrosis and Pediatric
  Pulmonary Diseases
University of Nebraska Hospital
42nd and Dewey Ave.
Omaha, NE 68105
(402) 559-6275
Center Director: John L. Colombo, M.D.

NEW HAMPSHIRE
New Hampshire Cystic Fibrosis Care and
  Teaching Center
c/o Mary Hitchcock Memorial Hospital
2 Maynard St.
Hanover, NH 03576
(603) 271-4513
Center Director: William E. Boyle, M.D.

New Hampshire Cystic Fibrosis Care and
  Teaching Center
Catholic Medical Center
100 McGregor St.
Manchester, NH 03103
(603) 668-1212
Center Director: Robert A. Joy, M.D.

NEW JERSEY
Cystic Fibrosis Center
Hackensack Medical Center
32 Prospect Ave.
Hackensack, NJ 07601
(201) 342-0922
Center Director: Lawrence J. Denson, M.D.

Cystic Fibrosis and Chronic Pulmonary
  Disease Center
Monmouth Medical Center
307 Third Ave.
Long Branch, NJ 07740
(201) 870-5106
Center Director: Ronald I. Platt, M.D.

Cystic Fibrosis Center
Morristown Memorial Hospital
Madison Ave.
Morristown, NJ 07960
(201) 540-5234
Center Director: Bayard Coggeshall, M.D.

NEW MEXICO
University of New Mexico
School of Medicine
Department of Pediatrics
Albuquerque, NM 87131
(505) 277-5551
Center Director: Shirley Murphy, M.D.

NEW YORK
Pediatric Pulmonary and Cystic Fibrosis Center
Albany Medical College of Union University
Department of Pediatrics, A108
47 New Scotland Ave.
Albany, NY 12208
(518) 445-5057
Center Director: Glenna B. Winnie, M.D.

Long Island College Hospital
340 Henry St.
Brooklyn, NY 11201
(718) 780-1025, 1026
Center Director: Daniel Mayer, M.D.

Children's Lung Center
Children's Hospital of Buffalo
State University of New York at Buffalo
219 Bryant St.
Buffalo, NY 14222
(716) 878-7524
Center Director: Gerd J. A. Cropp, M.D.,
  PR.D.

United Health Services
33 Harrison St.
Johnson City, NY 13790
(607) 770-6159
Center Director: John A. Manzari, M.D.

North Shore University Hospital
300 Community Drive
Manhasset, NY 11030
(516) 562-4641
Center Director: Laura S. Inselman, M.D.

Cystic Fibrosis and Pediatric Pulmonary Center
Long Island Jewish–Hillside Medical Center
Health Science Center
State University of New York at Stony Brook
New Hyde Park, NY 11042
(718) 470-3250
Center Director: Jack D. Gorvoy, M.D

Pediatric Pulmonary Center
Babies Hospital and Columbia University
  College of Physicians and Surgeons
630 W. 168th St.
New York, NY 10032
(212) 305-5122
Center Director: Robert B. Mellins, M.D.

Cystic Fibrosis and Pediatric Pulmonary Center
Mount Sinai Medical Center
One Gustave L. Levy Place
Fifth Ave. at 100th St.
New York, NY 10029
(212) 650-7788
Center Director: Richard J. Bonforte, M.D.

Cystic Fibrosis, Pediatric Pulmonary and
  Gastrointestinal Center
St. Vincent's Hospital and Medical Center of
  New York
36 Seventh Ave., Suite 509
New York, NY 10011
(212) 790-8899
Center Director: Carolyn R. Denning, M.D.

Strong Memorial Hospital
Box 667
Department of Pediatrics
University of Rochester School of Medicine
  and Dentistry
601 Elmwood Ave.
Rochester, NY 14642
(716) 275-5611
Center Director: John J. McBride, M.D.

Robert C. Schwartz Cystic Fibrosis Center
State University Hospital
Upstate Medical Center
750 E. Adams St.
Syracuse, NY 13210
(315) 473-5834
Center Director: Phillip T. Swender, M.D.

Cystic Fibrosis Center
Westchester Medical Center
New York Medical College
Valhalla, NY 10595
(914) 631-3283
Center Director: Armond V. Mascia, M.D.

Cystic Fibrosis Center
House of The Good Samaritan Hospital
830 Washington St.
Watertown, NY 13601
(315) 785-4072
Center Director: Ronald G. Perciaccante, M.D.

Cystic Fibrosis Clinical Center
Good Samaritan Hospital
1000 Montauk Highway
West Islip, NY 11795
(516) 957-4092
Center Director: Walter J. O'Connor, M.D.

NORTH CAROLINA
U.N.C. Cystic Fibrosis Center
University of North Carolina
School of Medicine/N.C. Memorial Hospital
Chapel Hill, NC 27514
(919) 966-1001
Center Director: Gerald W. Fernald, M.D.

Cystic Fibrosis and Pediatric Pulmonary Center
Duke University Medical Center
PO Box 2994
Durham, NC 27710
(919) 681-3402 or 684-3364
Center Director: Alexander Spock, M.D.

NORTH DAKOTA
Cystic Fibrosis Center
St. Alexius Hospital
9th and Thayer St.
Bismarck, ND 58501
(701) 224-7500
Center Director: Margaret E. Morgan, M.D.

OHIO
Pediatric Pulmonary Center
Children's Hospital Medical Center of Akron
281 Locust St.
Akron, OH 44308
(216) 379-8530
Center Director: Robert S. Stone, M.D.

The Children's Hospital Medical Center
Chest-CF Division
Department of Pediatrics
Bethesda at Elland Ave.
Cincinnati, OH 45229
(513) 559-4511
Center Director: Frank W. Kellogg, M.D.

Cystic Fibrosis and Pediatric Pulmonary
    Institute and Center
Rainbow Babies and Children's Hospital
Case Western Reserve University
2101 Adelbert Rd.
Cleveland, OH 44106
(216) 844-3269
Center Director: Carl F. Doershuk, M.D.

Children's Hospital
700 Children's Drive
Columbus, OH 43205
(614) 461-2216
Center Director: Gordon A. Young, M.D.

Pediatric Pulmonary Center
Children's Medical Center
One Children's Plaza
Dayton, OH 45404-1815
(513) 226-8376
Center Director: Martha N. Franz, M.D.

Northwest Ohio Cystic Fibrosis and Pediatric
    Pulmonary Center
The Toledo Hospital
2142 N. Cove Blvd.
Toledo, OH 43608
(419) 471-4549
Center Director: Pierre A. Vauthy, M.D.

OKLAHOMA
Cystic Fibrosis-Pediatric Pulmonary Center
Oklahoma Children's Memorial Hospital
University of Oklahoma Health Science Center
940 N.E. 13th St.
Oklahoma City, OK 73190
(405) 271-6390
Center Director: Owen Rennert, M.D.

Tulsa Ambulatory Pediatric Center
2815 S. Sheridan Rd.
Tulsa, OK 74129
(918) 749-6458
Center Director: John C. Kramer, M.D.

OREGON
Cystic Fibrosis Care, Teaching and Research
  Center
University of Oregon Medical School
3181 S.W. Sam Jackson Park Rd.
Portland, OR 97201
(503) 225-8023
Center Director: Michael Wall, M.D.

PENNSYLVANIA
Cystic Fibrosis Center
Polyclinic Medical Center
Third and Polyclinic Ave.
Harrisburg, PA 17110
(717) 232-9774
Center Director: James E. Jones, M.D.

Cystic Fibrosis and Pediatric Pulmonary Center
Hahnemann Medical College and Hospital
230 N. Broad St.
Philadelphia, PA 19102
(215) 448-7766
Center Director: Douglas S. Holsclaw, Jr.,
  M.D.

St. Christopher's Hospital for Children
Temple University School of Medicine
5th St. and Lehigh Ave.
Philadelphia, PA 19133
(215) 427-5183
Director: Daniel V. Schidlow, M.D.

Cystic Fibrosis Center for Care, Teaching and
  Research
Children's Hospital of Philadelphia
University of Pennsylvania School of Medicine
34th and Civic Center Blvd.
Philadelphia, PA 19104
(215) 596-9582
Center Director: Thomas F. Scanlin, M.D.

Cystic Fibrosis Center
Children's Hospital of Pittsburgh
University of Pittsburgh Medical School
3705 Fifth Ave. at DeSoto St.
Pittsburgh, PA 15213
(412) 647-5630
Center Director: David M. Orenstein, M.D.

PUERTO RICO
Cystic Fibrosis Care and Teaching Center
University of Puerto Rico Medical Sciences
  Campus
GPO Box 5067
Rio Piedras, PR 00936
(809) 763-4966
Center Director: Pedro M. Mayol, M.D.

RHODE ISLAND
Cystic Fibrosis Center
Rhode Island Hospital
593 Eddy St.
Providence, RI 02902
(401) 277-5685
Center Director: Mary Ann Passero, M.D.

SOUTH CAROLINA
Cystic Fibrosis Center
Medical University of South Carolina
171 Ashley Ave.
Charleston, SC 29425
(803) 792-3561
Center Director: Margaret Q. Jenkins, M.D.

Cystic Fibrosis Clinical Center
Ambulatory Care Center
701 Grove Rd.
Greenville, SC 29605
(803) 242-6160, x296
Center Co-Directors: Thomas Tiller, M.D.
  Fred Laffert, M.D.

SOUTH DAKOTA
South Dakota Cystic Fibrosis Center
Sioux Valley Hospital
1100 S. Euclid Ave.
Sioux Falls, SD 57117-5039
(605) 333-7189
Center Director: Guy A. Carter, M.D.

TENNESSEE
Memphis Cystic Fibrosis Center
LeBonheur Children's Medical Center
University of Tennessee Center for the Health
  Sciences
One Children's Plaza
Memphis, TN 38103
(901) 522-3302
Center Director: Philip George, M.D.

Vanderbilt University Medical Center
C-1200 Medical Center N.
Nashville, TN 37232
(615) 322-2244
Center Director: William D. Donald, M.D.

TEXAS
Cystic Fibrosis Care, Teaching and Research
  Center
Children's Medical Center
1935 Amelia St., Room 316
Dallas, TX 75235
(214) 920-2361
Center Director: Robert I. Kramer, M.D.

Cystic Fibrosis Center
Cook Children's Hospital
1212 W. Lancaster
Fort Worth, TX 76102
(817) 336-5521, x278
Center Director: William Wheeler, M.D.

Cystic Fibrosis Center
Department of Pediatrics
Baylor College of Medicine
One Baylor Plaza
Houston, TX 77030
(713) 665-3312
Center Director: Daniel K. Seilheimer, M.D.

Cystic Fibrosis Center
Santa Rosa Children's Hospital
University of Texas Health Science Center at
  San Antonio
519 W. Houston St.
San Antonio, TX 78207
(512) 271-0321
Center Director: Ricardo Pinero, M.D.

UTAH
Intermountain Cystic Fibrosis Pediatric
  Gastrointestinal Center
Department of Pediatrics
University of Utah Medical Center
50 N. Medical Drive
Salt Lake City, UT 84132
(801) 581-8227
Center Director: Philip Black, M.D.

VERMONT
Cystic Fibrosis and Pediatric Pulmonary Center
Medical Center Hospital of Vermont
University of Vermont
52 Timber Lane
South Burlington, VT 05401
(802) 658-2320
Center Director: Donald R. Swartz, M.D.

VIRGINIA
Cystic Fibrosis Care, Teaching and Research
  Center
University of Virginia
School of Medicine
Charlottesville, VA 22908
(804) 924-2613
Center Director: Robert F. Selden, Jr., M.D.

Eastern Virginia Medical School
Children's Hospital of the King's Daughters
800 W. Olney Rd.
Norfolk, VA 23507
(804) 628-7238
Center Director: Thomas Rubio, M.D.

Cystic Fibrosis Program
Medical College of Virginia
Box 271, MCV Station
Richmond, VA 23298
(804) 786-9445
Center Director: David A. Draper, M.D.

WASHINGTON
Pulmonary Disease and Cystic Fibrosis Center
Children's Orthopedic Hospital and Medical
  Center
PO Box C5371
Seattle, WA 98105
(206) 526-2024
Center Director: Bonnie W. Ramsey, M.D.

Pediatric Pulmonary and Cystic Fibrosis Center
Deaconess Hospital
W. 800 Fifth Ave.
Spokane, WA 99204
(509) 458-7300
Center Director: Michael M. McCarthy, M.D.

WEST VIRGINIA
Cystic Fibrosis Center for Care, Teaching and
  Research
West Virginia University Medical Center
Morgantown, WV 26506
(304) 293-4452
Center Director: Henry L. Abrons, M.D.

WISCONSIN
University of Wisconsin
Cystic Fibrosis/Pediatric Pulmonary Center
Clinical Sciences Center—H4/430
600 Highland Ave.
Madison, WI 53792
(608) 263-8555
Center Director: Elaine Mischler, M.D.

Children's Hospital of Wisconsin
Medical College of Wisconsin
1700 W. Wisconsin Ave.
Milwaukee, WI 53233
(414) 931-1010, x4352
Center Director: W. Theodore Bruns, M.D.

SOURCE: *Cystic Fibrosis Foundation.*

ORGANIZATION

The Cystic Fibrosis Foundation
6000 Executive Blvd., Suite 510
Rockville, MD 20852
(301) 881-9130
(800) Fight CF

A nationwide nonprofit, voluntary health organization, dedicated to improving the outlook for cystic fibrosis patients and their families. Supports basic research to find the cause, treatment and cure for cystic fibrosis. Has 64 state and local chapters, where families can find mutual support and guidance. Helps maintain the centers for health care to cystic fibrosis patients throughout the country at major medical centers. Publishes a quarterly newsletter and numerous brochures on all aspects of cystic fibrosis. Will provide more information and the name of a local chapter near you upon request.

BOOKS

Alex: The Life of a Child, **Frank Deford,** New York: Viking, 1983.
CF in His Corner, **Gail Radley,** New York: Four Winds Press, 1984.
Child in a White Fog, **Jann D. Jansen,** New York: Vantage Press, 1982.

Faith, Hope and Luck, a Sociological Study of Children Growing up with a Lifethreatening Illness, **Charles Waddell,** Washington: University Press of America, 1983.
The Time of Her Life, **Meg Woodson,** Grand Rapids, MI: Zondervan Publishing, 1982.

FREE MATERIALS

Single copies are free

The Commitment, a quarterly newsletter.
Cystic Fibrosis Facts and Figures, 32 pages, updated yearly.
Cystic Fibrosis: Questions Frequently Asked by Parents, 14 pages.
The Genetics of Cystic Fibrosis, 8 pages.
Living With Cystic Fibrosis: A Guide for Adolescents, 12 pages.
Research Highlights, 1982–1983

Cystic Fibrosis Foundation
6000 Executive Blvd., Suite 309
Rockville, MD 20852
(301) 881-9130

Cystic Fibrosis: The Puzzle and the Promise, 10 pages.

National Institute of Diabetes, Digestive and Kidney Diseases
9000 Rockville Pike
Building 31, Room 9A04
Bethesda, MD 20892
(301) 496-3583

DEPRESSION

Depression is so widespread that it is frequently called the "common cold" of mental illness. Often the symptoms are mild and recovery swift. But for 5 percent of the population, the depression is deep and lingering, what experts call a "major depression." Most susceptible are young adults between the ages of 18 and 24. Women of all ages are about twice as likely as men to be victims of a major depression. The illness can be devastating, disrupting family and work life and sometimes leading to suicide. About 30,000 Americans commit suicide every year, an increasing number of them children and young adults.

Fortunately, because of new diagnoses, treatments and understanding of the biological causes of the disorder, depression is one of the most effectively treated mental disorders. However, many cases go undiagnosed and untreated. According to one study, only one-fourth of all victims of major depression seek professional help.

Doctors usually distinguish between two main types of major depression: "unipolar" depression, which comes in a single episode or recurs intermittently with normal or near-normal states of mind; and "bipolar," or classic manic-depression, in which deep lows alternate with severe or mild highs. The more common unipolar depression usually comes on in midlife, although new evidence shows it is increasingly occurring in younger adults. It accounts for about 90 percent of the cases of major depression. Manic-depressives usually have their first episodes in their twenties. Unipolar depression is more commonly diagnosed in women, although there is some evidence that such depression is declining in middle-aged women; manic-depression shows up in both sexes equally. Both types of depression can be extremely serious; contrary to common belief, unipolar depression is not a less severe disorder than bipolar or manic-depression.

Cause: Like many other mental and physical conditions, depression is regarded as not one illness, but a constellation of disorders, ranging in type and severity. Doctors believe depression almost always has a combination of psychological and physical causes. For example, it may be brought on by an event, such as a death in the family, but the fact that it persists to become a major debilitating depression may be due to biological factors.

There is growing and compelling evidence that the susceptibility to depression, primarily manic-depression, is inherited. Studies show that those who have inherited a specific abnormality in brain-chemical processing may be more susceptible to major depression and other mood disorders, alcoholism, and drug abuse. In other words, bipolar depression does run in families; new research suggests that one-third of those with manic-depression may have inherited a biological susceptibility. This does not mean that depression is entirely a biological disorder. Even in susceptible individuals, experts believe that an episode of depression is triggered by severe psychological or physical stress.

Some researchers also believe that one subtype of unipolar depression is related to a kind of malfunctioning of the biological clock. Additionally, there is considerable evidence that some depressed persons have a dramatic reaction to the amount of sunlight available. Shorter days of sunlight and longer periods of darkness in winter send some people into deep depression. One researcher estimates that for every person who suffers a major depression from light-deprivation, there may be 10 others who go into less severe depressions for the same reason. Certain drugs—including some blood pressure medications, cortisone, alcohol, barbiturates and estrogen—can bring on depression in some persons, often those with a past personal or family history of depression.

Symptoms: Symptoms of major depression include sleep and appetite disturbance, loss of energy, reduced sexual drive—a physical and mental slowing down. Loss of self-esteem, guilt, self-blame, and recurrent thoughts of death and suicide are common. There is a significant loss of ability to function normally and loss of interest or pleasure in almost all usual activities. To be classified as major depression, such symptoms must last at least two weeks, but generally they persist for months.

Diagnosis: Doctors can usually detect depression by interviewing a person. Biochemical tests are being developed that provide great promise in detecting those who are at risk for major depression, but none has been sufficiently tested or yet proved totally reliable. Some experts do use biochemical tests in confirming a diagnosis, but still rely most heavily on a clinical examination. It is especially important to look for depression in elderly people. Sometimes their depression is mistaken for neurological diseases, such as Alzheimer's disease.

Treatment: The past few years have seen a revolution in the treatment of depression, so much so that most people, although not technically cured, can function normally thanks to various kinds of therapies, including short-term psychotherapy and drug therapy. It is estimated that about 90 percent of all depression can be effectively treated. Unquestionably, the drug of choice for effectively controlling manic-depression is lithium, a potent drug that prevents the up-and-down mood cycles.

Drugs are also used to treat unipolar major depressions. Lithium is sometimes used, but more common are the so-called tricyclic antidepressants. It usually takes at least two weeks for the antidepressants to take effect. These drugs are reportedly effective in warding off future bouts of depression in about two-thirds of those with unipolar depression. The drugs do have side effects, especially over the long-term, such as weight gain and possible heart problems. Some-

times another class of antidepressants, known as MAO inhibitors, are often used if the tricyclics don't work. Depression specialists follow a sequence of drugs until they find the right one.

Drugs do not necessarily eliminate the need for psychotherapy. Many patients need both to recover. Several studies show that a combination of drugs and psychotherapy is superior to either alone. But long-term psychoanalysis or other conventional talk-therapies are not the most effective. The newer therapies are very short-term, usually about four months or less. They do not concentrate on deep probes into the psyche, but on relieving symptoms and building new patterns of coping.

A major study recently showed two relatively new forms of short-term psychotherapy, cognitive behavior therapy and interpersonal therapy, to be as effective in curing depression as antidepressants.

In cases that do not respond to drugs or any other kind of therapy, electroconvulsive treatments are often recommended. Although electroshock has been discredited in the past, advances make the technique safer and much less frightening to patients. It is increasingly used in cases of deep depression as a last resort to prevent suicide.

Recent experiments also show that some persons recover from depression for short periods when their biological clocks are readjusted; that is, if they are forced to go to bed earlier or are deprived of sleep. This apparently puts them back into a normal night-day cycle for awhile. Others, whose depressions may be related to seasonal darkness in winter, have responded to prolonged exposure to artificial solar light. Researchers at the National Institute of Mental Health have found that some persons become severely depressed in the winter months, when daylight periods are shorter. By using artificial high intensity lights that simulate daylight, many of these people avoid their typical wintertime depressions. Apparently, the increased daylight produces beneficial changes in brain hormones.

Depression in children

Only recently has it been recognized that depression can be as serious and chronic in children as it is in adults. Depression has been diagnosed in children as young as five, and some psychiatrists believe it can affect infants. Some experts suspect that depression in youngsters from 6 to 12 is massively underdiagnosed.

The symptoms are often the same as in adults: sleep problems, lack of activity, inability to eat, suicidal thoughts. The number of childhood and teenage suicides has risen dramatically recently. Mild antidepressant drugs are sometimes suc-cessfully used on children, but many therapists believe psychotherapy should be the first line of treatment. Unless childhood depression is dis-covered and treated, it is likely to extend into adulthood. There is evidence that children of depressed parents are more vulnerable to depres-sion, suggesting a biological or environmental cause or, most likely, both.

SOME LEADING DEPRESSION TREATMENT CENTERS AND SPECIALISTS

ALABAMA
John Smythies, M.D.
University of Alabama
School of Medicine
University Station
Birmingham, AL 35294
(205) 934-2011

University of Southern Alabama
College of Medicine
Department of Psychiatry
307 University Blvd.
Mobile, AL 36688
(205) 471-7476

ARIZONA
Roger Steenland, Ph.D.
Southern Arizona Mental Health Center
1930 E. Sixth St.
Tucson, AZ 85719
(602) 628-5221

ARKANSAS
William G. Reese, M.D.
University of Arkansas for Medical Sciences
4301 W. Markham
Suite 506
Little Rock, AR 72205
(501) 661-5266

CALIFORNIA
Dr. Kay Jamison
Dr. Michael Gitlin
University of California at Los Angeles
Affective Disorders Clinic
760 Westwood Plaza–Box 18
Los Angeles, CA 90024
(213) 825-0764, 0271, 0491

Larry Sporty, M.D.
University of California at Irvine
Medical Center
Department of Psychiatry and Human Behavior
101 City Drive S.
Orange, CA 92668
(714) 634-5886

Sidney Zisook, M.D.
Steve Shuchter, M.D.
UCSD Gifford Mental Health Clinic
3427 Fourth Ave.
San Diego, CA 92103
(619) 299-3510

Victor Reus, M.D.
Langley Porter Neuropsychiatric Institute
401 Parnassus Ave.
San Francisco, CA 94143
(415) 476-7478

Philip Berger, M.D.
Stanford University
Department of Psychiatry and Behavioral
  Science
Stanford, CA 94305
(415) 493-5000, x5141

Robert Rubin, M.D., Ph.D.
Harbor—UCLA Medical Center
Building F-5
Torrance, CA 90509
(213) 533-3775, 3776

COLORADO
Robert Freedman, M.D.
University of Colorado Medical Center
4200 E. Ninth Ave.
Denver, CO 80220
(303) 394-8403

CONNECTICUT
Myrna Weissman, Ph.D.
University School of Medicine
Depression Research Unit
350 Congress Ave.
New Haven, CT 06519
(203) 785-5550

FLORIDA
Burton Goldstein, M.D.
University of Miami Medical Center
Box 016960
Miami, FL 33101
(305) 547-6755

Brian Weiss, M.D.
Mount Sinai Medical Center
4300 Alton Road
Miami Beach, FL 33140
(305) 674-2194

Eric Pfeiffer, M.D.
Director, Suncoast Gerontology Center
University of South Florida
Department of Psychiatry
12901 N. 30th St.–Box 50
Tampa, FL 33612
(813) 974-4355

Walter Wellborn, Jr., M.D.
Anclote Manor Hospital
PO Box 1224
Tarpon Springs, FL 33589
(813) 937-4211

GEORGIA
Marvin Brantley, M.D.
Emory University School of Medicine
Emory Outpatient Clinic
1365 Clifton Rd., N.E.
Atlanta, GA 30322
(404) 321-0111

HAWAII
John McDermott, M.D.
University of Hawaii
Department of Psychiatry
1356 Lusitana St.
Honolulu, HI 96813
(808) 548-3420

ILLINOIS
John M. Davis, M.D.
Illinois State Psychiatric Institute
1601 W. Taylor St.
Chicago, IL 60612
(312) 996-1065

Jan Fawcett, M.D.
Rush Medical College
1720 W. Polk St.
Chicago, IL 60612
(312) 942-5372

INDIANA
Iver Small, M.D.
Joyce Small, M.D.
LaRue D. Carter Memorial Hospital
1315 W. 10th St.
Indianapolis, IN 46202
(317) 634-8401

IOWA
George Winokur, M.D.
University of Iowa
Department of Psychiatry
500 Newton Rd.
Iowa City, IA 52242
(319) 353-3719

KANSAS
Sheldon Preskorn, M.D.
University of Kansas
School of Medicine
Department of Psychiatry
Kansas City, KS 67214
(913) 261-2647

Stuart Averill, M.D.
Director
Menninger Clinic
PO Box 829
Topeka, KS 66601
(913) 273-7500

KENTUCKY
Hugh Storrow, M.D.
University of Kentucky
Department of Psychiatry
Lexington, KY 40536
(606) 233-6005

LOUISIANA
Donald M. Gallant, M.D.
Tulane Medical Center
Department of Psychiatry
1415 Tulane Ave.
New Orleans, LA 70112
(504) 588-5236

Joel Steinberg, M.D.
Louisiana State University
School of Medicine
Department of Psychiatry
PO Box 33932
Shreveport, LA 71130
(318) 674-6040

MARYLAND
Elliott Gershon, M.D.
National Institute of Mental Health
9000 Rockville Pike
Building 10, Room 3N-218
Bethesda, MD 20892
(301) 496-3465

William Potter, M.D.
National Institute of Mental Health
9000 Rockville Pike
Building 10, Room 4S-239
Bethesda, MD 20892
(301) 496-5755, 2141

MASSACHUSETTS
Joseph Lipinski, M.D.
Alan Schatzberg, M.D.
McLean Hospital
115 Mill St.
Belmont, MA 02178
(617) 855-2255, 2201

Joseph Schildkraut, M.D.
Massachusetts Mental Health Center
74 Fenwood Rd.
Boston, MA 02115
(617) 731-2921

MICHIGAN
John Francis Greden, M.D.
Professor and Chairman
Department of Psychiatry
University Hospital
7500 E. Medical Center Drive
B2964, Box 0704
Ann Arbor, MI 48109
(313) 763-9629

Samuel Gershon, M.D.
Lafayette Clinic
951 E. Lafayette
Detroit, MI 48207
(313) 256-9418

Robert Bielski, M.D.
Michigan State University
Psychiatry Clinics
Affective Disorders Clinic
East Lansing, MI 48824
(517) 353-3070

MINNESOTA
Paula Clayton, M.D.
University of Minnesota
Medical School
Minneapolis, MN 55455
(612) 373-8869

MISSISSIPPI
William Johnson, Ph.D.
University of Mississippi
School of Medicine
Department of Psychiatry and Human Behavior
2500 N. State St.
Jackson, MS 39216
(601) 984-5805

MISSOURI
John Helzer, M.D.
Washington University
School of Medicine
4940 Audubon Ave.
St. Louis, MO 63110
(314) 362-2474

NEBRASKA
Jim Davis, M.D.
University of Nebraska
Nebraska Psychiatric Institute
602 S. 45th St.
Omaha, NE 68106
(402) 559-5019

Merrill Eaton, M.D.
6901 N. 72nd St.
Omaha, NE 68105
(402) 572-2955

NEVADA
Grant Miller, M.D.
University of Nevada School of Medicine
Department of Psychiatry and Behavioral
 Sciences
Reno, NV 89557
(702) 784-4917

NEW HAMPSHIRE
Mrs. Elizabeth Hunt
Dartmouth-Hitchock Medical Center
Community Mental Health Center
Hanover, NH 03755
(603) 646-5000, x5855

NEW JERSEY
Robert K. Davies, M.D.
Fair Oaks Hospital
19 Prospect St.
Summit, NJ 07901
(201) 522-7000

NEW MEXICO
Robert Kellner, M.D.
University of New Mexico
School of Medicine
Department of Psychiatry
2400 Tucker, N.E.
Albuquerque, NM 87131
(505) 277-2223

NEW YORK
Arthur Rifkin, M.D.
Mt. Sinai Services
City Hospital at Elmhurst
Department of Psychiatry
7901 Broadway
Elmhurst, NY 11373
(718) 830-2335

Anastase Georgotas, M.D.
New York University Medical Center
560 First Ave.
New York, NY 10016
(212) 340-5707

Ronald Fieve, M.D.
Alexander Glassman, M.D.
Frederic Quitkin, M.D.
Psychiatric Institute
722 W. 168th St.
New York, NY 10032
(212) 960-2200, 5882, 5787, 5750, 5784

Donald Klein, M.D.
Psychiatric Institute Annex
722 W. 168th St.
New York, NY 10032
(212) 960-2307

Boghos Yerevanian, M.D.
Susan Medoff, C.S.N., A.C.S.W.
University of Rochester
Department of Psychiatry
Affective Disorders Clinic
300 Crittenden Blvd.
Rochester, NY 14642
(716) 275-7818

Gerald L. Klerman, M.D.
Cornell University Medical Center
New York Hospital
Payne Whitney Clinic–Westchester Division
21 Bloomingdale Rd.
White Plains, NY 10605
(914) 997-5965

NORTH CAROLINA
Arthur Prange, Jr., M.D.
University of North Carolina
School of Medicine
Division of Health Affairs
Chapel Hill, NC 27514
(919) 966-1480

NORTH DAKOTA
Richard Stadter, M.D., M.P.H.
University of North Dakota
Medical Education Center
1919 N. Elm
Fargo, ND 58102
(701) 293-4113

OHIO
Allen Daniels, A.M.
Associate Director, Adult Division
Central Psychiatric Clinic
3259 Elland Ave.
Mail Location 539
Cincinnati, OH 45267
(513) 872-5856

Herbert Meltzer, M.D.
Case Western Reserve University
Department of Psychiatry
2040 Abington Rd.
Cleveland, OH 44106
(216) 844-8750

OKLAHOMA
William R. Leber, Ph.D.
University of Oklahoma
Health Sciences Center and Behavioral
  Sciences
Department of Psychiatry
PO Box 26901
Oklahoma City, OK 73190
(405) 271-5251

OREGON
Dan Casey, M.D.
Portland Division V.A.
3710 S. West U.S.
Veterans Hospital Rd.
PO Box 1034
Portland, OR 97207
(503) 222-9221, x2500

PENNSYLVANIA
Aaron Beck, M.D.
Center for Cognitive Therapy
133 S. 36th St.
Philadelphia, PA 19104
(215) 898-4102

Jay Amsterdam, M.D.
Larry Potter, Research Coordinator
Hospital of the University of Pennsylvania
Depression Research Unit
1-Gibson
36th and Spruce Sts.
Philadelphia, PA 19104
(215) 662-2844, 3462

George Simpson, M.D.
Medical College of Pennsylvania at Eastern
  Pennsylvania
Psychiatric Institute
3200 Henry Ave.
Philadelphia, PA 19129
(215) 825-4000

Robert Greenstein, M.D.
V.A. Ambulatory Care Center
Mental Hygiene Clinic 116A
1421 Cherry St.
Philadelphia, PA 19102
(215) 597-7168, 7169

David R. Burns, M.D.
111 N. 49th St.
Philadelphia, PA 19139
(215) 471-2415

David J. Kupfer, M.D.
Western Psychiatric Institute and Clinic
University of Pittsburgh
School of Medicine
3811 O'Hara St.
Pittsburgh, PA 15213
(412) 624-1000

RHODE ISLAND
Walter Brown, M.D.
V.A. Hospital of Providence
Providence, RI 02908
(401) 273-7100

SOUTH CAROLINA
Thomas Steele, M.D.
Medical University of South Carolina
Psychiatric Outpatient Department
171 Ashley Ave.
Charleston, SC 29425
(803) 792-4037

TENNESSEE
Barbara Chamberlain, M.D.
6027 Walnut Grove Rd.
Suite 306
Memphis, TN 38119
(901) 683-3770

Miles Crowder, M.D.
Vanderbilt University
Department of Psychiatry
Nashville, TN 37232
(615) 322-4927

TEXAS
Augustus J. Rush, M.D.
University of Texas
Health Science Center
Department of Psychiatry
5323 Harry Hines
Dallas, TX 75235
(214) 688-3992

Robert Rose, M.D.
University of Texas, Medical Branch
Department of Psychiatry and Behavioral
  Science
1200 Graves Building
Galveston, TX 77550
(409) 761-3901

Robert L. Williams, M.D.
Baylor College of Medicine
Texas Medical Center
Department of Psychiatry
1 Baylor Plaza
Houston, TX 77030
(713) 799-4889

Charles L. Bowden, M.D.
The University of Texas
Health Science Center at San Antonio
Medical School
Department of Psychiatry
7703 Floyd Curl Drive
San Antonio, TX 78284
(512) 691-7315

UTAH
Bernard I. Grosser, M.D.
University of Utah
College of Medicine
Department of Psychiatry
50 N. Medical Drive
Salt Lake City, UT 84132
(801) 581-4888

VERMONT
Richard Bernstein, M.D.
2 Church St.
Burlington, VT 05401
(802) 658-0255

VIRGINIA
Robert Vidaver, M.D.
Eastern Virginia Medical School
Chairman
Department of Psychiatry and Behavioral
  Sciences
PO Box 1980
Norfolk, VA 23501
(804) 446-5888

WASHINGTON
David Dunner, M.D.
Harbor View Medical Center
Psychiatry Department
2H Harbor View Hall
325 Ninth Ave.
Seattle, WA 98104
(206) 223-3404

WISCONSIN
James W. Jefferson, M.D.
John H. Griest, M.D.
Clinical Sciences Center
Department of Psychiatry
600 Highland Ave.
Madison, WI 53792
(608) 263-6078, 6075

CANADA
Yvon La Pierre, M.D.
Royal Ottawa Hospital
1145 Carling Ave.
Ottawa, Ontario
Canada K12 7K4
(613) 722-6521 x6227

Harvey Stancer, M.D.
Clark Institute of Psychiatry
250 College St.
Toronto, Ontario
Canada M5T 1R8
(416) 979-2221

SOURCE: *Mental Health Clinical Research Center for Affective Disorders, Western Psychiatric Institute and Clinic, University of Pittsburgh School of Medicine.*

RESEARCH AND TREATMENT AT THE NATIONAL INSTITUTE OF MENTAL HEALTH

The National Institute of Mental Health (NIMH) is conducting a wide range of studies on the psychobiology of mood and depression with particular attention to those who are manic-depressive. NIMH has on its staff many leading authorities on depression; some see private patients.

Patients are admitted to the National Institutes of Health Clinical Center on both an inpatient and outpatient basis. Treatment may include drugs, such as lithium and antidepressants; individual, family, and group psychotherapy; and milieu therapy. Investigators may also provide a definitive diagnosis of depression.

Participation is by physician referral. For more information your physician can contact:

Office of the Director
The Clinical Center
Building 10, Room 2C146
National Institutes of Health
Bethesda, MD 20892
(301) 496-1337

Antidepression Lights

More information about the artificial lights (Vitalite lamps) used to relieve wintertime depression can be obtained from:

Duro-Test Corporation
2321 Kennedy Blvd.
North Bergen, NJ 07047

ORGANIZATION

National Depressive and Manic-Depressive
  Association (NDMDA)
Merchandise Mart
Box 3395
Chicago, IL 60654

National voluntary, nonprofit advocacy group formed to help patients and their families. Will provide more information upon request.

BOOKS

The Book of Hope, **Helen A. DeRosis, M.D.,** and **Victoria Y. Pellegrino,** New York: Bantam, 1977.

Conquering Depression, **Wina Sturgeon,** New York: Cornerstone Library, 1981.

Coping with Teenage Depression, **Dr. Richard MacKenzie,** New York: New American Library, 1982.

The Courage to Live, **Ari Kiev, M.D.,** Crowell, 1979; Bantam, 1982.

Depression and Its Treatment, **John R. Greist, M.D.,** and **James Jefferson, M.D.,** Washington: American Psychiatric Press, 1984.

Depression: What We Know, **Brana Lobel** and **Robert M. A. Hirschfeld,** Bethesda, MD: National Institute of Mental Health, 1984; for sale by the Superintendent of

Documents, Government Printing Office, Washington, D.C.

End of a Dark Road, **Crystal Thrasher,** New York: Atheneum, 1982.

How to End Mental Depression, **Carl** and **Ray Weiss,** New York: Arco, 1978.

Moodswing, **Dr. Ronald R. Fieve, M.D.,** New York: Morrow, 1975.

Recovery from Depression, **Ari Kiev, M.D.,** New York: E.P. Dutton, 1982.

Suicide and Depression Among Adolescents and Young Adults, **edited by Gerald L. Klerman,** Washington, DC: American Psychiatric Press, 1986.

Why Isn't Johnny Crying? Coping with Depression in Children, **Dr. Leon Cytryn, Dr. Donald H. McKnew, Jr.,** and **Herbert Yahraes,** New York: W.W. Norton & Co., 1983.

FREE MATERIALS

Depression and Manic-Depressive Illness:
  Medicine for the Layman
Depression: What We Know, monograph.

National Institute of Mental Health
Alcohol, Drug Abuse and Mental Health
  Administration
5600 Fishers Lane
Rockville, MD 20857

SUICIDE

Depression can often lead to suicide. Studies show that the vast majority—from 60 to 80 percent—of those who commit suicide suffered from depression or alcoholism. Therefore, in cases where ideas of suicide are present, it is essential to pursue an aggressive diagnosis and treatment of depression.

There are a number of suicide prevention centers around the country, and studies show mixed results on their effectiveness in reducing the sui-

cide rate. Many experts believe that suicide prevention centers can be helpful in talking people through a crisis—allowing their suicidal thoughts to dissipate. However, severely depressed, potentially suicidal people should always get proper treatment. If a person actually attempts suicide, it should be regarded as a medical emergency, attended to in a hospital emergency room, and followed up by proper treatment.

SUICIDE PREVENTION CENTERS

The following centers are certified by the American Association of Suicidology. The Association also has for sale a directory listing other suicide prevention and crisis intervention centers around the country. You can contact them at 2459 S. Ash, Denver, CO 80222.

ALABAMA
Crisis Center of Jefferson County
3600 Eighth Ave. S.
Birmingham, AL 35222
Crisis Phone: (205) 323-7777
Business Phone: (205) 323-7782
Hours Available: 24

ALASKA
Fairbanks Crisis Clinic Foundation
PO Box 832
Fairbanks, AK 99707
Crisis Phone 1: (907) 452-4403
Business Phone: (907) 479-0166
Hours Available: 24

Suicide Prevention and Crisis Center
2611 Fairbanks St.
Anchorage, AK 99503
Crisis Phone 1: (907) 276-1600
Business Phone: (907) 272-2496
Hours Available: 24

CALIFORNIA
Suicide Prevention Crisis Center of San Mateo
  County
1811 Trousdale Drive
Burlingame, CA 94010
Crisis Phone 1: (415) 877-5600
Crisis Phone 2: (415) 367-8000
Crisis Phone 3: (415) 726-5228
Business Phone: (415) 877-5604
Hours Available: 24

Los Angeles Suicide Prevention Center
1041 S. Menlo
Los Angeles, CA 90006
Crisis Phone 1: (213) 381-5111
Business Phone: (213) 386-5111
Hours Available: 24

COLORADO
Pueblo Suicide Prevention, Inc.
229 Colorado Ave.
Pueblo, CO 81004
Crisis Phone 1: (303) 544-1133
Business Phone: (303) 545-2477
Hours Available: 24

CONNECTICUT
The Wheeler Clinic, Inc.
Emergency Services
91 Northwest Drive
Plainville, CT 06062
Crisis Phone 1: (203) 747-3434
Crisis Phone 2: (203) 524-1182
Business Phone: (203) 747-6801
Hours Available: 24

FLORIDA
Alachua County Crisis Center
730 N. Waldo Rd., Suite #100
Gainesville, FL 32601
Crisis Phone 1: (904) 376-4444
Crisis Phone 2: (904) 376-4445
Business Phone: (904) 372-3659
Hours Available: 24

Suicide & Crisis Center of Hillsborough
   County
2214 E. Henry Ave.
Tampa, FL 33610
Crisis Phone 1: (813) 238-8821
Business Phone: (813) 238-8411
Hours Available: 24

ILLINOIS
Call For Help
Suicide & Crisis Intervention Service
500 Wilshire Drive
Belleville, IL 62223
Crisis Phone 1: (618) 397-0963
Business Phone: (618) 397-0968
Hours Available: 24

KENTUCKY
Seven Counties Services
Crisis & Information Center
600 S. Preston St.
Louisville, KY 40202
Crisis Phone 1: (502) 589-4313
Business Phone: (502) 583-3951, x284
Hours Available: 24

LOUISIANA
Baton Rouge Crisis Intervention Center
PO Box 80738
Baton Rouge, LA 70898
Crisis Phone 1: (504) 924-3900
Business Phone: (504) 924-1595
Hours Available: 24

Mental Health Association of New
   Orleans
Crisis Line Program
2515 Canal St., Suite 200
New Orleans, LA 70119
Crisis Phone 1: (504) 523-2673
Business Phone: (504) 821-1024
Hours Available: 24

MARYLAND
Montgomery County Hotline
10920 Connecticut Ave.
Kensington, MD 20795
Crisis Phone 1: (301) 949-6603
Business Phone: (301) 949-1255
Hours Available: 24

MASSACHUSETTS
The Samaritans
500 Commonwealth Ave.
Boston, MA 02215
Crisis Phone 1: (617) 247-0220
Business Phone: (617) 536-2460
Hours Available: 24

South Norfolk Screening & Emergency
   Team
91 Central St.
Norwood, MA 02062
Crisis Phone 1: (617) 769-6060
Business Phone: (617) 769-6060
Hours Available: 24

MICHIGAN
Suicide Prevention Center/Detroit
220 Bagley, Suite 626
Detroit, MI 48226
Crisis Phone 1: (313) 224-7000
Business Phone: (313) 963-7890

MINNESOTA
Crisis Intervention Center
Hennepin County Medical Center
701 Park Ave. S.
Minneapolis, MN 55415
Crisis: (612) 347-3161
Suicide: (612) 347-2222
Crisis Home Program: (612) 347-3170
Sexual Assault Service: (612) 347-5838
Business Phone: (612) 347-3164
Hours Available: 24

MISSOURI
Life Crisis Services, Inc.
1423 S. Big Bend Blvd.
St. Louis, MO 63117
Crisis Phone 1: (314) 647-4357
Business Phone: (314) 647-3100
Hours Available: 24

NEW HAMPSHIRE
Intake/Crisis/Evaluation Unit
Counseling Center of Sullivan County
18 Bailey Ave.
Claremont, NH 03743
Crisis Phone 1: (603) 542-2578
Business Phone: (603) 542-2578
Hours Available: 24

Emergency Services/Concord
CNHCMS, Inc.
PO Box 2032
Concord, NH 03301
Crisis Phone 1: (603) 228-1551
Business Phone: (603) 228-1551
Hours Available: 24

Greater Manchester Mental Health Center
401 Cypress St.
Manchester, NH 03103
Crisis Phone 1: (603) 668-4111
Business Phone: (603) 668-4111

Center for Life Management
Salem Professional Park
44 Stiles Rd.
Salem, NH 03079
Crisis Phone 1: (606) 432-2253
Business Phone: (603) 893-3548
Hours Available: 24

NEW YORK
Suicide Prevention & Crisis Service
PO Box 312
Ithaca, NY 14850
Crisis Phone 1: (607) 272-1616
Business Phone: (607) 272-1505
Hours Available: 24

NORTH CAROLINA
Suicide & Crisis Service/Alamance County
PO Box 2573
Burlington, NC 27215
Crisis Phone 1: (919) 227-6220
Business Phone: (919) 228-1720
Hours Available: 24

OHIO
Support, Inc.
1361 W. Market St.
Akron, OH 44313
Crisis Phone 1: (216) 434-9144
Business Phone: (216) 864-7743
Hours Available: 24

Crisis Intervention Center of Stark County
2421 13th St., N.W.
Canton, OH 44708
Crisis Phone 1: (216) 452-6000
Business Phone: (216) 452-9812
Hours Available: 24

Suicide Prevention Center, Inc.
184 Salem Ave.
Dayton, OH 45406
Crisis Phone 1: (513) 223-4777
Business Phone: (513) 223-9096
Hours Available: 24

Help Hotline, Inc.
PO Box 46
Youngstown, OH 44501
Crisis Phone 1: (216) 747-2696
Crisis Phone 2: (216) 424-7767
Crisis Phone 3: (216) 426-9355
TTY: (216) 744-0579
Business Phone: (216) 747-5111
Hours Available: 24

PENNSYLVANIA
Contact Pittsburgh, Inc.
PO Box 30
Glenshaw, PA 15116
Crisis Phone 1: (412) 782-4023
Business Phone: (412) 487-7712

TENNESSEE
Crisis Intervention Center, Inc.
PO Box 120934
Nashville, TN 37212
Crisis Phone 1: (615) 244-7444
Business Phone: (615) 298-3359
Hours Available: 24

TEXAS
Suicide Prevention/Crisis Intervention Center
PO Box 3250
Amarillo, TX 79106
Crisis Phone 1: (806) 376-4251
Toll Free In-State: (800) 692-4039
Business Phone: (806) 353-7235
Hours Available: 24

Suicide & Crisis Center
2808 Swiss Ave.
Dallas, TX 75204
Crisis Phone 1: (214) 828-1000
Business Phone: (214) 824-7020
Hours Available: 24

Tarrant County Crisis Intervention
C/O Family Service, Inc.
716 Magnolia
Fort Worth, TX 76104
Crisis Phone 1: (817) 336-3355
Business Phone: (817) 336-0108
Hours Available: 24

Crisis Intervention of Houston, Inc.
PO Box 13066
Houston, TX 77219
Central: (713) 228-1505
Bay Area: (713) 333-5111
Business Phone: (713) 527-9426
Hours Available: 24

VIRGINIA
Northern Virginia Hotline
PO Box 187
Arlington, VA 22210
Crisis Phone 1: (703) 527-4077
Business Phone: (703) 522-4460
Hours Available: 24

WASHINGTON
Crisis Clinic
1530 Eastlake E.
Seattle, WA 98102
Crisis Phone 1: (206) 447-3222
Business Phone: (206) 447-3210

SOURCE: *American Association of Suicidology.*

SUICIDE ORGANIZATION AND MATERIALS

American Association of Suicidology
2459 S. Ash
Denver, CO 80222
(303) 692-0985

Membership professional organization of psychologists, psychiatrists, social workers, and others interested in "life-threatening behavior and suicide." Also an information source for the public. Publishes pamphlets, brochures, a quarterly newsletter, *Newslink,* a research journal, and a national directory of suicide prevention centers. Will send more information upon request by telephone or mail. Special services include certification of suicide prevention centers. The following publications are free of charge:

Before It's Too Late; What To Do When Someone You Know Attempts Suicide, 10 pages, booklet.
Suicide in Young People, 10 pages, booklet.
Suicide—It Doesn't Have to Happen, 14 pages.

DIABETES

See also Eye Diseases and Vision Problems, page 215.

Diabetes is a disorder of the pancreas, the gland that produces insulin. It affects an estimated 10 million Americans and contributes to the deaths of about 130,000 people yearly. Diabetes is the seventh leading cause of death by disease in the United States. Some 500,000 new cases are diagnosed each year. Today the average American has a one out of five chance of developing diabetes. According to the American Diabetes Association, about five million Americans have diabetes and don't know it. Women are about twice as likely as men to have diabetes.

There are several types of diabetes, but two distinct types are most common: Type I (insulin-dependent) and Type II (non-insulin-dependent). People with Type I must take insulin injections to live; this type usually becomes apparent in childhood (it used to be called juvenile-onset diabetes), although the risk extends up to age 40 or so. However, insulin-dependent diabetes is far less common, accounting for about 10 percent of all cases of diabetes. Type II diabetes, by far the most prevalent type, used to be called adult-onset diabetes because it usually develops after age 40. The two types of diabetes have some similar characteristics and symptoms, but their causes may be slightly different, and the treatment is generally different.

In cases of insulin-dependent diabetes, the pancreas does not produce enough insulin, and the hormone insulin must be replaced. In non-insulin-dependent diabetes, the pancreas produces insulin, but the body for some reason cannot properly utilize it. Non-insulin-dependent diabetes more often occurs in adults who are overweight.

In both cases, the lifespan of the person with diabetes may be shortened, largely because of complications in the circulatory system that affect primarily the kidneys, heart, and eyes. Diabetic patients are at high risk for heart disease, kidney failure, and circulatory problems, as well as vision problems or blindness caused by diabetic retinopathy (*see* page 216). The long-range complications typically show up 10 or more years after diagnosis. The toll from diabetes is considerable: It causes about half of all amputations of the foot and leg among adults, 20 percent of the cases of kidney failure, 15 percent of the blindness. Twenty-five percent of all diabetics have cardiovascular diseases. In pregnant women, diabetes can be risky, causing a miscarriage or a loss of the infant soon after birth. Birth defects are about five times more common in youngsters of diabetic mothers.

Cause: Only a few of the causes of both insulin-dependent and non-insulin-dependent diabetes are known. Research indicates that both types are hereditary to some degree. If one identical twin has non-insulin-dependent diabetes, the other twin will have it 100 percent of the time. The chances are 50-50 in twins with insulin-dependent diabetes. How the disease is transmitted genetically is not understood. There is also evidence that a virus and a malfunctioning immune system may be involved in insulin-dependent diabetes, and one theory is that an unknown virus may cause the disease in certain individuals who are genetically susceptible.

On the other hand, obesity is the prime factor in non-insulin-dependent diabetes and may for unknown reasons trigger the disease in individuals who are genetically predisposed to that type of diabetes. More than 80 percent of people diag-

177

nosed with the disease are overweight at the time, and about 50 to 60 percent of all obese people have abnormal glucose tolerance or other signs of non-insulin-dependent diabetes. How being overweight is related to diabetes is not clear; it is thought that it somehow alters the body's metabolism and reduces the body's response to insulin. When persons with non-insulin-dependent diabetes lose weight, their carbohydrate metabolism often improves, and their diabetic symptoms may disappear. Emotional or physical stress, including the stress of pregnancy, loss of a spouse, loss of a job, an injury, or serious illness, can also be related to the onset of diabetes.

Symptoms: Insulin-dependent diabetes (Type I) produces symptoms that are sudden and severe: extreme thirst, frequent urination, constant hunger, weight loss. Also, the body, unable to properly utilize food, begins raiding stored fat and protein, releasing certain acid by-products in the blood. This may produce a crisis called ketoacidosis, which is potentially fatal, and requires prompt treatment. A person with insulin-dependent diabetes also may have weakness and fatigue, nausea and vomiting, and irritability.

The symptoms of non-insulin-dependent diabetes (Type II) are more subtle and come on gradually. Some common signs are drowsiness, blurred vision, tingling, numbness in hands and feet, skin infections, slow healing of cuts (especially on the feet) and itching. Sometimes this type of diabetes is not recognized until complications, such as vision problems, appear.

Diagnosis: In some cases diabetes is easily diagnosed; for example, when the blood-sugar level is very high and there are other clear signs of diabetes. But when blood-sugar levels are "borderline," the diagnosis is more difficult. Recently, criteria for diagnosing diabetes have been clarified, so that slightly fewer people may be labeled as being diabetic. Formerly, a slightly elevated blood sugar (a fasting plasma glucose level of 120–140 mg/dl or two-hour plasma glucose level of 140 mg/dl) was considered evidence of a diagnosis of "mild diabetes." Such a diagnosis, although it did not imply a shorter life span or many of the complications attributed to diabetes, could prejudice some employers and insurance companies, causing unwarranted hardship to the person.

Consequently, experts have adopted less strict diagnostic criteria: a fasting plasma glucose level of at least 140 mg/dl on two or more occasions, or a plasma glucose level of 200 mg/dl or greater two hours after a high sugar intake. Patients with such slightly elevated blood sugar are now said to have "impaired glucose tolerance," instead of borderline diabetes. Experts warn that the glucose-tolerance test should be positive more than one time for a diagnosis of diabetes because the test can give false-positive results in some cases; for example, if the person has recently been on a very-low-calorie diet or extremely inactive.

Treatment: For the insulin-dependent diabetic person, whose pancreas produces little or no insulin, the mainstay of treatment is injections of insulin. In the absence of such insulin, a Type I diabetic person cannot survive more than days or weeks. Regulating the diet to prevent sudden surges of blood-glucose levels is also important, as is exercise for insulin-dependent diabetic persons.

Since so many non-insulin-dependent (Type II) diabetes sufferers are overweight, the most important treatment in such cases is weight loss. Apparently weight loss somehow results in a better production of insulin. If the person loses weight and keeps it off, no other treatment may be necessary. Drugs (oral hypoglycemic agents) are also often used to treat non-insulin-dependent diabetes, although some experts do not recommend drugs unless diet and exercise fail to control the diabetes. If Type II diabetes cannot be controlled any other way, insulin injections may be necessary. In addition, all diabetic patients should monitor their blood-sugar levels in attempts to keep them stable, mainly to try to prevent long-term complications such as diabetic retinopathy.

One of the most exciting advances in the treatment of insulin-dependent diabetes is the battery-driven insulin pump, which the diabetic patient can wear externally and which automatically injects doses of insulin continuously throughout the day. Before meals, the user can push a button to deliver an increased amount of insulin necessary to handle metabolism of the food. These so-called "open loop" pumps have allowed many patients much better control of their sugar; they have replaced the numerous daily insulin injections for some patients. However, when using the pump, people still have to take several daily measurements of their blood-sugar levels.

Some experts consider the pumps especially valuable during pregnancy to keep the blood sugar close to normal, and some studies show that diabetic women who use the pump during pregnancy can significantly reduce the risk of birth defects in their infants. Still, there can be problems with the pumps, such as delivering too much or too little insulin and causing swelling and abscesses in the skin where the needle is inserted.

A small number of diabetic patients have also received surgically implanted insulin pumps. Implantable insulin pumps were developed at the University of Minnesota by Dr. Henry Buchwald, professor of surgery and bioengineering. Neither of these pumps both monitors blood-glucose levels and automatically delivers the proper dose of insulin. Hospitals, on the other hand, have large machines, like an artificial pancreas, that do measure glucose levels and relay the information to an internal computer, which then triggers the release of the right amount of insulin. These machines are used in crisis situations and during pregnancy. Researchers are working to miniaturize that so-called "closed loop" system, creating an implantable artificial pancreas.

Another important development is devices that allow diabetic people to easily monitor their blood-sugar levels at home. Such tests are more accurate than urine tests because they reveal the precise amount of glucose in the blood at the time of the test. The diabetic patient takes a single drop of blood from fingertip or earlobe with a simple device called a lancet, and then puts the blood on a chemical strip. The blood-sugar level can then be read from the strip by an electronic device or by eye from a comparison chart. This type of monitoring allows the person with diabetes to keep a tight control over his or her blood-sugar levels. Some experts believe that "tight control" over the blood sugar levels reduces the risk of long-term complications, but proof of that is yet to come.

Pancreas transplants

Surgical transplantation of the pancreas, whole or in segments, or the critical pancreatic islet cells alone, has been done, but the procedure is still rare and has achieved only limited success. The technique is improving constantly, and in cases where it has succeeded the diabetic recipient has been able to stop insulin injections for a period of time. However, the transplant surgery is expensive, risky, and may be unsuccessful not only because of the chance of rejection of the new pancreatic tissue by the body but also because of the failure of other functions the new pancreas must perform. The surgery is still experimental, although promising, and new research victories in animals as well as humans are bringing it closer to becoming a reality. However, even if the operation succeeds, scientists would not know for many years whether the transplanted pancreas could prevent the long-term complications of diabetes.

SOME CENTERS FOR PANCREAS TRANSPLANTS

University of California at Los Angeles School of Medicine
Josiah Brown, M.D.
Department of Medicine
Los Angeles, CA 90024

University of Miami School of Medicine
Joshua Miller, M.D., Head of Transplant Division
George Kyriakides, M.D., Dan Mintz, M.D.
Department of Surgery
PO Box 016310
Miami, FL 33101

University of Minnesota Medical School
John S. Najarian, M.D.
Department of Surgery
516 Delaware St., S.E.
Minneapolis, MN 55455

Washington University School of Medicine
David Scharp, M.D.
Paul Lacy, M.D.
600 Euclid Ave.
St. Louis, MO 63110

Thomas E. Starzl, M.D.
Transplant Surgeon
Falk Clinic, Room 218
3601 Fifth Ave.
Pittsburgh, PA 15213

University of Wisconsin Clinical Sciences
  Center
Hans W. Sollinger, M.D.
Department of Surgery
600 Highland Place
Madison, WI 53792

WHERE TO FIND TREATMENT FOR DIABETES

Specialists in diabetes are called diabetologists and are endocrinologists or internists with a special interest in diabetes. (Endocrinologists deal with diseases and disorders related to hormone-secreting glands.) There is no medically designated specialty for diabetes, as there is for cardiology, neurology, and so forth; therefore, you will not find physicians who are board certified in treating diabetes. Many general practitioners handle diabetes successfully, but you will certainly want a specialist in some cases, for example, during pregnancy or if complications occur. And you may want to participate in research on diabetes that is going on at numerous centers throughout the country. Most medical schools have diabetes clinics, and there are some excellent private ones. One of the preeminent diabetes treatment and research centers is a private institution, the Joslin Diabetes Center in Boston, Massachusetts. The Center conducts extensive research on diabetes, produces much educational material on the subject, including a monthly newsletter, and does not require a physician referral.

Joslin Diabetes Center
15 Joslin Place
Boston, MA 02215
(617) 732-2400

For a list of endocrinologists who are heads of departments or divisions of endocrinology at leading medical colleges, *see* page 594.

GOVERNMENT-SPONSORED DIABETES CENTERS

In addition to financing research in diabetes throughout the country, the National Institute of Diabetes, and Digestive and Kidney Diseases supports diabetes centers at institutions known to have high-quality diabetes research and treatment. The government programs are not directed at patient care, but at research and the spread of the latest scientific developments to the rest of the medical community. Nevertheless, the centers are headed and staffed by experts in diabetes, and their designation as government-sponsored research centers identifies them as centers of excellence in treating and studying diabetes.

Diabetes research and training centers

ILLINOIS
Dr. Howard Tager
Diabetes Research & Training Center
University of Chicago
950 E. 59th St.
Chicago, IL 60637
(312) 962-9653

INDIANA
Dr. Charles M. Clark, Jr.
Department of Medicine
Indiana University Medical Center
1100 W. Michigan St.
Indianapolis, IN 46202
(317) 635-7401, x2266 or 264-3574

MICHIGAN
Dr. Stefan Fajans
Endocrinology & Metabolism Division
University of Michigan
School of Medicine
Ann Arbor, MI 48104
(313) 764-4155 or 763-5256

MISSOURI
Dr. William H. Daughaday
Washington University Diabetes Research and
  Training Center
660 S. Euclid
St. Louis, MO 63110
(314) 361-4808

NEW YORK
Dr. Norman S. Fleischer
Albert Einstein College of Medicine
1300 Morris Park Ave.
Bronx, NY 10461
(212) 430-2908

TENNESSEE
Dr. Oscar Crofford
Diabetes Research & Training Center
Vanderbilt University
School of Medicine
Nashville, TN 37232
(615) 322-2197

VIRGINIA
Dr. Joseph Larner
Diabetes Research & Training Center
University of Virginia
Charlottesville, VA 22903
(804) 924-5207, 5869

Diabetes-endocrinology research centers

IOWA
Dr. John MacIndoe (Acting Director)
Professor of Medicine and Biochemistry
Department of Internal Medicine
College of Medicine
University of Iowa
Iowa City, IA 52242
(319) 356-2883

MASSACHUSETTS
Dr. William L. Chick
University of Massachusetts
Medical School
Department of Biochemistry
55 Lake Ave. N.
Worcester, MA 01605
(617) 856-3047

PENNSYLVANIA
Dr. Franz Matschinsky
Diabetes-Endocrinology Center
University of Pennsylvania
School of Medicine
Philadelphia, PA 19104
(215) 898-4365

TEXAS
Dr. James B. Field
Diabetes Research Center
Baylor College of Medicine
1200 Moursund Ave.
Houston, TX 77030
(713) 799-4084
Juvenile Diabetes
Kenneth Gabbay, M.D.

WASHINGTON
Dr. Daniel Porte, Jr.
Diabetes-Endocrinology Center
University of Washington
1131 14th Ave. S., QR8
Seattle, WA 98195
(206) 762-1010, x2138 or 396-1431

SOURCE: *National Institute of Diabetes, and Digestive and Kidney Diseases*

SOME LEADING DIABETES RESEARCHERS

An important question for people with diabetes is whether controlling their blood glucose—keeping it within normal limits—helps prevent or lessen the well-known later complications of the disease, such as cardiovascular and kidney problems and diabetic retinopathy. Some leading diabetic research and treatment centers are now conducting a long-term investigation on insulin-dependent diabetic patients—ages 13 to 39—under the auspices of the National Institute of Diabetes, and Digestive and Kidney Diseases to find the answer.

These centers can be considered well-respected institutions of diabetes information and up-to-date patient treatment. Even if you are not in a patient research project, you can expect the center and its staff to be leaders in diabetes treatment.

Diabetes control and complications trial

The following researchers and centers are part of a long-term study of the treatment of insulin-dependent diabetes. Patients are given either standard insulin treatment or an experimental treatment regimen on a random-selection basis to see whether the experimental treatment prevents the occurrence of diabetes complications.

CONNECTICUT
William V. Tamborlane, M.D.
Yale University School of Medicine
PO Box 333
New Haven, CT 06510
(203) 436-4771

IOWA
Helmut G. Schrott, M.D.
University of Iowa
Department of Preventive Medicine and
    Environmental Health
Westlawn S.—212
Iowa City, IA 52242
(319) 356-1616

MASSACHUSETTS
Lawrence I. Rand, M.D.
Joslin Diabetes Center, Inc.
W. P. Beetham Eye Unit
1 Joslin Place
Boston, MA 02215
(617) 732-2400

David M. Nathan, M.D.
Massachusetts General Hospital
Diabetes Unit, Bulfinch 4
Fruit St.
Boston, MA 02114
(617) 726-8722

MICHIGAN
Fred W. Whitehouse, M.D.
Henry Ford Hospital
2799 W. Grand Blvd.
Detroit, MI 48202
(313) 876-2600

MINNESOTA
Donnell D. Etzwiler, M.D.
Diabetes Education Center
4959 Excelsior Blvd.
Minneapolis, MN 55416
(612) 927-3393

John Bantle, M.D.
University of Minnesota
Mayo Building—Box 91
420 Delaware St., S.E.
Minneapolis, MN 55455
(612) 373-2851

F. John Service, M.D.
Mayo Clinic
200 First St., S.W.
Rochester, MN 55905
(507) 284-2511

MISSOURI
Julio V. Santiago, M.D.
St. Louis Children's Hospital
PO Box 14871
St. Louis, MO 63178
(314) 454-6000

David E. Goldstein, M.D.
University of Missouri at Columbia
School of Medicine
807 Stadium Rd., Room, M770
Columbia, MO 65212
(314) 882-2923

NEW YORK
Robert Campbell, M.D.
Cornell University Medical College
1300 York Ave.
New York, NY 10021
(212) 628-1995

OHIO
Saul Genuth, M.D.
Case Western Reserve University
Mount Sinai Medical Center
1800 E. 105th St.
Cleveland, OH 44106
(216) 421-4000

PENNSYLVANIA
Lester Baker, M.D.
University of Pennsylvania
Children's Hospital of Philadelphia
34th St. and Civic Center Blvd.
Philadelphia, PA 19104
(215) 596-9100

Allan L. Drash, M.D.
Children's Hospital of Pittsburgh
5th Ave. and DeSoto St.
Pittsburgh, PA 15213
(412) 647-2345

Douglas Greene, M.D.
University of Pittsburgh
230 Lothrop St.
Pittsburgh, PA 15261
(412) 647-3740

SOUTH CAROLINA
John A. Colwell, M.D.
Medical University of South Carolina
171 Ashley Ave.
Charleston, SC 29425
(803) 792-2300

TENNESSEE
Abbas E. Kitabchi, M.D.
University of Tennessee Center for the Health
  Sciences
951 Court Ave., Room 327B
Memphis, TN 38163
(901) 528-5500

Rodney A. Lorenz, M.D.
Vanderbilt University School of Medicine
21st Ave. S. & Garland St.
Nashville, TN 37232
(615) 322-7311

TEXAS
Philip Raskin, M.D.
University of Texas Health Science Center at
  Dallas
5323 Harry Hines Rd.
Dallas, TX 75235
(214) 688-3111

WASHINGTON
Jerry P. Palmer, M.D.
University of Washington
Seattle Public Health Hospital
1131 14th Ave. S., Quarters 8
Seattle, WA 98144
(206) 543-3300

SOURCE: *National Institute of Diabetes, and Digestive and Kidney Diseases.*

DIABETES RESEARCH AT THE NATIONAL INSTITUTES OF HEALTH

Several research projects involving both adults and children with diabetes are being conducted at the Clinical Center of the National Institutes of Health in Bethesda, Maryland. One study is of patients with diabetes mellitus who have never received insulin or received it for less than four weeks. Treatment is by referral of a physician. For more information your physician can contact:

Office of the Director
The Clinical Center
Building 10, Room 2C146
National Institutes of Health
Bethesda, MD 20892
(301) 496-4891
Physicians with severely ill patients can call:
  (301) 496-4181 or (301) 495-4658.

ORGANIZATIONS

American Diabetes Association
1660 Duke Street
Alexandria, VA 22314
(703) 549-1500
(800) 232-3472

A national voluntary membership organization for people with diabetes, their families, physi-
cians, health professionals, and other interested persons. Funds extensive diabetes research. Has about 700 local affiliates and chapters throughout the country. A major source of information and patient services. Discussion groups, education programs in hospitals, camps, seminars. Numerous publications, booklets, pamphlets, books,

a quarterly newsletter, a bimonthly magazine for diabetics, *Diabetes Forecast* (free with membership); also journals for physicians. Will provide more information and name of local chapters upon request. Local affiliates and chapters are also usually listed in the white pages of your local directory.

Juvenile Diabetes Foundation International
60 Madison Ave.
New York, NY 10010
(212) 889-7575
(800) 223-1138

A national voluntary membership organization for people with juvenile or insulin-dependent diabetes. Has about 160 local affiliates throughout the country that do fund raising for research into insulin-dependent diabetes and provide educational materials and support services in the com-

munity. The Foundation is a major source of information on this type of diabetes and publishes numerous booklets and brochures and a quarterly magazine, *Diabetes Countdown*. Will provide more information upon request.

The National Diabetes Information
    Clearinghouse
Box NDIC
Bethesda, MD 20892
(301) 468-2162

A federal government service within the Department of Health and Human Services concerned with medical aspects of diabetes. The Clearinghouse answers questions from the public and provides referrals to other agencies as well as bibliographies, and government publications on diabetes.

SOME MANUFACTURERS OF PRODUCTS FOR DIABETICS

Lifescan
1025 Terra Bella Ave.
Mountain View, CA 94043
Glucose-monitoring equipment

Ames Division, Miles Laboratories, Inc.
PO Box 70
Elkhart, IN 46515
Chemical strips and other glucose-monitoring products

Bio-Dynamics
9115 Hague Rd.
Indianapolis, IN 46250
Chemical strips and other glucose-monitoring products

Derata Corporation
7380 32nd Ave.
Minneapolis, MN 55427
Automatic insulin injectors

Ulster Scientific, Inc.
PO Box 902
Highland, NY 12528
(800) 431-8233
(800) 522-2257—New York State
Glucose-monitoring equipment

Teledyne Avionics
PO Box 6098
Charlottesville, VA 22906
Glucose-monitoring equipment

CAMPS FOR YOUNGSTERS WITH DIABETES

The American Diabetes Association sponsors two-week camps in the summer and skiing weekends in the winter for youngsters with diabetes. At the camps, the youngsters, ages 8 to 14, learn how to be independent, how to monitor their blood-sugar levels and how to give themselves injections. They also take part in rap sessions

and mutual support sessions, sometimes led by psychiatrists. Contact the national organization, 1660 Duke Street, Alexandria, VA 22314, or your local American Diabetes Association affiliate for more details. They are listed in the white pages of local phone directories.

BOOKS

General

Diabetes: The Comprehensive Self-Management Handbook, **John F. Aloia,** New York: Doubleday, 1984.

The Diabetes Fact Book, **Theodore G. Duncan,** New York: Scribner, 1982.

Diabetes: A Guide to Self Management for Patients and Their Families, **Terri Kivelowitz,** Englewood Cliffs, NJ: Prentice-Hall, 1981.

Diabetes in the Family, **Dorothy Born,** New York: American Diabetes Association, 1982.

Diabetes: Reach for Health and Freedom, New York: American Diabetes Association, 1984.

The Diabetes Self-Help Method, **C. M. Peterson,** New York: Simon & Schuster, 1984.

Diabetics and Exercise, **Dr. Robert C. Cantu,** New York: Dutton, 1982.

The Diabetic's Total Health Book, **June Biermann** and **Barbara Toohey,** Los Angeles: J.P. Tarcher, Inc., 1980.

Kiss the Candy Days Goodbye, **Vincent T. Dacquino,** New York: Delacorte Press, 1982.

No Time to Lose, **Gary Kleiman,** New York: Morrow, 1983.

The Peripatetic Diabetic, **June Biermann,** Los Angeles: J.P. Tarcher, Inc. 1984.

Diet

The Comprehensive Diabetic Cookbook, **Dorothy J. Kaplan,** New York: Greenwich House, 1984.

Diabetes, a Practical Guide to Healthy Living, **Dr. James W. Anderson,** New York: Arco, 1981. The value of a high-fiber diet in controlling diabetes; by a leading nutrition researcher and professor of medicine at the University of Kentucky.

The Diabetes Brand Name Food Exchange Handbook, **Andrea Barrett,** Philadelphia: Running Press, 1984.

The Family Cookbook, Englewood Cliffs, NJ: Prentice-Hall, 1980. Also available from the American Diabetes Association, Alexandria, VA.

Gourmet Recipes for Diabetics, **Francine Prince,** New York: Cornerstone Library, 1983.

MATERIALS, FREE AND FOR SALE

Free (single copies)

Children: What You Need to Know About Diabetes, 16 pages.

Exchange Lists for Meal Planning, booklet.

In the Later Years: What You Need to Know About Diabetes, 36 pages.

In the Middle Years: What You Need to Know About Diabetes, 32 pages.

Teens/Young Adults: What You Need to Know About Diabetes, 28 pages.

What You Need to Know About Diabetes, 24 pages.

American Diabetes Association
National Service Center
1660 Duke St.
Alexandria, VA 22314
(800) 232-3472

Blindness and Diabetes, 16 pages.

American Foundation for the Blind
15 W. 16th St.
New York, NY 10011

Diabetes, 12-page booklet.

Today's Topics in Diabetes, 12-page booklets: *Insulin Pump, Artificial Pancreas, New Insulins, The Eye, Biomedical Research: An Overview, Diabetes and the Family*

Joslin Diabetes Center
One Joslin Place
Boston, MA 02215
(617) 732-2400

Joslin Tapes
111 French Ave.
Braintree, MA 02184

What the Teacher Should Know About the Student with Diabetes, booklet.

What You Should Know About the Child With Diabetes, booklet.
What You Should Know About Insulin, booklet.
What You Should Know About Juvenile Diabetes, booklet.
What You Should Know About Self Blood Glucose Monitoring, booklet.

Juvenile Diabetes Foundation International
60 Madison Ave.
New York, NY 10010
(212) 889-7575
(800) 223-1138

Diabetes and Your Eyes, 20-page booklet.
Facts About Insulin-Dependent Diabetes, 12-page booklet.

National Diabetes Information Clearinghouse
Box NDIC
Bethesda, MD 20892

For sale

The Diabetes Dictionary, 50-page illustrated booklet.

National Diabetes Information Clearinghouse
Box NDIC
Bethesda, MD 20892

Managing Your Diabetes: A Patient Handbook, **Jean Ranch, R.N.,** and **Mae McWeeny, R.N.,** 32 pages, book-size format, 1980.

Sister Kenny Institute
800 E. 28th St.
Minneapolis, MN 55407

Diabetes Teaching Guide, a manual for coping with diabetes, staff of Joslin Diabetes Center. Mail order:

Joslin Diabetes Center
One Joslin Place
Boston, MA 02215

Audiotapes

A set of three one-hour audiocassette tapes by medical experts in diabetes. Information to help diabetics cope with everyday living. Produced by Joslin Diabetes Center. Mail order:

Joslin Tapes
111 French Avenue
Braintree, MA 02184

DIGESTIVE DISEASES

See also Cancer, page 124.

Digestive diseases are one of the least recognized and discussed maladies, yet about 20 million Americans suffer from them. Many diseases of the digestive system can be debilitating and potentially fatal. Often they require surgery. In fact, digestive diseases, including colon cancer and liver problems, are the leading cause of surgery, accounting for one-fourth of all operations.

BOWEL DISEASES

Some of the most serious and baffling digestive diseases are the inflammatory bowel diseases, including ulcerative colitis and Crohn's disease, also called ileitis and regional enteritis. Ulcerative colitis affects the inner lining of the entire colon, the five-foot stretch of intestine including the last portion, the rectum. The rectum is almost always inflamed. Crohn's disease can affect the colon, but is most commonly found in the ileum or small intestine that stretches from the stomach to the colon. The inflammation in Crohn's disease usually involves not only the inner lining but all layers of the intestinal wall.

Inflammatory bowel disease can be a major cause of disability. It strikes at least one-half million Americans, and some estimates put that figure as high as one or two million. Most are children and young adults between ages 12 and 28. About three-quarters of the cases show up before age 40; then, for some mysterious reason, the disease levels off and launches a second attack on those between the ages of 50 and 70, although the risk is much lower at that age.

Cause: Unknown. Several causes are suspected, including infectious agents (viruses or bacteria), hereditary factors (the disease is not considered definitively genetic but sometimes does "run in families"), and some form of abnormality of the immune functions. Some experts believe ulcerative colitis and Crohn's disease persist because of an immunodeficiency in which the body produces antibodies that attack the lining of the intestine. Experts in gastroenterology say emotional stress does not initiate the disease, but it does precipitate attacks and aggravates their severity once the disease is present.

Symptoms: Abdominal pain, diarrhea (sometimes with blood), bowel obstruction, weight loss, and fever. Pus or mucus is often present in the stool of those with ulcerative colitis. Additionally, since both of these diseases are considered systemic diseases (affecting many bodily processes), one-third of those with inflammatory bowel disease typically develop mild to moderate complications, such as aching joints, inflammation of the eyes and mouth, and skin and liver problems. The risk of colon and rectal cancer is greater in those who have chronic ulcerative colitis for 10 or more years. Inflammatory bowel disease also often has periods of intense flare-ups and remissions and sometimes may "burn itself out." Growth and sexual development can be retarded in children with inflammatory bowel disease, and in rare cases the disease can be fatal. The course of the disease is erratic and unpredictable.

187

Diagnosis: Generally, physicians can spot inflammatory bowel disease through physical examination, both external and internal, and laboratory tests. Often a sigmoidoscope, a fiber optic tube with a light, is inserted into the rectum; this allows a physician to detect inflammation in the intestinal lining. A barium X-ray may confirm the diagnosis and indicate the severity and extent of the disease. In some cases, a more accurate diagnosis comes from an intestinal examination by a colonoscope, a flexible fiberglass instrument with a tiny lens on the tip, which allows the doctor to take photos of the colon wall.

Treatment: Treatment is first focused on trying to control the inflammation in an attempt to reduce the symptoms and produce remission. Flare-ups of both diseases are commonly treated with anti-inflammatory drugs, namely sulfasalazine and corticosteroids. Sometimes antibodies and immunosuppressive drugs are added. Sulfasalazine has proved most effective in keeping ulcerative colitis under control in many cases, and physicians frequently use the drug on patients with Crohn's disease, although the evidence of its effectiveness for that disease is less clear. Scientific studies have found corticosteroids, such as prednisone and prednisolone, effective in acute attacks of Crohn's disease. However, there is evidence that low-dose maintenance levels of steroid drugs do not prevent the flare-ups or recurrences of either Crohn's disease or ulcerative colitis over periods of more than a year or two. Diet is sometimes changed, although the role of diet in managing the disease is controversial. Another form of therapy for seriously ill patients is total parenteral nutrition (an intravenous infusion of nutrients through a catheter), which provides adequate nutrition while allowing the bowel to rest; this therapy alone sometimes brings about remission. Some sufferers of ulcerative colitis improve for no known reason.

If medical therapy cannot combat the symptoms, and severe complications develop, such as *persistent* obstruction, colon cancer, abscesses, perforations, massive hemorrhage, or formation of fistulas (abnormal channels), surgery may be called for. In most cases, a diseased portion of the intestine is surgically removed, and the ends of the healthy bowel reattached. (This procedure is resection and anastomosis.)

However, in some cases more radical surgery may be necessary. Such surgery in ulcerative colitis removes the entire diseased colon and cures the disease. Surgery is not considered a cure for Crohn's disease. Even though the diseased part of the bowel is cut out, the disease may later attack other parts of the intestine. The small intestine cannot be totally removed, because it is necessary for the absorption of food. The surgical strategy for Crohn's disease has changed; experts now believe surgery is indicated only to cure complications of Crohn's disease, but that the disease itself is best treated medically and not with surgery. It has been discovered that the loss of long stretches of the ileum may put the patient with Crohn's disease at risk in later years.

Removal of the colon or a portion of the small intestine is almost always a traumatic experience, although afterward many patients live long, symptom-free, physically active lives. In a typical operation for ulcerative colitis, the entire colon and rectum are removed, and the lower part of the small intestine (ileum) protrudes through a hole in the abdomen. A pouch or bag worn on the outside of the body is fitted over the end of the ileum to collect body waste. Obviously, the pouches must be changed regularly.

Some people find the consequences of this surgery so distressing they refuse to have it performed, even in life-threatening situations. Thus, in the past 10 years, physicians have experimented increasingly with surgery that is not so emotionally devastating. In many cases, choices other than the standard ileostomy are available through newer surgical techniques.

One such operation is called the Kock pouch (continent ileostomy) technique, named for the Swedish physician who developed it. The surgeon removes the colon and then fashions the ileum into an *internal* pouch in the abdomen. To dispose of the waste, the patient inserts a plastic tube into the pouch through a tiny hole in the abdominal wall. Advocates proclaim the procedure successful in about 95 percent of the cases. Many physicians do not recommend this surgery for patients with Crohn's disease.

In still another surgical advancement for ulcerative colitis, the colon is removed, and the ileum is pulled through the muscular part of the lower rectum and attached to the anus. This procedure allows defecation through normal routes. This surgery, too, is said to be 85–90 percent successful; however, it works only in those patients without severe rectal disease. The patient with such surgery usually has to be extensively trained to learn to control bowel movements. Again, this surgery is not suitable for patients with Crohn's disease, and although more people are having it, some physicians still consider it experimental.

The National Foundation for Ileitis and Colitis can provide more information on the newer surgery and the names of physicians doing the procedures.

National Foundation for Ileitis and Colitis
444 Park Ave.
New York, NY 10017
(212) 685-3440

ULCERS

A peptic ulcer is a tiny hole usually one-quarter- to three-quarter-inch in diameter in the lining of the stomach or duodenum (first part of the small intestine), which forms when the stomach's secretion of hydrochloric acid and a digestive enzyme goes awry. A person may produce excessive acid or be unable to tolerate normal amounts of acid secretions. Two percent of Americans—roughly four million—have ulcers at any one time. Another six million have ulcers that flare up, heal, and then flare up again. The pattern can go on for years. Ulcers of the duodenum are about *four* times more common than gastric or stomach ulcers.

Even infants and children can have ulcers, although the disease most commonly strikes people between ages 25 and 40. Twice as many men as women have ulcers. An estimated 7,000 Americans die every year from ulcer complications; many of them are older people with gastric ulcers. Duodenal ulcers are more common among young adults (the incidence rises until about age 30); gastric ulcers are more commonly found in older people (the rate rises until about age 50).

Cause: Unknown. Genetic susceptibility is partly to blame. A person whose close relatives have ulcers are about three times more likely to develop ulcers—generally of the same kind. Also, ulcers occur more often and heal more slowly in people who smoke. Cigarette smokers are nearly twice as likely to have ulcers as nonsmokers. Certain drugs, including aspirin, may also lead to stomach ulcers. Despite popular myths about ulcers, there is only inconclusive evidence that day-to-day emotional stress causes ulcers. The studies are contradictory, although

some experts believe that stress does contribute to the disease in some individuals.

Symptoms: The most common initial symptom is gnawing or burning pain in the upper middle of the abdomen; the pain usually occurs one or two hours after eating. The pain can be severe, then go away, then return. It is usually worse between meals. A serious ulcer may result in bloody stools and vomiting of blood and perforation of the stomach or intestinal wall, which can be fatal if untreated.

Diagnosis: A family history is important. Also, a barium X-ray detects about 80–90 percent of active ulcers. If symptoms persist, use of a fiber optic tube, an endoscope, enables a doctor to visually examine the upper gastrointestinal tract for signs of ulcers.

Treatment: The purpose of treatment is to reduce the amount of acid in the stomach, promoting healing of the ulcer. This is often accomplished by antacids that neutralize the acid or by the drug cimetidine (Tagamet), which decreases the secretion of acid by the stomach. Newer drugs, based on natural substances called prostaglandins, are also proving effective. In perhaps 15 percent of ulcer cases, surgery may be necessary, although the type recommended is somewhat controversial. One type of surgery cuts selected branches of the vagus nerve, which stimulates the stomach to secrete acid. Another type of surgery removes a part of the stomach that promotes secretion of acid. Lasers have also been used to stop bleeding. Ulcer diets go in and out of fashion; certain foods do not cause ulcers, but many people report they feel better when they adjust their diets to avoid certain acidic or acid-producing foods. Still, the subject of diet is highly controversial; some experts say it makes no difference in ulcer healing, others advocate a bland diet or eating several small meals during the day.

Gastroenterologists, hepatologists (liver specialists), and colon and rectal surgeons specialize in the treatment of digestive diseases.

LIVER DISEASES

There are about 100 different diseases of the liver, ranging from genetic defects that strike the very young to alcohol-induced cirrhosis, which usually strikes the old. The toll from liver disease is considerable, and rising: 50,000 deaths annually. Still, much of the population is ill-informed about the problem. In the public mind, liver disease is too often synonymous with alcoholism. And although alcohol is a major cause of cirrhosis, there are many other causes of acute and chronic liver disease, such as viruses, chemicals and metabolic disorders. There is increasing awareness that infants may suffer from liver diseases. Some victims may be saved by liver transplants.

Hepatitis: Hepatitis simply means "inflammation of the liver," and can be caused by a number of agents, including chemicals and parasites, but the most common cause is viral. Symptoms may be mild or severe and may or may not include jaundice, the tell-tale yellow cast of the whites of the eyes and skin. Hepatitis is often difficult to distinguish because of its vague symptoms of fatigue, nausea and generalized aching, similar to those for flu and other common diseases. Most hepatitis, however, can be spotted by blood analyses. Type A hepatitis is acute, of short duration, and usually causes no lasting damage. Type B hepatitis, on the other hand, and so-called Non-A, Non-B type hepatitis (which means it is neither of the other two) can become chronic and go on to cause permanent liver damage and liver failure. Type B can even cause liver cancer. Liver biopsy may be necessary to spot chronic hepatitis. Powerful cortisone-like drugs may be prescribed to try to check the disease in some cases.

Primary biliary cirrhosis: A chronic, slowly progressive liver disease of the bile ducts with a name that is somewhat of a misnomer. Only in the last stages, sometimes more than 20 years after diagnosis, does the disease progress to the malfunctioning and scarred liver of true cirrhosis. The progression can sometimes be slowed down by drugs, but it can be life-threatening if complications from cirrhosis develop. The disease is 10 times more likely to show up in women, usually beginning between the ages of 30 and 60. Its cause is unknown; it is probably not genetic, but does "run in families," and may result from a disturbed immune system.

Biliary atresia: A potentially fatal inflammation and obstruction of the bile ducts of the liver, usually diagnosed within six weeks of birth. It is thought to be caused by an infection around the time of birth. Drugs may work to stimulate bile flow; if not, surgery is usually necessary. If all efforts cannot stimulate bile flow, the infant may survive only a year. The disease affects about one in 20,000 newborn.

Alpha 1 antitrypsin deficiency: An inherited incurable enzyme deficiency that appears most often in the newborn, causing jaundice and abdominal swelling. It can also show up in adolescents. About 75 percent of the victims develop cirrhosis; typically, however, one in four youngsters who makes it through infancy without cirrhosis survives with little or no liver damage.

Hemochromatosis: This is an inherited iron-overload disease, in which iron builds up in the liver, pancreas and other organs. Early diagnosis is essential, so the abnormal stores of iron in the liver can be depleted. This is done by regular removal of blood from the body, as needed. Such treatment, instituted early enough, usually means a normal life span. Still, a possible complication, in about one out of four cases, is liver cancer, although this occurs only in those who have developed cirrhotic scarring of the liver. Close relatives of those with hemochromatosis should also be screened for evidence of the disorder.

Wilson's disease: An inherited, potentially fatal disease in which excessive amounts of copper accumulate in the liver and other organs, including the brain and cornea of the eye. Although the disease begins at birth, it may not become apparent for two or even three decades. Symptoms are similar to those for hepatitis, namely jaundice; neurological or psychiatric symptoms may also develop from the toxic effect of copper in the brain. Fortunately, the rare disease, although fatal if untreated, can usually be reversed even in advanced cases. The copper is removed from the body by drugs.

Cirrhosis: Cirrhosis is the term applied to the end-stage, severe damage from a number of liver diseases, including all of the above. The word cirrhosis simply means a liver that is distorted, scarred, sometimes shrunken and often so damaged it is unable to function. Early signs of such severe damage may be liver enlargement, loss of appetite, nausea, weight loss and jaundice (yellow discoloration of eyes and skin). But since signs of the disease are well hidden, many cases of cirrhosis remain undiagnosed during routine examinations. The complications of advanced cirrhosis are: ascites (or a swelling up of the abdominal area), hemorrhaging from the esophagus and rectum, sometimes coma. Unfortunately, by the time symptoms of cirrhosis, especially alcohol-induced cirrhosis appear, the disease is often extensive. Cirrhosis kills about 30,000 Americans each year.

Cirrhosis can result from some forms of chronic viral hepatitis, congenital defects of metabolism, abnormal handling of iron or copper (hemochromatosis and Wilson's disease), toxic chemicals, drug reactions, some forms of heart disease and parasites. However, alcohol abuse is by far the leading cause of cirrhosis in the United States.

It is established that alcohol is a poison that works directly on the liver. Even heavy social drinkers can end up with so-called fatty liver, signifying some liver damage, although it is usually reversible if alcohol consumption decreases. About 15 percent of all alcoholics develop cirrhosis, even with adequate nutrition. It is not known why some alcoholics are susceptible to cirrhosis while others are not, but new tests to identify drinkers who are vulnerable to cirrhosis are being developed.

Early diagnosis and treatment of cirrhosis have improved, and if discovered early enough, the disease progression can be halted—by drugs, by diet and by avoiding the damage-causing poisons. Fortunately, the liver can function despite damage and can regenerate to a degree. Some infants and adults with cirrhosis have been rescued from death by liver transplants, which are becoming more common and successful after nearly a quarter of a century of experimentation.

LIVER TRANSPLANTS

Removing and implanting a liver is a dramatic endeavor that has become much more successful since the more widespread use of powerful immunosuppressant drugs, including cyclosporine. Liver transplants have been done since 1963; at first, 30 percent of the patients could expect to survive for one year. Some, however, did survive much longer. With the introduction of cyclosporine, and further technical advances, one-year survival rates for liver transplants in the hands of some experts nearly doubled to about 55 percent and are sometimes as high as 85 percent. Three-year survival rates are about fifty/fifty.

Only those with potentially fatal and incurable liver disease are candidates for a transplant. The best candidates are children with birth defects, such as biliary atresia, those with Wilson's disease and those with nonalcoholic cirrhosis. People with chronic hepatitis who are drug and alcohol abusers are not often considered as recipients for liver transplants because it has been found that the disease frequently recurs in the transplanted liver. Alcoholic-cirrhosis victims who abstain from alcohol might also be considered for liver transplants. The heartbreaking fact, of course, is that many more people could benefit from liver transplants than there are livers available.

How to donate your liver

Livers for transplant are in great demand. There are far more potential recipients than donors, and in most cases death is imminent without a liver to transplant. To donate your liver after death, you can get a ''gift of life donor card,'' which is legal in all states, from:

American Liver Foundation
998 Pompton Ave.
Cedar Grove, NJ 07009
(201) 857-2626
(800) 223-0179

SOME LEADING LIVER TRANSPLANT CENTERS AND SPECIALISTS

As with other surgery, your chances of survival and success for a liver transplant increase with the experience of your surgical team. Newer centers, some at prestigious medical centers, are opening. Following are some of the leading pioneering centers.

ALABAMA
University Hospital
619 S. 19th St.
Birmingham, AL 35233
(205) 934-4011
Transplant Director: Arnold Dietheim, M.D.

ARIZONA
Good Samaritan
1111 E. McDowell Rd.
Phoenix, AZ 85006
(602) 239-2000
Surgeon: Lawrence Koep, M.D.

CALIFORNIA
UCLA Medical Center
Department of Surgery
Room 77-132
10833 LeConte Ave.
Los Angeles, CA 90024
(213) 825-7651 or 852-9111
Surgeon: R. Busuttil, M.D.

UC Sacramento Davis Medical Center
2315 Stockton
Sacramento, CA 95817
(916) 453-2011
Transplant Coordinator: Judy Gruber
Surgeon: Richard Ward, M.D.

CONNECTICUT
Hartford Hospital
80 Seymour St.
Hartford, CT 06115
(203) 524-3011 or 534-2256
Transplant Coordinator: Mary Rovelli
Surgeon: Robert Schweitzer, M.D.

ILLINOIS
University of Chicago Hospitals and Clinics
5841 S. Maryland Ave.
Box 77A
Chicago, IL 60637
(312) 962-6424
Chief of Hepatibiliary Surgery and
    Transplantation: Christopher E. Broelsch,
    M.D.

University of Illinois at Chicago
Department of Surgery
Division of Transplantation
840 S. Wood St.
Chicago, IL 60612
(312) 996-3500, 6771
Transplant Coordinator: Martin Mozes, M.D.

IOWA
University of Iowa Hospitals and Clinics
Iowa City, IA 52242
(319) 353-2121
Transplant Coordinator: Barbara Schaubacher

LOUISIANA
School of Medicine in Shreveport
Louisiana State University Medical Center
1501 Kings Highway
PO Box 33932
Shreveport, LA 71130-3932
(318) 674-6100
Transplant Coordinator: Louise M. Jacobbi
Surgeons: John D. McDonald, M.D., Michael
    S. Ruhn, M.D.

MASSACHUSETTS
Children's Hospital
300 Longwood
Boston, MA 02115
(617) 735-6000, 7641, 8268
Transplant Coordinator: Fran Lytz
Surgeon: Joseph P. Vacanti, M.D.

Massachusetts General Hospital
Fruit St.
Boston, MA 02114
(617) 726-2000
Transplant Director: Paul S. Russell, M.D.

New England Deaconess
185 Pilgrim Rd.
Boston, MA 02215
(617) 732-7000
Surgeon: Roger Jenkins, M.D.

Tufts Medical School/New England Medical
  Center
171 Harrison
Boston, MA 02111
(617) 956-7000
Transplant Coordinator: Eileen Donovan
Surgeon: Sang Chow, M.D.

MINNESOTA
Mayo Clinic
200 First St., S.W.
Rochester, MN 55905
(507) 284-2511
Surgeon: Ruud Krom, M.D.

University of Minnesota Medical Center
420 Delaware S.E.
Minneapolis, MN 55455
(612) 373-8808, 8883; Donor #: 1-(800)-247-
  4273
Transplant Coordinator: Barbara Elick
Transplant Director: John S. Najorian, M.D.

MISSISSIPPI
University of Mississippi
Transplant Program
2500 N. State
Jackson, MS 39216
(601) 987-3500

MISSOURI
St. Luke's Hospital
308 Medical Plaza
4320 Wornall Rd.
Kansas City, MO 64111
(816) 753-7460
Surgeon: Thomas Helling, M.D.

NEBRASKA
University of Nebraska Medical Center
Department of Surgery
42nd & Dewey Ave.
Omaha, NE 68105
(402) 559-6022
Transplant Coordinator: Laurel Williams,
  R.N., M.S.N.
Transplant Director: Byers Shaw, M.D.

NEW YORK
Montefiore Hospital
111 E. 210th St.
Bronx, NY 10467
(212) 920-4712, 4716
Frank Veith, M.D.

NORTH CAROLINA
Duke Medical Center
Box 3354
Durham, NC 27710
(919) 684-8111
Transplant Coordinator: R. Randal Bollinger,
  M.D.

OHIO
Cleveland Clinic Foundation
9500 Euclid Ave.
Cleveland, OH 44106
(216) 444-2549

The Ohio State University
University Hospitals Clinic
456 Clinic Dr.
Columbus, OH 43210-1228
(614) 421-8746

PENNSYLVANIA
St. Christopher's Hospital for Children
Department of Surgery
2600 N. Lawrence St.
Philadelphia, PA 19133
(215) 427-5292
Surgeon: Charles Wagner, M.D.

Thomas Jefferson University
11th & Walnut
Philadelphia, PA 19107
(215) 928-6000
Transplant Coordinator: Betsy Mallon
Surgeons: Bruce Jarrele, M.D., Francis
  Rosato, M.D.

Children's Hospital
125 DeSoto
Pittsburgh, PA 19213
(412) 647-5016
Staff from University of Pittsburgh Hospital

University of Pittsburgh
Presbyterian Hospital
DeSoto at O'Hara St.
Pittsburgh, PA 15213
(412) 647-3016
Transplant Coordinator: Bob Duckworth, Brian
  Boznick
Surgeon: Thomas Starzl, M.D.

TENNESSEE
University of Tennessee Center for Health
  Sciences
951 Court Ave.
Memphis, TN 38163
(901) 528-5923
Transplant Coordinator: Gary Hall
Surgeon: James Williams, M.D.

TEXAS
Baylor University Hospital
3500 Gaston
Dallas, TX 75246
(214) 820-0111
Transplant Coordinator: Goran Klintmaln,
  M.D.

Children's Hospital Medical Center
1935 Amelia
Dallas, TX 75235
(214) 920-2000 or 688-4720
Transplant Coordinator: Betsy Brunetti Fyock,
  R.N.
Surgeon: Walter Andrews, M.D.

Hermann Hospital
Liver Transplant Center
Houston, TX 77030
(713) 797-4011

VIRGINIA
Medical College of Virginia
Box 499/MCV Station
Richmond, VA 23298
(804) 786-9000, 0465, 9313
Transplant Coordinator: Ann Martin
Surgeon: H.M. Lee, M.D.

WISCONSIN
University of Wisconsin Hospital
600 Highland
Madison, WI 53792
(608) 263-6400, 1384
Transplant Coordinator: Doug Miller
Surgeon: Munci Kalayoglue, M.D.

Froedtert Memorial Lutheran Hospital
9200 W. Wisconsin
Milwaukee, WI 53226
(414) 259-3000
Transplant Coordinator: Pete Walczak, R.N.
Surgeon: Mark B. Adams, M.D.

SOURCE: *American Liver Foundation.*

NATIONAL DIGESTIVE DISEASE RESEARCH CENTERS

The National Institute of Diabetes, and Digestive and Kidney Diseases supports 13 Digestive Disease Research Centers. The centers are staffed by outstanding clinicians and basic scientists committed to finding the causes, treatments, and prevention of a variety of gastrointestinal disorders. Each of the centers has special areas of interest.

CURE (Center for Ulcer Research and
  Education)
University of California
Los Angeles, CA 90024
(Ulcers)

Liver Core Research Center
University of California
San Francisco, CA 94143
Dr. Robert Ockner, Director
(Liver diseases)

Digestive Diseases Research Center
Harbor-UCLA Medical Center
Torrance, CA 90509
Dr. William J. Snape, Director
(Inflammatory bowel disease)

Digestive Diseases Research Center
University of Colorado
Denver, CO 80262
Dr. Francis R. Simon, Director
(Liver diseases)

Digestive Diseases Research Center
Yale University
New Haven, CT 06510
Dr. James L. Boyer, Director
(Liver diseases)

Digestive Diseases Research Center
University of Iowa
Iowa City, IA 52242
Dr. James Christensen, Director
(Gastrointestinal disorders)

Digestive Disease Research Center
Harvard University
Boston, MA 02115
Dr. William Silen, Director
(Intestinal diseases and ulcers)

Digestive Diseases Research Center
Tufts/New England Medical Center
Boston, MA 02111
Dr. Mark Donowitz, Director
(Gastrointestinal disorders)

Digestive Diseases Research Center
University of Michigan
Ann Arbor, MI 48109-0010
Dr. Tadataka Yamada, Director
(Gastrointestinal disorders and ulcers)

Digestive Diseases Research Center
University of Minnesota
Minneapolis/St. Paul, MN 55455
Dr. Joseph R. Bloomer, Director
(Liver disease)

Digestive Diseases Research Center
Mayo Clinic
Rochester, MN 55905
Dr. Sidney F. Phillips, Director
(General digestive diseases)

Digestive Diseases Research Center
University of North Carolina
Chapel Hill, NC 27514
Dr. Don W. Powell, Director
(Inflammatory bowel disease)

Digestive Diseases Research Center
Albert Einstein College of Medicine
New York, NY 10461
Dr. David Shafritz, Director
(Liver diseases)

SOME LEADING CENTERS AND SPECIALISTS IN GASTROENTEROLOGY

For some leading centers and specialists in gastroenterology, *see* page 577. The physicians listed there are heads of departments or divisions of gastroenterology at leading medical schools. These are not the only excellent centers and physicians specializing in the field, but they are considered to be among the most knowledgeable and experienced. They can be an excellent source of treatment and/or medical referrals to others specializing in various types of gastrointestinal disorders.

HELP BY TELEPHONE

An anonymous gastroenterologist (a physician specializing in digestive diseases) will answer your questions about any facet of digestive diseases—including symptoms and latest treatments. The information line, called Gutline, is an educational service of the American Digestive Disease Society. In operation Tuesday nights from 7:30 to 9:00, Eastern time.

(301) 652-9293

ORGANIZATIONS

American Digestive Disease Society
7720 Wisconsin Ave.
Bethesda, MD 20014
(301) 652-9293

A national membership organization, designed to help people deal with their digestive disorders. A source of information, offering personal counseling, specialist physician referral service. Provides pamphlets, a monthly magazine, *Living Healthy,* and a series of special dietary plan books for digestive diseases. Operates an information hotline at certain hours. Will provide more information upon request.

American Liver Foundation
998 Pompton Ave.
Cedar Grove, NJ 07009
(201) 857-2626
(800) 223-0179

A national nonprofit membership organization dedicated to disseminating information about liver diseases. Chapters and mutual self-help groups in many parts of the country. A major source of information for the public. Supports research. Provides pamphlets, fact sheets and a newsletter for youngsters with liver disease, *Sharing Cares and Hopes.* Conducts a Gift of Life Organ Donor Program and supplies the names of liver specialists in most regions of the country. Will provide more information upon request.

Iron Overload Diseases Association, Inc.
224 Datura Street, Suite 912
West Palm Beach, FL 33401
(305) 659-5616

A national, voluntary organization, serves patients with hemochromatosis and their families. It acts as a clearinghouse for information and medical referrals and sponsors conferences and symposia. A bimonthly newsletter. Will provide more information upon request.

National Digestive Disease Education and
  Information Clearinghouse
1255 23rd Street, N.W., Suite 275
Washington, DC 20037
(202) 296-1138

A clearinghouse for all kinds of information on digestive diseases. Supported by the federal government. Answers questions from the public, physicians, and health professionals and provides fact sheets. Other information is given upon request.

National Foundation for Ileitis and Colitis, Inc.
444 Park Ave.
New York, NY 10016
(212) 685-3440

A national nonprofit research-oriented organization dedicated to finding the cause of and cure for, ileitis and colitis. Supports research. Also has local mutual support chapters in many states. Answers questions from the public, and medical referrals usually through local chapters. Publishes pamphlets, booklets, and a quarterly scientific newsletter. Will provide more information and the name of a local chapter near you upon request.

United Ostomy Association
2001 W. Beverly Blvd.
Los Angeles, CA 90057-2491
(213) 413-5510

A national membership organization of mutual aid, moral support, and education for people with colostomy, ileostomy, or urostomy surgery. More than 600 local chapters in the United States and Canada provide person-to-person contact for new colostomy patients. Answers questions and gives advice. Offers pamphlets, booklets, and a magazine, *Ostomy Quarterly.* Will provide more information and a directory of local chapters upon request.

BOOKS

*The Bowel Book: A Practical Guide to Good
  Health.* New York: Schocken Books, 1981.
The Crohn's Disease and Ulcerative Colitis

Fact Book, **National Foundation for Ileitis
  and Colitis,** New York: Scribners, 1983.
The Great American Stomach Book, **Maureen**

Mylander, New York: Ticknor and Fields, 1982.
These Special Children: The Ostomy Book for Parents of Children with Colostomies, Ileostomies and Urostomies, **Katherine F.**

Jeter, Los Angeles: Bull Publishing Co., 1982. Also available from the United Ostomy Association, 2001 W. Beverly Blvd., Los Angeles, CA 90057-2491.

MATERIALS, FREE AND FOR SALE

Free (single copies)

Person to Person brochures about:
    Acid Reflux, Colon Cancer, Gall Bladder, Inflammatory Bowel Disease, Irritable Bowel Syndrome

American Digestive Disease Society
7720 Wisconsin Ave.
Bethesda, MD 20014
(301) 652-9293

Biliary Atresia, leaflet.
Cirrhosis: Many Causes, leaflet.
Diet and Your Liver, leaflet.
Gallstones and Other Gallbladder Disorders, leaflet.
How Can You Love Me—If You Don't Know Me, leaflet.
Liver Disease: A Problem for the Child?, leaflet.
Liver Diseases, leaflet.
Viral Hepatitis, leaflet.
Your Liver Lets You Live, leaflet.

Information sheets:
Alpha 1-Antitrypsin Deficiency
Cancer of the Liver
Chronic Hepatitis
Cystic Disease of the Liver
Drug-Induced Liver Injury
Fatty Liver
Galactosemia
Hemochromatosis
Neonatal Hepatitis
Porphyria
Primary Biliary Cirrhosis
Primary Sclerosing Cholangitis
Sarcoidosis
Type 1 Glycogen Storage Disease
Wilson's Disease

American Liver Foundation
998 Pompton Ave.
Cedar Grove, NJ 07009

Fact sheets:
Bleeding in the Digestive Tract
Cirrhosis of the Liver
Facts and Fallacies About Digestive Diseases
Gallstone Disease

National Digestive Disease Education and Information Clearinghouse
1233 23rd St., N.W.
Washington, DC 20037
(202) 296-1138

Coping with Crohn's and Ulcerative Colitis, for children and teenagers, 10 pages.
Crohn's Disease, Ulcerative Colitis and Your Child, 12 pages.
Questions and Answers About the Complications of Ileitis and Colitis, 6 pages.
Questions and Answers About Diet and Nutrition in Ileitis and Colitis, 15 pages.
Questions and Answers About Emotional Factors in Ileitis and Colitis, 8 pages.
Questions and Answers About Ileitis and Colitis, 15 pages.
Questions and Answers About Pregnancy in Ileitis and Colitis, 6 pages.

National Foundation for Ileitis and Colitis
444 Park Ave., S.
New York, NY 10016
(212) 685-3440

For sale

The "Gallbladder" Diet, 64 pages.
The "Inflammatory Bowel" Diet, 64 pages.
The "Gas" Diet, 64 pages.
The Irritable Bowel Diet, 64 pages.
The Lactose Intolerance Diet, 64 pages.

American Digestive Disease Society
7720 Wisconsin Ave.
Bethesda, MD 20014
(301) 652-9293

Living Comfortably with Your Colostomy,
  Minneapolis, MN: Sister Kenny Institute, 22
  pages, book-size format.
Living Comfortably with Your Ileostomy,
  Minneapolis, MN: Sister Kenny Institute, 38
  pages, book-size format.

Also, you may want to subscribe to a quarterly
newsletter, *Crohn's Colitis Update*, Educational
Insights, Inc., 150 W. Carob St., Compton, CA
90220.

DRUG ABUSE

Drug abuse is a major health problem in the United States. More than 57 million Americans over age 12—or 31 percent—say they have smoked marijuana. Twenty-two million say they have used cocaine. Yet, figures on single drug use do not document the extent or nature of the problem. Drug abuse is rarely restricted to one drug. Most youngsters who abuse drugs have multiple-drug habits—the average youngster who enters treatment is on five different drugs. Most youngsters who end up in drug-treatment centers are also heavy users of alcohol. Although many youngsters experiment with drugs, just as other generations experimented with alcohol, there is now a fairly large population of so-called "dedicated" or serious drug users among the young population.

In addition, the use of certain drugs is expanding to include all socioeconomic classes and older age groups. Some who used drugs extensively in the 1960s and 1970s have now carried drug abuse into older generations. The use of drugs has spread to become a problem among workers in all occupations, on assembly lines, in the mines, as well as in corporate offices and in the entertainment industry. A drug such as heroin, while still primarily a street drug, is more frequently being used by the well-educated, successful middle class. It is no longer unheard of for professionals, like computer programmers, and children of the rich to frequent urban "shooting galleries" for injections of heroin.

TYPES AND EFFECTS OF DRUGS

Narcotics: Include heroin, opium, morphine, codeine, methadone, and hydromorphine (Dilaudid). They are physically and psychologically addictive, produce euphoria, drowsiness, respiratory depression, constricted pupils, and in overdose can produce convulsion, coma, and death. Signs of use: scars ("tracks") on arms or backs of hands from injecting the drugs, constricted pupils and loss of appetite.

Depressants: Include barbiturates, benzodiazepines (such as Valium, Ativan, Librium), methaqualone (better known as Quaaludes or "ludes"), and chloral hydrate. They produce various degrees of dependence, both physical and psychological. Effects are slurred speech,

disorientation, and drunken behavior without odor of alcohol. They can cause withdrawal symptoms and death both from the withdrawal and from an overdose. Signs of use: staggering, stumbling, apparent drunkenness, dilated pupils, and falling asleep at work or school.

Stimulants: Include cocaine, (although it is erroneously designated a narcotic under federal law), amphetamines (or speed), phenmetrazine (Preludin), methylphenidate (Ritalin). Psychological dependence on these drugs is high, but there is controversy over the physical dependence. Some experts say there is a physical addiction or build-up of tolerance to cocaine, for example. Others disagree. But there is evidence that those addicted to cocaine, whether the reason is psychological or physical, desire more and more of it and feel compelled to use it when it is available. Effects are increased alertness, talkativeness, excitation, euphoria, and increased pulse rate and blood pressure. An overdose can produce hallucinations, convulsions, and possible death. Some signs of use: dilated pupils and long periods without eating or sleeping (the drugs depress the appetite and keep the user awake).

Hallucinogens: Include LSD, mescaline and peyote, and phencyclidine (PCP, "Angel Dust"). There is little evidence of a physical or psychological dependence for these drugs, except for phencyclidine, which creates a high risk of psychological addiction. Effects can be illusions, hallucinations, and poor perception of time and distance. Overdoses induce longer, more intense "trip" episodes, psychosis, and possible death. It is unusual for people to use these in public places or at work because the behavior changes are so great; use is generally in small groups or with friends in controlled environments.

Cannabis: Includes marijuana, hashish, hashish oil, and tetrahydrocannabinol, or THC, the active ingredient in marijuana and hash. The degrees of physical or psychological dependence are unknown, although a tolerance to the drugs can be built up. They cause euphoria, relaxed inhibitions, increased appetite, and disoriented behavior. Overdoses can cause fatigue, paranoia, and possible psychosis. Some signs of use: dilated pupils, bloodshot eyes, distortions of perception of time, and bursts of laughter. Long-time heavy use can be associated with mental deterioration.

TREATMENT FOR ADOLESCENTS

Our knowledge about and resources for effective treatment lag behind the national concern. Most people find treatment programs through word-of-mouth or nationwide publicity in the media. Surprisingly few treatment programs exist solely or primarily for adolescent drug abusers—seemingly our most critical problem—and few treatment programs have been subjected to scientific scrutiny to discover which ones work best.

Traditionally, drug-treatment programs have been aimed at adults, notably the street users of heroin. Consequently, most youngsters with drug problems are put into the traditional treatment programs designed for adults, with adults. Of more than 3,000 drug rehabilitation centers nationwide, according to a survey by the National Institute on Drug Abuse, only about 160 said they primarily treated adolescents.

Unfortunately, since there have been no definitive follow-up studies, no one really knows which drug programs work best over long periods of time. Since drug-rehabilitation programs are rarely evaluated for effectiveness, even professionals are hard put to point out the best drug-treatment centers for youngsters. However, some experts believe that adolescents with severe drug dependency—who are more than mere experimenters—have special problems that demand a different kind of treatment from the standard treatment for adult drug abusers. For one thing, many adolescents are poorly motivated to accept treatment, because they do not believe they have a drug problem. Unlike adult drug abusers, adolescents almost always go back to the same environment after they leave treatment—the same family, friends, and school situation. Thus, many experts believe that family involvement has to be part of successful drug treatment. Certainly critical is "aftercare" group support, as in Alcoholics Anonymous or Narcotics Anonymous, half-way houses, and family counseling.

Other experts believe that drug-abuse problems, although tough to handle, can be treated with dramatic success. They say that even though a youngster or adult with a drug problem does not recover immediately or at a certain treatment center does not mean he or she is doomed to a life of drugs. Often, they say, several treatment efforts may be necessary to kick the drug habit, and they encourage both families and addicts to keep trying to find the key to success.

Most experts say there is no panacea—no one program that is effective for all types of adolescent drug users. Parents should try to find one that they think best suits their youngster. Some experts believe the chances of success are greater in programs geared to adolescents. One of the best ways to get information is to simply spend several hours making phone calls to drug therapists in your area to check out the various types of programs.

In any event, if you have a problem, or suspect that someone in your family or among your friends does, you may find help from an increasing number of sources, both private and public.

HOTLINES AND HELPLINES

(800) 662-HELP
Operated by the National Institute of Drug Abuse.

(800) 554-KIDS
Operated by the National Federation of Parents for Drug-Free Youth. Open 9 A.M. to 5 P.M., Eastern time. Answers questions and sends information to parents who call about their youngsters' drug problems. Does not do counseling. Not a crisis line.

800-241-7946
Operated by the National Parents' Resource Institute for Drug Education (PRIDE). Open 9 A.M. to 5 P.M. Eastern time. Answers drug-related questions and provides referral services for those with drug problems. Taped messages on drugs and drug issues are available from 5 P.M. to 9 A.M.

(800) COCAINE
Operated by the nonprofit Fair Oaks Hospital in Fair Oaks, New Jersey. Trained operators answer questions and make referrals to treatment centers, hospitals, and physicians around the country. Does not do counseling. Open 24 hours a day.

Narcotics Anonymous maintains hotlines in every state. Consult your local phone directory or directory assistance for the number in your area.

DRUG TREATMENT PROGRAMS

You can find a list of state agencies that can refer you to drug treatment centers on page 19. A national directory *Drug Abuse and Alcoholism Treatment and Prevention Programs* (about 7,500 across the country), is also available from the Superintendent of Documents, Government Printing Office, Washington, DC 20402; document number: S/N 01702401252-1.

SOME DRUG TREATMENT PROGRAMS FOR ADOLESCENTS

The following programs report that all or the major part of their drug treatment is geared to adolescents.

ALABAMA
Eufaula Adolescent Adjustment Center Drug
  Treatment Program
Drug Abuse Treatment Unit
PO Box 270
Eufaula, AL 36027
(205) 687-5741, x259

Alternatives Inc.
Drug Abuse Treatment Unit
PO Box 341
Wetumpka, AL 36092
(205) 567-7083

ARIZONA
Prehab of Mesa Inc.
Alcoholism/Drug Abuse Treatment Units
PO Drawer G
Mesa, AZ 85201
(602) 969-4024

The New Foundation
Drug Abuse Treatment Unit
6401 S. Eighth Place
Phoenix, AZ 85040
(602) 268-3421

Phoenix South Community Mental Health
  Service
North Clinic, Substance Abuse
1424 S. Seventh Ave.
Phoenix, AZ 85007
(602) 258-0011

CALIFORNIA
Turning Point
Family Services Program
Drug Abuse Treatment Unit
12832 Garden Grove Blvd.
Room 240
Garden Grove, CA 92643
(714) 636-3823

Chabad Drug Rehabilitation Program
Chabad Residential Clinic
Drug Abuse Treatment Center
1952 S. Robertson Blvd.
Los Angeles, CA 90034
(213) 204-3196

The House of Uhuru
Drug Abuse Treatment Center
8005 S. Figueroa
Los Angeles, CA 90003
(213) 778-5290

Neighborhood Youth Association Youth
  Services
Drug Abuse Treatment Center
3877 Grandview Blvd.
Los Angeles, CA 90066
(213) 390-6641

Sunrise Youth Community
1001 S. Westmoreland
Los Angeles, CA 90006
(213) 384-1937

New Morning Youth and Family Services
460 Main St.
Placerville, CA 95667
(916) 622-1515

Sacramento County Drug Alternatives Program
Drug Abuse Treatment Unit
1708 Q St.
Sacramento, CA 95816
(916) 446-0117

Awareness Program
Drug Abuse Treatment Center
1153 Oak St.
San Francisco, CA 94115
(415) 431-9000

Santa Cruz Community Counseling Center—
  Youth Services North
Drug Abuse Treatment Center
117 Union St.
Santa Cruz, CA 95060
(408) 429-8350

CONNECTICUT
Vitam Center Inc.
Drug Abuse Treatment Unit
57 W. Rocks Rd.
Norwalk, CT 06851
(203) 846-2091

Regional Network Program
171 Golden Hill St.
Bridgeport, CT 06604
(203) 333-4105

FLORIDA
The Starting Place, Inc.
State Drug Abuse Program
Drug Abuse Treatment Unit
2057 Coolidge St.
Hollywood, FL 33020
(305) 925-2225

Starting Place Residential
Drug Abuse Treatment Unit
5925 McKinley St.
Hollywood, FL 33021
(305) 925-2225

Metatherapy Institute Inc.
27200 Old Dixie Highway
Naranja, FL 33032
(305) 247-4515

Straight Incorporated
Drug Abuse Treatment Unit
3100 Gandy Blvd.
PO Box 1577
Pinellas Park, FL 34290-1577
(813) 577-6011

Brevard County MHC Inc.
Substance Abuse Services
Alcoholism/Drug Abuse Treatment Unit
1770 Cedar St.
Rockledge, FL 39255
(305) 632-9480

Turnabout
2531 W. Tharpe St.
PO Box 13488
Tallahassee, FL 32303
(904) 385-5179

Dacco Family Outpatient Program
Drug Abuse Treatment Unit
3200 Henderson Blvd.
Tampa, FL 33609
(813) 870-2905

Disc Village
Drug Abuse Treatment Unit
PO Box 568
Woodville, FL 32362
(904) 421-4115

GEORGIA
Alchemy Therapeutic Community
Drug Abuse Treatment Unit
8134 Blythe St.
Columbus, GA 31904
(404) 324-7241

Clayton Outpatient Program
Drug Abuse Treatment Unit
6315 Don Hastings Drive
Flint River Center
Riverdale, GA 30274
(404) 991-0111

HAWAII
Awareness House Inc.
Alcoholism/Drug Abuse Treatment Unit
305 Wailuku Drive
Hilo, HI 96720
(808) 961-4771

ILLINOIS
Northwest Youth Outreach Drug Abuse
    Treatment
Alcoholism/Drug Abuse Treatment Unit
6417 W. Irving Park Rd.
Chicago, IL 60634
(312) 777-7112

Tapestry Youth Center
Drug Abuse Treatment Unit
950 E. 61st St.
Chicago, IL 60637
(312) 324-2551

Omni House
Drug Abuse Treatment Unit
222 E. Dundee Rd.
Wheeling, IL 60090
(312) 541-0190

Interventions/Contact
400 Anderson Rd., Box 341
Wauconda, IL 60084
(312) 526-0404

INDIANA
Intensive Outpatient Program (IOP)
The Center for Mental Health
Alcoholism/Drug Abuse Treatment Unit
2020 Brown St.
PO Box 1258
Anderson, IN 46015
(317) 649-8161

Aquarius House
Alcoholism/Drug Abuse Treatment
413 S. Liberty
Muncie, IN 47305
(317) 282-2257

LOUISIANA
Education and Treatment Council Inc.
Alcoholism/Drug Abuse Treatment Unit
1146 Hodges
Lake Charles, LA 70601
(318) 433-1062

MAINE
Bath-Brunswick Mental Health Association
Drug Abuse Treatment Unit
Full Circle Program
24 Jordan Ave.
Brunswick, ME 04011
(207) 729-8706

Saco Unit
Alcoholism/Drug Abuse Treatment Unit
265 North St.
Saco, ME 04072
(207) 282-7504

MARYLAND
Youth Services Program
Harbel Drug Abuse
5807 Harford Rd.
Baltimore, MD 21214
(301) 444-2100

Focus on Family
650 Ritchie Highway
Severna Park, MD 21146
(301) 647-8121

Substance Abuse Treatment
Family Therapy Services
8500 Colesville Rd.
Silver Spring, MD 20910
(301) 565-7729

Somerset County Health Department Addiction
  Program
Alcoholism/Drug Abuse Treatment Unit
PO Box 129
Westover, MD 21871
(301) 651-0822, x72

MASSACHUSETTS
Project Concern, Inc.
Drug Abuse Treatment Unit
1000 Harvard St.
Boston, MA 02126
(617) 298-0106

New Perspective School Inc.
Drug Abuse Treatment Unit
74 Green St.
Brookline, MA 02146
(617) 232-1958

Burlington Community Life Center
Drug Abuse Treatment Unit
Center School
Center St.
Burlington, MA 01803
(617) 273-1300

Chicopee Adolescent Program
99 Main St.
Chicopee Falls, MA 01020
(413) 594-2141

Peabody Council on Youth Needs
Drug Abuse Treatment Unit
30 Central St.
Peabody, MA 01960
(617) 532-3839

Youth and Family Services of Greater
  Westfield
Drug Abuse Treatment Unit
41 Church St.
Westfield, MA 01085
(413) 568-3368

MICHIGAN
Ann Arbor Community Center Project
Alcoholism/Drug Abuse Treatment Unit
625 N. Main St.
Ann Arbor, MI 48104
(313) 662-3128

Substance Abuse Services to Special Youth
  (SASSY)
Woodland Counseling Center
314 S. Main St.
Cheboygan, MI 49721
(616) 347-6063

Project Rehab Siloh Family
Alcoholism/Drug Abuse Treatment Unit
750 Cherry St., S.E.
Grand Rapids, MI 49503
(616) 774-9536

The Center for Human Resources
1113 Military St.
Port Huron, MI 48060
(313) 985-5168

Mackinac County Youth Services Bureau
Drug Abuse Treatment Unit
PO Box 155
Saint Ignace, MI 49781
(906) 643-9550, x31

MINNESOTA
Warren Eustis House
720 O'Neill Drive
Eagan, MN 55121
(612) 452-6908

NEVADA
Bridge Counseling Associates
Alcoholism/Drug Abuse Treatment Unit
1785 E. Sahara, Suite 130
Las Vegas, NV 89104
(702) 734-6070

NEW HAMPSHIRE
Southeastern New Hampshire Services
PO Box 978
50 Chestnut St.
Dover, NH 03820
(603) 749-3981

Odyssey House Inc.
Drug Abuse Treatment Unit
New Hampshire Unit
30 Winnacunnet Rd.
PO Box 474
Hampton, NH 03842
(603) 926-6702

Office of Youth Services
36 Lowell St.
Manchester, NH 03101
(603) 624-6470

Nashua Youth Council
19 Chestnut St.
Nashua, NH 03060
(603) 889-1090

NEW JERSEY
Woodbridge Action for Youth
Drug Abuse Treatment Unit
73 Green St.
Woodbridge, NJ 07095
(201) 634-7910

NEW MEXICO
San Felipe Pueblo Drug Program
PO Box A
San Felipe
Albuquerque, NM 87001
(505) 867-3381

Behavioral Health Services of Acoma
Substance Abuse Prevention Program
PO Box 328
Pueblo of Acoma, NM 87034
(505) 552-6663

Eight Northern Indian Pueblo
Drug Council Program
Drug Abuse Treatment Unit
PO Box 969
San Juan Pueblo, NM 87566
(505) 852-4265, x139

NEW YORK
Hospitality House
Therapeutic Community, Inc.
271 Central Ave.
Albany, NY 12206
(518) 434-6468

Saint Anne's Institute Program
Drug Abuse Treatment Unit
160 N. Main Ave.
Albany, NY 12206
(518) 489-7411

Bethpage Adolescent Development Association
936 Stewart Ave.
Bethpage, NY 11714
(516) 433-5344

Argus Community Inc.
Drug Abuse Treatment Unit
760 E. 160th St.
Bronx, NY 10456
(212) 993-5300

Addiction Research & Treatment Corp.
(ARTC)
Drug Abuse Treatment Unit
564 Hopkinson Ave.
Brooklyn, NY 11212
(718) 636-6742

District III Youth and Adult Inc.
Drug Abuse Treatment Unit
271 Melrose St.
Brooklyn, NY 11206
(718) 821-7710

The Family Youth Center
Downstate (Kings Co.) Medical Center
600 Albany Ave.
Box 9, Building K1
Code 26
Brooklyn, NY 11203
(718) 735-2844

Volunteer Family Counseling Service
36 Main St.
Marine Midland Building
Cortland, NY 13045
(607) 753-9349

Northport/East Northport Youth Development
Association
Drug Abuse Treatment Unit
7 Diane Court
East Northport, NY 11731
(516) 261-7901

Daytop Village Inc.
Drug Abuse Treatment Unit
Queens Daycare and Outpatient
166-10 91st Ave.
Jamaica, NY 11432
(718) 523-8288

Manhasset Day Care Center
1355 Northern Blvd.
Manhasset, NY 11030
(516) 627-5002

Daytop Village Inc.
Route 44
PO Box 607
Millbrook, NY 12545
(914) 677-5335

Phase Piggy Back Inc.
Youth Intervention and Development
Drug Abuse Treatment Unit
458 W. 145th St.
New York, NY 10031
(212) 234-1660

Tioga County Alcohol and Drug Services
Alcoholism/Drug Abuse Treatment Unit
175 Front St.
Owego, NY 13827
(607) 687-5555

Threshold
115 S. Clinton Ave.
Rochester, NY 14604
(716) 454-7530

Saratoga Springs Office of Abused Substances
   & Intervention Services Inc. (OASIS)
117 Vandam St.
Saratoga Springs, NY 12866
(518) 587-2992

Syosset's Concern About its Neighborhood
   (SCAN)
184 Jackson Ave.
Syosset, NY 11791
(516) 921-3740

OHIO
Catholic Counseling Center
Outpatient Adolescent–409 Hispanic Division
2012 W. 25th St., Room 615
Cleveland, OH 44113
(216) 696-6650

Choices
Westside CMHC
8711 Dennison Ave.
Cleveland, OH 44102
(216) 631-8686

Family Health Association
3737 Lander Rd.
Cleveland, OH 44124
(216) 831-6960

Shawnee Mental Health
225 Carlton Davidson Lane
Coalgrove, OH 45638
(614) 533-0648

Alcohol and Drug Dependency Services of
   Medina County
Drug Abuse Treatment Unit
246 Northland Drive
Medina, OH 44256
(216) 723-3641, x321

Straight Inc.
6074 Branch Hill/Guinea Pike
Milford, OH 45150
(513) 575-2673

Parmadale Family Treatment Program
6753 State Rd.
Parma, OH 44134
(216) 845-7700

Wayne County Human Resource Center
Drug Abuse Treatment Unit
2692 Akron Rd.
Wooster, OH 44691
(216) 264-9597

PENNSYLVANIA
Genesis Ministries Inc.
115 Cocoa Ave.
Hershey, PA 17033
(717) 534-2823

Abraxas Foundation Inc., Abrax I
Alcoholism/Drug Abuse Treatment Unit
Blue Jay Village
PO Box 59
Marienville, PA 16239
(814) 927-6615

The Bridge
Therapeutic Center at Fox Chase
8400 Pine Rd.
Philadelphia, PA 19111
(215) 342-5000

Cora Services
Drug Abuse Treatment Unit
733 Susquehana Rd.
Philadelphia, PA 19111
(215) 342-7660

Philadelphia Psychiatric Center
Wurzel Clinic
Ford Road and Monument Ave.
Philadelphia, PA 19131
(215) 581-3757

RHODE ISLAND
Caritas House Inc.
Drug Abuse Treatment Unit
166 Pawtucket Ave.
Pawtucket, RI 02860
(401) 722-4644

TEXAS
United Medical Centers
610 S. Monroe
Eagle Pass, TX 78852
(512) 773-9271

Tropical Texas Center
Drug Treatment
1208 N. Seventh St.
Harlingen, TX 78550
(512) 425-7080

Vernon Center South
Adolescent Drug Abuse & Addiction Service
FM 433 and SH283
PO Box 2231
Vernon, TX 76384
(817) 552-9901

VIRGINIA
Chesapeake Substance Abuse Program
4715 Bainbridge Blvd.
Chesapeake, VA 23320
(804) 494-0533

Loudon County Mental Health Center
Alcoholism/Drug Abuse Treatment Unit
8 South St., S.W.
Leesburg, VA 22075
(703) 777-0320

Shalom et Benedictus Inc.
Alcoholism/Drug Abuse Treatment Unit
PO Box 309
Stephenson, VA 22656
(703) 667-0875

Bacon Street, Inc.
Drug Abuse Treatment Unit
105 Bacon Ave.
Williamsburg, VA 23185
(804) 253-0111

WASHINGTON
Youth Eastside Services
Drug Abuse Treatment Unit
257 100th Ave., N.E.
Bellevue, WA 98004
(206) 454-5502

Highline Youth Service Bureau
15631 Des Moines Way S.
Seattle, WA 98166
(206) 243-5544
Crisis Clinic: (206) 447-3222

WEST VIRGINIA
Western District Guidance Center
Alcoholism/Drug Abuse Treatment Unit
2121 Seventh St.
Parkersburg, WV 26101
(304) 485-1721

WISCONSIN
Community Impact Programs, Inc.
Alcoholism/Drug Abuse Treatment Unit
2106 63rd St.
Kenosha, WI 53140
(414) 654-1004

The Recovery Center
County Highway Z
Parkland East Building Box 58A
Wentworth, WI 54894
(715) 398-7646

SOURCE: *National Institute on Drug Abuse.*

INFORMATION AND ORGANIZATIONS

Families Anonymous
PO Box 528
Van Nuys, CA 91408
(818) 989-7841

Self-help, mutual support group for families and friends of those with drug abuse problems. Modeled after Alcoholics Anonymous, with over 300 local groups throughout the country. Offers pamphlets, booklets and a bimonthly newsletter. Will send more information, including where to find a local group in your area or how to establish one.

Hazelden Foundation
PO Box 11
Center City, MN 55012
(800) 328-9000
(612) 257-4010

A nonprofit organization for chemical dependency rehabilitation. Maintains several programs in Minnesota, including the Hazelden Rehabilitation Center, a large private treatment center accommodating about 1,600 people a year. Also operates a rehabilitation program in West Palm Beach, Florida, a live-in 5-day program for families. A major publisher and distributor of materials on drug and alcohol abuse: numerous books, booklets, pamphlets, audiotapes, videotapes, films. Quarterly newsletter. Will provide more information and a catalogue of materials upon request.

Narcotics Anonymous
16155 Wyandotte Street
Van Nuys, CA 91406
(818) 780-3951

National self-help, mutual support group for those with drug abuse problems, modeled on Alcoholic Anonymous. Local groups throughout the country. Pamphlets, quarterly newsletter. Will send more information on how to find or form local groups upon request. Listed in telephone directories of major cities. Hotlines in major cities.

National Clearinghouse for Drug Abuse
   Information
5600 Fishers Lane, Room 10 A-43
Rockville, MD 20857
(301) 443-6500

To order specific publications through the mail, the address is PO Box 416, Kensington, MD 20795.

An information source sponsored by the federal government. Provides information to the public and professionals working in the field of drug rehabilitation on all aspects of drug abuse. Will answer questions over the phone and send detailed information upon request. Can also tell you how to set up parent-peer groups in your community to fight drug abuse.

National Federation of Parents for Drug Free
   Youth
PO Box 722
Silver Spring, MD 20901
(301) 585-5437

A national voluntary organization of parents concerned about drug abuse and alcohol use by children and teens. A source of information, with local groups throughout the country. Helps parents and community leaders set up local programs. Special service: operates a telephone info line, and Reach America training program for drug-free youth peer leaders. Will provide more information upon request.

National Institute on Drug Abuse
Prevention Branch
Room 11A-33
5600 Fishers Lane
Rockville, MD 20857

The agency within the federal government's Department of Health and Human Services most concerned with the problems of drug abuse. Sponsors research on drug abuse. Publishes numerous materials. Provides information on how to organize communities to combat drug abuse.

Parents' Resource Institute for Drug Education,
   Inc. (PRIDE)
100 Edgewood Ave., Suite 1216
Atlanta, GA 30303
(800) 241-9746

A private nonprofit organization for parents, educators, and others interested in adolescent drug abuse. A source of information, it sponsors an annual conference and helps parents organize local networks and educational programs on drug abuse. Referrals are provided for those needing help with drug problems. More information upon request.

TOUGHLOVE
PO Box 1069
Doylestown, PA 18901
(215) 348-7090

A national alcohol and drug abuse prevention program geared toward helping parents, families and friends cope with individuals who are chemi-cally dependent or potentially chemically dependent. Has a listing of about 1,500 local groups for parents and kids. Helps parents organize local groups. Provides books, audiocassettes, a bimonthly newsletters. Makes referrals to local groups. Will provide more information upon request.

Also *see* page 50 for Alcoholics' Self-Help groups that deal with drug abuse.

BOOKS

Daytop Village, **Barry Sugarman,** New York: Irvington Publishers, 1983.

Drug Use and Misuse, New York: St. Martin's Press, 1983.

Evaluation of Drug Treatment Programs, New York: Haworth Press, 1983.

The Female Fix, **Muriel Nellis,** New York: Penguin, 1981, (tranquilizers).

Getting Off the Hook, **Meg Patterson,** Wheaton, IL: Harold Shaw, 1983.

Getting Tough on Gateway Drugs: A Guide for the Family, **Robert L. Dupont, Jr., M.D.,** Washington, D.C., American Psychiatric Press, 1984.

Managing the "Drugs" In Your Life: A Personal and Family Guide to the Responsible Use of Drugs, Alcohol,

Medicine, **Stephen J. Levy,** New York: McGraw Hill, 1983.

Narcotics Anonymous, Van Nuys, CA: World Service Office, 1982.

Pot Safari: A Visit to the Top Marijuana Researchers in the U.S., **Peggy Mann,** New York: Woodmere Press, 1983.

Stopping Valium, **Eve Bargmann,** New York: Warner Books, 1983, (covers other tranquilizers also).

Toughlove, **Phyllis and David York,** New York: Doubleday, 1982, Bantam Books, 1983.

Toughlove Solutions, **Phyllis and David York,** New York: Doubleday, 1984, Bantam Books, 1985.

MATERIALS, FREE AND FOR SALE

Free (single copies)

Are You a Drug Quiz Whiz?, 8 pages.

Communities: What You Can Do About Drug and Alcohol Abuse, 16 pages.

Hallucinogens and PCP: Just Say No, 5 pages.

Marijuana: Just Say No, 5 pages.

Opiates: Just Say No, 5 pages.

Parents, Peers and Pot, a handbook for parents on how to form a parent network against drugs.

Sedative-Hypnotics: Just Say No, 4 pages.

Stimulants and Cocaine: Just Say No, 6 pages.

National Clearinghouse for Drug Abuse Information
PO Box 416
Kensington, MD 20795
(301) 443-6500

What Parents Must Learn, pamphlet series.

National Federation of Parents for Drug-Free Youth
PO Box 722
Silver Spring, MD 20901

For sale

A Father Faces Drug Abuse
A Guide for the Family of the Drug Abuser
Tough Love: Alternative to Enabling

Families Anonymous
PO Box 528
Van Nuys, CA 91408
(818) 989-7841

Learn About Cocaine, 16 pages.
Learn About Marijuana, 16 pages.

Hazelden Foundation
PO Box 11
Center City, MN 55012
(800) 328-9000

Toughlove: A Self-Help Manual for Parents
  Troubled by Teenage Behavior, 98 pages.
Toughlove: A Self-Manual for Kids, 134 pages.
Toughlove Cocaine: Help for People Who
  Care About a Cocaine User

Toughlove
PO Box 1069
Doylestown, PA 18901

EPILEPSY

Epilepsy is a brain disorder that affects about 1 percent of the population—more than two million Americans. The condition is characterized by recurrent seizures induced by temporary brain changes. About 100,000 new cases show up each year, three-quarters of them in children under age 18. In about 30 percent of the cases epilepsy appears before school age. It can strike in middle age (5 percent of the cases) and old age (2 percent of the cases) as well.

Cause: Unknown in about half the cases, even after extensive examination and testing by neurological specialists. When no brain damage can be found, it is theorized that the epilepsy may be caused by some unknown chemical brain abnormality. Epilepsy has been linked to fetal damage, such as infections and oxygen deprivation; birth traumas; brain tumors; lead poisoning; infectious diseases, such as meningitis and encephalitis, even severe cases of measles; strokes; head injuries, for example, from auto accidents; and inherited diseases, such as phenylketonuria (PKU). There is a slight genetic predisposition to some forms of epilepsy. Epilepsy can also develop without a family history.

Some children outgrow epilepsy, although there is no sure way to predict which children will. Children with *petit mal* (''absence'') epilepsy have a good chance of outgrowing the disorder. There is also a benign childhood epilepsy, called Rolandic, in which the seizures almost always disappear after adolescence.

Symptoms: The type and severity of seizures vary greatly. They may range from a *grand mal* or convulsive seizure, in which the person becomes unconscious, to simple nonconvulsive brief staring or ''blanking out'' spells. Epileptic seizures may also be characterized by stiffening or jerking motions or abnormal physical movements.

Diagnosis: Most physicians diagnose epilepsy after a comprehensive medical history detailing the seizures, along with certain diagnostic tests. Epilepsy is often detected by an electroencephalogram (EEG) that records abnormal electrical brain wave activity. An EEG, however, may not reveal epilepsy, often making other diagnostic procedures necessary. These might include brain scan, skull X-rays, CAT scan, or an angiogram.

Treatment: Drugs are by far the most common treatment and have been amazingly successful in keeping epilepsy under control for most people. Drugs bring total control of seizures for about half of all people with epilepsy and reduce the number of seizures for another 30 percent. Drugs are not effective for about 20 percent of those with epilepsy. Usually, the drugs must be taken regularly over a lifetime, but recent research has shown that some children who have been free of seizures for a few years may no longer need medication. The drugs have been cautiously withdrawn from them with no recurrence of seizures. However, this drug withdrawal must be done under a physician's supervision. Withdrawing medication from children with epilepsy is potentially dangerous and could result in continuous seizures and even death if not done under medical supervision.

Surgery is usually performed to relieve epilepsy if the cause is a tumor. Surgery may also be called for if medication does not work, or if the seizures are traced to a very small area of the brain that can be removed without impairing

211

mental or physical function. Special high-fat diets, which produce a chemical condition called ketosis, sometimes help control epilepsy in children. Biofeedback, in which patients learn to produce certain brain-wave patterns to prevent seizures, has also been used successfully in a small number of cases, although some experts fear that the effect wears off and the seizures return.

WHERE TO FIND TREATMENT FOR EPILEPSY

Neurologists, pediatric neurologists, pediatricians, and family physicians can treat epilepsy. People whose seizures are difficult to control can find help from leading experts in epilepsy at medical centers, from neurological clinics at university and other hospitals, and from neurological specialists in private practice.

For the names of neurologists who head departments of neurology at leading medical colleges, *see* page 621. The physicians can be an excellent source of treatment and/or referrals to others specializing in epilepsy.

NATIONAL EPILEPSY PROGRAMS

There are four comprehensive epilepsy programs and six research centers, supported by the National Institutes of Health. The physicians and other specialists at these clinics are among the country's most respected authorities in epilepsy.

Clinical Epilepsy Programs

UCLA School of Medicine, University of
  California
Los Angeles, CA 90024
Paul H. Crandall, M.D.
(213) 824-4303

University of Minnesota–Minneapolis Medical
  School
1360 Mayo Memorial Building
Minneapolis, MN 55455
Robert J. Gumnit, M.D.
(612) 376-1260

University of Virginia
Charlottesville, VA 22908
Fritz E. Dreifuss, M.D.
(703) 924-5401

University of Washington School of Medicine
Seattle, WA 98195
Arthur A. Ward, Jr., M.D.
(206) 223-3557

Epilepsy Research Centers

Stanford University Medical Center
300 Pasteur Drive
Stanford, CA 94305
David A. Prince, M.D.
(415) 723-5522

Yale University School of Medicine
333 Cedar St.
New Haven, CT 06516
Gilbert H. Glaser, M.D.
(203) 785-4086

Washington University School of Medicine
660 S. Euclid Ave.
St. Louis, MO 63110
James Ferrendelli, M.D.
(314) 362-7815

Duke University School of Medicine
PO Box 3005
Durham, NC 27710
James McNamara, M.D.
(919) 681-2659

Baylor College of Medicine
1200 Moursund Ave.
Houston, TX 77025
Peter Kellaway, M.D.
(713) 790-3105

University of Utah College of Medicine
50 N. Medical Drive
Salt Lake City, UT 84132
Dixon Woodbury, M.D.
(801) 581-6780

SOURCE: *National Institute of Neurological and Communicative Disorders and Stroke.*

ORGANIZATIONS

Epilepsy Foundation of America
4351 Garden City Drive
Suite 406
Landover, MD 20785
(301) 459-3700

A national nonprofit charitable organization and major source of information on epilepsy, with local affiliates around the country. Information and referral system that answers all types of questions from the public about epilepsy, including sources of medical and rehabilitation help. Operates the National Library and Resource Center on Epilepsy. Pamphlets, booklets, books and bibliographies. Will provide more information upon request, including the name of a local affiliate near you.

National Easter Seal Society, Inc.
2023 W. Ogden Ave.
Chicago, IL 60612
(312) 243-8400/Voice
(312) 243-8880/TDD

A national organization, state and local societies formed to give services to people with disabilities from many causes, including epilepsy, cerebral palsy, stroke, speech and hearing disorders, geriatric problems, fractures, arthritis, learning and developmental disorders, heart disease, spina bifida, accidents, and multiple sclerosis. It maintains about 200 rehabilitation centers nationwide, with various services depending upon the local unit. A major source of information and self-help. Publishes pamphlets and booklets. Referrals to services are made through local Easter Seal affiliates listed in local phone directories. Will provide more information and location of Easter Seal affiliate near you upon request.

BOOKS

The Epilepsy Fact Book, **Harry Sands** and **Frances C. Minters,** New York: Charles Scribner's Sons, 1979.
The Epilepsy Handbook, **Robert J. Gumnit,** New York: Raven Press, 1983.
Epilepsy: A Handbook, **Allen H. Middleton, Arthur A. Attwell,** and **Gregory Walsh,** Boston: Little Brown, 1982.

Seizures, Epilepsy and Your Child, **Joreg C. Lagos, M.D.,** New York: Harper & Row, 1974.
What If They Knew?, **Patricia Hermes,** New York: Harcourt Brace Jovanovich, 1980.

FREE MATERIALS

Single copies are free

Epilepsy: Medical Aspects, 6 pages.
Medications for Epilepsy, 15 pages.
Questions and Answers About Epilepsy, 16
  pages.

Epilepsy Foundation of America
4351 Garden City Drive
Suite 406
Landover, MD 20785

Epilepsy: Hope Through Research

National Institute of Neurological and
  Communicative Disorders and Stroke
Building 31, Room 8A06
Bethesda, MD 20892

EYE DISEASES AND VISION PROBLEMS

About 11.5 million Americans have visual impairments that cannot be corrected by eyeglasses or contact lenses. One and one-half million of these people cannot read ordinary newspapers or books. One-half million are legally blind; that is, even their best eye cannot be corrected by contact lenses or glasses to 20/200 vision. Vision problems strike all ages, but older people are a prime target. Every year more than a million Americans are hospitalized for an eye disorder. Eye disorders and blindness take an annual economic toll of $14 billion.

MAJOR DISEASES OF THE EYE

Glaucoma: Glaucoma is an incurable but usually controllable disease in which fluid pressure builds up within the eyeball. It causes the progressive loss of peripheral vision and, in some cases, blindness due to irreversible damage to the optic nerve. The progression of glaucoma can be stopped or slowed by relieving the pressure with drugs, laser treatment, or surgery. That is why it is essential to have glaucoma diagnosed as early as possible. Once damage occurs, the visual loss cannot be reversed.

Glaucoma is generally a disease of aging; it occurs most often after age 40, although there are some types that occur in infants. Glaucoma affects between one and two million Americans and accounts for blindness in more than 60,000, making it the leading cause of blindness. The disease tends to run in families and is more common among black Americans. There are two dominant types of glaucoma: One is called open-angle, a progressive form that accounts for 80 percent of the cases; the other is called closed-angle, which strikes suddenly, causing pain, blurriness, and halos. There are few early signs of progressive open-angle glaucoma, so many people have the disease without knowing it, and it is often not discovered until damage has been done.

The cause of glaucoma is unknown, although it is more common among those with a family history of the disease. It is rather easily detected by a competent ophthalmologist through physical examination and measurement of eye pressure. Usually drugs are used to reduce the pressure, and lately there have been exciting developments in the use of lasers for treatment of both open- and closed-angle glaucoma. Certainly, anyone with glaucoma should seek top-notch medical treatment from a glaucoma specialist and may want to participate in experimental research now being conducted at several centers and at the National Institutes of Health.

Age-related macular degeneration: The macula is the tiny central part of the retina that produces sharp central vision. If the macula deteriorates, a person loses the ability to read and see fine detail. Macular degeneration is a serious but little-known disease that is the second leading cause of blindness. It affects more than 10 million people over age 50 and is the number-one cause of new blindness in people age 65 and over. In some people the disease progresses slowly and may never cause much difficulty; in others it causes rapid vision deterioration and may lead to blindness. This type is characterized by the growth of abnormal blood vessels in the eye, and typical symptoms are the perception of straight lines as wavy or crooked. Later, a blind spot may be noticeable in the central field of vision. Early treatment is essential because irreversible damage can occur in a short period of time. If the rapidly progressing form of the disease is detected, however, new techniques of treating it with lasers can be amazingly successful in preventing macular damage and blindness.

Cataracts: The lenses of the eyes become clouded and opaque, making it difficult to see. Although cataracts primarily affect older people, the disease can occur at any age, even very occasionally in infants. However, cataracts are definitely an older person's disease: About 60 percent of Americans between the ages of 65 and 74 have signs of cataracts and more than three million are visually impaired. About 42,000 are blind because of cataracts, making cataracts the third leading cause of blindness.

Fortunately, cataracts, though serious, are rather routinely removed by a simple surgical procedure that can be done by a qualified ophthalmologist. Good vision is restored in about 95 percent of the cases by contact lenses, glasses, or artificial implants called intraocular lenses. Even though the cataract removal is usually simple, successful, and safe, the implantation of an artificial lens is best done by a skilled eye surgeon, preferably at a leading eye center if one is nearby. Serious complications and even blindness have resulted when the surgery is not done properly. Even when the surgery is done properly, some people will develop serious complications. Thus, it is important to have good follow-up care after cataract surgery so any complications can be detected and treated.

Diabetic retinopathy: This disease is a complication of diabetes, resulting from problems with the vascular system that damage the retina. It is the leading cause of new cases of blindness for persons aged 20 to 74. The majority of people who have had diabetes for seven or more years

show at least mild signs of diabetic retinopathy. As long as the disease remains mild, there is no immediate danger of visual loss. The type of diabetic retinopathy that can lead to blindness affects less than 10 percent of all diabetics. However, doctors are unable to predict which diabetics will develop that serious disease and how rapidly it will progress. Diabetic retinopathy results in the hemorrhaging of small blood vessels in the eye and the growth of new blood vessels, which can cause scarring and possibly retinal detachment. All diabetics should be aware of the possibility of developing this disease, and it is recommended that diabetics have two eye examinations yearly.

If diabetic retinopathy is diagnosed early, it can be effectively treated. One treatment is vitrectomy, a surgical technique that restores sight in some diabetics. Another highly successful treatment is the use of an argon laser to seal off the newly formed blood vessels and prevent further vessel growth. Now research shows that laser treatment is effective against an early form of diabetic retinopathy called diabetic macular edema.

Retinitis pigmentosa: Retinitis pigmentosa is an incurable genetic disease causing deterioration of the retina. The disease may cause a marked reduction in vision or legal blindness. It usually shows up in children and adolescents; the first symptom is "night blindness" that gradually worsens. Side vision is also diminished, leaving the person with "tunnel vision." The rate at which the disease progresses varies greatly. Although many sufferers of the disease retain some vision, including their reading vision, for a lifetime, the disease is a leading cause of blindness, accounting for about 24,000 cases.

Victims of retinitis pigmentosa may also have other vision problems, such as cataracts, retinal edema, and glaucoma, and frequently hearing loss as well. The disease is usually diagnosed by an ophthalmologist who detects black pigment deposits scattered throughout the retina. This pigment characterizes the disease and gives it its name. In rare cases the pigment may be absent.

There is no treatment for the disease, but early diagnosis is recommended, so the individual can take advantage of devices and aids when vision decreases. Also, the appearance of retinitis pigmentosa calls for genetic counseling to determine how future offspring will be affected. (*See* Genetic Counseling, page 226.)

Other eye diseases: Some other eye diseases that call for specialized treatment and management are optic nerve atrophy (the optic nerve shrinks or wastes away, leading to blindness); uveitis (an inflammation of the middle layer of the eye); detachment of the retina; ocular histoplasmosis syndrome (a potentially blinding disease related to histoplasmosis, a fungal infection).

If you have anything seriously wrong with your eyes that necessitates drugs, surgery, or other medical procedures, you will want to make sure you're in the hands of a competent ophthalmologist (a physician who specializes in eye treatment). There are many excellent special eye hospitals, centers, and ophthalmologists around the country; some are affiliated with medical schools. Such centers treat all kinds of eye disorders and usually have specialists in major eye diseases. For a list of specialists who head departments of ophthalmology at leading medical schools, *see* page 603. They can be excellent sources of treatment and/or referrals to other specialists.

DIABETIC RETINOPATHY RESEARCH SPECIALISTS

The following eye centers were selected to conduct government-sponsored research to test the effectiveness of various early treatments for diabetic retinopathy.

CALIFORNIA
Estelle Doheny Eye Foundation
University of Southern California
School of Medicine
1355 San Pablo Ave.
Los Angeles, CA 90033
B. John Hodgkinson, M.D.
(213) 226-5232

Jules Stein Eye Institute
Center for the Health Sciences
UCLA Medical Center
Room 3-114
800 Westwood Plaza
Los Angeles, CA 90024
Stanley M. Kopelow, M.D.
(213) 206-6093

Zweng Memorial Retinal Research Foundation
1225 Crane St.
Menlo Park, CA 94025
Hunter L. Little, M.D.
(415) 323-0231

Department of Ophthalmology
Pacific Medical Center
2340 Clay St.
San Francisco, CA 94115
Everett Ai, M.D.
(415) 563-4321, x2923

FLORIDA
Bascom Palmer Eye Institute
Department of Ophthalmology
School of Medicine
University of Miami
900 N.W. 17th St.
Miami, FL 33136
Harry Flynn, M.D.
(305) 326-6118

ILLINOIS
University of Illinois
Abraham Lincoln School of Medicine
Room 2224
1855 W. Taylor St.
Chicago, IL 60612
Jose Cunha-Vaz, M.D.
(312) 996-7843

Ingalls Memorial Hospital
Retinal Vascular Service
One Ingalls Drive
Harvey, IL 60426
David H. Orth, M.D.
(312) 333-2300, x5927

LOUISIANA
LSU Eye Center
136 S. Roman St.
New Orleans, LA 70112
Rudolph M. Franklin, M.D.
(504) 568-6766

MARYLAND
Johns Hopkins University
The Wilmer Ophthalmological Institute
School of Medicine
Wilmer, Room 116
600 N. Wolfe St.
Baltimore, MD 21205
Robert P. Murphy, M.D.
(301) 955-2840

MASSACHUSETTS
Joslin Diabetes Foundation
William P. Beecham Eye Unit
One Joslin Place
Boston, MA 02215
Lloyd M. Aiello, M.D.
(617) 732-2554

Eye Research Institute of Retina Foundation/
  Retina Associates, Inc.
100 Charles River Plaza
Boston, MA 02114
Sheldon M. Buzney, M.D.
(617) 523-7810

MICHIGAN
Kresge Eye Institute
Wayne State University
School of Medicine
3994 John R. St.
Detroit, MI 48201
Robert M. Frank, M.D.
(313) 577-1320

Associated Retinal Consultants
3535 W. 13 Mile Rd.
Suite 507
Royal Oak, MI 48072
Raymond R. Margherio, M.D.
(313) 288-2280

MINNESOTA
University of Minnesota
Department of Ophthalmology
Medical School
Box 493
Mayo Memorial Building
Minneapolis, MN 55455
William H. Knobloch, M.D.
(612) 373-8425

NEW YORK
Department of Ophthalmology
Albany Medical College of Union University
Retina Division—K328
47 New Scotland Ave.
Albany, NY 12208
Aaron Kassoff, M.D.
(518) 445-5246

OREGON
Devers Eye Clinic
Good Samaritan Hospital and Medical Center
1200 N.W. 23rd Ave.
Portland, OR 97210
Michael L. Klein, M.D.
(503) 229-7459

PENNSYLVANIA
Retina Service
Wills Eye Hospital
9th and Walnut Sts.
Philadelphia, PA 19107
William Tasman, M.D.
(215) 233-4300

PUERTO RICO
University of Puerto Rico
Department of Ophthalmology
Room A904, GPO Box 5067
San Juan, PR 00936
Jose Berrocal, M.D.
(809) 725-9315

TEXAS
University of Texas Medical School at
  Houston
Hermann Eye Center
1203 Ross Sterling Ave.
Houston, TX 77030
Charles A. Garcia, M.D.
(713) 792-7677

UTAH
Holy Cross Hospital
1045 E. First St. S.
Salt Lake City, UT 84102
F. Tempel Riekhof, M.D.
(801) 532-7406

WASHINGTON
University of Washington
Department of Ophthalmology
Seattle, WA 98195
James L. Kinyoun, M.D.
(206) 543-2599

WISCONSIN
University of Wisconsin
Department of Ophthalmology
Medical School
D4-219 Clinical Science Center
600 Highland Ave.
Madison, WI 53706
George H. Bresnick, M.D.
(608) 263-7169

Medical College of Wisconsin
Department of Ophthalmology
8700 W. Wisconsin Ave.
Milwaukee, WI 53226
George A. Williams, M.D.
(414) 475-0701

SOURCE: *National Eye Institute.*

SCREENING CENTERS FOR NIGHT VISION AID

The Night Vision Aid is a binocular-like device to help people with retinitis pigmentosa regain some vision at night. It is made for those who still have functioning daylight vision. The aid was developed by the International Telephone and Telegraph Company in cooperation with the Retinitis Pigmentosa Foundation. The aid does not arrest retinitis pigmentosa or cure it; it merely allows a person to use his or her best daylight vision in darkness. It cannot be used for driving at night. If you want to know more about it, contact the Retinitis Pigmentosa Foundation (Rolling Park Building, 8331 Mindale Circle, Baltimore, MD 21207) or one of the screening centers listed below.

ARIZONA
Harold E. Cross, M.D., Ph.D.
Tucson Medical Park West
5200 E. Grant Rd., Suite 101
Tucson, AZ 85712
(602) 881-8544

CALIFORNIA
Kenneth E. Brookman, O.D., Ph.D.
Chief, Low Vision Services
Optometric Center of Fullerton
Southern California College of Optometry
2001 Associated Rd.
Fullerton, CA 92631
(714) 870-7226

Bill Mattingly, Low Vision Specialist
Scripps Clinic Medical Facility
10666 N. Torrey Pines Rd.
LaJolla, CA 92037
(619) 455-9100

Alan J. Reizman, O.D.
Loma Linda University
Department of Ophthalmology
11370 Anderson St., Suite 3900
Loma Linda, CA 92354
(714) 825-6513

Kenneth R. Diddie, M.D.
Estelle Doheny Eye Foundation
1355 San Pablo St.
Los Angeles, CA 90033
(213) 224-7701

John Heckinlively, M.D.
Jules Stein Eye Institute
800 Westwood Plaza
Los Angeles, CA 90024
(213) 825-6089

Wayne W. Hoeft, O.D.
Coordinator, Low Vision Services
Southern California College of Optometry
3916 S. Broadway
Los Angeles, CA 90037
(213) 234-9137

Samuel M. Genensky, Ph.D.
Director
Center for the Partially Sighted
919 Santa Monica Blvd.
Suite 200
Santa Monica, CA 90401
(213) 458-3501

FLORIDA
Sam G. Jacobson, M.D.
Bascom Palmer Eye Institute
PO Box 016880
Miami, FL 33101
(305) 326-6032

LOUISIANA
J.T. Rumage, M.D.
Gertrude Bernhauer, Visual Aids
Clinic Coordinator
Louisiana State University Eye Center
136 South Roman St.
New Orleans, LA 70112
(504) 586-6700

MARYLAND
Daniel Finkelstein, M.D.
The Johns Hopkins Hospital
Wilmer Institute, Room B27
601 N. Broadway
Baltimore, MD 21205
(301) 955-5033

Richard C. Edlow, O.D.
The Katzen Eye Group
333 St. Paul Place
Baltimore, MD 21202
(301) 727-8380

MASSACHUSETTS
Eliot L. Berson, M.D.
Professor of Ophthalmology
Harvard Medical School
Massachusetts Eye & Ear
Infirmary
243 Charles St.
Boston, MA 02114
(617) 523-7900, x388

Clifford Scott, O.D.
Optometric Clinic
VA Medical Center
1400 VFW Parkway
West Roxbury, MA 02132
(617) 323-7700, x5139
(Practice limited to veterans only.)

MINNESOTA
Jonathin D. Wirtschaefer, M.D.
Professor, Neuro-Ophthalmology
University of Minnesota
516 Delaware St., S.E.
Minneapolis, MN 55455
(612) 373-8425

MISSOURI
Mitchell L. Wolf, M.D.
Jewish Hospital of St. Louis
Department of Ophthalmology
4910 Forest Park, #220
St. Louis, MO 63108
(314) 454-7885

NEW JERSEY
Gerald Fonda, M.D.
Director, Low Vision Rehabilitation Service
St. Barnabas Medical Center
Old Short Hills Rd.
Livingston, NJ 07039
(201) 533-5000

Donald Greenfield, M.D.
Coordinator, Low Vision Service
The Eye Institute of New Jersey
15 S. Ninth St.
Newark, NJ 07107
(201) 268-8036

NEW YORK
Peter Gouras, M.D.
Department of Ophthalmology
Columbia University College of Physicians &
  Surgeons
160 Fort Washington Ave.
New York, NY 10032
(212) 694-3468

NORTH CAROLINA
Howard T. Lewis, O.D.
Department of Ophthalmology
School of Medicine
University of North Carolina at Chapel Hill
617 Clinical Science Building, 229H
Chapel Hill, NC 27514
(919) 966-5296

OHIO
Robert V. Spurney, M.D.
Chief Consultant, Low Vision Clinic
The Cleveland Society for the Blind
PO Box 1988, 1909 E. 101st St.
Cleveland, OH 44106
(216) 791-8118

Jerald A. Bovino, M.D.
Daniel F. Marcus, M.D.
St. Vincent Hospital & Medical Center
Retina Unit
2213 Cherry St.
Toledo, OH 43608
(419) 259-4367

OKLAHOMA
Wayne E. March, M.D.
LV Center
Dean A. McGee Eye Institute
608 Stanton L. Young Drive
Oklahoma City, OK 73104
(405) 271-6060

SOUTH CAROLINA
William W. Vallotton, M.D.
Director, Storm Eye Institute
Medical University of South Carolina
171 Ashley Ave.
Charleston, SC 29403
(803) 792-2492

TENNESSEE
Robert W. Ebbers, M.S., O.D.
Chief, Low Vision/Electrodiagnostic Clinics
Southern College of Optometry
1245 Madison Ave.
Memphis, TN 38104
(901) 725-0180

TEXAS
David G. Birch, Ph.D.
Research Director
Retina Foundation of the Southwest
8220 Walnut Hill Lane, Suite 012
Dallas, TX 75231
(214) 363-3911

Franklin I. Porter, O.D.
Low Vision Clinic
Department of Ophthalmology
Baylor College of Medicine
1 Baylor Plaza
Houston, TX 77030
(713) 799-5933

WASHINGTON
Terry Porter, O.D.
Lions Low Vision Clinic
1401 Madison
Seattle, WA 98104
(206) 386-2025

WISCONSIN
Rod Kossick
Wisconsin Workshop for the Blind
5316 State St.
Milwaukee, WI 53208
(414) 257-7887

SOURCE: *Retinitis Pigmentosa Foundation.*

EYE DONATION HOTLINE

(800) 638-1818 (toll-free, 24 hour)
(301) 269-4031—Maryland, call collect

This hotline is especially for those who have retinitis pigmentosa or their families. This is the number to call immediately after a donor's death because the eyes must be specially prepared immediately after death. The Retinitis Pigmentosa Foundation also has wallet cards for those with the genetic retinal disease, instructing family members and physicians of their wishes to donate.

FREE CAMPS FOR THE BLIND

National Camps for Blind Children sponsors about 360 camps around the country, including a winter camp with skiing, tobogganing, sleighing, snowmobiling, ice-skating, and swimming. Summer camps have activities such as archery, boating, canoeing, crafts, hiking, horseback riding, sailing, swimming, waterskiing, and bicycling.

Any legally blind person is eligible; there is no cost to the blind for the week of camp. It is funded by private donations to the Christian Record Braille Foundation, Inc., an institution of the General Conference of Seventh-Day Adventists. There are also adult camps for people age 20 and over. For more information, locations, and schedules contact:

National Camps for Blind Children
4444 S. 52nd St.
Lincoln, NE 68506
(402) 488-0981

RECORDINGS AND LARGE-PRINT MATERIALS

Your public library may have a section devoted to large-print books, periodicals, and other materials, or "talking" books and magazines recorded on tape. You can also contact any of the following organizations. All of them produce and distribute large-print and recorded materials for the visually handicapped.

American Foundation for the Blind, Inc.
15 W. 16th St.
New York, NY 10011
(212) 620-2000
(National Headquarters)
Regional Offices:
New York: (212) 620-2039
Washington: (202) 429-0358
Chicago: (312) 269-0095
Atlanta: (404) 525-2303
Dallas: (214) 630-8035
San Francisco: (415) 392-4845

American Printing House for the Blind
1839 Frankfort Ave.
Louisville, KY 40206
(502) 895-2405

Christian Record Braille Foundation
4444 S. 52nd St.
Lincoln, NE 68506
(402) 488-0981

National Association for the Visually
  Handicapped, Inc.
305 E. 24th St.
New York, NY 10010
(212) 889-3141

Regional Office:
3201 Balboa St.
San Francisco, CA 94121
(415) 221-3201

National Library Service for the Blind and
  Physically Handicapped
Library of Congress
1291 Taylor St., N.W.
Washington, DC 20542
(202) 287-5100

The Library of Congress has a large collection of books and magazines in braille and records on disks and cassettes, which are circulated without charge to eligible persons. You can borrow these recordings and publications through a network of regional libraries. You must complete an application for free library services, which can be obtained from any regional library or by contacting the Library of Congress.

New York Times Large Type Weekly
The New York Times
Times Square
New York, NY 20036
(212) 556-1234

Reader's Digest Fund for the Blind, Inc.
Subscription Department
Pleasantville, NY 10570
(914) 769-7000
Publishes large-print Reader's Digest and the
  Large-Print Reader.

Recorded Periodicals
919 Walnut St.
Eighth Floor
Philadelphia, PA 19107
(215) 627-4230

Recording for the Blind, Inc.
213 E. 58th St.
New York, NY 10022
(212) 751-0860

Regional Office:
5022 Hollywood Blvd.
Los Angeles, CA 90027
(213) 664-5525

Vision Foundation
2 Mt. Auburn St.
Watertown, MA 02172
(617) 926-4232

GUIDE DOGS

All of the following groups provide guide dogs and training to qualified blind persons free of charge, unless noted. However, since not all blind people are good candidates for coping with Seeing Eye dogs, it is best to consult a health professional before inquiring about a guide dog.

Guide Dogs for the Blind
PO Box 1200
San Rafael, CA 94915
(415) 479-4000

International Guiding Eyes
13445 Glenoaks Blvd.
Sylmar, CA 91342
(213) 362-5834

Leader Dogs for the Blind
1039 S. Rochester Rd.
Rochester, MI 48063
(313) 651-9011

The Seeing Eye, Inc.
PO Box 375
Morristown, NJ 07960
(201) 539-4425

Guide Dog Foundation for the Blind
Administrative Offices
109–19 72nd Ave.
Forest Hills, NY 11375
(718) 263-4885

Guiding Eyes for the Blind
611 Granite Springs Rd.
Yorktown Heights, NY 10598
(914) 245-4024
Provides guide dogs for a fee, which is waived if a person cannot afford to pay.

Pilot Guide Dog Foundation
625 W. Town St.
Columbus, OH 43215
(614) 221-6367

EYE DISEASE RESEARCH AND TREATMENT AT THE NATIONAL INSTITUTES OF HEALTH

Several research studies on eye diseases are ongoing at the Clinical Center at the National Institutes of Health in Bethesda, Maryland. Subjects are patients with various kinds of cataracts, especially congenital ones; adults and children with glaucoma and congenital glaucoma; patients with congenital and genetic eye diseases, including night blindness; familial macular disease; color vision deficiencies; patients with age-related macular degeneration; patients with retinitis pigmentosa; patients with uveitis. Participation is by physician referral. For more information your physician can contact:

Office of the Director
Clinical Center
Building 10, Room 2C-146
National Institutes of Health
Bethesda, MD 20892

or:

Clinical Director of the National Eye Institute
Building 10, Room ION 202
(301) 496-3123

ORGANIZATIONS

American Council of the Blind
1211 Connecticut Ave., N.W.
Washington, DC 20036
(202) 833-1251

Membership organization, state affiliates, for blind and visually impaired persons. A national clearinghouse for information on blindness. Publishes *The Braille Forum* monthly in braille, large print, audiocassette and disk.

American Foundation for the Blind
15 W. 16th St.
New York, NY 10011
(212) 620-2000

A national nonprofit organization for the blind, their families, and professionals. A major source of information and referral. Six regional offices. Publishes talking books, monographs, magazines, leaflets in large type, recorded and in braille. Manufactures and sells special aids and appliances for the visually impaired. Maintains a special library on blindness. Designs self-help programs for blind persons and their families. Will supply more information upon request.

Blind Outdoor Leisure Development
533 E. Main St.
Aspen, CO 81611
(303) 925-8922

Volunteer nonprofit organization to set up leisure vacations for the blind (financed by donations). 14 local clubs help the blind participate in outdoor sports, such as skiing, skating, golfing, swimming, camping, etc. Supplies guides and instructors. Will provide more information upon request.

Christian Record Braille Foundation
4444 S. 52nd St.
Lincoln, NE 68506
(402) 488-0981

A nonprofit publishing house for the blind, affiliated with the Seventh-Day Adventists. Lending library of books and magazines in recorded media, large print and braille, free to all legally blind persons. Also sponsors free national camps for blind youth and adults. Maintains some glaucoma screening clinics. Will provide more information upon request.

National Society to Prevent Blindness
500 E. Remington Rd.
Schaumburg, IL 60173
(312) 843-2020

National voluntary health agency. 26 state affiliates. A source of information to the public about visual disorders, prevention, available treatments, and techniques in eye care. Sponsors research and screening programs. Pamphlets, booklets, audiovisual materials. Will provide more information upon request.

RP Foundation Fighting Blindness
1401 Mt. Royal Ave.
Baltimore, MD 21217
(301) 225-9400, 9409 (TDD)
(800) 638-2300

A national nonprofit organization to disseminate information about retinitis pigmentosa and allied inherited retinal degenerations. About 60 affiliates nationwide. Supports research. Pamphlets, audiovisual materials. Supports screening centers around the country, some self-help programs. Answers questions from the public. Will provide more information upon request.

BOOKS

American Foundation for the Blind Directory of Agencies Serving the Visually Handicapped in the United States. **American Foundation for the Blind,** 15 W. 16th St., New York, NY 10011. A state-by-state listing of rehabilitation agencies, with descriptions of the services they provide.

Cataracts, What You Must Know About Them, **Charles D. Kelman, M.D.,** New York: Crown, 1982.

Eyes Only, **Kenneth B. Kauvar, M.D.,** Norwalk, CT: Appleton-Century-Crofts, 1982.

Eye Wise: Eye Disorders and Their Treatment, **Kenneth P. Wolf, M.D.,** New York: Harper & Row, 1982.

Insight Into Eyesight: The Patient's Guide to Visual Disorders, **Paul E. Michelson, M.D.,** Chicago: Nelson-Hall, 1980.

Making Life More Livable, **Irving R. Dickman,** New York: American Foundation for the Blind, 1983. A handbook for the visually impaired older person.

FREE MATERIALS

Single copies are free

Blindness and Diabetes, 16 pages.
Cataracts and Their Treatment, 24 pages.
Dog Guides for the Blind, 6 pages.
Environmental Modifications for the Visually Impaired, 14 pages.
Facts About Blindness and Visual Impairment, 113 pages.
Glaucoma: Diagnosis, Treatment, Prevention, 29 pages.
Living with Blindness, 28 pages.
Parenting Preschoolers, 28 pages.
Products for People with Vision Problems, catalog.
Recreation for Disabled Persons, 28 pages.
Touch the Baby, 16 pages.

American Foundation for the Blind
15 W. 16th St.
New York, NY 10011
(212) 620-2000

Fact sheets:
Age-related Macular Degeneration
Age-related Macular Degeneration Study Results

Diagram of the Eye
Early Treatment Diabetic Retinopathy Study (ETDRS)
Low Vision
Ocular Histoplasmosis
Retinitis Pigmentosa
Cataract, 24 pages.
Diabetes and Your Eyes, 16 pages.

National Eye Institute
National Institutes of Health
Building 31, Room 6A32
Bethesda, MD 20892
(301) 496-5248

Age-related Macular Degeneration, 8 pages.
The Aging Eye: Facts on Eye Care for Older Persons, 16 pages.
Cataracts, 8 pages.
Diabetic Retinopathy, 6 pages.
Glaucoma: Sneak Thief of Sight, 6 pages.

National Society to Prevent Blindness
500 E. Remington Rd.
Schaumburg, IL 60173
(312) 843-2020

GENETIC COUNSELING

No other area of medicine is taking such a giant leap into the future as is medical genetics. As biologists increasingly break the mysterious codes of how our genes cause birth defects and inherited diseases and influence our susceptibility to diseases in later life, genetic counseling becomes increasingly important. Currently, genetic disorders occur in about one out of 20 births. According to some estimates, about 250,000 American infants are born every year with physical or mental damage of some kind.

Some common genetic diseases: Cystic fibrosis, Duchenne muscular dystrophy, hemophilia, Huntington's disease, brittle bone disease (osteogenesis imperfecta), sickle-cell anemia, and Tay-Sachs.

Many physicians do simple reproductive counseling, for example, advising pregnant women, especially those age 35 and over, to have a test (amniocentesis) mainly to determine if their fetus has Down syndrome. But as the potential for spotting and repairing birth defects becomes more complex, the need for specialized genetic counseling grows. Amniocentesis, done only after the sixteenth week of pregnancy, was until recently the only test for fetal damage. Amniocentesis is used mainly to screen for Down syndrome fetuses and is considered 99.4 percent reliable. In 1983 the federal government approved widespread use of another biomedical test, alpha fetoprotein screening (AFP), that can

help detect abnormalities in the embryo's spinal cord and brain—so-called neural tube defects—including spina bifida.

In the future, amniocentesis may give way to widespread use of a new experimental technique, chorionic villus biopsy, that can be done in the first trimester of pregnancy. The technique is being tested in only a few institutions, and there are still important questions about its safety and reliability. Virtually risk-free screening tests for sickle-cell anemia have been developed. Many other screening tests, some involving the identification of genetic "markers," are on the horizon for prenatal detection of Huntington's disease and other inherited neurological and neuromuscular disorders. In addition, there are a number of screening tests that can identify those who are carrying genes—for Tay-Sachs, for example—putting them at risk of having genetically defective youngsters. More of these types of tests are expected in the next few years.

Genetic counselors primarily help their clients to understand the complexities of gene transmission, provide information about the latest screening tests and the chances of having a genetically defective child, give psychological support (the diagnosis of a genetic disease is often emotionally traumatic), and help the family make choices involving the risks of having children. Most families who seek genetic counseling want to know more about prenatal diagnosis and monitoring.

As it becomes more sophisticated, the field of genetic counseling is expanding to provide education and advice about diseases with genetic components that show up later in life, such as Alzheimer's disease (a form of senile dementia) and even various kinds of cancer. If scientists find they can perhaps eliminate certain disorders prior to birth and even influence other traits in the unborn, prospective parents will be faced with more options and decisions during pregnancy.

Families with a genetic disorder, or who are in a high-risk part of the population for such disorders, may need the help of genetic counselors. Sometimes such genetic counseling requires only a single visit, but it can continue for a period of years and involve many members of the family.

Genetic counselors do not actually treat disease; they leave that up to your physician. Nor do they advise couples whether to have children. They simply make sure you have accurate information with which to make decisions, and that you know what genetic tests are available. They then offer support regardless of what decision you make. They can help you make some complex medical decisions.

LEADING COMPREHENSIVE GENETIC COUNSELING AND TESTING CENTERS

Most of the centers listed below also have prenatal testing.

ALABAMA

University of Alabama at Birmingham Medical
  Center
University Station
1720 Seventh Ave. S.
Birmingham, AL 35294
Laboratory of Medical Genetics
Director: Wayne H. Finley, M.D., Ph.D.
(205) 934-4973

University of South Alabama College of
  Medicine
U.S.A. Medical Center
Moorer Building
2451 Fillingim St.
Mobile, AL 36617
Department of Medical Genetics
Director: Wladimir Wertelecki, M.D.
(205) 476-6305

ALASKA

Genetics and Birth Defects Clinic
March of Dimes Birth Defects Foundation
4600 Shelikof St.
Anchorage, AK 99507
Department of Health and Social Services
Division of Public Health
Director: Virginia Sybert, M.D.
(206) 526-2056

ARIZONA

The Genetics Center of Southwest Biomedical
  Research Institute
123 E. University Drive
Tempe, AZ 85281
Director: Frederick Hecht, M.D.
(602) 894-1104

University of Arizona Health Science Center
College of Medicine
1401 N. Campbell Ave.
Tucson, AZ 85724
Department of Obstetrics and Gynecology
Director: Louis Weinstein, M.D.
(602) 626-6324

ARKANSAS

University of Arkansas Medical Sciences
  Center
4301 W. Markham
Little Rock, AR 72205
Department of Pediatrics Slot 512B
Director: Florence Char, M.D.
(501) 661-5991

CALIFORNIA

The Genetics Institute
1708 W. Huntington
Alhambra, CA 91801
Director: Omar S. Alfi, M.D.
(818) 281-0954

Southern California Permanente Medical Group
Anaheim Medical Arts Building
1188 N. Euclid
Anaheim, CA 92801
Department of Genetics Services
Director: Diane L. Broome, M.D.
(714) 778-8624

City of Hope National Medical Center
1500 E. Duarte Rd.
Duarte, CA 91010
Department of Medical Genetics
Director: David E. Comings, M.D.
(818) 359-8111, x2631

Valley Children's Hospital
3151 N. Millbrook
Fresno, CA 93703
Department of Medical Genetics and Prenatal
   Detection
Director: Cynthia J. Curry, M.D.
(209) 225-3000, x1437

Kaiser-Permanente Medical Center
1100 W. Pacific Coast Highway
Harbor City, CA 90710
Department of Pediatrics
Division of Medical Genetics
Director: E. David Weinstein, M.D.
(213) 539-7050

University of California San Diego
Basic Science Building, M-013-F
La Jolla, CA 92093
Department of Medicine
Division of Medical Genetics
Director: Oliver W. Jones, M.D.
(619) 452-4307

Loma Linda University Medical Center
11234 Anderson St., Room A-527
Loma Linda, CA 92350
Department of Pediatrics
Division of Genetics
Director: Constance J. Sandlin, M.D.
(714) 796-7311, x2838

Children's Hospital of Los Angeles
4650 Sunset Blvd.
Los Angeles, CA 90027
Department of Pediatrics
Division of Medical Genetics
Director: Richard Koch, M.D.
(213) 699-2152

Kaiser-Permanente Medical Center
6041 Cadillac Ave.
Los Angeles, CA 90034
Department of Pediatrics
Division of Medical Genetics
Director: Nancy Shinno, M.D.
(213) 419-3322

Los Angeles County–University of Southern
   California Medical Center
1129 N. State St.
Los Angeles, CA 90033
Department of Pediatrics
Division of Genetics–Cytogenetics Laboratory
Director: Miriam G. Wilson, M.D.
(213) 226-3816

Martin Luther King Jr. General Hospital
12021 S. Wilmington Ave.
Los Angeles, CA 90059
Department of Pediatrics
Director: Robert J. Schlegel, M.D.
(213) 603-4641
Department of Obstetrics and Gynecology
Director: Rosetta Willis, M.D.
(213) 603-4624

University of California Los Angeles
Center for Health Sciences
Los Angeles, CA 90024
Department of Pediatrics
Division of Medical Genetics
Director: Robert S. Sparkes, M.D.
(213) 825-5720

Children's Hospital
747 52nd St.
Oakland, CA 94609
Medical Genetics Unit
Director: Sanford Sherman, M.D.
(415) 428-3550

Kaiser-Permanente Medical Care Program
280 W. MacArthur Blvd.
Oakland, CA 94611
Department of Genetics
Director: Ronald Backman, M.D.
(415) 428-5964, 5816

University of California at Irvine
Irvine Medical Center
101 City Drive S.
Orange, CA 92668
Department of Pediatrics
Division of Clinical Genetics and
  Developmental Disabilities
Director: Kenneth W. Dumars, M.D.
(714) 634-5791

Kaiser-Permanente Medical Center
13652 Cantara St.
Panorama City, CA 91402-5497
Department of Pediatrics
Division of Genetic Services
Director: Harold N. Bass, M.D.
(818) 908-2582

Kaiser-Permanente Medical Care Program
2025 Morse Ave.
Sacramento, CA 95825
Department of Genetics
Director: Mark Lipson, M.D.
(916) 486-6521

University of California at Davis
School of Medicine and Medical Center
4301 X St.
Sacramento, CA 95817
Department of Pediatrics
Medical Genetic Services
Acting Director: Elinor Zorn, M.D.
(916) 453-3721

Children's Hospital and Health Center San
  Diego
8001 Frost St.
San Diego, CA 92123
Department of Dysmorphology and Genetics
Birth Defects and Genetic Counseling Clinic
Director: Marilyn C. Jones, M.D.
(619) 576-5840

San Diego Regional Center for the
  Developmentally Disabled
4355 Ruffin Rd.
San Diego, CA 92123
Director: Raymond M. Peterson, M.D.
(619) 576-2996

University Hospital
University of California, San Diego Medical
  Center
225 Dickinson St., H-814
San Diego, CA 92103
Department of Pediatrics
Division of Genetics and Dysmorphology
Directors: Kenneth Lyons Jones, M.D.,
  William L. Nyhan, M.D.
(714) 294-6992

University of California San Francisco
Third and Parnassus Ave.
San Francisco, CA 94143
Department of Pediatrics U-100
Division of Medical Genetics
Director: Charles J. Epstein, M.D.
(415) 666-2757

Kaiser-Permanente Medical Care Program
260 International Circle
San Jose, CA 95119
Department of Genetics
Director: John Mann, M.D.
(408) 972-3300

Stanford University Medical Center
300 Pasteur Drive, Room A335A
Stanford, CA 94305
Department of Pediatrics
Birth Defects/Genetics Center
Director: Luigi Luzzatti, M.D.
(415) 497-6858

Harbor UCLA Medical Center
1000 W. Carson St.
Torrance, CA 90509
Department of Pediatrics
Division of Medical Genetics
Director: David L. Rimoin, M.D., Ph.D.
(213) 533-3673

COLORADO
The Children's Hospital
1056 E. 19th Ave.
Denver, CO 80218
Department of Pediatric Medicine
Division of Genetic Services
Director: James E. Strain, M.D.
(303) 861-6395

Rose Medical Center
University of Colorado School of Medicine
4567 E. Ninth Ave.
Denver, CO 80220
Department of Genetics
Director: James J. Nora, M.D.
(303) 320-2955

University of Colorado Health Sciences Center
School of Medicine, B-160
4200 E. Ninth Ave.
Denver, CO 80262
Department of Pediatrics
Genetics Unit
Director: Eva Sujansky, M.D.
(303) 394-8742, 8808, 8777

CONNECTICUT
University of Connecticut Health Center
School of Medicine
Farmington, CT 06032
Department of Pediatrics
Division of Genetics
Director: Suzanne B. Cassidy, M.D.
(203) 674-2676

Yale University School of Medicine
333 Cedar St.
New Haven, CT 06510
Department of Human Genetics
Genetic Consultation Service
Director: Margretta R. Seashore, M.D.
(203) 785-2660

DELAWARE
Medical Center of Delaware
Christiana Hospital
PO Box 6001
Newark, DE 19718
Department of Pediatrics
Cytogenetics Laboratory
Director: Digamber S. Borgaonkar, Ph.D.
(302) 733-3530

Alfred I. duPont Institute
PO Box 269
Wilmington, DE 19899
Department of Medical Genetics
Director: Charles I. Scott, Jr., M.D.
(302) 651-5916

DISTRICT OF COLUMBIA
Children's Hospital National Medical Center
111 Michigan Ave., N.W.
Washington, DC 20010
Department of Clinical Genetics
Director: Kenneth N. Rosenbaum, M.D.
(202) 745-2187

Columbia Hospital for Women
2425 L St., N.W.
Washington, DC 20037
Department of Obstetrics and Gynecology
Division of Maternal-Fetal Medicine
Director: Sergio E. Fabro, M.D., Ph.D.
(202) 293-5135

George Washington University Medical Center
Wilson Genetics Unit
Ross Hall 455
2300 I St., N.W.
Washington, DC 20037
Department of Obstetrics and Gynecology
Director: John W. Larsen, Jr., M.D.
(202) 676-4096

Georgetown University Medical Center
3800 Reservoir Rd., N.W.
Washington, DC 20007
Department of Obstetrics and Gynecology
Division of Medical Genetics
Director: Robert C. Baumiller, Ph.D.
(202) 625-7852
Department of Pediatrics
Center for Genetic Counseling and Birth
     Defect Evaluation
Director: Nina Scribanu, M.D.
(202) 625-2348

Howard University
College of Medicine
Box 75
520 W St., N.W.
Washington, DC 20059
Department of Pediatrics and Child Health
Division of Medical Genetics
Director: Robert F. Murray, Jr., M.D.
(202) 636-6340, 6341, 6342

FLORIDA

University of Florida
College of Medicine, Box J-296
J. Hillis Miller Health Center
Gainesville, FL 32610
Department of Pediatrics
Division of Genetics
Director: Jaime L. Frias, M.D.
(904) 392-3388

University Hospital of Jacksonville
655 W. Eighth St.
Jacksonville, FL 32209
Department of Pediatrics
Division of Genetics
Director: Charlotte Z. Lafer, M.D.
(904) 350-6872

University of Miami
School of Medicine
Department of Medicine
Division of Genetic Medicine
PO Box 016960
1500 N.W. 12th Ave.
Miami, FL 33101
Director: Karl H. Muench, M.D.
(305) 547-6652

University of Miami
School of Medicine
Department of Pediatrics
Mailman Center for Child Development
Division of Endocrinology, Genetics and
  Metabolism
PO Box 016820
1601 N.W. 12th Ave.
Miami, FL 33101
Director: William Cleveland, M.D.
(305) 547-6364

University of South Florida
College of Medicine
Box 15-G
12901 N. 30th St.
Tampa, FL 33612
Department of Pediatrics
Division of Medical Genetics
Director: Boris Kousseff, M.D.
(813) 974-3310

GEORGIA

Emory University School of Medicine
2040 Ridgewood Drive
Atlanta, GA 30322
Department of Pediatrics
Division of Medical Genetics
Director: Louis J. Elsas, II, M.D.
(404) 329-5840

Human Genetics Institute
Medical College of Georgia
1120 15th St., CJ-263
Augusta, GA 30912
Acting Director: Paul G. McDonough, M.D.
(404) 828-2828

HAWAII

Kapiolani Children's Hospital
University of Hawaii
1319 Punahou St.
Honolulu, HI 96826
Department of Genetics and Pediatrics
Division of Medical Genetic Services
Director: Y. Edward Hsia, M.D.
(808) 948-6872, 6834

IDAHO

Idaho Department of Health and Welfare
2220 Old Penitentiary Rd.
Boise, ID 83712
Department of Health and Welfare
Bureau of Laboratories
Director: Mary Jane Webb, B.S., Coordinator
(208) 334-4778

ILLINOIS

Children's Memorial Hospital
2300 Children's Plaza
Chicago, IL 60614
Division of Genetics
Acting Director: John Charrow, M.D.
(312) 880-4462

Cook County Children's Hospital
700 S. Wood St.
Chicago, IL 60612
Department of Pediatrics
Division of Genetics and Metabolism
Director: Catherine Harris, M.D.
(312) 633-5580

Illinois Masonic Medical Center
836 W. Wellington
Chicago, IL 60657
Department of Pediatrics
Division of Medical Genetics
Director: George F. Smith, M.D.
(312) 883-7053

Michael Reese Hospital and Medical Center
Lakeshore Drive at 31st St.
Chicago, IL 60616
Department of Pathology
Division of Medical Genetics
Director: Eugene Pergament, M.D., Ph.D.
(312) 791-3848

Mount Sinai Hospital
Medical Center of Chicago
California Ave. at 15th St.
Chicago, IL 60608
Department of Pediatrics
Division of Genetics
Director: Jeannette Israel, M.D.
(312) 650-6472

Prentice Women's Hospital
Northwestern University Medical School
333 E. Superior St.
Chicago, IL 60611
Department of Obstetrics and Gynecology
Division of Human Genetics
Director: Joe Leigh Simpson, M.D.
(312) 649-7441

Rush-Presbyterian–St. Luke's Medical Center
1753 W. Congress Parkway
Chicago, IL 60612
Department of Pediatrics
Section of Genetics
Director: Paul Wong, M.D.
(312) 942-6298

University of Chicago Hospital and Clinics
Pritzker School of Medicine
South Maryland Ave.
Chicago, IL 60637
Department of Obstetrics and Gynecology
Division of Sciences Division
Director: Anthony P. Amarose, Ph.D.
(312) 962-6122
Department of Pediatrics-Box 413
Director: Allen Horwitz, M.D., Ph.D.
(312) 962-6174

University of Illinois
College of Medicine at Chicago
840 S. Wood St.
Chicago, IL 60612
Department of Pediatrics
Division of Genetics and Metabolism
Director: Reuben Matalon, M.D., Ph.D.
(312) 996-6714

Evanston Hospital
2530 Ridge Ave.
Evanston, IL 60201
Department of Pediatrics
Division of Genetics
Director: Ira Salafsky, M.D.
(312) 492-6771

Lutheran General Hospital
1775 Dempster
Park Ridge, IL 60068
Department of Pediatrics
Division of Medical Genetics
Directors: Carol W. Booth, M.D., Celia Kaye,
    M.D., Ph.D.
(312) 696-7705

Southern Illinois University
School of Medicine
PO Box 3926
Springfield, IL 62708
Department of Pediatrics
Division of Genetics Program
Director: Kyrieckos A. Aleck, M.D.
(217) 782-8460

Genetic Counseling Service and Laboratory
Regional Health Resource Center
1408 W. University Ave.
Urbana, IL 61801
Director: William Daniel, Ph.D.
(217) 333-8172

INDIANA
Tri-State Regional Genetics Services Center
The Rehabilitation Center, Inc.
3701 Bellemead Ave.
Evansville, IN 47715
Director: Ronald L. Haun, M.D.
(812) 424-0953

Northeastern Indiana Genetics Counseling
  Center
Parkview Memorial Hospital
2200 Randalia Drive
Fort Wayne, IN 46805
Director: Patricia I. Bader, M.D.
(219) 484-6636, x4145

Riley Hospital, RR 129
Indiana University School of Medicine
702 Barnhill Drive
Indianapolis, IN 46223
Department of Medical Genetics
Director: Joe C. Christian, M.D., Ph.D.
(317) 264-2241

North Central Indiana Regional Genetics
  Counseling Center
Memorial Hospital
615 N. Michigan St.
South Bend, IN 46601
Director: Harvey A. Bender, Ph.D.
(219) 239-7075

IOWA
University of Iowa Hospitals and Clinics
Iowa City, IA 52242
Department of Obstetrics and Gynecology
Prenatal Diagnosis Program
Director: Roger A. Williamson, M.D.
(319) 356-4119
Department of Pediatrics
Division of Medical Genetics
Director: James W. Hanson, M.D.
(319) 356-2674
Department of Pediatrics
Regional Genetic Consultation Service
Director: James A. Bartley, M.D., Ph.D.
(319) 356-2674

KANSAS
University of Kansas Medical Center
39th and Rainbow Blvd.
Kansas City, KS 66103
Department of Medicine-Room 4023-C
Division of Metabolism, Endocrinology, and
  Genetics
Director: R. Neil Schimke, M.D.
(913) 588-6022

University of Kansas
School of Medicine–Wichita
1010 N. Kansas
Wichita, KS 67214

Wesley Medical Center
Prenatal Diagnosis and Genetic Clinic
550 N. Hillside
Wichita, KS 67214
Departments of Pediatrics and Obstetrics and
  Gynecology
Division of Medical Genetics
Director: Sechin Cho, M.D.
(316) 261-2622 or 688-2360

KENTUCKY
University of Kentucky School of Medicine
800 Rose St.
Lexington, KY 40536
Department of Pediatrics
Division of Genetics and Dysmorphology
Director: Bryan D. Hall, M.D.
(606) 233-5558

University of Louisville Medical School
334 E. Broadway
Louisville, KY 40202
Department of Pediatrics
Child Evaluation Center
Clinical Genetics and Dysmorphology Clinic
Genetic Outreach Clinics
Director: Bernard Weisskopf, M.D.
(502) 588-5331

LOUISIANA
Louisiana State University Medical Center
1542 Tulane Ave.
New Orleans, LA 70112
Department of Pediatrics
Division of Genetics
Director: Theodore F. Thurmon, M.D.
(504) 568-6225

Tulane University School of Medicine
1430 Tulane Ave.
New Orleans, LA 70112
The Hayward Genetics Center
Human Genetics Program
Director: Emmanuel Shapira, M.D., Ph.D.
(504) 588-5229

University Hospital
Louisiana State University
School of Medicine
1501 Kings Highway
Shreveport, LA 71130
Department of Pediatrics
Birth Defects Center
Director: Harold Chen, M.D.
(318) 226-3210

MAINE
Eastern Maine Medical Center
489 State St.
Bangor, ME 04401
Department of Pediatrics
Genetics Program
Director: Laurent J. Beauregard, Ph.D.
(207) 945-7354

Foundation for Blood Research
PO Box 428
Scarborough, ME 04074
Division of Clinical Genetics
Director: Thomas G. Brewster, M.D.
(207) 883-4131

MARYLAND
Johns Hopkins University
School of Medicine
Department of Medicine
Division of Medical Genetics
The Moore Clinic
600 N. Wolfe St.
Baltimore, MD 21205
Director: Reed E. Pyeritz, M.D., Ph.D.
(301) 955-3122

Johns Hopkins University
School of Medicine
Department of Obstetrics and Gynecology,
   CMSC-1001
Prenatal Diagnostic Center
601 N. Broadway
Baltimore, MD 21205
Director: Haig Kazazian, Jr., M.D.
(301) 955-6327

Johns Hopkins University
School of Medicine
Department of Pediatrics, CMSC-1004
Division of Pediatric Genetics
601 N. Broadway
Baltimore, MD 21205
Director: David Valle, M.D.
(301) 955-3071, 3075

University of Maryland School of Medicine
655 W. Baltimore St.
Baltimore, MD 21201
Departments of Obstetrics and Gynecology and
   Pediatrics
Division of Human Genetics
Director: Maimon M. Cohen, Ph.D.
(301) 528-3480

National Institutes of Health
Building 10, Room 9C-436
Bethesda, MD 20205
Inter-Institute Clinical Genetics Program
Directors: John J. Mulvihill, M.D., Dilys M.
   Parry, Ph.D.
(301) 496-4947

MASSACHUSETTS
Boston University Medical Center
80 E. Concord St.
Boston, MA 02118
Department of Pediatrics
Division of Human Services
Director: Aubrey Milunsky, M.B., B., D.C.H.
(617) 247-5720

Brigham and Women's Hospital
721 Huntington Ave.
Boston, MA 02115
Department of Medicine
Genetics Clinic
Director: Peter V. Tishler, M.D.
(617) 732-5981

Children's Hospital Medical Center
300 Longwood Ave.
Boston, MA 02115
Department of Pediatric Medicine
Genetics Division
Director: Samuel A. Latt, M.D., Ph.D.
(617) 735-7577

Massachusetts General Hospital
Children's Service
Genetics Unit
Boston, MA 02114
Director: Richard W. Erbe, M.D.
(617) 726-3826, 3827, 3828

Tufts New England Medical Center
171 Harrison Ave.
Boston, MA 02111
Department of Pediatrics
Center for Birth Defects and Genetic
   Counseling
Acting Director: Sidney S. Gellis, M.D.
(617) 956-5454

Eunice Kennedy Shriver Center
200 Trapelo Rd.
Waltham, MA 02154
Division of Genetics
Director: Wayne Miller, M.D.
(617) 893-4909

University of Massachusetts Medical Center
55 Lake Ave. N.
Worcester, MA 02105
Department of Pediatrics
Genetics Clinic
Director: Philip L. Townes, M.D., Ph.D.
(617) 856-3949

MICHIGAN
University of Michigan Medical School
C. S. Mott Children's Hospital
Department of Pediatrics
Section of Pediatric Genetics
D1225 Medical Professional Building
Box 46
Ann Arbor, MI 48109-0010
Director: Robert P. Erickson, M.D.
(313) 764-0579

University of Michigan Medical School
Department of Internal Medicine and Human
  Genetics
Division of Medical Genetics
Box 015
1137 Catherine St.
Ann Arbor, MI 48109-0010
Director: Thomas Gelehrter, M.D.
(313) 764-1352

Children's Hospital of Michigan
Wayne State University
3901 Beaubien Blvd.
Detroit, MI 48201
Department of Pediatrics
Division of Clinical Genetics and Metabolic
  Disorders
Director: Henry L. Nadler, M.D.
(313) 577-1335

Henry Ford Hospital
2799 W. Grand Blvd.
Detroit, MI 48202
Medical Genetics and Birth Defects Center
Director: Lester Weiss, M.D.
(313) 876-3116

Hutzel Hospital
Wayne State University School of Medicine
4707 St. Antoine Blvd.
Detroit, MI 48201
Department of Gynecology and Obstetrics
Director: Mark Evans, M.D.
(313) 577-3529 or 484-7066

Michigan State University
B240 Life Sciences Building
East Lansing, MI 48824
Department of Pediatrics and Human
  Development
Division of Human Genetics, Immunology,
  and Toxicology
Director: James V. Higgins, Ph.D.
(517) 355-2871

Blodgett Memorial Medical Center
1840 Wealthy St., S.E.
Grand Rapids, MI 49506
Genetics/Birth Defects/Neurology Clinic
Director: Donald F. Waterman, M.D.
(616) 774-1898

William Beaumont Hospital
3601 W. 13 Mile Rd.
Royal Oak, MI 48072
Department of Anatomic Pathology
Birth Defects and Genetic Counseling Clinic
Director: A. Al Saadi, Ph.D.
(313) 288-8050

MINNESOTA
University of Minnesota Hospital
Mayo Memorial Building
Box 485
420 Delaware St., S.E.
Minneapolis, MN 55455
Department of Medicine
Division of Genetics
Director: Richard A. King, M.D., Ph.D.
(612) 373-4999

Mayo Clinic
200 First St., S.W.
Rochester, MN 55905
Department of Genetics
Director: Hymie Gordon, M.D.
(507) 284-2170

MISSISSIPPI
U.S. Air Force Medical Center
Keesler Air Force Base
Biloxi, MS 39534
Department of Medical Genetics
Director: David T. Ringdon, M.D.
(601) 377-6393

University of Mississippi Medical Center
2500 N. State St.
Jackson, MS 39216
Department of Preventive Medicine
Division of Medicine Genetics
Director: John F. Jackson, M.D.
(601) 987-5611

MISSOURI
University of Missouri Health Sciences Center
One Hospital Drive
Columbia, MO 65212
Department of Child Health
Division of Medical Genetics
Director: Judith Miles, M.D., Ph.D.
(314) 882-6992

Children's Mercy Hospital
University of Missouri at Kansas City
24th and Gillham Rd.
Kansas City, MO 64108
Genetic Counseling Center
Director: David J. Harris, M.D.
(816) 234-3290

Cardinal Glennon Children's Hospital
1465 S. Grand Blvd.
St. Louis, MO 63104
Department of Pediatrics
Genetics Section
Director: Patricia L. Monteleone, M.D.
(314) 577-5639

Jewish Hospital of St. Louis
Washington University Medical School
216 S. King's Highway
St. Louis, MO 63110
Department of Obstetrics and Gynecology
Division of Genetics
Director: James P. Crane, M.D.
(314) 454-7700

St. Louis Children's Hospital
Washington University Medical School
500 S. King's Highway
St. Louis, MO 63110
Department of Pediatrics
Division of Medical Genetics
Director: Richard Hillman, M.D.
(314) 454-6093

MONTANA
Shodair Children's Hospital
PO Box 5539
840 Helena Ave.
Helena, MT 59604
Department of Medical Genetics
Director: John M. Opitz, M.D.
(406) 442-1980, x302

NEBRASKA
Clinical Genetics Center
8111 Dodge St., Suite 248
Omaha, NE 68114
Clinical Genetics Center
Director: Mark S. Lubinsky, M.D.
(402) 390-1170

University of Nebraska Medical Center
Hattie B. Monroe Pavilion
4420 Dewey
Omaha, NE 68105
Meyers Children's Rehabilitation Institute
Center for Human Genetics
Directors: Bruce Buehler, M.D., Warren
    Sanger, Ph.D.
(402) 559-5070

NEVADA
The Genetics Center of Southwest Biomedical
    Research Institute
901 Rancho Lane, Suite 104
Las Vegas, NV 89106
Director: Frederick Hecht, M.D.
(702) 384-5515 or (800) 521-8247

Southern Nevada Mental Retardation Services
1300 S. Jones Blvd.
Las Vegas, NV 89158
Director: Charlotte Crawford, M.A.
(702) 870-0220

Northern Nevada Mental Retardation Services
605 S. 21st St.
Sparkes, NV 89431
Director: David Luke, Ph.D.
(702) 789-0550

NEW HAMPSHIRE
Dartmouth-Hitchcock Medical Center
Dartmouth Medical School
Hanover, NH 03755
Department of Maternal and Child Health
Dysmorphology/Genetics Unit
Director: John Graham, M.D.
(603) 646-5478

NEW JERSEY
University of Medicine and Dentistry of New
 Jersey
School of Osteopathic Medicine
401 Haddon Ave.
Camden, NJ 08103
Department of Pediatrics
Division of Genetics
Director: Michael K. McCormack, Ph.D.
(609) 757-7809

University of Medicine and Dentistry of New
 Jersey
100 Bergen St., MSB-F534
Newark, NJ 07103
Department of Pediatrics
Division of Human Genetics
Director: Franklin Desposito, M.D.
(201) 456-4499

University of Medicine and Dentistry of New
 Jersey
Rutgers Medical School, CN-19
New Brunswick, NJ 08903
Department of Pediatrics
Division of Medical Genetics
Director: Ming-Liang Lee, M.D., Ph.D.
(201) 937-7891

NEW MEXICO
University of New Mexico School of Medicine
2701 Frontier, N.E.
Albuquerque, New Mexico 87131
Department of Obstetrics and Gynecology
Director: Kent Arqubright, M.D.
(505) 277-4051
Department of Pediatrics
Dysmorphology Unit
Director: Jon M. Aase, M.D.
(505) 277-5551

NEW YORK
Albany Medical College Hospital
New Scotland Ave.
Albany, NY 12208
Department of Pediatrics, Obstetrics, and
 Gynecology
Division of Medical Genetics
Director: Ian H. Porter, M.D.
(518) 445-5120

Albert Einstein Medical Center
Rose Kennedy Center, Room 211
College of Medicine
1410 Pelham Parkway
Bronx, NY 10461
Department of Pediatrics
Genetic Counseling Program
Director: Harold M. Nitowsky, M.D.
(212) 430-2510

Brookdale Hospital Medical Center
Linden Blvd. at Brookdale Plaza
Brooklyn, NY 11212
Department of Pediatrics
Division of Genetics
Director: Edward J. Schutta, M.D.
(718) 240-5883

Brooklyn Hospital/Caledonian Hospital
121 Dekalb Ave.
Brooklyn, NY 11201
Department of Obstetrics/Gynecology and
 Pediatrics
Division of Genetics
Director: Karen L. David, M.D.
(718) 403-8032

Downstate Medical Center
450 Clarkson Ave.
Brooklyn, NY 11203
Department of Pediatrics
Division of Clinical Genetics
Director: Qutub H. Qazi, M.D., Ph.D.
(718) 270-1691

Long Island College Hospital
350 Henry St.
Brooklyn, NY 11201
Department of Obstetrics and Gynecology
Genetics Center
Director: George I. Solish, M.D., Ph.D.
(718) 780-1772

The Buffalo General Hospital
100 High St.
Buffalo, NY 14203
Department of Medicine
Division of Medical Genetics
Acting Director: John A. Edwards, M.D.
(716) 862-2820

The Children's Hospital of Buffalo
219 Bryant St.
Buffalo, NY 14222
Department of Pediatrics
Division of Human Genetics
Acting Director: Elizabeth McPherson, M.D.
(716) 878-7530

Nassau County Medical Center
2201 Hempstead Turnpike
East Meadow, NY 11554
Department of Pediatrics
Division of Medical Genetics
Director: Morris Angulo, M.D.
(516) 542-3148

Queens Hospital Center
Long Island Jewish Hillside Medical Center
82-68 164th St.
Jamaica, NY 11432
Center for Developmentally Disabled
Director: Alan Shanske, M.D.
(718) 990-3167

North Shore University Hospital
Cornell University College of Medicine
300 Community Drive
Manhasset, NY 11030
Child Development Center
Division of Genetics
Director: Jessica G. Davis, M.D.
(516) 562-4610

Schneider Children's Hospital of Long Island
   Jewish–Hillside Medical Center
271-16 76th Ave.
New Hyde Park, NY 11042
Department of Pediatrics
Division of Human Genetics
Director: Lewis Waber, M.D.
(718) 470-3010

Beth Israel Medical Center
10 Nathan D. Perlman Place
New York, NY 10003
Department of Pediatrics
Division of Medical Genetics
Director: Hyon Ju Kim, M.D.
(212) 420-4178

Columbia-Presbyterian Medical Center
622 W. 168th St.
New York, NY 10032

Division of Genetics
Babies' Hospital
Director: Arthur D. Bloom, M.D.
(212) 305-3901
Department of Obstetrics and Gynecology
Genetic Counseling Service
Director: Georginia M. Jagiello, M.D.
(212) 305-4066

Mt. Sinai Medical Center
Annenberg Building
Fifth Ave. and 100th St.
New York, NY 10029
Department of Pediatrics
Division of Genetics
Director: Robert J. Desnick, Ph.D., M.D.
(212) 650-6947

New York Hospital
Cornell Medical Center
525 E. 68th St.
New York, NY 10021
Genetic Counseling Program
Director: Phyllis Klass, M.A., M.S.
(212) 472-6825

New York University Medical Center–Bellevue
   Hospital
550 First Ave.—MSB 136
New York, NY 10016
Department of Pediatrics
Division of Human Genetics
Acting Director: Marcia M. Wishnick, Ph.D.,
   M.D.
(212) 340-5746

University of Rochester Medical Center
Box 777
601 Elmwood Ave.
Rochester, NY 14642
Department of Pediatrics
Division of Genetics and Dysmorphology
Rochester Regional Genetics Services Program
Director: Richard A. Doherty, M.D.
(716) 275-3304

New York State Institute for Basic Research in
   Developmental Disabilities
1050 Forest Hill Rd.
Staten Island, NY 10314
Department of Human Genetics
Director: W. Ted Brown, M.D., Ph.D.
(718) 494-5230

Health Sciences Center
S.U.N.Y. at Stony Brook
Stony Brook, NY 11794
Department of Obstetrics and Gynecology
Genetics Unit
Director: Carolyn Trunca, Ph.D.
(516) 444-2790

Upstate Medical Center
State University of New York
766 Irving Ave.
Syracuse, NY 13210
Department of Pediatrics
Regional Genetics Center
Director: Lytt I. Gardner, M.D.
(315) 473-5834

Letchworth Village
Thiells, NY 10984
Regional Medical Genetic Services and
  Laboratory
Director: Lawrence R. Shapiro, M.D.
(914) 947-3487

Westchester County Medical Center
Valhalla, NY 10595
Medical Genetics Unit
Director: Lawrence R. Shapiro, M.D.
(914) 347-7627

NORTH CAROLINA
Genetics Associates of North Carolina, Inc.
Estes Office Park, Suite 107
104 S. Estes Drive
Chapel Hill, NC, 27514
Director: Philip D. Buchanan, Ph.D.
(919) 942-0021

University of North Carolina at Chapel Hill
School of Medicine
Biological Sciences Research Center #220H
Chapel Hill, NC 27514
Department of Medicine
Division of Medical Genetics
Director: Michael Swift, M.D.
(919) 966-2266
Department of Pediatrics
Division of Genetics and Metabolism
Director: Henry N. Kirkman, M.D.
(919) 966-4202

Charlotte Memorial Hospital and Medical
  Center
PO Box 32861
Charlotte, NC 28232
Department of Pediatrics
Clinical Genetics Program
Director: James C. Parke, Jr., M.D.
(704) 331-3156

Duke University Medical Center
Durham, NC 27710
Department of Obstetrics and Gynecology
Division of Perinatal Medicine
Director: Allen P. Killam, M.D.
(919) 684-2876
Department of Pediatrics
Division of Genetics and Metabolism
Director: Charles R. Roe, M.D.
(919) 684-2036

East Carolina University
School of Medicine
Greenville, NC 27834
Department of Pediatrics
Division of Medical Genetics
Director: Theodore Kushnick, M.D.
(919) 757-2525

Bowman Gray School of Medicine
300 S. Hawthorne Rd.
Winston-Salem, NC 27103
Department of Pediatrics
Genetic Counseling Program
Director: Harold O. Goodman, Ph.D.
(919) 748-4321

NORTH DAKOTA
University of North Dakota
School of Medicine
501 Columbia Rd.
Grand Forks, ND 58201
Department of Pediatrics
Division of Medical Genetics
Director: John T. Martsolf, M.D.
(701) 777-4277

OHIO
The Children's Hospital Medical Center of
  Akron
281 Locust St.
Akron, OH 44308
Genetics Clinic
Director: John Waterson, M.D., Ph.D.
(216) 379-8792

Cincinnati Center for Developmental Disorders
3300 Elland Ave.
Cincinnati, OH 45229
Department of Human Genetics
Cincinnati Regional Genetic Center
Director: Peter St. John Dignan, M.D.
(513) 559-4760, 4471

Case Western Reserve University
School of Medicine
Wearn Building-Room 150
2058 Abington Rd.
Cleveland, OH 44106
Department of Pediatrics
Genetics Center
Director: Walter E. Johnson, Ph.D.
(216) 844-3936

Cleveland Metropolitan General Hospital
3395 Scranton Rd.
Cleveland, OH 44109
Department of Pediatrics
Division of Medical Genetics
Director: Irwin A. Schafer, M.D.
(216) 459-4323

Children's Hospital
700 Children's Drive
Columbus, OH 43205
Genetics Section
Director: Annemarie Sommer, M.D.
(614) 461-2663

Children's Medical Center
One Children's Plaza
Dayton, OH 45404
Department of Medical Genetics and Birth
  Defects
Division of Genetics
Director: Meinhard Robinow, M.D.
(513) 226-8408

Medical College of Ohio at Toledo
Department of Pediatrics, C.S. 10008
Genetics Center
Toledo, OH 43699
Director: Thaddeus W. Kurczynski, M.D.,
  Ph.D.
(419) 381-4435

OKLAHOMA
Presbyterian Hospital
N.E. 13th St. at Lincoln Blvd.
Oklahoma City, OK 73104
Genetics Diagnostic Center
Director: J. Rodman Seely, M.D., Ph.D.
(405) 271-6777

University of Oklahoma Health Science Center
Children's Memorial Hospital
Department of Pediatrics
Division of Genetics, Endocrinology, and
  Metabolism
Regional Genetic Diagnosis and Counseling
  Center
940 N.E. 13th St.–PO Box 26901
Oklahoma City, OK 73190

Oklahoma Memorial
Department of Medicine
Division of Genetics
800 N.E. 13th St.
Oklahoma City, OK 73190
Director: Owen M. Rennert, M.D.
(405) 271-3468

Children's Medical Center
5300 E. Skelly Drive
Tulsa, OK 74135
Regional Genetics Center
Director: Burhan Say, M.D.
(918) 664-6600, x268

OREGON
Emanuel Hospital
2801 N. Gantenbein Ave.
Portland, OR 97227
Department of Pediatrics
Oregon Medical Genetics and Birth Defects
  Center
Director: John H. DiLiberti, M.D.
(503) 280-3042

Kaiser-Permanente
Division Medical Office
7705 S.E. Division St.
Portland, OR 97206
Department of Pediatrics
Director: Jacob Reiss, M.D.
(503) 777-3311, x3223

Oregon Health Sciences University
3181 S.W. Sam Jackson Park Rd.
Portland, OR 97201
Department of Medical Genetics, L-103
Director: Robert D. Koler, M.D.
(503) 225-7703

PENNSYLVANIA
Hershey Medical Center
PO Box 850
Hershey, PA 17033
Department of Pediatrics
Division of Genetics
Director: Roger L. Ladda, M.D.
(717) 534-8412

Children's Hospital of Philadelphia
34th and Civic Center Blvd.
Philadelphia, PA 19104
Clinical Genetics Center
Director: Elaine H. Zackai, M.D.
(215) 596-9800

Pennsylvania Hospital
8th and Spruce Sts.
Philadelphia, PA 19107
Division of Perinatology
Section of Medical Genetics
Director: Linda K. Dunn, M.D.
(215) 829-5633

St. Christopher's Hospital for Children
2600 N. Lawrence St.
Philadelphia, PA 19133
Department of Pediatrics
Division of Genetics
Director: Hope H. Punnett, Ph.D.
(215) 427-5289

Thomas Jefferson University
10th St., Suite 425, Main Building
Philadelphia, PA 19107
Department of Medicine
Division of Medical Genetics
Director: Laird G. Jackson, M.D.
(215) 928-6955

University of Pennsylvania Hospital
3400 Spruce St.
Philadelphia, PA 19104
Department of Obstetrics and Gynecology
Prenatal Genetic Diagnosis Program
Director: Michael Mennuti, M.D.
(215) 662-3232

Children's Hospital of Pittsburgh
125 De Soto St.
Pittsburgh, PA 15213
Department of Pediatrics
Division of Medical Genetics
Director: Mark W. Steele, M.D.
(412) 647-5070

Magee Women's Hospital
Forbes Avenue and Halket St.
Pittsburgh, PA 15213
Department of Reproductive Genetics
Director: Kenneth L. Garver, M.D., Ph.D.
(412) 647-4168

RHODE ISLAND
Rhode Island Hospital
593 Eddy St.
Providence, RI 02902
Department of Pediatrics
Genetic Counseling Service
Director: Diane N. Abuelo, M.D.
(401) 277-8361

SOUTH CAROLINA
Medical University of South Carolina
171 Ashley Ave.
Charleston, SC 29425
Department of Diagnostic Science
Division of Craniofacial Genetics
Director: Carlos F. Salinas, D.D.S.
(803) 792-2489
Department of Pediatrics
Division of Medical Genetics
Director: Shashidhar Pai, M.D.
(803) 792-2620

University of South Carolina
School of Medicine
3321 Medical Park Rd., Suite 301
Columbia, SC 29203
Department of Obstetrics and Gynecology
Division of Clinical Genetics
Director: S. Robert Young, Ph.D.
(803) 765-7316

Greenwood Genetic Center
Gregor Mendel Circle
Greenwood, SC 29646
Director: Roger E. Stevenson, M.D.
(803) 223-9411

SOUTH DAKOTA
University of South Dakota
School of Medicine
Julian Hall, Room 208
Clark and 414 E.
Vermillion, SD 57069
Birth Defects/Genetics Center
Director: Virginia P. Johnson, M.D.
(605) 677-5623

TENNESSEE
Regional Clinical Genetics Center
Suite 400, Professional Building
112 E. Myrtle St.
Johnson City, TN 37614
Department of Pediatrics
Division of Genetics and Dysmorphology
Director: Terry L. Myers, M.D., Ph.D.
(615) 926-3188

University of Tennessee
Memorial Research Center and Hospital
1924 Alcoa Highway
Knoxville, TN 37920
Birth Defects and Human Development Center
Director: Carmen B. Lozzio, M.D.
(615) 544-9030

University of Tennessee
Center for Health Sciences
711 Jefferson Ave.
Memphis, TN 38163
Division of Genetics
Child Development Center, Room 523
Director: R. Sid Wilroy, M.D.
(901) 528-6595

Meharry Medical College
1005 18th Ave.
Nashville, TN 37208
Department of Pediatrics
Division of Medical Genetics
Director: Dharmdeo N. Singh, Ph.D.
(615) 327-6786, 6399

Vanderbilt University School of Medicine
Room T-2404 Medical Center N.
Nashville, TN 37232
Department of Pediatrics
Director: John A. Phillips, M.D.
(615) 322-7601

TEXAS
University of Texas Health Science Center at
   Dallas
Southwestern Medical School
5323 Harry Hines Blvd.
Dallas, TX 75235
Department of Obstetrics/Gynecology and
   Pediatrics
Division of Clinical Genetics
Director: Jan M. Friedman, M.D.
(214) 688-2143

Texas Department of Mental Health and
   Mental Retardation
404 W. Oak St.
Denton, TX 76201
Genetic Screening and Counseling Service
Director: Donald Day, M.D.
(817) 383-3561

University of Texas Medical Branch at
   Galveston
Child Health Center
Galveston, TX 77550
Department of Pediatrics
Division of Cytogenetics
Director: Lillian Lockhart, M.D.
(409) 761-3466

Texas Children's Hospital
Baylor College of Medicine
6621 Fannin
Houston, TX 77030
Birth Defects/Genetics Clinic
Director: Frank Greenberg, M.D.
(713) 791-4774

University of Texas Medical School at
   Houston
Texas Medical Center
PO Box 20708
Houston, TX 77225
Department of Pediatrics
Medical Genetics Program
Director: William A. Horton, M.D.
(713) 797-4557

Santa Rosa Medical Center
PO Box 7330, Station A
San Antonio, TX 78285
Birth Defects Evaluation Center
Director: Robert J. Clayton, M.D.
(512) 228-2386

University of Texas Health Science Center at San Antonio
7703 Floyd Curl Drive
San Antonio, TX 78284
Department of Cellular and Structural Biology
Division of Human Genetics
Director: Barbara Bownam, Ph.D.
(512) 691-6441
Department of Pediatric Dentistry
Division of Clinical Genetics
Director: Ronald J. Jorgenson, D.D.S., Ph.D.
(512) 691-7587

UTAH
University of Utah Medical Center
50 N. Medical Drive
Salt Lake City, UT 84132
Department of Pediatrics
Division of Medical Genetics
Director: John C. Carey, M.D.
(801) 581-8943

VERMONT
University of Vermont
College of Medicine
A115 Medical Alumni Building
Burlington, VT 05405
Department of Pediatrics
Vermont Regional Genetics Center
Director: H. Eugene Hoyme, M.D.
(802) 656-4024

VIRGINIA
University of Virginia Medical School
PO Box 386
Charlottesville, VA 22908
Department of Pediatrics
Division of Medical Genetics
Director: Thaddeus E. Kelly, M.D., Ph.D.
(804) 924-2665

Genetics and IVF Institute
3020 Javier Rd.
Fairfax, VA 22031
Director: Joseph D. Schulman, M.D.
(703) 698-7355

Eastern Virginia Medical School
PO Box 1980, Lewis Hall
Norfolk, VA 23501
Department of Pediatrics
Division of Genetics
Director: Jack M. Rary, Ph.D.
(804) 623-1500

Medical College of Virginia
Virginia Commonwealth University
PO Box 33, MCV Station
Richmond, VA 23298
Department of Human Genetics
Director: Walter E. Nance, M.D., Ph.D.
(804) 786-9632

WASHINGTON
Children's Orthopedic Hospital and Medical Center
University of Washington
4800 Sand Point Way N.E.
PO Box C5371
Seattle, WA 98105
Department of Pediatrics
Division of Medical Genetics
Director: Roberta Pagon, M.D.
(206) 526-2056

Swedish Hospital Medical Center
747 Summit Ave.
Seattle, WA 98104
Attn: Perinatal Medicine
Department of Obstetrics and Gynecology
Director: Laurence Karp, M.D.
(206) 386-2101

University of Washington
Seattle, WA 98195
Department of Medicine, RG-25
Division of Medical Genetics
Director: Arno Motulsky, M.D.
(206) 548-4030
Department of Obstetrics and Gynecology, RH-20
Division of Perinatology
Director: Thomas J. Benedetti, M.D.
(206) 543-3753

Deaconess Medical Center
W. 800 Fifth Ave.
Spokane, WA 99210
Inland Empire Genetic Counseling Service
Director: Michael Donlan, M.D.
(509) 458-7115

Mary Bridge Children's Health Center
311 S. "L" St.
Tacoma, WA 98405
Genetics Clinic
Director: Robert G. Scherz, M.D.
(206) 594-1415

St. Mary Medical Center
401 W. Poplar, PO Box 1477
Walla Walla, WA 99362
Blue Mountain Genetics Counseling Service
Director: Dale E. Dietzman, M.D.
(509) 525-3320, x2495

Yakima Valley Memorial Hospital
2811 Tieton Drive
Yakima, WA 98902
Department of Child Health Services
Central Washington Genetics Program
Directors: Cherie Howry, M.D., Joseph
  Markee, M.D.
(509) 575-8160

WEST VIRGINIA
West Virginia University Medical Center
Morgantown, WV 26500
Department of Pediatrics
Genetics Evaluation and Counseling Center
Director: R. Stephen Amato, M.D., Ph.D.
(304) 293-7331, 7334

WISCONSIN
University of Wisconsin at Madison
337 Waisman Center
1500 Highland Ave.
Madison, WI 53705-2280
Department of Medical Genetics
Clinical Genetics Center
Director: Renata Laxova, M.D., Ph.D.
(608) 263-5918

Marshfield Genetics and Birth Defects Center
Marshfield Clinic
1000 N. Oak St.
Marshfield, WI 54449
Director: Stephen F. Wagner, M.D.
(715) 387-5089

Milwaukee Children's Hospital
1700 W. Wisconsin Ave.
Milwaukee, WI 53233
Department of Pediatrics
Birth Defects Center
Director: Jurgen Herrmann, M.D.
(414) 931-4039

Mt. Sinai Medical Center
University of Wisconsin Medical School
Milwaukee Clinical Campus
950 N. 12th St.
Milwaukee, WI 53201
Department of Obstetrics and Gynecology
Genetics Section
Director: B. Rafael Elajalde, M.D.
(414) 289-8236

Great Lakes Genetics
2600 N. Mayfair Rd.
Wauwatosa, WI 53226
Director: Jurgen Herrmann, M.D.
(414) 475-7400

SOURCE: *National Center for Education in Maternal and Child Health.*

ORGANIZATIONS

National Maternal and Child Health
  Clearinghouse
3520 Prospect St., N.W.
Washington, DC 20057
(202) 625-8410

A government-supported service to supply information and answer questions for the public. Pamphlets, booklets, single copies free of charge. Will provide information on phone or mail request. Difficult questions or requests for more specific information are referred to genetic specialists or health educators at the National Center for Education in Maternal and Child

Health at the same address. The Center's phone number is (202) 625-8400.

March of Dimes Birth Defects Foundation
1275 Mamaroneck Ave.
White Plains, NY 10605
(914) 428-7100

A national organization dedicated to preventing and treating birth defects. About 275 local chapters nationwide. A major source of information on birth defects and genetic counseling. Pamphlets, booklets, books, including an International Directory of Genetic Services. Answers questions from the public. Refers individuals to comprehensive service centers for birth defects. Refers individuals to genetic counseling services in their area. Some local chapters make the services of certified midwives available for normal pregnancies and facilitate prenatal home care for high risk women. Will provide more information and location of local chapters upon request. Local March of Dimes Chapters are also listed in the white pages of phone directories.

BOOKS

The Heredity Factor: Genes, Chromosomes and You, **William L. Nyhan, M.D.,** with **Edward Edelson,** New York: Grosset & Dunlap, 1976.
International Directory of Genetic Services, White Plains, NY: March of Dimes Defects Foundation, 1983.

Know Your Genes, **Aubrey Milunsky, M.D.,** Boston: Houghton Mifflin Co., 1977.
New Hope for Problem Pregnancies: Helping Babies Before They're Born, **Dianne Hales** and **Robert K. Creasy, M.D.,** New York: Harper & Row, 1982.

FREE MATERIALS

Single copies are free

Genetic Screening for Inborn Errors of Metabolism, 106 pages.
Learning Together: A Guide for Families with Genetic Disorders, 24 pages.
Prenatal Care, 98 pages, illustrated.

National Maternal and Child Health Clearinghouse
3520 Prospect St., N.W.
Washington, DC 20057
(202) 625-8410

Birth Defects: Tragedy and Hope, 16 pages.
Family Health Tree. Family project to trace health histories over four generations.
Genetic Counseling. Booklet explaining the why and how of tests for genetic counseling.

Information sheets:
Achondroplasia
AIDS

Cleft Lip and Palate
Clubfoot
Congenital Heart Defects
Down Syndrome
Genital Herpes
Low Birthweight
Marfan Syndrome
Neurofibromatosis
PKU
Polio
Rh Disease
Rubella
Sickle-Cell Anemia
Spina Bifida
Tay-Sachs
Thalassemia

March of Dimes Birth Defects Foundation
1275 Mamaroneck Ave.
White Plains, NY 10605
(914) 428-7100

HEADACHES

See also Pain, page 427.

Although everyone has a headache now and then, an estimated 42 million Americans suffer from severe, recurring headaches. These are different from the common "tension" headache that can usually be alleviated by aspirin, acetaminophen, or other nonprescription drugs. Headaches—especially those that appear suddenly and for the first time—may be a symptom of underlying disease, such as a brain tumor or cerebral hemorrhage. A very small percentage of chronic headaches—only 2 percent, according to one estimate—are caused by life-threatening organic causes. Chronic headaches may also stem from inflamed sinuses, poor dental alignment, TMJ disorders (temporomandibular joint of the jaw), and eye, ear, and neck diseases.

The vast majority of chronic headaches are classified as either vascular (including migraine and cluster headaches) or muscle-contraction headaches. In a vascular headache, the blood vessels inside and outside the skull swell up, producing pain. Muscle contraction headaches result from a constant tightening of the jaw, face, and neck muscles over a long period of time and are often referred to as "psychogenic" headaches, having a psychological cause. Both types can be quite serious and debilitating.

Migraine headaches: A migraine attack is an intermittent and excruciating throbbing headache, sometimes preceded by neurological warning signs, such as a partial obliteration of vision, an aura, or other visual disturbances. Once triggered, it typically lasts for several hours, a day, or even longer. It is also characterized by a sensitivity to light and by nausea. About 70 percent of migraine sufferers are women.

Cause: Unquestionably, migraine headaches have a physical basis—perhaps a genetic defect in the way the brain handles the chemical serotonin. About 70 percent of migraine sufferers report a family history of the disorder. Precipitating factors, such as certain foods, emotional stress, a head injury, or birth control pills, can trigger migraines in susceptible individuals. Many women cease having migraines at menopause, when the body's supplies of estrogen drop—that is, unless they take estrogen replacement (doses of estrogen to prevent weakening of bones and to alleviate symptoms of menopause).

Treatment: Migraines can often be effectively treated by drugs and by relaxation techniques, including biofeedback. Sometimes drugs and biofeedback are used together. The drug ergotamine tartrate is often given to help relieve the symptoms of an acute attack. During such an attack, it may help to lie quietly in a dark room. An individual may learn to reduce the pain by using biofeedback to redirect the blood flow, causing the dilated blood vessels in the scalp to constrict. In some cases, regular doses of drugs, such as propranolol (Inderal), taken over a period of months may prevent the onset of migraines in about 80 percent of the cases, according to some studies.

Cluster headaches: These headaches affect mostly males (85 to 90 percent of the patients are men). The pain, generally concentrated around one eye, is described as pounding, stabbing, burning, like a "hot poker in the eye." During a typical attack, the pain comes regularly, almost like clockwork, in intervals of one to three hours, each attack lasting about half an hour. This series of attacks or "cluster" may go on for weeks or months, and then disappear for a similar length of time. The pain is so severe that some sufferers pound their heads against the wall. A few have committed suicide.

Cause: The cause is unknown. It is not thought to be inherited nor particularly sensitive to emotional factors, such as stress. However, cluster headaches have been precipitated by alcohol, by smoking, and by eating foods containing the chemical sodium nitrite, such as hotdogs and other cured meats.

Treatment: Cluster headaches respond to a variety of medications, including ergotamine tartrate and dihydroergotamine. Sometimes other drugs are used to try to prevent the cluster attacks, such as methysergide maleate (Sansert), propranolol (Inderal), lithium, and corticosteroids, when other drugs fail. Reportedly, biofeedback is not an effective treatment for cluster headaches.

Muscle-contraction headaches: This is by far the most common type of headache physicians are asked to treat. It comes from the constant tightening of muscles in the neck and head. The pain is usually on both sides of the head and is said to feel like a band around the head. Often, the neck and facial muscles are stiff or tender to the touch. These headaches can strike frequently, for example, once a week for two or three hours, or be constant, day after day, for years. Both men and women have muscle-contraction headaches, although women seem to be slightly more susceptible. The headaches frequently come in early morning, early evening, and on the weekends and holidays.

Cause: Most muscle-contraction headaches are attributed to psychological causes, such as emotional stress, chronic anxiety, frustration, suppressed anger, and depression. There is no evidence that they are inherited or accompanied by neurological abnormalities. Experts believe that an emotional factor usually triggers muscle-contraction headaches, even though the person is not aware of a psychological problem. The type of mental tension determines the frequency and pattern of the headaches. Muscle-contraction headaches can also result from physical causes, such as arthritis and disorders in the muscles or bones of the neck, spinal cord, and face.

Treatment: In many cases, physicians try to find the psychological problem triggering the headaches. Drugs, such as antidepressants and tranquilizers, are sometimes used to relieve some of the symptoms temporarily. Common analgesics, such as aspirin and Tylenol, usually do not combat muscle-contraction headaches. Sufferers often need a combination prescription drug to relieve pain. Heat, exercise to relax the muscles, and massage of the neck muscles may help. Biofeedback can help sufferers learn how to relax the tense muscles and has proved dramatically successful in many cases.

Experts believe that you may need medical attention if you have chronic and serious headaches that occur as frequently as a few times a month. Although in many cases headaches are adequately treated by a family physician, many sufferers need specialized care. Some experts advise that persistent headaches should be treated not only by specialists in pain but by clinics and physicians that specialize in relieving *headache* pain. Since chronic headache is a special kind of pain, it may require the special kind of expertise found at a headache clinic. A reputable headache clinic will also give you a thorough work-up, including a neurological examination, to rule out any other organic causes, such as a brain tumor.

WHERE TO FIND TREATMENT FOR HEADACHES

Here are some of the leading clinics devoted exclusively or primarily to the treatment of headaches. For additional physicians knowledgeable about headache treatment, contact the National Migraine Foundation, 5252 N. Western Ave., Chicago, IL 66025; (312) 878-7715.

SOME LEADING HEADACHE CLINICS

CALIFORNIA
Donald J. Dalessio, M.D.
Scripps Clinic Medical Group
10666 N. Torrey Pines Rd.
La Jolla, CA 92037
(619) 455-9100

Barbara Jessen, M.D.
351 Hospital Rd., #316
Newport Beach, CA 92663
(714) 642-1437

N. Vijayan, M.D.
Headache and Neurology Clinic
2600 Capitol Ave., #211
Sacramento, CA 95816
(916) 442-7807

John Sterling Ford, M.D.
4501 Mission Bay Drive
San Diego, CA 92109
(619) 273-3300

Jerome Goldstein, M.D.
San Francisco Headache Clinic
909 Hyde St., Suite 314
San Francisco, CA 94109
(415) 673-4600

Gary W. Jay, M.D.
Valley Multispecialty Pain Center
14624 Sherman Way, #303
Van Nuys, CA 91405
(213) 787-7800

COLORADO
Richard L. Stieg, M.D.
Medical Director
Boulder Memorial Hospital
Pain Control Center and Headache Clinic
311 Mapleton Ave.
Boulder, CO 80302
(303) 441-0506

Charles S. Adler, M.D.
955 Eudora St., #1605
Denver, CO 80220
(303) 333-0505

CONNECTICUT
Fred P. Sheftell, M.D.
New England Center for Headache
40 E. Putnam Ave.
Cos Cob, CT 06807
(203) 661-3900

DISTRICT OF COLUMBIA
Margaret Abernathy, M.D.
Associate Professor of Neurology
Director, Headache Treatment Center
Georgetown University Medical Center
3800 Reservoir Rd.
Washington, DC 20007
(202) 625-0100

FLORIDA
Allan Herskowitz, M.D.
Cedars Medical Center, Inc.
Headache Treatment Center
1295 N.W. 14th St.
Miami, FL 33125
(305) 325-4520

Robert A. Davidoff, M.D.
Department of Neurology D4-5
University of Miami School of Medicine
1501 N.W. Ninth Ave.
Miami, FL 33103
(305) 284-2211

Larry S. Eisner, M.D.
The Neurological Center for Headache
1135 Kane Concourse
Miami Beach, FL 33154
(305) 865-1995

Russell C. Packard, M.D.
5225 Carmel Heights Drive
Pensacola, FL 32504
(904) 474-0740

ILLINOIS
Seymour Diamond, M.D.
Diamond Headache Clinic, Ltd.
5252 N. Western Ave.
Chicago, IL 60625
(312) 878-5558

INDIANA
Howard E. Burg, M.D.
801 St. Mary's Drive
Suite 509
Evansville, IN 47715
(812) 473-4394

KANSAS
Dewey K. Ziegler, M.D.
Department of Neurology
Kansas University College of Health Sciences
Kansas City, KS 66103
(913) 588-5000

Joseph D. Sargent, M.D.
Department of Internal Medicine
Menninger Foundation
Box 829
Topeka, KS 66601
(913) 273-7500

MARYLAND
William G. Speed, III, M.D.
Speed Headache Center
11 E. Chase St.
Baltimore, MD 21202
(301) 727-1615

David Satinsky, M.D.
9715 Medical Center Drive
Rockville, MD 20850
(301) 424-5630

MASSACHUSETTS
John Graham, M.D.
The Headache Research Foundation
Patient Care Division
Professional Office Suite at Faulkner Hospital
  (#5975)
Centre at Allendale Sts.
Jamaica Plain, MA 02130
(617) 522-7900

MICHIGAN
Joel R. Saper, M.D.
Michigan Headache and Neurological Institute
3120 Professional Drive
Ann Arbor, MI 48104
(313) 973-1155

Kamal Sadjadpour, M.D.
4005 Orchard Drive
Midland, MI 48640
(517) 835-8744

MINNESOTA
C. Camak Baker, M.D.
Minnesota Headache Institute
5851 Duluth St., Suite 204
Minneapolis, MN 55422
(612) 588-0661

MISSOURI
James D. Dexter, M.D.
Department of Neurology
University of Missouri
Health Science Center
Columbia, MO 65212
(314) 822-8788

NEW JERSEY
R. Michael Gallagher, D.O.
Medical Center for Headache
513 S. Lenola Rd.
Moorestown, NJ 08057
(609) 234-7421

NEW MEXICO
Ruth A. Atkinson, M.D.
Department of Neurology
University of New Mexico
2 S. BCMC
2211 Lomas, N.E.
Albuquerque, NM 87131
(505) 843-2241

NEW YORK
Seymour Solomon, M.D.
Montefiore Hospital Headache Unit
111 E. 210th St.
Bronx, NY 10467
(212) 920-4636

Arthur Elkind, M.D.
20 Archer Ave.
Mount Vernon, NY 10550
(914) 667-2230

David R. Coddon, M.D.
1031 Fifth Ave.
Mt. Sinai Headache Clinic
New York, NY 10028
(212) 650-7691

OHIO
Robert Smith, M.D.
Department of Family Medicine
University of Cincinnati School of Medicine
231 Bethesda Ave.
Cincinnati, OH 45267
(513) 872-5491

Robert S. Kunkel, M.D.
Department of Internal Medicine
The Cleveland Clinic
9500 Euclid Ave.
Cleveland, OH 49094
(216) 444-5665

A. David Rothner, M.D.
Department of Pediatric Neurology
The Cleveland Clinic
9500 Euclid Ave.
Cleveland, OH 49094
(216) 444-5519

Robert B. Daroff, M.D.
Department of Neurology
University Hospital
Cleveland, OH 44106
(216) 444-5567

Robert L. Hazelrigg, M.D.
The Toledo Headache Clinic
4235 Secor Rd.
Toledo, OH 43623
(419) 473-3561

SOUTH CAROLINA
Hiram B. Curry, M.D.
Department of Family Practice
College of Medicine
Medical University of South Carolina
171 Ashley Ave.
Charleston, SC 29425
(803) 792-3451

TEXAS
Ninan T. Mathew, M.D.
Houston Headache Clinic
1213 Hermann Drive
Houston, TX 77004
(713) 528-1916

WISCONSIN
J. D. Kabler, M.D.
University of Wisconsin
1551 University Ave.
Madison, WI 53705
(608) 263-6400

SOURCE: *American Association for the Study of Headache.*

ORGANIZATIONS

American Association for the Study of
  Headache
5252 N. Western Ave.
Chicago, IL 60625
(312) 878-8977

Professional association of physicians, dentists, and other scientists interested in headaches. Publishes bimonthly journal, *Headache.*

The National Migraine Foundation
5252 N. Western Ave.
Chicago, IL 66025
(312) 878-7715

Voluntary membership organization of patients who suffer from headaches and their families. Provides information, answers questions from the public, and makes medical referrals. Publishes a quarterly newsletter. Will send a list of physicians in local areas who are interested in the treatment of headache and are members of the American Association for the Study of Headache upon request.

BOOKS

Advice from the Diamond Headache Clinic,
  Seymour Diamond, M.D., and **Judi**

Diamond-Falk, New York: International
Universities Press, 1982.

Coping With Your Headaches, **Seymour Diamond, M.D.,** and **Mary Franklin Epstein, R.N.,** New York: Delair Publishing Company, 1982.

Dealing With Headaches, **Wendy B. Murphy,** Alexandria, VA: Time-Life Books, 1982.

Free Yourself From Neck Pain and Headache, **David F. Fardon,** Englewood Cliffs, NJ: Prentice-Hall, 1983.

Freedom from Headaches, **Joel R. Saper, M.D.,** and **Kenneth R. Magee,** New York: Simon and Schuster, 1978.

Migraine and Headaches: Understanding, Controlling and Avoiding the Pain, **Marcia Wilkinson,** New York: Arco Publishers, 1982.

Migraine and Other Headaches, **James W. Lance,** New York: Charles Scribner's Sons, 1986.

Migraine: Understanding a Common Disorder, **Oliver Sacks, M.D.,** Berkeley, CA: University of California Press, 1985.

No More Headaches, **Lillian Rowen,** New York: Putnam, 1982.

No More Headaches, **Alan C. Turin,** Boston: Houghton Mifflin, 1981.

The Woman's Holistic Headache Relief Book, **June Biermann** and **Barbara Toohey,** Los Angeles: Tarcher, 1979.

MATERIALS, FREE AND FOR SALE

Free

Headache: Hope Through Research, 18 pages.

National Institute of Neurological and Communicative Disorders and Stroke
Building 31, Room 8A06
Bethesda, MD 20892

For sale

What We Know About Headaches, **Arthur S. Freese,** 20 pages.

Public Affairs Pamphlets
381 Park Ave. S.
New York, NY 10016

HEARING PROBLEMS AND HEARING LOSS

Hearing problems and hearing loss affect millions of Americans. More than 200,000 youngsters alive today were born deaf or developed severe hearing loss in early childhood. Many also have related speech and language difficulties. Diseases and injuries later in life also rob people of hearing. About 2 million Americans are deaf or so significantly impaired they cannot hear ordinary sounds, such as the ringing of a telephone or conversation. Another 15 million Americans have moderate to severe hearing loss or problems.

TYPES OF HEARING LOSS

Essentially, there are two distinct types of hearing loss: conductive and sensorineural; some people have a combination of both. The first is concerned with the transmission of airborne sound from outside the ear, through the ear canal and eardrum to an important snail-shaped bony structure called the cochlea. Any impairment in this first part of the trip through the ear is called a conductive problem. This is frequently caused by wax build-up, other obstructions in the ear canal, perforated eardrum, or congenital deformities of the outer or middle ear. The most common cause is a middle-ear disease, called otitis media, which most often strikes children, causing inflammation and swelling of the middle ear; it can lead to temporary or sometimes permanent hearing loss. Another disease, otosclerosis, is hereditary and shows up in adults. It is characterized by an overgrowth of bone in the inner ear, and can often be easily corrected by removing the excess bone and implanting a partial or complete artificial stapes; this operation, called a stapedectomy, is fairly common, and can restore hearing to a remarkable degree in about 90 per-cent of the cases. However, after a period of time, hearing loss may return, and doses of sodium fluoride may be recommended to arrest progressive deterioration.

The second cause of hearing loss is by far more complicated, serious, and mysterious. It involves the inner ear, including the cochlea. The cochlea, less than one-half-inch across at the base, is the structure that translates the sound waves to electrical nerve signals that are eventually transmitted through the auditory nerve to the brain. The transformed electrical signals reach the nerve centers concerned with hearing and, eventually, the brain cortex, where they are interpreted as music, speech, and so forth. Any malfunction in this sensory neurological transmission at any location can produce hearing problems and deafness.

Damage to the inner ear mechanism can be inherited, and youngsters can be born deaf or develop inherited hearing deficiencies later in life. Of the 4,000 infants born deaf in the United States every year, 2,000 have genetic defects. Also, deafness can result from insults to the fetus in the womb. A common cause of such birth defects is infection; rubella, German measles, was once a common cause of deafness before the development of a vaccine against the disease. There is a form of herpes that, if contracted by pregnant women, is thought to cause children to be born deaf. Drugs that reach the fetus can also cause hearing damage. Impaired hearing may be one of a cluster of birth defects associated with such congenital conditions as cerebral palsy and mental retardation. Other causes of sensorineural hearing loss are accidents, blows to the head, tumors (called acoustic neuromas, which can sometimes be removed by surgery preventing hearing loss if discovered soon enough), and certain pharmaceutical drugs. Well-documented causes of hearing loss are certain antibiotics, such as streptomycin. High doses of aspirin can also cause temporary and possibly permanent hearing damage.

Diagnosis: There are essentially three groups of professionals who diagnose hearing loss— physicians called otologists (ear specialists), otolaryngologists (ear, nose, and throat specialists), and audiologists, who conduct hearing tests. Physicians usually diagnose ear disorders by physical examinations, medical histories, blood tests, and CAT scans.

Audiologists, on the other hand, are specialists in the science of hearing and conduct actual hearing tests in soundproof rooms. They sometimes use an ''EEG for hearing,'' which picks up and records brain-wave patterns related to hearing nerve centers. Infants can be tested this way for hearing losses. In general, the earlier a hearing deficiency is detected, the better. Though it may not be curable, there may be ways to prevent further deterioration and to prevent other developmental difficulties such as abnormal or delayed speech and language in young children.

Treatment: Minor ear infections and temporary hearing loss may not need the services of a specialist, but anything more serious does. Those who are candidates for a hearing aid should certainly have a physical examination to be sure the hearing loss is not due to a medical problem that may be treatable or progressive.

Tinnitus

Tinnitus is a mysterious type of sensorineural disorder. It is the perception of a continuous ringing or buzzing in the ear. No one is sure of the cause, although recent research suggests it may be a biological defect. It most often affects those who are also hard of hearing. Sometimes it can become so severe that it interferes with normal activity, even sleep; psychologically, it can be devastating. However, it is often mild and not necessarily progressive.

To combat severe cases, some people can successfully use a ''tinnitus masker,'' which looks a little like a hearing aid. It helps drown out the noise associated with tinnitus. The only way to tell if masking will help is to have your tinnitus properly evaluated. If you do not respond to masking, other therapies may help. Biofeedback, relaxation therapy, drug therapy, electrical stimulation, and alteration of air pressure in the ear canal have all had some success. Drugs, however, give only temporary improvement and may have serious side effects.

Increasing numbers of researchers are investigating tinnitus and increasing numbers of sufferers are forming self-help groups to deal with it. It is important to be adequately evaluated in order to rule out organic causes of the internal noise, such as a brain tumor, and to consult an experienced specialist who can properly assess and treat the disorder.

Age-related hearing loss

The most common cause of hearing loss comes with aging. Formally, it is called presbycusis. It is generally classified as a sensorineural defect and is impossible to cure. Hearing aids, growing ever smaller and more sophisticated, offer the best help to date. The loss invariably occurs in the high-frequency range and becomes noticeable around the ages of 40 to 50. About 25 percent of all Americans in their sixties and seventies—an estimated six million people— have difficulty hearing. The cause of this gradual hearing loss is unknown, and scientists are unclear about its relationship to aging. Some believe it may have something to do with our environment.

Meniere's disease

Meniere's is a disease of the inner ear that can cause severe attacks of dizziness. It is estimated to affect as many as four million Americans. It occurs most often in men and women between the ages of 30 and 60. The dizziness and other symptoms apparently result from the pressure due to a build-up of fluid in the inner ear. The cause is unknown. Scientists speculate it may be caused by injury, infection, or by an immune malfunctioning in which the body attacks its own tissues.

Symptoms: An early warning sign is a sense of fullness or deep pressure in the affected ear. Later, there are sudden attacks of dizziness, which may last for minutes or hours. At the same time, there may be nausea, ringing in the ear (tinnitus), or hearing loss. The attack usually stops without treatment, and then recurs, unpredictably, perhaps several times a year. There is

almost always nerve-deafness or hearing impairment in at least one ear.

Diagnosis: The diagnosis may be made by a general physician, but should be confirmed by an otologist or otolaryngologist.

Treatment: There is no standard treatment, and no curative medication or prevention. Doctors sometimes recommend cutting down on salt, fats, smoking, alcohol, or coffee. If the attacks are severe, frequent, and uncontrollable by medications such as diuretics and vasodilators, a physician may recommend surgery. Surgery usually controls the dizziness, but may cause deafness in the affected ear. Even though treatment is not certain, it can halt the progression to permanent hearing loss if applied in time.

SPECIALISTS IN EAR DISEASES AND HEARING PROBLEMS

Physicians who specialize in the treatment of ear (as well as nose and throat) diseases and hearing impairment are called otolaryngologists. For a list of the heads of departments of otolaryngology at leading medical colleges, *see* page

586. These physicians can be excellent sources of treatment and/or medical referrals to others who specialize in all kinds of ear diseases and hearing problems.

HEARING AND SPEECH HOTLINES

(800) 638-TALK (8255)
(301) 897-8682—Maryland, Alaska, and
  Hawaii
(301) 897-8682—TTY (call collect)

Answers a variety of hearing and speech questions, such as what to do if your spouse cannot hear or cannot talk normally after a stroke, where to find resources and information about any hearing or speech problem. Operates during regular weekday business hours. Will provide literature

and tell you where to find an accredited audiology or hearing clinic. Operated by the National Association for Hearing and Speech Action, the consumer affiliate of the American Speech-Language-Hearing Association.

(800) 424-8576

Operated by the Better Hearing Institute, answers all kinds of questions about hearing for the public and professionals.

INFORMATION ABOUT HEARING AIDS

Buying and maintaining a hearing aid is often tricky because hearing aids are usually distrib-

uted by hearing-aid dealers who have a vested interest in selling them. The following procedure is recommended: First, have a physical exam to rule out a medical cause; then see a clinical audiologist (a person with graduate professional training who specializes in hearing problems) to test your hearing to see if you will benefit from a hearing aid. Audiologists can then tell you what type of hearing aid you need, if any, and refer you to a reputable supplier.

INFORMATION ON AUDIOLOGISTS

Almost all medical centers, medical schools, and large urban hospitals have speech and hearing centers that can be expected to be of high quality. They usually have both audiologists and speech-language pathologists. You may also find qualified clinical audiologists at rehabilitation centers, in private practice, in state and federal governmental agencies, in industry, in nursing-care facilities, and in health departments and community clinics.

For a list of audiology and speech-language pathology centers accredited by the American Speech-Language-Hearing Association, *see* Speech and Language Problems, page 510. For names of other accredited audiologists in your area contact the American Speech-Language-Hearing Association at 10108 Rockville Pike, Rockville, MD 20852; (800) 638-8255 or (301) 897-5700.

HEARING-AID DEALERS

After you have had a physical exam and a hearing test, you may need to find a hearing-aid dealer if your audiologist does not recommend one. The hearing-aid specialist will first take an impression of your ear for the mold, order the hearing aid, show you how to use it, and, if necessary, do follow-up adjustments.

The National Hearing Aid Society, a trade association for hearing-aid dealers, puts out a directory of "certified hearing-aid audiologists" throughout the country, which you can get without cost. The hearing-aid specialists must pass a Society course and test, have at least two years' experience fitting hearing aids, have references, and agree to abide by the Society's code of ethics.

National Hearing Aid Society
20361 Middlebelt
Livonia, MI 48152
(313) 478-2610

Or you can call:

HEARING AID HOTLINE
(800) 521-5247
(313) 478-2610—Michigan

Answers questions about hearing aids and hearing-aid specialists, identifies possible sources of financial assistance (but does not provide financial assistance), and acts to help resolve problems with individual hearing aid dealers. Also provides without charge a Better Business Bureau booklet, *Facts About Hearing Aids;* does not give medical advice, recommend specific hearing aids or quote prices. Operated by the National Hearing Aid Society.

HEARING DOGS

Just as dogs have been trained to act as eyes for the blind, they have also been trained to act as ears for the deaf. The dogs are trained to hear such sounds as a baby crying, a smoke alarm, an alarm clock, a security buzzer, a ringing telephone, a knock at the door, and unfamiliar sounds that may indicate danger or an emergency.

Many dogs are provided free of charge through contributions from the Lions Club International.

Lions Club International
300 22nd St.
Oak Brook, IL 60570

Hearing Dog, Inc.
5901 E. 89th Ave.
Henderson, CO 80640
(303) 287-EARS—voice and TTY for hearing impaired.

EAR DONATION AND EAR BANKS

Just as there are eye banks and brain tissue banks, there are ear banks. The banks are in need of the part of the hearing apparatus called the temporal bone, which includes the eardrum, the entire middle ear, the entire inner ear, and nerve tissues. The banks distribute the temporal bones after death and are sponsored by the Deafness Research Foundation.

If you pledge the temporal bone structures, they may be used in the following ways: as transplants to help restore hearing to persons who have lost their hearing through infection, injury, or congenital imperfections; for the education of young physicians specializing in ear medicine; or in basic research to help answer questions about nerve deafness and other ear disorders. The temporal bone banks need donations from all kinds of people—those who have documented hearing impairments, secondary hearing loss from other health problems, and those who have normal hearing (to be used for comparisons).

To find out how to register your intended donation and get a donor card, contact the Deafness Research Foundation, 55 E. 34th St., New York, NY 10016; (212) 684-6556, TTY (212) 684-6559—or contact one of the regional ear banks.

Ear banks (regional centers)

Eastern and National Center
Massachusetts Eye & Ear Infirmary
243 Charles St.
Boston, MA 02114
Harold F. Schuknecht, M.D., Director
Linda M. Joyce, Coordinator
(617) 523-7900, x2711

Serves Connecticut, Maine, Massachusetts, New Hampshire, New Jersey, New York, Pennsylvania, Rhode Island and Vermont.

Midwestern Center
University of Minnesota
Box 396–Mayo
Minneapolis, MN 55455
Michael M. Paparella, M.D., Director
Marilyn Matheny, Coordinator
(612) 373-5466

Serves Illinois, Indiana, Iowa, Kansas, Michigan, Minnesota, Missouri, Nebraska, North Dakota, Ohio, Oklahoma, South Dakota and Wisconsin.

One Southern Center
Baylor College of Medicine
Neurosensory Center
Room A523
Houston, TX 77030
Bobby R. Alford, M.D., Director
Rosalyn Guess, Coordinator
(713) 790-5470

Serves Alabama, Arkansas, Delaware, Florida, Georgia, Kentucky, Louisiana, Maryland, Mississippi, North Carolina, South Carolina, Puerto Rico, Tennessee, Texas, Virginia, Washington, DC and West Virginia.

Western Center
UCLA School of Medicine
31-24 Rehabilitation Center
Los Angeles, CA 90024
Paul H. Ward, M.D., Director
Jane Greenstein, Coordinator
(213) 825-4710
Serves Alaska, Arizona, California, Colorado, Hawaii, Idaho, Montana, Nevada, New Mexico, Oregon, Utah, Washington and Wyoming.

SOURCE: *Deafness Research Foundation.*

ORGANIZATIONS

The Alexander Graham Bell Association for the Deaf
3417 Volta Place, NW
Washington, DC 20007-2778
(202) 337-5220 (voice/TDD)

Nonprofit, membership organization. Affiliates throughout the country. Information source on all aspects of hearing impairment for adults, children, and professionals. Pamphlets, brochures, textbooks, audiovisual materials, newsletter, *Newsounds,* professional journal, *The Volta Review.* Answers questions from the public on all kinds of hearing problems, including questions about tinnitus, cochlear implants, teacher training programs, oral interpreting services, lipreading and signalling devices for the home. Will send more information and name of local affiliate in your area upon request.

American Speech-Language-Hearing Association
10801 Rockville Pike
Rockville, MD 20852
(301) 897-5700 (voice/TDD)

National professional membership organization for speech language pathologists and audiologists concerned with communication behavior and disorders. A major source of information for anyone with hearing problems. Pamphlets, booklets, audiovisual materials, scientific journals, monographs, reports, directories. Provides the names of certified audiologists, speech pathologists and clinical centers. Will answer questions from the public and send more information upon request.

American Tinnitus Association
PO Box 5
Portland, OR 97207
(503) 248-9985

National membership association for those who suffer from tinnitus, and for physicians and health professionals. Over 100 local self-help groups. Answers questions from the public. Makes referrals of specialists. Pamphlets, brochures. Will send more information and the name of a local group in your area upon request.

Better Hearing Institute
1430 K St., NW, Suite 600
Washington, DC 20005
(202) 638-7577, 2848 (TTY)

National nonprofit educational organization for the hearing impaired, their friends and relatives and the general public about hearing loss and rehabilitation. Booklets, a newsletter, audiovisual materials. Answers questions from the public about all aspects of hearing impairment. Special service: Maintains a toll-free Hearing Helpline for professionals and consumers. Will send more information upon request.

American Society for Deaf Children
814 Thayer Ave.
Silver Spring, MD 20910
(301) 585-5400

A national information, mutual-support membership organization, dedicated to parent-to-parent support and networking among parents, professionals and friends. A source of information for parents and other interested persons. Pamphlets, booklets, bimonthly newsletter, and a summer camp directory. Maintains a resource library on all topics of concern to families with deaf children. Special services: sponsors a nationwide self-help program for new parents of deaf children, "Two Years of Love." Will send more information upon request.

National Association for Hearing and Speech Action
10801 Rockville Pike
Rockville, MD 20852
(800) 638-8255 (voice/TDD)
(301) 897-8682 (voice/TDD)

A national organization which is the consumer affiliate of the American Speech-Language-Hearing Association. Provides information about all speech, language and hearing disorders. Publishes a bimonthly newsletter, pamphlets and packets on a variety of communication disorders. Maintains a hotline. Answers questions on all aspects of hearing and speech disorders and provides professional referrals throughout the world.

National Association of the Deaf
814 Thayer Ave.
Silver Spring, MD 20910
(301) 587-1788 (voice/TTY)

A national nonprofit, membership consumer organization. 50 affiliated state associations and local chapters that act as advocates for the deaf. An information source about deafness. Books, booklets, audiovisual materials, *Deaf American* magazine and the *Broadcaster,* a tabloid. Answers questions from the public. Will send more information upon request.

National Hearing Aid Society
20361 Middlebelt Rd.
Livonia, MI 48152
(313) 478-2610

A national trade association for hearing aid dealers. Pamphlets, brochures for the public. Certifies hearing aid dealers as "certified hearing aid audiologists." Operates a hearing aid Helpline for consumers with questions about hearing aids, hearing loss and for help in resolving a problem with a hearing-aid transaction. Publishes an annual directory of certified hearing aid audiologists, available to the public. Will send more information upon request.

National Hearing Association
PO Box 8897
Metairie, LA 70011
(504) 888-HEAR

National membership organization for the hearing impaired, physicians and professionals interested in hearing loss. An information source for the public. Pamphlets, a newsletter, *Hear, Hear.* Supports research. Will provide more information upon request.

Self-Help for Hard of Hearing People, Inc.
4848 Battery Lane
Suite 100
Bethesda, MD 20814
(301) 657-2248 (voice)
(301) 657-2249 (TTY)

A national nonprofit membership educational organization of hard of hearing people, relatives and friends. Local chapters throughout the country. Information source for those who cannot hear well, but are not deaf. Special reports and a journal about hearing loss, *Shhh,* with articles directed toward issues of interest to the hearing impaired. Makes referrals. Answers questions. Acts as an advocacy organization for the hard of hearing. Will send more information upon request.

BOOKS

Access: The Guide to a Better Life for Disabled Americans, **Lilly Bruck,** New York: Random House, 1978.

American Sign Language: A Comprehensive Dictionary, **Martin Sternberg,** New York: Harper and Row, 1981.

A Basic Course in Manual Communication, **T. J. O'Rourke,** Silver Spring, MD: National Association of the Deaf, 1973 (beginning sign language book).

Can't Your Child Hear? **Roger Freeman, Clifton Carbin,** and **Robert Boese,** Baltimore: University Park Press, 1981.

Dancing Without Music, **Beryl Lieff Benderly,** New York: Anchor Press, 1980.

Deaf Like Me, **Thomas S. Spraley** and **James P. Spradley,** New York: Random House, 1978.

A Difference in the Family, **Helen Featherstone,** New York: Viking-Penguin, 1981.

For Parents of Deaf Children, **Jerome Schein** and **Doris Naiman,** Silver Spring, MD: National Association of the Deaf, 1977.

Legal Rights of Hearing Impaired People, National Center for Law and the Deaf, Washington, DC: Gallaudet Press, 1982.

A Show of Hands: Say It in Sign Language,
Mary Beth Sullivan and **Linda Bourke,**
Boston: Addison Wesley, 1980.

The Silent Garden, **Paul Ogden** and **Suzanne
Lipsett,** New York: St. Martin's Press,
1982.

They Grow in Silence, **Eugene Mindel, M.D.,**
and **McCay Vernon, Ph.D.,** Silver Spring,
MD: National Association of the Deaf,
1971.

Tinnitus: Facts, Theories, and Treatments,
Washington: National Academy Press,
National Academy of Sciences, 2101
Constitution Ave., NW, Washington, DC,
1982.

Children's books

Just Like Everybody Else, **Lillian Rosen,** New
York: Harcourt Brace Jovanovich, 1981.

Sesame Street Sign Language Fun, with **Linda
Bove,** New York: Random House/Children's
Television Workshop, 1980.

Silent Dancer, **Bruce Hlibok,** New York:
Simon and Schuster, 1981.

MATERIALS, FREE AND FOR SALE

Free (single copies)

Sounds or Silence?, booklet.
Tinnitus or Head Noises, brochure.
Nerve Deafness and You, brochure.

Better Hearing Institute
1430 K St., NW
Washington, DC 20005

Facts About Hearing Aids

Council of Better Business Bureaus
1515 Wilson Blvd.
Arlington, VA 22209

A Discussion of Acoustic Neuromas
A Discussion of Chronic Ear Infection
A Discussion of the Cochlear Implant
A Discussion of Dizziness
A Discussion of Otosclerosis

House Ear Institute
256 S.Lake St.
Los Angeles, CA 90057
(213) 483-4431

Assistive Listening Devices
Communication Disorders and Aging
*Do Your Health Insurance Benefits Cover
Speech, Language and Hearing Services?*
Hearing Aids and Hearing Help
How Does Your Child Hear and Talk?
*NAHSA Answers Questions About: Noise and
Hearing Loss; Otitis Media and Language
Development; Recognizing Communication
Disorders; Tinnitus*

The National Association for Hearing and
Speech Action
10801 Rockville Pike
Rockville, MD 20852

Dizziness, 22 pages; includes Meniere's
Disease.
Hearing Loss: Hope Through Research, 36
pages.

National Institute of Neurological and
Communicative Disorders and Stroke
900 Rockville Pike
Building 31, Room 8A06
Bethesda MD 20892

For sale

Deafness and Adolescence, a monograph.
A Parent Kit. With brochures on various
aspects of children and hearing impairment,
information on children's rights, a sample of
the organization's newsletter, journal, and
10 reprints from the journal.

The Alexander Graham Bell Association for
the Deaf
3417 Volta Place, NW
Washington, DC 20007
(202) 337-5220 (voice/TDD)

Directory of Assistive Listening Devices. A list
of more than 4,000 public places in the
United States and Canada equipped with
assistive listening devices.

Getting the Most out of Your Hearing Aid, 40
    pages.
Lip Reading Made Easy, 32 pages.
Raising Your Hearing Impaired Child, 256
    pages.

The National Association for Hearing and
    Speech Action
10801 Rockville Pike
Rockville, MD 20852
(800) 638-8255

HEART AND CARDIOVASCULAR DISEASES

Heart disease, along with blood vessel disease, is the number-one killer of Americans, accounting for an astounding one-half of all deaths each year—nearly one million, three times more than from cancer. More than 43 million Americans, about one in four adults, have cardiovascular disease. On the average, three Americans suffer heart attacks every minute.

Heart disease is the deadliest of the chronic diseases. It is also largely preventable, with current knowledge. The death rate from heart disease and stroke has been declining significantly in the past 15 years, presumably because of better medical treatment, including the control of blood pressure, and changes in life-style, such as lower-fat diets, more exercise, and less smoking. At the same time, there have been dramatic new advances in dealing with the clogged and hardened arteries that cause heart attacks, strokes, and amputations of the legs. As grim as heart and other vascular diseases are, they are beginning to yield to prevention and high technology.

The underlying cause of most cardiovascular disease is atherosclerosis. Over many years, the arteries and blood vessels build up deposits of fat and minerals, causing arteries to lose their elasticity (become hard) and too narrow, allowing less blood to pass through them. This sets the stage for the development of blood clots that can then block off blood flow. When the disease is in the artery of the heart itself it is called coronary artery disease, or CAD. If the blood flow is interrupted in the coronary arteries, a heart attack can occur, causing in some cases potentially fatal fibrillation (abnormal rhythms of the heart beat), and damage to the heart muscle.

Since the entire body is fed by a network of blood vessels, it is difficult to consider heart disease without including other conditions resulting from diseased arteries and blood vessels. Thus, if a blood vessel develops a clot or restricts blood flow in the brain (cerebrovascular disease), a stroke may result. If blockage occurs in the femoral artery of the leg, tissue below may be starved of blood and oxygen, gangrene may set in, and amputation of the foot or leg may be necessary. If blood pressure is high, heart disease or stroke may follow. Heart and other blood vessel diseases are often considered together, under the term cardiovascular disease. There are other causes of heart disease, such as coronary artery spasm, rheumatic fever (exceedingly rare today), and congenital defects, but by far the major cause is diseased coronary arteries.

HEART DISEASE

The major danger of heart disease is heart attack—when the obstructions in the arteries of the heart shut down the supply of blood and oxygen to the heart muscle, damaging or killing heart tissue. Heart attacks kill about 550,000 Americans a year, accounting for about half of all deaths from heart and blood vessel diseases. Generally, blood and the oxygen it carries to the heart are interrupted by a permanent blockage in the arteries themselves. Recently, scientists have turned considerable attention to coronary artery spasm, which can cause a temporary shutdown of the artery, also resulting in heart attack.

Cause: The factors that put a person at high risk for cardiovascular disease are well known and many can be altered, significantly reducing the chances of heart attack. Men are more susceptible, although the risk rises in women after menopause. Twenty-five percent of all heart attacks occur before age 65, and there is an inherited susceptibility to heart disease and atherosclerosis. The main preventable causes of heart disease are cigarette smoking, high blood pressure, and high blood cholesterol levels. Diabetics and obese people are also prime heart attack candidates. In addition, the more risk factors a person has, the greater the chances of cardiovascular disease. For example, middle-aged men who smoke and have high blood pressure are three-and-one-half times more likely to have cardiovascular disease than men who do not have these risk factors.

Stopping smoking, getting exercise, controlling diabetes, and reducing blood cholesterol levels can help prevent heart disease. A recent major study shows for the first time that lowering elevated blood cholesterol levels resulted in a lowering of the risk of heart disease. In the study, middle-aged men who lowered their cholesterol by 25 percent through drugs and other means reduced their risk of heart attack by 50 percent. Studies show that diet can reduce cholesterol by 10–15 percent in most people. Stress also plays a part in bringing on heart attack and may be especially linked to spontaneous spasms in the coronary artery.

Symptoms: Classic symptoms of heart attack are a heavy, squeezing sensation, known as angina, in the middle of the chest and pain that radiates to the shoulder, arm, neck, or jaw. There may also be sweating, nausea, vomiting, shortness of breath, dizziness, and fainting. Often, the symptoms go away and then recur; however, when warning signs appear, it is essential to get emergency medical help immediately, for minutes or even seconds often mean the difference between life and death. About one-half of all first heart attacks are fatal, frequently because of treatment delay.

Diagnosis: Heart disease is not difficult to diagnose; often the risk can be determined by obtaining a medical history of the individual and his or her ancestors, plus an assessment of current life-style and habits. The diagnosis may be confirmed by routine tests that include blood tests, electrocardiograms (to reveal irregular heart rhythms), and chest X-rays. More specialized diagnostic procedures include exercise electrocardiograms (stress tests), echocardiograms (ultrasound tests), angiography (the viewing of the heart on a monitor, involving insertion and manipulation of a catheter through the veins or arteries), and the use of radioactive isotopes, which can be traced as they make their way through the blood vessels and heart. This procedure can reveal the extent and location of damaged heart muscle after a heart attack.

Treatment: Because life-style plays a major role in the development of heart disease, there is a great deal a person can do to prevent it—adhering to a low-saturated-fat and low-cholesterol diet, getting regular exercise, and quitting smoking. But when heart disease does develop, medicine offers an array of modern lifesaving techniques that may relieve symptoms and prolong life. Drugs, including beta- and calcium-blockers, are a mainstay of heart-disease treatment; aspirin is sometimes recommended as an anticoagulant to prevent heart attack and especially stroke. Newer drugs are being infused directly into the coronary artery to dissolve a clot within hours after heart attack pain begins. There is little question that such drugs dissolve the clot, but whether this happens in time to prevent heart-muscle damage and prolong life is controversial. Increasingly recognized as a part of treatment is cardiac rehabilitation, a systematic program of exercise and life-style changes to strengthen the heart and prevent future heart attacks.

Some coronary problems may require surgery and other "invasive techniques." A common one is coronary bypass surgery, in which a snippet of vein, usually from the leg, is attached to the heart in such a way as to detour blood around the obstructed heart artery. When more than one artery is involved, the procedure is called double, triple, or even quadruple, bypass.

There is evidence that coronary bypass surgery can relieve angina—chest pain—and, in some studies, prolong life, although the same process of atherosclerosis that created blockage in the original arteries can attack the new bypass vessels, causing them to close up too. So, as a result, coronary bypass often does not give permanent relief, and many experts believe that the procedure is performed too frequently and often prematurely. Recent evidence shows that about 25,000 coronary bypass operations, or approximately 15 percent of bypasses done every year, can at least be postponed for a considerable time and possibly avoided. Often, the heart-disease symptoms could just as effectively be treated with drugs or other means.

Some experts believe that the first question to ask about coronary bypass is not *who* should perform it but *whether* it should be done at all. Once the need for bypass surgery is established, any number of heart surgeons can successfully operate; it is no longer an esoteric procedure. At the same time, an experienced surgeon is clearly desirable. It is important to choose an experienced physician and a hospital in which many of these procedures are performed. Despite the fact that many small hospitals now do heart bypass surgery, it is still a complex, potentially fatal operation. Look for a topnotch hospital and a practiced surgeon with an excellent safety record.

For some people, a recent alternative to bypass surgery, called percutaneous transluminal angioplasty, can be less painful and less expensive. The procedure involves inserting a catheter, with an uninflated balloon on the tip, into the artery of an arm or leg and guiding it to the blockage in the heart vessel. At the point of obstruction, the balloon is inflated, compressing the arterial plaque and opening the passage. This procedure is successful in opening and keeping the arteries open about 70–80 percent of the time in selected cases. But not everyone with coronary arterial obstruction is a candidate for this type of procedure; it has been generally recommended for those with obstructions in only one coronary artery. However, some physicians are now expanding and refining the technique to include multiple arteries. The use of balloon angioplasty is becoming much more common, although its wide application is still controversial. Some experts maintain balloon angioplasty can successfully replace coronary bypass surgery in 20 percent of the cases.

However, as with coronary bypass, the opened arteries can close up again, and in a small percentage of cases, the person experiences a heart attack during balloon catheterization and has to undergo emergency bypass surgery. For best results and your safety, do not let anyone but an experienced physician perform balloon angioplasty; government studies show that success rates rise along with the number of procedures done.

HEART TRANSPLANT CENTERS

If all attempts to repair the heart fail, some patients may receive a new heart. Heart transplants are growing at an astounding rate, largely due to the ability of drugs to suppress rejection of the transplanted hearts. In rare cases, surgeons are transplanting both heart and lungs.

The number of heart transplants has quadrupled since 1976. Some surgeons, who had shunned heart transplants because of their failure rate, have resumed such surgery. The heart transplant success rate is reportedly about 78 percent for one-year survival, and 50 percent for five years. But heart transplants are hardly a panacea; they may fail, are exceedingly expensive, and are restricted by a shortage of hearts for transplant.

ARTIFICIAL HEART RESEARCH

Even more avant-garde than the heart transplant is the artificial heart implant, a mechanical device that duplicates the functions of pumping blood through the circulating system. It is still highly experimental and in the initial testing stages.

Dr. William DeVries, formerly chief of cardiothoracic surgery at the University of Utah School of Medicine, implanted the first artificial hearts in Barney Clark in 1982 and William Schroeder in 1984. The heart was invented by Dr. Robert Jarvik and developed by Willem J. Kolff, a pioneer in research on artificial organs. The Humana Heart Institute is part of a for-profit hospital chain.

Dr. William DeVries
Humana Heart Institute International
1 Audubon Plaza
Louisville, KY 40217
(502) 636-7135

WHERE TO FIND TREATMENT FOR HEART DISEASE

Often an internist with a subspecialty in cardiology is quite competent to manage heart disease. In many cases, however, you may need a specialist called a cardiologist. For a list of cardiologists who head the departments or divisions of cardiology at leading medical schools accredited by the American Association of Medical Colleges, *see* page 612. These physicians can be excellent sources of treatment and/or referrals to other specialists in cardiovascular disease. They are not the only outstanding cardiologists in the country, but they are among the best and are assumed to be extremely knowledgeable about the latest treatments for heart disease. They are a starting point in finding the right specialist when you need one.

GOVERNMENT CARDIOVASCULAR DISEASE RESEARCH CENTERS

The National Heart, Lung, and Blood Institute supports specialized centers of research in ischemic heart disease (blood deficiency due to blood-vessel constriction or obstructions), atherosclerosis, hypertension, and thrombosis (blood clotting). These centers do basic as well as clinical (patient) research and are also committed to educational activities on the prevention of heart disease and rehabilitation of patients. The staffs at these centers are connected with universities, and are unquestionably leading authorities in cardiovascular disease.

ALABAMA
Harriet P. Dustan, M.D.
Cardiovascular Research and Training Center
University of Alabama at Birmingham
Birmingham, AL 35294
(205) 934-2580
(Hypertension)

Albert L. Waldo, M.D.
Department of Medicine
University of Alabama at Birmingham
University Station—336 LHR
Birmingham, AL 35294
(205) 934-2351
(Ischemic heart disease)

CALIFORNIA
John Ross, Jr., M.D.
University of California, San Diego
Basic Science Building, Room 2022
La Jolla, CA 92093
(619) 452-3347
(Ischemic heart disease)

James S. Forrester, M.D.
Cedars-Sinai Medical Center
8700 Beverly Blvd.
Los Angeles, CA 90028
(213) 855-3884
(Ischemic heart disease)

Richard J. Havel, M.D.
University of California
1315 Moffitt Hospital
San Francisco, CA 94143
(415) 476-2226
(Arteriosclerosis)

ILLINOIS
Godfrey S. Getz, M.D.
Department of Pathology
University of Chicago
950 E. 59th St.
Chicago, IL 60637
(312) 962-1265
(Arteriosclerosis)

IOWA
Melvin L. Marcus, M.D.
Department of Internal Medicine
Cardiovascular Division
University of Iowa Hospitals
Iowa City, IA 52242
(319) 356-3420
(Ischemic heart disease)

LOUISIANA
Gerald S. Berenson, M.D.
LSU Medical Center
1542 Tulane Ave.
New Orleans, LA 70112
(504) 568-5845
(Arteriosclerosis)

MARYLAND
Myron L. Weisfeldt, M.D.
Robert L. Levy, Professor of Cardiology
Johns Hopkins Hospital
600 N. Wolfe St.
Baltimore, MD 21205
(301) 955-3097
(Ischemic heart disease)

MASSACHUSETTS
Aram V. Chobanian, M.D.
Boston University School of Medicine
80 E. Concord St.
Boston, MA 02118
(617) 247-6220
(Hypertension)

Gordon H. Williams, M.D.
Brigham and Women's Hospital
75 Francis St.
Boston, MA 02115
(617) 732-5661
(Hypertension)

Edgar Haber, M.D., Chief, Cardiac Unit
Massachusetts General Hospital
32 Fruit St.
Boston, MA 02114
(617) 726-2887
(Ischemic heart disease)

MISSOURI
Burton E. Sobel, M.D., Director,
 Cardiovascular Division
Washington University
660 S. Euclid Ave.
St. Louis, MO 63110
(314) 362-8902
(Ischemic heart disease)

Philip W. Majerus, M.D.
Washington University
660 S. Euclid Ave.
St. Louis, MO 63110
(314) 362-8801
(Thrombosis)

NEW YORK
DeWitt S. Goodman, M.D.
Columbia University
630 W. 168th St.
New York, NY 10032
(212) 305-4055
(Arteriosclerosis)

John H. Laragh, M.D.
Cornell University Medical College
1300 York Ave.
New York, NY 10021
(212) 472-5464
(Hypertension)

Ralph L. Nachman, M.D.
Cornell University
1300 York Ave.
New York, NY 10021
(212) 472-6140
(Thrombosis)

NORTH CAROLINA
Harold C. Strauss, M.D.
Duke University
Department of Medicine
Durham, NC 27710
(919) 684-3962
(Ischemic heart disease)

Thomas B. Clarkson, M.D.
Bowman Gray School of Medicine
Wake Forest University
Winston-Salem, NC 27103
(919) 748-4528
(Arteriosclerosis)

OHIO
Robert C. Tarazi, M.D.
Research Division
Cleveland Clinic Foundation
9500 Euclid Ave.
Cleveland, OH 44106
(216) 444-5832
(Hypertension)

PENNSYLVANIA
Robert W. Colman, M.D.
Temple University
3400 N. Broad St.
Philadelphia, PA 19140
(215) 221-4665
(Thrombosis)

TENNESSEE
Tadashi Inagami, Ph.D.
Department of Biochemistry
Vanderbilt University School of Medicine
Nashville, TN 37232
(615) 322-3315
(Hypertension)

TEXAS
James T. Willerson, M.D.
University of Texas
Director of Cardiology Division
5323 Harry Hines Blvd.
Dallas, TX 75235
(214) 688-2615
(Ischemic heart disease)

Antonio M. Gotto, M.D.
Baylor College of Medicine
6555 Fannin Mail Station A601
Houston, TX 77030
(713) 799-4126
(Arteriosclerosis)

SOURCE: *National Heart, Lung, and Blood Institute.*

PERIPHERAL VASCULAR DISEASE

Atherosclerosis takes its toll not only in blood vessels of the heart and brain, but throughout the body, including the main vessels of the legs. Such narrowing or blockage of arteries in the extremities is called peripheral vascular disease and is often responsible for amputations in the aged. Every year about 30,000 leg amputations are performed, and about 50,000 patients are hospitalized for peripheral vascular disease. Unlike coronary artery disease, peripheral vascular disease rarely occurs before age 50 and is most common in people age 70 and older. Signs of peripheral vascular disease are pain in the calf or foot, pale skin when the foot is elevated and abnormally red skin when the leg is put down, loss of hair on toes, leg ulcers or sores, and gangrene. Fortunately, amputation is not the only solution. Many limbs can be saved by removing an obstruction through surgery or balloon angioplasty (insertion of a catheter and inflation of a balloon to widen the arterial opening). Sometimes drugs are injected to eliminate the blood-clotting factor, and bypass surgery to prevent leg amputation is fairly common.

Bypass surgery is reportedly 85 percent successful when the bypass is above the knee and 70 percent successful when the bypass is below the knee. It is similar to coronary bypass surgery—a human or synthetic vein is spliced into the arterial system to detour blood around the clogged section and feed starved tissue in the lower leg or foot. This technique may prevent many amputations, but not everyone is a candidate for it.

HIGH BLOOD PRESSURE (HYPERTENSION)

About 55 million adults and about three million children aged six through seventeen have chronic high blood pressure. Experts consider blood pressure high when three different readings are above 140/90.

High blood pressure is a mysterious, symptomless disease, often called a "silent killer." It is the number-one cause of stroke and contributes heavily to heart and kidney disease. Black Americans are more likely to have high blood pressure than whites; men are more susceptible generally than women; and high blood pressure often becomes more apparent with age. Even mild or moderate elevated blood pressure over a period of time increases your risk of catastrophic illness and death, many experts believe.

Causes: There are two types of high blood pressure. One is called "secondary," in which the cause, such as an adrenal tumor or a kidney problem, is known, but such conditions account for only about 5 percent of all hypertension. The remaining 95 percent fall into the category of "essential hypertension," in which the exact causes are unknown. High blood pressure may be influenced by heredity and environmental factors, such as chronic repeated stress and a high-fat or high-salt diet. Although new research shows that calcium and potassium may be somehow associated with high blood pressure, it appears that some, but not all, Americans with high blood pressure are extra sensitive to salt. Still, scientists do not fully understand the underlying physiological abnormalities that produce high blood pressure. They believe that the delicate biochemical mechanisms that regulate arterial pressure and ordinarily protect against high blood pressure fail.

Symptoms: High blood pressure is unusual in that there are few symptoms unless damage becomes severe, resulting in hemorrhaging, heart attack, stroke, kidney failure, or other severe problems.

Diagnosis: Hypertension is easily measured by a device called a sphygmomanometer, although there is some disagreement about when blood pressure is high enough to warrant treatment, especially by drugs.

Although the classifications are arbitrary, blood pressure in which the diastolic (lower) reading is below 90 is considered normal. Diastolic pressures ranging from 90 to 104 signify mild high blood pressure, 105 to 114 signify moderately high blood pressure, and a diastolic pressure of 115 or more is considered severe high blood pressure. Physicians know that as a group people with high blood pressure are at a higher risk for stroke and heart disease. However, it is impossible to determine which individuals are at risk. In general, the higher the blood pressure, the greater the chance of developing cardiovascular disease.

Treatment: The treatment of hypertension was revolutionized a quarter of a century ago by the introduction of diuretics (drugs that increase the flow of urine and excretion of sodium). Diuretics for years were the first choice of treatment for high blood pressure. Now physicians often try either a diuretic or beta-blocker drug, such as Inderal, first. If one of these drugs doesn't work, the other one is used. Sometimes, both of these drugs, plus other antihypertensive drugs, are used together. Physicians sometimes find that several drugs in lower doses control high blood pressure and produce fewer side effects than high doses of one or two drugs. Physicians may try several before finding the most effective ones.

When drug treatment should begin is controversial. Some physicians say drugs are not necessary unless the diastolic pressure measures 95 or more; others start drug therapy if the diastolic blood pressure is consistently above 90.

There is also evidence that a restricted sodium diet for some (up to half of those with hypertension, according to research) and weight loss for the obese will generally lower blood pressure. For some, changing to a low-fat diet may reduce blood pressure by approximately 10 percent. Vigorous exercise will lower "resting" blood pressure; that is, blood pressure measured not during a stress test. Some health professionals also have used biofeedback and other relaxation techniques to relieve stress and lower blood pressure. Thus, there are many effective techniques for lowering blood pressure besides drugs.

Ordinarily, a family physician, internist, or cardiologist (a person specializing in heart disease) is well qualified to treat hypertension.

STROKE

See also Neurology Specialists, page 621, Rehabilitation, page 460, Speech and Language Problems, page 510.

Stroke strikes about 400,000 Americans each year and kills about 165,000 annually. Black Americans and men are most susceptible. Deaths from strokes have declined dramatically in recent years: Many experts believe that the control of blood pressure is mainly responsible for that decline. Also, more people survive a stroke today than in previous years, and rehabilitation techniques have vastly improved. A stroke occurs when vascular disease in the brain's blood vessels causes an interruption in the supply of blood and oxygen to the brain.

A stroke can occur in several ways. The most common cause is a blood clot that forms in a cerebral artery due to arteriosclerosis. A clot also can travel through the blood stream from another part of the body and lodge in a vessel supplying blood to the brain. The most severe type of stroke is caused by hemorrhaging, when a defective blood vessel bursts, leaking blood into the brain. These ruptures can also occur in an aneurysm— a weak spot ballooning out from an artery. Aneurysms can be congenital defects, and the rupture is often associated with high blood pressure.

Cause: Atherosclerosis—narrowed, hardened arteries—is the underlying cause of stroke, often aggravated by high blood pressure.

Symptoms: A massive stroke can leave a person paralyzed on one side of the body and with brain damage, limiting the ability to think, speak, remember, or understand. However, there are quite often warning signs of impending stroke; these are called "little strokes," or TIAs (transient ischemic attacks), signaling temporary lack of blood and oxygen to the brain. The appearance of any of these warning signs, especially in the elderly, should send a person immediately to a physician, preferably a neurologist, for help. Prompt attention may forestall a major stroke.

The warning signs include: any type of neurological disturbance, such as trouble talking or understanding; temporary loss of vision (particularly in one eye); weakness or numbness of the face, arm, or leg on one side of the body; dizziness or unsteadiness. Signals that the blood supply to the brain is being interrupted may appear days, weeks, or even months before a massive stroke. Drugs, surgery, or other methods may be able to correct the blood insufficiency. Prevention is essential, for once stroke occurs, dead brain tissue cannot be revived.

Diagnosis: Physical examination, history of symptoms, and specialized tests, such as arteriography (radioactive dyes to detect obstructions), CAT and PET scans (a sophisticated X-ray of the brain), and ultrasound recordings can confirm stroke, the cause of damage, and its extent.

Treatment: Surgery to remove a blood clot in the neck artery or drugs to try to dissolve clots are sometimes used, especially to ward off further strokes. The treatment immediately after stroke is growing increasingly aggressive. Since there is no effective treatment for stroke, the philosophy used to be "just put them to bed and hope they recover." The initial damage from stroke often worsens in the first few hours or days in at least one-third of the cases; therefore, physicians are now trying to intervene in those first hours and days. There is some experimentation with drugs to help prevent brain damage once a stroke is in progress. Some of these drugs even promise reversal of paralysis and neurological problems several days after the stroke has occurred. However, their success is far from proved.

A person who survives a stroke may need extensive rehabilitation. Damage to the body depends on which side of the brain the stroke has affected. If, for example, damage is on the left side of the brain, the right side of the body may be paralyzed. A common after-effect of stroke is aphasia, the loss of ability to make sense of words. Speech may be jumbled and incoherent, and a stroke victim may not be able to read, even though intelligence is unaffected. Aphasia is a symptom of brain injury and afflicts approximately one million Americans, usually stroke victims. Aphasia, one of the most frustrating consequences of stroke, can often be effectively treated with rehabilitative language therapy.

A person who survives stroke damage will need rehabilitation, often both physical and mental. Most hospitals have rehabilitation facilities, and there are many excellent rehabilitation centers around the country.

Specialists who handle the treatment and prevention of stroke are neurologists. For a roster of some leading neurologists, *see* page 621.

CEREBROVASCULAR RESEARCH CENTERS

The National Institute of Neurological and Communicative Disorders and Stroke supports 12 centers that do research on cerebrovascular problems. All of these centers have physicians and other personnel who are leading specialists in treating and managing stroke, and although the centers are not specifically treatment centers, many patients are treated as part of research. Some of the physicians on the staffs also see private patients and may be available for consultations.

ALABAMA
James H. Halsey, Jr., M.D.
Chairman, Department of Neurology
University of Alabama
School of Medicine
Birmingham, AL 35294
(205) 934-2400

FLORIDA
Myron D. Ginsberg, M.D.
Department of Neurology
University of Miami School of Medicine
  (D4-5)
PO Box 016960
Miami, FL 33101
(305) 547-6449

MARYLAND
Thomas R. Price, M.D.
Department of Neurology
University of Maryland School of Medicine
Baltimore, MD 21201
(301) 528-5080

MASSACHUSETTS
Nicholas T. Zervas, M.D.
Chief, Neurosurgery Service
Massachusetts General Hospital
Boston, MA 02114
(617) 726-8382

MICHIGAN
Kenneth M. A. Welsh, M.D.
Chairman, Department of Neurology
Henry Ford Hospital
2799 W. Grand Blvd.
Detroit, MI 48202
(313) 876-3396

MINNESOTA
Jack P. Whisnant, M.D.
Department of Neurology
Mayo Clinic
Rochester, MN 55901
(507) 284-4035

MISSOURI
Marcus E. Raichle, M.D.
Washington University
School of Medicine
St. Louis, MO 63110
(314) 454-3596

NEW YORK
Fred Plum, M.D.
Chairman, Department of Neurology
Cornell University Medical College
New York, NY 10021
(212) 472-5744

NORTH CAROLINA
James N. Davis, M.D.
Duke University Medical Center
PO Box 3813
Durham, NC 27710
(919) 286-0411

James F. Toole, M.D.
Chairman, Department of Neurology
300 S. Hawthorne Rd.
Bowman Gray School of Medicine
Winston-Salem, NC 24103
(919) 748-4536

OREGON
Bruce Coull, M.D.
Director, Comprehensive Stroke Center
University of Oregon Health Sciences Center
3181 S.W. Sam Jackson Park Rd.
Portland, OR 97201
(503) 225-7321

PENNSYLVANIA
Martin Reivich, M.D.
Department of Neurology
Hospital of the University of Pennsylvania
Philadelphia, PA 19104
(215) 662-2632

TEXAS
Kenneth K. Wu, M.D.
Division, Hematology/Oncology
University of Texas Medical School
6431 Fannin St.
Houston, TX 77030
(713) 792-5450

SOURCE: *National Institute of Neurological and Communicative Disorders and Stroke.*

CARDIOVASCULAR RESEARCH AND TREATMENT AT THE NATIONAL INSTITUTES OF HEALTH

Several studies are ongoing at the NIH Clinical Center in Bethesda, Maryland, on various aspects of cardiovascular disease involving selected patients with the following disorders:

Congenital heart diseases, which are potentially correctable—of special interest are infants, children, and adults with interventricular septal defects and congenital narrowing of the aorta;

Coronary artery disease, under age 65 with angina for diagnostic and treatment research;

Essential hypertension for experimental treatments;

Renalovascular (kidney-related) hypertension for therapy.

Consideration for participation in such research is by physician referral. For more information your physician can contact:

Office of the Director
The Clinical Center
Building 10, Room 2C-146
National Institutes of Health
Bethesda, MD 20892
(301) 496-4891

ORGANIZATIONS AND AGENCIES

American Heart Association
7320 Greenville Ave.
Dallas, TX 75231
(214) 750-5300

A national voluntary membership organization for the public, health professionals and other interested persons, with state and local groups throughout the country. These groups are a source of information on all aspects of heart disease. Pamphlets, booklets, various publications and audiovisual materials. The groups offer many special services to heart patients and their families. Many sponsor Stroke Clubs, mutual support groups for those recovering from a stroke and their families. Consult the white pages of your telephone directory for an AHA group near you.

Association of Heart Patients
PO Box 54305
Atlanta, GA 30308
(800) 241-6993
(404) 523-0826

A nationwide voluntary membership organization for people with cardiovascular diseases, their families and other interested persons. A source of information for the public. Operates a toll-free information hotline. Booklets, brochures, a magazine. Answers questions on all aspects of cardiovascular disease, pacemakers, diet, exercise. Will provide more information upon request.

The Coronary Club, Inc.
Cleveland Clinic Educational Foundation
9500 Euclid Ave.
Cleveland, OH 44120
(216) 292-7120

A national voluntary membership organization for people with heart disease and their families. About 20 chapters in several cities, mostly in the midwest. An information, mutual support source emphasizing prevention, treatment, and rehabilitation. Booklets and *Heartline*, a monthly newsletter on the latest heart disease information, written by cardiovascular specialists. Will provide more information upon request.

High Blood Pressure Information Center
120/80 National Institutes of Health
Bethesda, MD 20892
(301) 496-1809

An information source for the public and health professionals. Makes referrals to state organizations for medical help. Distributes booklets, leaflets, other publications. Will answer all kinds of general questions on high blood pressure.

The Mended Hearts, Inc.
7320 Greenville Ave.
Dallas, TX 75231
(214) 750-5442

A nationwide support group for patients who have heart disease. Trained members answer questions and give moral support to patients. About 120 chapters, usually connected with heart surgical centers. Quarterly magazine, *Heartbeat*. Will give more information upon request and refer you to a chapter in your area.

National Heart, Lung, and Blood Institute
National Institutes of Health
9000 Rockville Pike, Building 31, Room 4A21
Bethesda, MD 20892
(301) 496-4236

This is the Institute within the National Institutes of Health most concerned with cardiovascular diseases. Supports research on heart disease, blood vessel disease, hypertension. Helps set national policy on all aspects of cardiovascular disease. Publishes numerous booklets, fact sheets. Will provide more information upon request as well as a catalogue of publications.

BOOKS

The American Way of Life May Be Harmful to Your Health, **John Farquhar,** New York: Norton, 1979.

Boston University Medical Center's Heart Risk Book: A Practical Guide to Preventing Heart Disease, **Aram V. Chobanian, M.D.,** New York: Bantam Books, 1982.

Cardiac Rehabilitation for the Patient and Family, **Judy A. David,** Reston, VA: Reston Publishing, 1980.

Change of Heart: The Bypass Experience, **Nancy Yanes Hoffman,** New York: Harcourt Brace Jovanovich, 1985.

Control Your High Blood Pressure—Without Drugs, **Cleaves M. Bennett,** Garden City, NY: Doubleday, 1984.

The Heart Attack Handbook, **Joseph S. Alptert,** Boston: Little, Brown and Co., 1978.

The Heartbook, **The American Heart Association,** New York: E.P. Dutton, 1980.

Heart ByPass: What Every Patient Must Know, **Gloria Hochman,** New York: St. Martin's Press, 1982.

Heart Care, **American Medical Association,** New York: Random House, 1982.

Heartsounds, **Martha Weinman Lear,** New York: Simon and Schuster, 1980; Pocket Books, 1981.

The Living Heart, **Michael Debakey** and **Antonio Gotto,** New York: McKay, 1977.

The Pritikin Promise: 28 Days to a Longer Life, **Nathan Pritikin,** New York: Simon & Schuster, 1983.

The Rutgers' Guide to Lowering Your Cholesterol, **Hans Fisher** and **Eugene Boe,** Baltimore: Rutgers University Press, 1985.

The Silent Disease, Hypertension, **Lawrence**

Galton, New York: New American Library, 1974.

Stroke: From Crisis to Victory: A Family Guide, **John H. Lavin,** New York: Franklin Watts, 1985.

Stroke: How to Prevent It/How to Survive It, **Gloria Jean Sessler,** Englewood Cliffs, NJ: Prentice-Hall, 1980.

Surgeon Under the Knife, **William A. Nolen, M.D.,** New York: Coward McCann & Geoghegan, 1976.

Surviving Your Heart Attack, **James V. Warren, M.D.,** and **Genell J. Subak-Sharpe,** Garden City, NY: Doubleday, 1984.

Treating Type A Behavior, **Dr. Meyer Friedman** and **Diane Ulmer,** New York: Knopf, 1984.

Type A Behavior and Your Heart, **Dr. Meyer Friedman** and **Dr. Ray Rosenman,** New York: Fawcett, 1978.

Cookbooks

The American Heart Association Cookbook, **Ruthe Eishelman** and **Mary Winston,** New York: McKay, 1979; Ballantine, 1979.

Craig Claiborne's Gourmet Diet, **Craig Claiborne** and **Pierre Franey,** New York: Times Books, 1980; low-calorie, low-salt recipes for hypertension.

Don't Eat Your Heart Out, **Joseph Piscatella,** 1983; Joseph Piscatella, PO Box 9882, Tacoma, WA 98499.

The Joy of Living Salt-Free, **Ralph E. Minear,** New York: Macmillan, 1984.

Living with High Blood Pressure—The Hypertension Cookbook, **Joyce Daly Margie** and **James C. Hunt,** Radnor, PA: Chilton, 1979.

Stroke rehabilitation

About Stroke, **Sister Kenny Institute Staff,** Minneapolis, MN: Sister Kenny Institute, 1978; 38 pages, booksize format.

Communication Problems After a Stroke, **Lillian Kay Cohen,** Minneapolis, MN: Sister Kenny Institute, 1978; 28 pages, booksize format.

Help the Stroke Patient to Talk, **Marie C. Crickmay,** Springfield, IL: Charles C. Thomas, 1977.

Home Care for the Stroke Patient: Living in a Pattern, **Margaret Johnstone,** New York: Churchill Livingstone, 1980.

Sourcebook for Aphasia: A Guide to Family Activities and Community Resources, **Susan H. Brubaker,** Detroit, MI: Wayne State University Press, 1982.

Speech After Stroke, **Stephanie Stryker,** Springfield, IL: Charles C. Thomas, 1981; a manual of drills.

Speech and Language Rehabilitation: A Workbook for the Neurologically Impaired and Language Delayed, **Robert L. Keith,** Danville, IL: Interstate Printers and Publishers, 1980; 19 N. Jackson, Danville, IL 61831.

Stroke: A Doctor's Personal Story of Recovery, **Charles Clay Dahlberg** and **Joseph Jaffe,** New York: W.W. Norton, 1977.

Stroke: How to Prevent It/How to Survive It, **Gloria Jean Sessler,** Englewood Cliffs, NJ: Prentice-Hall, 1981.

Stroke: The New Hope and the New Help, **Arthur S. Freese,** New York: Random House, 1980.

MATERIALS, FREE AND FOR SALE

Free (single copies)

After a Heart Attack, 20 pages.
E is for Exercise, 8 pages.
Facts About Stroke, 4 pages.
High Blood Pressure, 4 pages.
Nutrition Labeling, 8 pages.

American Heart Association
Box DIR
7320 Greenville Ave.
Dallas, TX 75231
(214) 750-5300

Blacks and High Blood Pressure, 8 pages.

High Blood Pressure, 8 pages.
High Blood Pressure and What You Can Do About It, 32 pages.
High Blood Pressure: Facts and Fiction, 4 pages.
Questions about Weight, Salt and High Blood Pressure, 8 pages.

High Blood Pressure Information Center
120/80 National Institutes of Health
Bethesda, MD 20892
(301) 496-1809

Arteriosclerosis, fact sheet.
Diabetes and Cardiovascular Disease, fact sheet.
Exercise and Your Heart, 44 pages, illustrated.
A Handbook of Heart Terms, 58 pages.
Heart Attacks: Medicine for the Layman, 28 pages.
High Blood Pressure: Medicine for the Layman, booklet.
How Doctors Diagnose Heart Disease, 17 pages.
Venous Thrombosis and Pulmonary Embolism, fact sheet.

National Heart, Lung, and Blood Institute
National Institutes of Health
Building 31
Room 4A21
Bethesda, MD 20892
(301) 496-4236

Stroke: Hope Through Research, 32 pages.

National Institute of Neurological and Communicative Disorders and Stroke
9000 Rockville Pike
Building 31, Room 8A06
Rockville, MD 20892

For sale

Current Cardiac Medications, Association of Heart Patients, book, 1984.

American Association of Heart Patients
PO Box 54305
Atlanta, GA 30308
(404) 523-0826 or (800) 241-6993

Anatomy of a Heart Attack, 6 pages.
Common Cardiac Drugs, 1986 edition, 22 pages.
Coronary Angioplasty, 6 pages.
How Do Angina Medicines Work?, 6 pages.
Stress Management, 6 pages.

The Coronary Club, Inc.
Cleveland Clinic Educational Foundation
9500 Euclid Ave.
Cleveland, OH 44120

Stroke: New Approaches to Prevention and Treatment, 20 pages.
Watch Your Blood Pressure, 28 pages.

Public Affairs Pamphlets
381 Park Ave. S.
New York, NY 10016

About Stroke, 38 pages.
Communication Problems After a Stroke, Lillian Cohen.

Sister Kenny Institute
Publications Office
800 E. 28th St.
Minneapolis, MN 55407

HEMOPHILIA

Hemophilia is an inherited disorder in which the blood fails to clot normally, resulting in excessive bleeding, sometimes internally. It is, except in very rare cases, a male disease. About 25,000 American males have hemophilia. It is usually spotted quickly in the newborn and almost always diagnosed by age two. However, if the condition is mild or moderate it may not be detected until much later, and sometimes only after an injury, surgery, or tooth extraction. Males with hemophilia lack a clotting factor and must have blood plasma infusions regularly. Although hemophilia used to mean death by age 20, with modern treatment, most hemophiliacs born today can expect to have an almost normal life span.

Cause: Hemophilia is a sex-linked genetic defect passed on through families, although in many cases a family history cannot be found, perhaps because the gene has remained hidden for generations. Women "carry" the gene without exhibiting signs of the disease. A carrier mother can expect that on the average half of her sons will have hemophilia and half of her daughters will be carriers. The daughters of a hemophiliac (male) will all be carriers, but he will not transmit hemophilia to his sons.

Symptoms: Hemophiliacs do not bleed faster; they bleed longer. Without their own clotting factor, they cannot stop bleeding. The bleeding is usually painful, spontaneous, and often occurs in the joints. Hemophiliacs can often detect the internal bleeding; they feel a "bubbling" or "tingling sensation." Repeated hemorrhages, with their biochemical side effects, can damage the joints; thus, hemophiliacs can develop an arthritis-like condition.

Diagnosis: Hemophilia is usually suspected by a family physician, who then refers the patient to a special center for confirming blood tests.

Treatment: Hemophilia cannot be "cured," but it can be controlled. The patient must replace the missing blood-clotting factor for a lifetime through infusions of blood plasma from blood banks. Such replacement is easier than in the past. The plasma is often freeze-dried, and patients can mix it with water, then inject it. Many hemophiliacs can be treated by family physicians, but since there are many complications of the disease, specialized care may be necessary.

Specialized, comprehensive care can be obtained at hemophilia centers throughout the United States. The centers have a team, usually made up of hematologists (blood experts), orthopedists, nurses, physical therapists (hemophiliacs often need special exercises), dentists, psychiatrists, social workers, and vocational counselors. Some hemophiliacs depend on local family physicians for general care and go to centers regularly for check-ups. Children may need treatment at a center initially to help them learn to deal with the disorder.

HEMOPHILIA TREATMENT CENTERS

The federal government supports the following comprehensive hemophilia treatment centers. Each of these centers has several affiliated centers that may be closer to you. Contact any of them for more information.

NEW ENGLAND AREA

New England Area Comprehensive Hemophilia
Center
Worcester Memorial Hospital
119 Belmont St.
Worcester, MA 01605
Peter H. Levine, M.D.
(617) 793-6488

NEW YORK AREA

Comprehensive Hemophilia Care Center
Middlesex General University Hospital
180 Somerset St.
New Brunswick, NJ 08901
Parvin Saidi, M.D., Director
(201) 937-8816

Comprehensive Hemophilia Treatment Center
Long Island Jewish–Hillside Medical Center
Lakeville Rd.
New Hyde Park, NY 11040
Richard A. Lipton, M.D., Director
(718) 470-2124, 2125

Regional Comprehensive Hemophilia
Diagnostic and Treatment Center
Department of Medicine
Mt. Sinai School of Medicine
Fifth Ave. and 100th St.
New York, NY 10029
Louis M. Aledort, M.D., Director
(212) 650-7971

Hemophilia Center–Rochester Region, Inc.
Rochester General Hospital
1425 Portland Ave.
Rochester, NY 14621
Mary M. Gooley, Executive Director
(716) 544-3630

EASTERN AREA

Comprehensive Hemophilia Diagnostic and
Treatment Center
Department of Hematology-Oncology
Children's Hospital National Medical Center
111 Michigan Ave., N.W.
Washington, DC 20010
Sanford L. Leikin, M.D., Director
(202) 745-2140

Comprehensive Care Program for
Hemophiliacs
Division of Hematology
Milton S. Hershey Medical Center
Pennsylvania State University College of
Medicine
500 University Drive
Hershey, PA 17033
M. Elaine Eyster, M.D., Director
(717) 534-8399

Regional Hemophilia Diagnostic and Treatment
Center
Cardeza Foundation Hemophilia Center
Jefferson Medical College
Main Building, Suite 249
11th and Walnut Sts.
Philadelphia, PA 19107
Sandor S. Shapiro, M.D., Director
(215) 928-7786

SOUTHEAST AREA

Comprehensive Hemophilia Diagnostic and
Treatment Center
Division of Hematology
North Carolina Memorial Hospital
433 Burnett–Womack Building, 229H
Chapel Hill, NC 27514
Campbell W. McMillan, M.D., Director
(919) 966-4736

Comprehensive Hemophilia Diagnostic and
Treatment Center
Department of Pediatrics
Bowman Gray School of Medicine
300 S. Hawthorne Rd.
Winston-Salem, NC 27103
Christine A. Johnson, M.D., Director
(919) 748-4324

GREAT LAKES AREA

Hemophilia Foundation of Michigan
401 N. Main
Ann Arbor, MI 48104
Sally Crudder
(313) 973-0350

Comprehensive Hemophilia Diagnostic and
Treatment Center
Great Lakes Hemophilia Foundation
1725 W. Wisconsin Ave.
Milwaukee, WI 53233
Janice Hand, Executive Director
(414) 344-0772

SOUTHWEST AREA

Arkansas Hemophilia Diagnostic and
  Treatment Center
Arkansas Children's Hospital
804 Wolfe St.
Little Rock, AR 72202-3591
Morris Kletzel, M.D.
(501) 370-1100

Oklahoma Hemophilia Center
State of Oklahoma Teaching Hospitals
PO Box 26307
Oklahoma City, OK 73126
Charles L. Sexauer, M.D.
(405) 271-3661

North Texas Comprehensive Hemophilia
  Center
University of Texas Health Sciences Center at
  Dallas
5323 Harry Hines Blvd.
Dallas, TX 75235
George Buchanan, M.D., Director
(214) 688-2647

Gulf States Hemophilia Center
Department of Internal Medicine/Hematology
University of Texas Medical School at
  Houston
Texas Medical Center
PO Box 20780
Houston, TX 77225
W. Keith Hoots, M.D., Director
(713) 792-6620

South Texas Comprehensive Hemophilia
  Center
Department of Pediatrics
University of Texas Health Sciences Center at
  San Antonio
7703 Floyd Curl Drive
San Antonio, TX 78284
Richard T. Parmley, M.D., Director
(512) 691-6197

MIDWEST AREA

Rural Comprehensive Care for Hemophilia
Department of Pediatrics
University of Iowa Hospitals and Clinics
2520 Colloton Pavilion
Iowa City, IA 52242
C. Thomas Kisker, M.D., Director
(319) 356-3422

WEST COAST AREA

Mountain States Regional Hemophilia Center
  Program
Department of Pediatrics
University of Arizona Health Sciences Center
College of Medicine
1501 N. Campbell Ave.
Tucson, AZ 85724
James J. Corrigan, Jr., M.D., Director
(602) 626-6527

Hemophilia Comprehensive Care Center
Division of Hematology/Oncology
Children's Hospital of Los Angeles
4650 Sunset Blvd.
Los Angeles, CA 90027
Edward D. Gomperts, M.D.

Comprehensive Hemophilia Center
Hemophilia Rehabilitation Center
Orthopaedic Hospital
2400 S. Flower St.
PO Box 60132 Terminal Annex
Los Angeles, CA 90060
Shelby L. Dietrich, M.D.
(213) 742-1357

CHMC-UCSF Northern Coastal California
  Hemophilia Program
Department of Hematology
Children's Hospital Medical Center of
  Northern California
51st and Grove Sts.
Oakland, CA 94609
Joseph E. Addiego, Jr., M.D., Director
(415) 428-3371

UCD Northern Central California Hemophilia
  Program
Department of Pediatrics
UCD Medical Center
4301 X St.
Sacramento, CA 95817
Charles F. Abildgaard, M.D., Director

Mountain States Regional Hemophilia Center
Department of Pediatrics (Container No. C220)
University of Colorado Health Sciences Center
4200 E. Ninth Ave.
Denver, CO 80262
William E. Hathaway, M.D., Director
(303) 399-1211

NORTHWEST AREA
Comprehensive Hemophilia Diagnostic and
    Treatment Center
University of Oregon Health Sciences Center
Crippled Children's Division
PO Box 574
707 Gains S.W. Rd.
Portland, OR 97207
Everett W. Lovrien, M.D., Director
(503) 225-8716

SOURCE: *National Heart, Lung, and Blood Institute.*

ORGANIZATIONS

National Hemophilia Foundation
19 W. 34th St.
New York, NY 10001
(212) 563-0211

A nonprofit, voluntary health organization dedicated to helping hemophiliacs. Fifty chapters nationwide, some with hotlines. Acts as a clearinghouse on information about hemophilia for all interested persons. Pamphlets; booklets for patients and professionals; a complete directory of hemophilia treatment centers; a guide to summer camps for hemophiliacs, *Hemophilia Camp Directory*, a quarterly newsletter, *Hemophilia Newsnotes*. Will send more information and name of a local chapter in your area upon request.

World Federation of Hemophilia
Suite 2902
1155 Dorchester Blvd., W.
Montreal, Quebec H3B 2L3
Canada

International voluntary membership organization, dedicated to helping hemophiliacs and advancing medical knowledge about the disease. Publishes *Passport,* an 86-page guide to hemophilia treatment centers throughout the world, with advice for the hemophiliac on traveling. Will provide more information upon request.

BOOKS

Journey, **Robert** and **Suzanne Massie,** New
    York: Warner Books, 1976.

Living with Hemophilia, **Peter Jones,**
    Philadelphia: Davis Company, 1974.

FREE MATERIALS

Single copies are free with postage

*Comprehensive Care for the Person with
    Hemophilia*
Control of Pain in Hemophilia
*Employment Issues in Hemophilia: Questions
    and Answers*

Hemophilia Camp Directory
What You Should Know about Hemophilia

National Hemophilia Foundation
19 W. 34th St.
New York, NY 10001

HOSPICES

Hospices, long popular in England and other parts of Europe, are now widely available in the United States. They offer specialized care to relieve the suffering of the terminally ill. Some hospices are associated with hospitals; some are run by community agencies; others are independent. At their best, they provide a more humane, family-oriented way of dying, allowing a person in the final phase of terminal illness to be as comfortable as possible.

At first the dying individual may remain at home and later be moved to a residential hospice for terminal care. Both outpatient and inpatient care are given by a hospice team. Teams usually include a physician; a supervisor; social workers; physical, occupational, or speech therapists; pastoral and bereavement counselors; nurses; and trained volunteers, who may act as home health-care aides. The hospice team helps patients retain a high quality of life by relieving physical pain, with narcotics if necessary, attending to the emotional and spiritual needs of the patient and family (with special attention to relieving feelings of isolation), and helping families through the bereavement period.

Hospices operate on a 24-hour, seven-day-per-week basis. Hospices usually accept patients who are expected to live no more than six months. Certain hospices that have sought and received certification by the federal government are covered by Medicare. There are an estimated 1,400 hospices in the United States.

Hospices are a relatively recent health-care option in this country, and many new ones have sprung up in response to the demand and to Medicare's willingness to pay. Consequently, you will want to look into a hospice thoroughly. There are no guarantees of quality, but here are three checkpoints: membership in the National Hospice Organization (the group represents hospices of all types), accreditation by the Joint Commission on Accreditation of Hospitals, and certification by Medicare. Lack of certification by Medicare, however, does not mean the hospice is not of high quality; some hospices, because of the strict criteria pertaining to payment and liabilities involved, did not seek certification.

HOW TO FIND A HOSPICE

Contact the National Hospice Organization. The group maintains lists of its members and will send you a list of hospices in your state.

The American Cancer Society chapters often have the names of hospices in a community. Such chapters are listed in the white pages of your local directory.

HOSPICES CERTIFIED BY MEDICARE

The following hospices are certified by Medicare. They are either based in a hospital or based with a skilled nursing facility (SNF-based), home health agency (HHA-based), the Visiting Nurse Association (VNA-based), or freestanding.

ALABAMA

Baptist Medical Center Montclair Hospice
800 Montclair Rd.
Birmingham, AL 35213
(Hospital-based)
(205) 592-1000

Villa Mercy, Inc.
101 Villa Drive
PO Box 1096
Daphne, AL 36526
(SNF-based)
(205) 626-2694

Hospice of Baptist Medical Center
2105 E. South Blvd.
Montgomery, AL 36198
(Hospital-based)
(205) 288-2100, x6670

ARIZONA

Marcus J. Lawrence Hospice
202 S. Willard St.
Cottonwood, AZ 85626
(Hospital-based)
(602) 634-2251

Valley of the Sun Hospice
214 E. Willetta St.
Phoenix, AZ 85004
(HHA-based)
(602) 258-1572

St. Mary's Hospice
1601 W. St. Mary's Rd.
Tucson, AZ 85745
(Hospital-based)
(602) 622-5833, x540

ARKANSAS

Washington Regional Medical Center Hospice
1125 N. College
Fayetteville, AR 72701
(Hospital-based)
(501) 442-1000

Hospice of the Ozarks
906 Baker
Mountain Home, AR 72653
(HHA-based)
(501) 425-2797

CALIFORNIA

Hospice of Monterey Peninsula
8900 Carmel Valley Rd.
Carmel, CA 93923
(SNF-based)
(408) 625-0666

Home Health Hospice
11266 Washington Blvd.
Culver City, CA 90230
(Freestanding)
(213) 390-7454

Comprehensive Community Home Health
  Agency and Hospice
PO Box 682
Daly City, CA 94017
(HHA-based)
(415) 994-9100

Kaiser Foundation
Hospital Hospice
9951 Sierra
Fontana, CA 92335
(Hospital-based)
(714) 829-5000

Visiting Nurse Association
3755 Beverly Blvd.
Los Angeles, CA 90004
(VNA-based)
(213) 667-1050

Kaiser Foundation Hospital–Norwalk Hospice
12500 S. Hoxie Ave.
Norwalk, CA 90650
(Hospital-based)
(213) 920-4525

VNA Complete Hospice, Inc.
5232 Claremont Ave.
Oakland, CA 94618
(Hospital-based)
(415) 654-8420

Hospice of North County
12709 Poway Rd. Suite E-2
Poway, CA 92004
(Freestanding)
(619) 271-0085

San Diego Hospice Corporation
243 Mission Village Drive
San Diego, CA 92123
(HHA-based)
(714) 560-0302

Hospice of San Francisco
2225 30th St.
San Francisco, CA 94131
(HHA-based)
(415) 668-2673

Hospice of the Valley
1150 S. Bascon Ave.
#7A
San Jose, CA 95128
(Freestanding)
(408) 356-6898

Vesper Hospice
311 MacArthur Blvd.
San Leandro, CA 94577
(HHA-based)
(415) 351-8686

Pacifica Home Care
1386 B–W. Seventh St.
San Pedro, CA 90732
(HHA-based)
(213) 832-3311

Hospice of Marin
77 Mark Drive
#17
San Rafael, CA 94903
(HHA-based)
(415) 472-6240

Visiting Nurse Association–Santa Clara
2216 The Alameda
Santa Clara, CA 95050
(HHA-based)
(408) 244-1280

Hospice Home Health Care Agency of
    California
23228 Hawthorne Blvd., #11
Torrance, CA 90505
(HHA-based)
(213) 373-6373

COLORADO
Boulder County Hospice, Inc.
2825 Marine
Boulder, CO 80303
(HHA-based)
(303) 449-7740

Pikes Peak Hospice
601 N. Tejon
Colorado Springs, CO 80903
(HHA-based)
(303) 633-3400

Denver Catholic Community Services
Hospice of Peace
200 Josephine St.
Denver, CO 80206
(HHA-based)
(303) 388-4435

Hospice of Metro Denver
1719 E. 19th Ave.
Denver, CO 80218
(HHA-based)
(303) 839-6256

Mt. Evans Hospice, Inc.
3709 S. Colorado Highway 74
PO Box 2770
Evergreen, CO 80439
(HHA-based)
(303) 674-6400

Hospice at the Prospect, Inc.
PO Box 585
18100 County Rd. One
Florissant, CO 80816
(HHA-based)
(303) 748-3611

Hilltop Hospice
1100 Patterson Rd.
Grand Junction, CO 81501
(HHA-based)
(303) 242-8980

Hospice of Weld County, Inc.
1801-16th St.
Greeley, CO 80631
(HHA-based)
(303) 352-8484

Lamar Area Hospice Association
1001 S. Main
Lamar, CO 81052
(HHA-based)
(303) 336-2100

Sangre de Cristo Hospice
102 W. Orman
Pueblo, CO 81004
(HHA-based)
(303) 542-0032

Lutheran Hospice Care
8300 W. 38th Ave.
Wheatridge, CO 80033
(Hospital-based)
(303) 425-4500

CONNECTICUT
The Connecticut Hospice
61 Burben Drive
Branford, CT 06405
(HHA-based)
(203) 481-6231

DELAWARE
Delaware Hospice Central Division
637 Governors Ave.
Dover, DE 19901
(HHA-based)
(302) 734-0569

Delaware Hospice Southern Division
Beebe Hospital, Room 104
Lewes, DE 19958
(Freestanding)
(302) 645-3300

Delaware Hospice
3509 Silverside Rd.
Wilmington, DE 19810
(Freestanding)
(302) 656-0807

FLORIDA
Hospice By The Sea, Inc.
1580 N.W. Second Ave.
Suite 6
Boca Raton, FL 33432
(Freestanding)
(305) 395-5031

Hospice Care of Broward County
3625 N. Andrews Ave.
Fort Lauderdale, FL 33309
(Freestanding)
(305) 467-7423

Hope Hospice
2635 Cleveland Ave.
Fort Myers, FL 33901
(Freestanding)
(813) 936-1157

Hospice of the Treasure Coast
131 N. Third St.
Fort Pierce, FL 33450
(Freestanding)
(305) 465-0504

North Central Florida Hospice, Inc.
801 S.W. Second Ave.
Gainesville, FL 32602
(Hospital-based)
(904) 372-4321

Hernando-Pasco Hospice
13825 U.S. Highway #19
Suite 401
Hudson, FL 33567
(Freestanding)
(813) 863-7971

Hospice of Northeast Florida
3599 University Blvd., S.
Suite 3
Jacksonville, FL 32216
(Freestanding)
(904) 398-4724

Methodist Hospital Hospice
580 W. Eighth St.
Jacksonville, FL 32209
(Hospital-based)
(904) 356-7008

Hospice, Inc. (Broward)
2331 N. State Rd.
Lauderhill, FL 33313
(Freestanding)
(305) 486-4085

Hospice of South Brevard
1350 S. Hickory St.
Melbourne, FL 32901
(Freestanding)
(305) 727-7000

Hospice, Inc. (Dade)
111 N.W. 10th Ave.
Miami, FL 33128
(Freestanding)
(305) 325-0245

Hospice Care, Inc.
3400-70th Ave., N.
North Pinelles Park, FL 33565
(Freestanding)
(813) 521-1199

Ocala Hospice, Inc.
3850 S.W. 58th Ave.
Building B
Ocala, FL 32678
(Freestanding)
(904) 694-1118

Hospice of Northwest Florida
1600 N. Palafox St.
Pensacola, FL 32501
(Freestanding)
(904) 944-2513

Hospice of Gold Coast Home Health Service
4699 N. Federal Highway
Pompano Beach, FL 33064
(HHA-based)
(304) 785-2990

Brevard Hospice, Inc.
110 Longwood Ave.
Rockledge, FL 32955
(Hospital-based)
(305) 636-2211

Hospice of Martin
925 Lincoln Ave.
Stuart, FL 33494
(Freestanding)
(305) 335-2244

Hospice of Hillsborough
6400 N. 15th St.
Tampa, FL 33610
(Freestanding)
(813) 237-1356

Hospice of Palm Beach County
444 Bunker Rd.
West Palm Beach, FL 33405
(Freestanding)
(305) 582-2205

Good Shepherd Hospice of Polk County
601 First St. N.
Winter Haven, FL 33882
(Freestanding)
(813) 293-5473

Hospice of Central Florida
500 N. Knowles Ave.
Winter Park, FL 32789
(Freestanding)
(305) 647-2523

GEORGIA
Grady Memorial Hospital Hospice Program
80 Butler St., S.E.
Atlanta, GA 30303
(Hospital-based)
(404) 588-4885

Hospice Atlanta
100 Edgewood Ave., N.E.
Suite 1500
Atlanta, GA 30303
(HHA-based)
(404) 256-7271

Northside Hospice
1000 Johnson Ferry Rd.
Atlanta, GA 30042
(Hospital-based)
(404) 851-8000

Peachtree Hospice
3123 Presidential Drive
Atlanta, GA 30340
(Freestanding)
(404) 457-0700

Hospice of the Golden Isles
1326 Union St.
Brunswick, GA 31520
(Freestanding)
(215) 265-4735

Hamilton Medical Center Hospice
PO Box 1168
Dalton, GA 30720
(Hospital-based)
(404) 278-2105

Hospice of Georgia
PO Box 37A
High Shoals, GA 30645
(SNF-based)
(404) 769-7738

Kennestone Regional Hospice
PO Box 1208
677 Church St.
Marietta, CA 30061
(Hospital-based)
(404) 424-8522, x3087

Hospice Savannah, Inc.
PO Box 23015
3025 Bull St.
Savannah, GA 31403
(Freestanding)
(912) 236-1182

HAWAII
St. Francis Hospital Hospice Program
2230 Liliha St.
Honolulu, HI 96817
(Hospital-based)
(808) 547-6011

IDAHO
Hospice of the Palouse
PO Box 9461
Moscow, ID 83843
(Freestanding)
(208) 882-1228

Idaho Home Health and Hospice
200 Second Ave., N.
Twin Falls, ID 83301
(HHA-based)
(208) 734-4061

ILLINOIS
Belleville Hospice
315 N. Church
Belleville, IL 62221
(Freestanding)
(618) 234-4410

Four Fountains Hospice
101 S. Belt W.
Belleville, IL 62221
(SNF-based)
(618) 277-1800

Hospice of Proviso-Leyden
330 Eastern Ave.
Bellwood, IL 60104
(HHA-based)
(312) 547-8282

West Town Nursing Service
2140 S. Wesley
Berwyn, IL 60402
(HHA-based)
(312) 749-7171

Home Health and Hospice of Illinois
Masonic Medical Center
836 W. Wellington Ave.
Chicago, IL 60657
(Hospital-based)
(312) 975-1600, x5654

St. Thomas Hospice, Inc.
7 Salt Creek Lane
Hinsdale, IL 60521
(Freestanding)
(312) 920-8300

Community Nursing Service of Oak Park
Home Hospice Care
124 S. Marion
Oak Park, IL 60302
(HHA-based)
(312) 383-1719

Hospice of Adams County
1005 Broadway
Quincy, IL 62301
(Hospital-based)
(217) 223-5811, x1717

St. John's Hospital Hospice Program
801 E. Carpenter
Springfield, IL 62702
(Hospital-based)
(217) 544-6464, x4572

IOWA
Hospice of Central Iowa
2116 Grand Ave.
Des Moines, IA 50312
(HHA-based)
(515) 277-7687

Holy Family Hospice
826 N. Eighth St.
Estherville, IA 51334
(Hospital-based)
(712) 362-2631

Hospice of Cerro Gordo
810 12th St. N.W.
Suite 23
Mason City, IA 50401
(HHA-based)
(515) 423-3508

Hospice of Siouxland
Marion Health Center
2101 Court St.
Sioux City, IA 51105
(Hospital-based)
(712) 279-2514

Cedar Valley Hospice
Kimbell & Ridgeway Drive
Waterloo, IA 50702
(Freestanding)
(319) 234-5705

KENTUCKY
Ashland Community Hospice
2201 Lexington Ave.
Ashland, KY 41011
(Freestanding)
(606) 329-2133, x468

Community Hospice of Lexington
1105 Nicholasville Rd.
Lexington, KY 40503
(Freestanding)
(606) 252-2308

Hospice of Louisville
101 W. Chestnut St.
Louisville, KY 40202
(Freestanding)
(502) 584-4834

LOUISIANA
Hospice of Acadiana
4010 W. Congress, #208
Lafayette, LA 70506
(HHA-based)
(318) 232-1234

Homehealth Agency–VNA of Southwestern
   Louisiana, Inc.
1520-18th St.
Lake Charles, LA 70601
(HHA-based)
(318) 478-3877

Hospice New Orleans
3535 Ridge Lake Drive
Metairie, LA 70002
(HHA-based)
(504) 838-8944

Hotel Dieu Community Hospice
2021 Perdido
New Orleans, LA 70112
(Freestanding)
(504) 588-3130

MARYLAND
Harford Home Health Agency/Hospice
52 E. Broadway
Belair, MD 21014
(HHA-based)
(301) 272-3490

Stella Maris Hospice Care
2300 Dulaney Valley Rd.
Towson, MD 21204
(SNF-based)
(301) 252-4500

MASSACHUSETTS
VNA of Greater Lawrence
Lawrence Hospice Program
451 Andover St.
Andover, MA 01845
(VNA-based)
(617) 689-0383

Hospice Care, Inc.
39 Hospital Rd.
Arlington, MA 02174
(Freestanding)
(617) 646-3770

Hospice Community Services of the VNA,
   Inc.
1100 High St.
Dedham, MA 02026
(HHA-based)
(617) 329-8603

VNA of South Middlesex, Inc.
Hospice Service
50 Lawrence St.
Framingham, MA 01701
(HHA-based)
(617) 875-3511

Hampshire County Hospice, Inc.
PO Box 1204
7 Denniston Rd.
Northampton, MA 01061
(Freestanding)
(413) 586-8288

Hospice of the Good Shepherd
PO Box 144
Waban, MA 02168
(Freestanding)
(617) 969-6130

Hospice Program of Watertown, Waltham, and
   Belmont
25 Curtis St.
Waltham, MA 02154
(Freestanding)
(617) 894-1100

Hospice at Home
266 Cochituate Rd.
Wayland, MA 01778
(Freestanding)
(617) 653-4217, 5111

VNA of Worcester, Inc.
50 Elm St.
Worcester, MA 01639
(VNA-based)
(617) 756-7176

MICHIGAN

Hospice of Washtenaw
2350 S. Main
Ann Arbor, MI 48104
(HHA-based)
(313) 995-1995

Good Samaritan Hospice
450 North Ave.
Battle Creek, MI 49017
(HHA-based)
(616) 965-1391

Hospice of the Straits
PO Box 419
748 S. Main St.
Cheboygan, MI 49721
(Hospital-based)
(616) 627-5601

Bay Valley Hospice
1014 Gilbert St.
Flint, MI 48504
(HHA-based)
(313) 733-3050

Hospice of Greater Grand Rapids
1901 Robinson Rd., S.E.
Grand Rapids, MI 49506
(HHA-based)
(616) 459-5976

Hospice of Livingston County
1333 W. Grand River
Howell, MI 48843
(Freestanding)
(517) 548-1900

Hospice of Greater Kalamazoo
247 W. Lovell St.
Kalamazoo, MI 49007
(HHA-based)
(616) 345-0273

Hospice of Muskegon County
313 W. Webster
Muskegon, MI 49440
(Freestanding)
(616) 728-3442

St. Mary's Hospital Hospice
830 S. Jefferson
Saginaw, MI 48601
(Hospital-based)
(517) 776-8120

Hospice of Southeastern Michigan
22401 Foster Winter Drive
Southfield, MI 48075
(SNF-based)
(313) 559-9209

Michigan Home Care, Inc.
955 E. Commerce Drive
Traverse City, MI 49684
(HHA-based)
(616) 943-8540

MINNESOTA

Pope County Hospice
10 Fourth Ave., S.E.
Glenwood, MN 56334
(Hospital-based)
(612) 634-4521

Immanuel–St. Joseph's Hospice
325 Garden Blvd.
Mankato, MN 56001
(Hospital-based)
(507) 625-4031

St. Cloud Hospital Hospice
1406 Sixth Ave., N.
St. Cloud, MN 56301
(Hospital-based)
(507) 255-5610

Hospice St. Paul of Bethesda Lutheran
 Medical Center
559 Capital Blvd.
St. Paul, MN 55103
(Hospital-based)
(612) 221-2298

St. Joseph's Hospital Hospice Program
69 W. Exchange St.
St. Paul, MN 55102
(Hospital-based)
(612) 291-3540

MISSISSIPPI

The Hospice of Home Health Agency Multi-
 County, Inc.
PO Box 3409
Hattiesburg, MS 39403-3409
(HHA-based)
(601) 583-2665

South Mississippi
Home Health-Hospice
120 N. 40th Ave.
PO Box 888
Hattiesburg, MS 39401
(HHA-based)
(601) 544-3148

North Mississippi Medical Center Hospice
1030 S. Madison
Tupelo, MS 38801
(Hospital-based)
(601) 841-3000

MISSOURI
Hospice of Care
Texas County Hospital
1333 S. Highway 63
Houston, MO 65483
(Hospital-based)
(417) 967-3311

Kansas City Hospice
8800 Blue Ridge Blvd., Suite 11
Kansas City, MO 64138
(Freestanding)
(816) 765-8023

Hospice of Southwest Missouri
2550-D S. Campbell
Springfield, MO 68507
(Freestanding)
(417) 869-7878

Lutheran Medical Center Hospice
2639 Miami St.
St. Louis, MO 63118
(Hospital-based)
(314) 577-5818

NEBRASKA
Bergan Mercy Health Services Hospice
Bergan Mercy Health Center
2410 S. 73rd St.
Suite 106
Omaha, NE 68124
(Hospital-based)
(402) 398-6060

NEW JERSEY
Community Health and Nursing Service
    Hospice Program
28 W. Collings Ave.
Collingswood, NJ 08108
(HHA-based)
(609) 854-0040

Community Care of Union County
354 Union Ave.
Elizabeth, NJ 07208
(HHA-based)
(201) 352-5694

Hackensack Medical Center Hospice
385 Prospect Ave.
Hackensack, NJ 07601
(HHA-based)
(201) 441-2050

Christ Hospital Home Health
149 Palisade Ave.
Jersey City, NJ 07306
(HHA-based)
(201) 795-8200

Hospice, Inc.
331 Claremont Ave.
Montclair, NJ 07042
(Freestanding)
(201) 783-7879

Hospice of Burlington County
214 W. Second St.
Moorestown, NJ 08057
(Freestanding)
(609) 778-8181

Hospice of Morris County
282 W. Hanover Ave.
Morristown, NJ 07960
(Freestanding)
(201) 539-6121

Karen A. Quinlan Center for Hope
175 High St.
Newton, NJ 07860
(Freestanding)
(201) 383-0115

Muhlenburg Hospital Hospice
Park Ave. and Randolph Rd.
Plainfield, NJ 07061
(HHA-based)
(201) 668-2253

Medical Center at Princeton
Supportive Care Program
253 Witherspoon St.
Princeton, NJ 08540
(HHA-based)
(609) 734-4626

Rahway Hospital Hospice
865 Stone St.
Rahway, NJ 07065
(Hospital-based)
(201) 381-4200

Center for Hope
219 E. Fourth Ave.
Roselle, NJ 07203
(Freestanding)
(201) 241-1132

Overlook Hospital Hospice
193 Morris Ave.
Summit, NJ 07901
(HHA-based)
(201) 522-2846

Holy Redeemer Hospice
280A Brooks Ave.
Swainton, NJ 08210
(HHA-based)
(609) 465-2082

Passaic Valley Hospice
50 Galesi Drive
Wayne, NJ 07470
(HHA-based)
(201) 256-4636

West Essex Hospice
3 Fairfield Ave.
West Caldwell, NJ 07006
(HHA-based)
(201) 228-5540

NEW MEXICO
Hospital Home Health Care Hospice
500 Walter, N.E.
Suite 316
Albuquerque, NM 87102
(HHA-based)
(505) 842-5967

Mesilla Valley Hospice, Inc.
2906 Hillrise
Las Cruces, NM 88001
(HHA-based)
(505) 523-4700

Roswell Hospice
1302 N. Kentucky
Roswell, NM 88201
(Freestanding)
(505) 347-5102

Visiting Nurse Service–Hospice
1316 Apache Ave.
Santa Fe, NM 87504
(HHA-based)
(505) 471-9201

NEW YORK
St. Peter's Hospice
315 S. Manning Blvd.
Albany, NY 12208
(Hospital-based)
(518) 454-1688

Our Lady of Lourdes
165 Riverside Drive
Binghamton, NY 13905
(Hospital-based)
(607) 798-5124

Beth Abraham Hospice
612 Allerton Ave.
Bronx, NY 10467
(SNF-based)
(212) 920-6048

Brooklyn Hospice
4915 10th Ave.
Brooklyn, NY 11219
(SNF-based)
(718) 853-2800, x364

Hospice of Buffalo
2929 Main St.
Buffalo, NY 14214
(HHA-based)
(716) 838-4438

Hospice Care of Tompkins County
1287 Trumansburg Rd.
Ithaca, NY 14850
(Freestanding)
(607) 274-4011

Hospice Care
1714-A Burrstone Rd.
New Hartford, NY 13413
(Freestanding)
(315) 798-6160

Cabrini Hospice
227 E. 19th St.
New York, NY 10003
(HHA-based)
(212) 725-6480

United Hospital and Hospice
406 Boston Post Rd.
Port Chester, NY 10573
(Hospital-based)
(914) 939-7000, x4400

Genesee Regional Home Care Association
311 Alexander St.
Rochester, NY 14604
(HHA-based)
(716) 325-1880

Capital District Hospice
514 McClellan St.
Schenectady, NY 12304
(Freestanding)
(518) 377-8846

Caring Coalition of New York
Box 6271
Syracuse, NY 13217
(Freestanding)
(315) 476-5552

NORTH CAROLINA
Mountain Area Hospice, Inc.
40 Church St.
PO Box 16
Asheville, NC 28802
(HHA-based)
(704) 255-0231

Hospice of Charlotte, Inc.
1609 E. Fifth St.
PO Box 221118
Charlotte, NC 28222
(HHA-based)
(704) 375-0100

Hospice at Greensboro
811 N. Elm St.
Greensboro, NC 27401
(Freestanding)
(919) 274-4592

Hospice of Winston-Salem/Forsyth County
3333 Silas Creek Parkway
Winston-Salem, NC 27103
(HHA-based)
(919) 768-3972

NORTH DAKOTA
Hospice of Red River Valley
PO Box 389
1325 S. 11th St.
Fargo, ND 58107
(Freestanding)
(701) 237-4629

OHIO
Intercommunity Hospice Program of Lutheran
    Medical Center
2609 Franklin Blvd.
Cleveland, OH 44113
(Hospital-based)
(216) 696-4300

Hospice of Columbus
181 Washington Blvd.
Columbus, OH 43215
(HHA-based)
(614) 222-6474

Hospice of Dayton, Inc.
2181 Embury Park Rd.
Dayton, OH 45414
(HHA-based)
(513) 278-0060

Hospice of Hancock County
1815 S. Main St.
Findley, OH 45840
(HHA-based)
(419) 424-0380

Hospice of Miami Valley
712 Dayton St.
Hamilton, OH 45013
(HHA-based)
(513) 867-2133

Hospice and Health Services of Fairfield
    County, Inc.
1231 E. Main St.
Lancaster, OH 43130
(HHA-based)
(614) 687-4410

Hospice of Lake County, Inc.
5976 Heisley Rd.
Mentor, OH 44060
(HHA-based)
(216) 974-8516

Hospice of Middletown
105 McKnight Drive
Middletown, OH 45042
(HHA-based)
(513) 424-2111, x951

Community Hospice Care
182 St. Francis Ave.
PO Box 160
Tiffin, OH 44883
(Freestanding)
(419) 447-4040

Northwest Ohio Hospice Association
3350 Collinwood Blvd.
Toledo, OH 43610
(Freestanding)
(419) 241-6609

Hospice of VNA
707 Fox Rd.
Van Wert, OH 45891
(VNA-based)
(419) 238-9223

OKLAHOMA
Judith Karman Hospice
720 S. Husband, Suite 10
Stillwater, OK 74074
(HHA-based)
(405) 377-8012

OREGON
Kaiser Foundation Hospitals Hospice
3414 N. Kaiser Center Drive
Portland, OR 97227
(Hospital-based)
(503) 285-9321

Providence Medical Center Hospice
4805 N.E. Glisan
Portland, OR 97213
(Hospital-based)
(503) 234-1111

McKenzie–Willamette Hospital Hospice
1460 "G" St.
Springfield, OR 97477
(Hospital-based)
(503) 726-4400

PENNSYLVANIA
Home Nursing Agency of Blair, Huntington,
  and Fulton Counties
201 Chestnut Ave.
Altoona, PA 16603
(HHA-based)
(814) 946-5411

McKean County
VNA Hospice Program
I.O.O.F. Building
Two Main St.
Bradford, PA 16701
(VNA-based)
(814) 362-7466

Hospice Services of VNA of Butler County
154 Hindman Rd.
Alameda Community Park
Butler, PA 16001
(VNA-based)
(412) 282-6806

Family Hospice of Indiana County
Route 3, Box 4
Airport Office and Professional Center
Indiana, PA 15701
(HHA-based)
(412) 463-8711

Hospice St. John
383 Wyoming Ave.
Kingston, PA 18704
(HHA-based)
(717) 288-5428

Home Hospice Agency of St. Francis
South Mercer at Phillips St.
New Castle, PA 16101
(Hospital-based)
(412) 658-3511

Chandler Hall Hospice
1502 Buck Rd., and Barclay St.
Newtown, PA 18940
(SNF-based)
(215) 968-4786

Hospice–Albert Einstein Medical Center
York and Tabor Rds.
Philadelphia, PA 19141
(Hospital-based)
(215) 456-7155

Wissahickon Hospice
8831 Germantown Ave.
Philadelphia, PA 19118
(HHA-based)
(215) 247-0277

North Chester County Community Nursing
  Services/Hospice Program
301 Gay St.
Phoenixville, PA 19460
(HHA-based)
(215) 933-1263

Forbes Hospice
6655 Frankstown Ave.
Pittsburgh, PA 15206
(SNF-based)
(412) 665-3553

Hospice of Pennsylvania, Inc.
916 Wyoming Ave.
Scranton, PA 18503
(HHA-based)
(717) 961-0725

Professional Home Health Care Agency
  Hospice Program
325 N. Second St.
Wormleysburg, PA 17043
(HHA-based)
(717) 761-2186

RHODE ISLAND
Hospice Care of Rhode Island
1240 Pawtucket Ave.
East Providence, RI 02916
(HHA-based)
(401) 434-4740

Hospice of Washington County, Inc.
93 Kenyon Ave.
Wakefield, RI 02879
(Freestanding)
(401) 789-5200

VNA of Greater Woonsocket
Northern Rhode Island Hospice
Marquette Plaza
Woonsocket, RI 02895
(VNA-based)
(401) 769-5670

SOUTH CAROLINA
Spartanburg General Hospital Hospice
101 E. Wood St.
Spartanburg, SC 29303
(Hospital-based)
(803) 573-6785

TENNESSEE
Home Health and Hospice Services of
  Memphis, Inc.
3100 Walnut Grove Rd.
Memphis, TN 38111
(HHA-based)
(901) 454-1333

Hospice of Murfreesboro
602 E. Bell
Murfreesboro, TN 37130
(HHA-based)
(615) 896-4663

Alive Hospice of Nashville, Inc.
PO Box 120033
1908 21st Ave., S.
Nashville, TN 37212
(HHA-based)
(615) 298-3351

Valley Ridge Hospice
128 Division Rd.
Box 822
Oak Ridge, TN 37830
(Freestanding)
(615) 482-9281

TEXAS
South Texas Home Health and Hospice
  Services, Inc.
County Rd. 242
Route 3, Box 21
Alice, TX 78332
(HHA-based)
(512) 664-0246

Spohn Hospice
600 Elizabeth St.
Corpus Christi, TX 78404
(Hospital-based)
(512) 881-3000

Dallas Hospice Care, Inc.
5722 Oram St.
Dallas, TX 75206
(Freestanding)
(214) 823-2891

Visiting Nurse Association of Texas Home
   Hospice
8200 Brookriver Drive
Suite 200 N
Dallas, TX 75247
(VNA-based)
(214) 689-0000

Hospice of El Paso
1900 N. Oregon
El Paso, TX 79902
(Freestanding)
(915) 532-5699

Community Hospice of St. Joseph
1401 S. Main St.
Fort Worth, TX 76104
(Hospital-based)
(817) 336-9371

Galveston Hospice
1111 36th St.
Galveston, TX 77553
(Freestanding)
(713) 765-5548

New Age Hospice of Houston, Inc.
7 Chelsea Place
Houston, TX 77006
(Freestanding)
(713) 528-2098

St. Benedict Home Health Hospice
323 E. Johnson
San Antonio, TX 78204
(HHA-based)
(512) 222-0171

VERMONT
Visiting Nurse Association
260 College St.
Burlington, VT 05401
(VNA-based)
(802) 658-1900

Lamoille HHA
Box 769, Washington Highway
Morrisville, VT 05661
(HHA-based)
(802) 888-4651

Orleans and North Essex HHA
103 Main St.
Newport, VT 05855
(HHA-based)
(802) 334-7897

Franklin County HHA
261 N. Main St.
St. Albans, VT 05478
(HHA-based)
(802) 527-7531

Caledonia Hospice of Caledonia HHA
12 Western Ave.
St. Johnsbury, VT 05819
(HHA-based)
(802) 748-8116

VIRGINIA
Hospice of Northern Virginia
4712 N. 15th St.
Arlington, VA 22205
(Hospital-based)
(703) 525-7070

Norfolk General Hospital Hospice
600 Gresham Drive
Norfolk, VA 23507
(Hospital-based)
(804) 628-3602

Wellspring Hospice
3636 High St.
Portsmouth, VA 23707
(Hospital-based)
(804) 398-2200

Medical College of Virginia Hospital's
   Continuing Care Program
401 N. 12th St., Box 30
Richmond, VA 23298
(Hospital-based)
(804) 786-0932

WASHINGTON
Hospice of Whatcom County
1111 Cornwall
Bellingham, WA 98225
(HHA-based)
(206) 734-9724

Tri Cities Chaplaincy Hospice, Inc.
7514 W. Yellowstone
Kennewick, WA 99336
(Freestanding)
(509) 783-2416

Sound Home Health Services of Thurston-
   Mason Counties
4502 Weorplace Drive, S.E.
Lacey, WA 98503
(HHA-based)
(206) 459-8311

Good Samaritan Hospice
407 14th Ave., S.E.
Puyallup, WA 98371-0118
(HHA-based)
(206) 848-6661

Community Hospice
200 W. Thomas
Seattle, WA 98119
(HHA-based)
(206) 285-5048

Highline Community Hospital Hospice
16200 Eighth, S.W.
Seattle, WA 98166
(Hospital-based)
(206) 244-9970

Hospice of Spokane
N. 1620 Monroe
Spokane, WA 99210
(Freestanding)
(509) 325-2536

Hospice of Tacoma
742 Market St.
Tacoma, WA 98402
(HHA-based)
(206) 383-1788

Hospice of Clark County
316 E. Fourth Plain Blvd.
Suite B
Vancouver, WA 98663
(HHA-based)
(206) 696-5000

Southwest Washington Hospital's Cancer
   Program/Hospice Services
600 N.E. 92nd
Vancouver, WA 98668
(Hospital-based)
(206) 256-2147

WISCONSIN
Appleton Community Hospice
120 W. Franklin
PO Box 1074
Appleton, WI 54912
(HHA-based)
(414) 734-2008

Jefferson Health Hospice Program
1350 Jefferson St.
Baraboo, WI 53913
(HHA-based)
(608) 356-7570

Bellin Memorial Hospital Hospice
744 S. Webster St.
Green Bay, WI 54305
(Hospital-based)
(414) 468-3480

Kenosha Hospice Alliance
625-57th St., Suite 600
Kenosha, WI 53140
(Freestanding)
(414) 658-8344

Hospice Care, Inc.
303 Lathrop St.
Madison, WI 53705
(HHA-based)
(608) 255-0915

Milwaukee Hospice Home Care
1022 N. Ninth St.
Milwaukee, WI 53233
(Freestanding)
(414) 271-3686

Rogers Memorial Hospital Inc.
34810 Pabst Rd.
Oconomowoc, WI 53066
(Hospital-based)
(414) 567-5535

SOURCE: *Health Care Financing Administration.*

CHILDREN'S HOSPICES

The following hospices provide hospice or palliative care services to children and/or minors from birth to 21 years.

ALABAMA
Hospice of the Baptist Medical Center–
   Montclair
800 Montclair Rd.
Birmingham, AL 35213
(205) 592-1059

ALASKA
Hospice of Anchorage
3605 Arctic Blvd., #555
Anchorage, AK 99504
(907) 272-0633

ARIZONA
Hospice of the Valley
214 E. Willetta
Phoenix, AZ 85004
(602) 258-1572

Hospice of Yuma
281 W. 24th St., Suite 120
Yuma AZ 85364
(602) 726-6844

CALIFORNIA
Auburn Faith Hospice
11795 Education St., Suite 218
Auburn, CA 95603
(916) 885-7201

Alta Bates Hospice
2905 Telegraph Ave.
Berkeley, CA 94705
(415) 834-7110, x2383

Mt. Diablo Hospital Medical Center
2540 East St.
Concord, CA 94520
(415) 682-8200, x7191

Hospice of Corona/Norco/Lake Elsinore
108 W. Eighth St.
Corona, CA 91720
(714) 737-4343, x6294

South Bay Hospice
20863 Stevens Creek Blvd.
Cupertino, CA 95014
(408) 252-3110

Yolo Hospice
PO Box 1014
Davis, CA 95617
(916) 758-5566

Hospice of Napa Valley
3 Woodland Ave.
Deer Park, CA 94576
(707) 963-3691

Hospice of Fresno
1303 E. Herndon
Fresno, CA 93710
(209) 449-3379

Valley Children's Hospital
3151 N. Millbrook
Fresno, CA 93703
(209) 225-3000

Town and Country Hospice
12681 Pala Drive
Garden Grove, CA 92680
(714) 891-0441

Hospice in the Home
Verdugo Hills Visiting Nurse Association
109 E. Harvard, #205
Glendale, CA 91205
(213) 956-1860

Hospice Service of Lake County
201 S. Smith St.
Lakeport, CA 95453
(707) 263-6222

Children's Hospital
4650 Sunset Blvd.
Los Angeles, CA 90266
(213) 660-2450

UCLA–Department of Pediatric Hematology/
  Oncology
10833 Leconte Ave.
Los Angeles, CA 90024
(213) 825-5041

Visiting Nurse Association of Los Angeles,
  Inc.
3755 Beverly Blvd.
Los Angeles, CA 90004
(213) 667-1050

Contra Costa County Hospice
2500 Alhambra Ave.
Martinez, CA 94553
(415) 372-4241

Community Hospice, Inc.
1112 Ferrari Drive
Modesto, CA 95350
(209) 577-0615

Clinishare Home Health
18420 Roscoe Blvd.
Northridge, CA 91328
(213) 885-5357

Visiting Nurse Association
5232 Claremont Ave.
Oakland, CA 94618
(415) 654-8420

Visiting Nurse Association of Orange County
1337 Braden Court
PO Box 1129
Orange, CA 92668-0129
(714) 771-1209

St. John's Mercy Hospice
333 N. F St.
Oxnard, CA 93030
(805) 487-7861, x2116

Hospice of Pasadena, Inc.
464 E. Walnut
Pasadena, CA 91103
(213) 577-8484

Hospice of Petaluma
400 N. McDowell
Petaluma, CA 94952
(707) 763-6054

Inland Hospice Association
1787 N. Gancy Ave.
Pomona, CA 91767
(714) 623-0771

Sutter/VNA Hospice Care
52nd and F Sts.
Sacramento, CA 95819
(916) 454-3333, x1280

San Diego Hospice Corp.
3243 Mission Village Drive
San Diego, CA 92123
(714) 560-0302

Hospice of San Francisco
225 30th St.
San Francisco, CA 94131
(415) 668-2673

Hospice of the Valley
1150 S. Bascom Ave., Suite 7A
San Jose, CA 95128
(408) 356-6898

Vesper Hospice
311 MacArthur Blvd.
San Leandro, CA 94577
(415) 351-8686

Hospice of San Luis Obispo County
PO Box 1342
559 Marsh
San Luis Obispo, CA 93406
(805) 544-2266

Hospice of Marin
77 Mark Drive, #17
San Rafael, CA 94903
(415) 472-6240

Hospice of Santa Barbara, Inc.
330 E. Carrillo St.
Santa Barbara, CA 93101
(805) 963-8608

Visiting Nurse Association
Home Health Care, Inc.
2216 The Alameda
Santa Clara, CA 95050
(408) 244-1280

Hospice Caring Project
115 Maple
Santa Cruz, CA 95060
(408) 426-1993

Home Hospice of Sonoma County
1811 Fourth St.
Santa Rosa, CA 95404
(707) 542-5045

Hospital Home Health Care Agency of
    California
23456 Hawthorne Blvd.
Torrance, CA 90505
(213) 373-6373

Tahoe Forest Hospital Hospice
PO Box 759
Truckee, CA 95734
(916) 587-6011

Home Health Hospice
1776 Solano Ave.
Vallejo, CA 94590
(707) 553-5571

National In-Home Health Services
14549 Archwood St., Suite 220
Van Nuys, CA 91405
(213) 988-7575

Livingston Memorial Visiting Nurse
    Association
1996 Eastman Ave., Suite 101
Ventura, CA 93003
(805) 642-0239

Hospice of Tulare County
208 W. Main St., Suite H
Visalia, CA 93279
(209) 733-7090

Community Visiting Nurses, Inc.
110 Petticoat Lane
Walnut Creek, CA 94596
(415) 937-8311

COLORADO
Boulder County Hospice
2825 Marine St.
Boulder, CO 80303
(303) 449-7740

The Pikes Peak Hospital, Inc.
601 N. Tegon
Colorado Springs, CO 80903
(303) 633-3400

Hospice of Metro Denver
1719 E. 19th Ave.
Denver, CO 80218
(303) 839-6256

Prospect Home Care-Hospice
PO Box 585
Florissant, CO 80816
(303) 748-3611

Parkview Episcopal Medical Center Hospice
400 W. 16th St.
Pueblo, CO 81003
(303) 584-4479

CONNECTICUT
Hospice Program of Greater Bridgeport
1054 North Ave.
Bridgeport, CT 06606
(203) 366-3821

Visiting Nurse and Home Care of Hartford
80 Coventry St.
Hartford, CT 06112
(203) 243-2511

DISTRICT OF COLUMBIA
The Washington Home Hospice
3720 Upton St., N.W.
Washington, DC 20016
(202) 966-3720
(16 years and older)

FLORIDA
Hospice by the Sea, Inc.
1580 N.W. Second Ave.
Boca Raton, FL 33432
(305) 395-5031

Halifax Hospital Medical Center
Hospice of Volusia
PO Box 1990
Daytona Beach, FL 32015
(904) 258-1611

Hospice Care of Broward County, Inc.
309 S.E. 18th St.
Fort Lauderdale, FL 33316
(305) 467-7423

North Central Florida Hospice
801 S.W. Second Ave.
Gainesville, FL 32601
(904) 372-4321

Hospice of Northeast Florida, Inc.
3599 University Blvd., S., Suite 3
Jacksonville, FL 32216
(904) 398-4724

Methodist Hospital Hospice
580 W. Eighth St.
Jacksonville, FL 32209
(904) 356-7008

Hospice of Osceola County
PO Box 1827
Kissimmee, FL 32741
(305) 846-7444

Holmes Regional Medical Center
1350 S. Hickory St.
Melbourne, FL 32903
(305) 727-7000

Hospice Care, Inc.
3400 70th Ave.
North Pinellas Park, FL 33565
(813) 521-1199

Brevard Hospice
110 Longwood
Rockledge, FL 32955
(305) 636-2211

All Children's Hospital
801 Sixth St., S.
St. Petersburg, FL 33701
(813) 898-7451

Good Shepherd Hospice of Polk County, Inc.
PO Box 1183
Winter Haven, FL 33882-1183
(813) 293-5473

GEORGIA
Albany Community Hospice
417 Third Ave.
Albany, GA 31703
(912) 888-4047

Hospice of Atlanta
100 Edgewood Ave., N.E.
Atlanta, GA 30303-3078
(404) 577-6989

Hospice of the Golden Isles, Inc.
1326 Union St.
Brunswick, GA 31520
(215) 265-4735

Hamilton Medical Center–HHC & Hospice
Box 1168
Dalton, GA 30720
(404) 278-2105

West Georgia Medical Center Hospice
    Program
1514 Vernon Rd.
LaGrange, GA 30240
(404) 882-1411

Kennestone Regional Hospice
PO Box 1208
Marietta, GA 30061
(404) 424-8522, x3087

Hospice of Savannah, Inc.
PO Box 23015
Savannah, GA 31403
(912) 236-1182

HAWAII
Kapiolani Women's & Children's Medical
    Center
1319 Punahou St.
Honolulu, HI 96826
(808) 947-8511

Hospice of Maui
95 Mahalani St.
Wailuku, HI 96732
(808) 244-4077

IDAHO
Hospice of North Idaho, Inc.
2003 Lincoln Way
PO Box 820
Coeur d'Alene, ID 83814
(208) 667-4537

Good Samaritan Hospice
840 E. Elva
Idaho Falls, ID 83401
(208) 523-4795

Intermountain Hospice
Memorial Drive
Pocatello, ID 83201
(208) 232-6150

ILLINOIS
Hospice of Proviso-Layden
330 Eastern Ave.
Bellwood, IL 60104
(312) 547-8282

West Towns Hospice
2140 S. Wesley
Berwyn, IL 60402
(312) 749-7171

Mid-Illinois Hospice
807 N. Main St.
Bloomington, IL 61701
(309) 827-4321

Cook County Hospital
Department of Pediatrics
Chicago, IL 60612
(312) 633-6000

Home Health and Hospice of Illinois
836 W. Wellington Ave.
Chicago, IL 60657
(312) 883-7048

Horizon Hospice, Inc.
2800 N. Sheridan
Chicago, IL 60657
(312) 871-3658

Lakeview Medical Center Hospice
812 N. Logan Ave.
Danville, IL 61832
(217) 443-5000

Cancer Home Health Care
2300 N. Edward
Decatur, IL 62526
(217) 877-8120

Sauk Valley Hospice
100 W. Second St.
Dixon, IL 61020
(815) 288-3673 or 284-6887

St. Thomas Hospice
7 Salt Creek Lane
Hinsdale, IL 60521
(312) 920-8300

Joliet Area Community Hospice
333 N. Hammes
Joliet, IL 60435
(815) 740-7012

Riverside Medical Center
350 N. Wall St.
Kankakee, IL 60901
(815) 933-1671

Hospice Volunteers of DuPage
1019 Maple Ave.
Lisle, IL 60532
(312) 810-9292

Care for the Terminally Ill
525 E. Grant St.
Macomb, IL 61455
(309) 833-4101, x416

Pathway Hospice–Lutheran Hospital
501-10th Ave.
Moline, IL 61265
(309) 757-2611

Home Hospice Care of Community Nursing
   Service
124 S. Marion
Oak Park, IL 60302
(312) 383-1719

Hospice of Adams County
Broadway & 11th St.
Quincy, IL 62301
(217) 223-5811, x1717

Hospice Program–St. John's Hospital
800 E. Carpenter
Springfield, IL 62729
(217) 544-6464, x4572

Fox Valley Hospice, Inc.
PO Box 1365
St. Charles, IL 60174
(312) 377-5433

Mercy Hospice Care Program
1400 W. Park
Urbana, IL 61801
(217) 337-2362

S.T.A.R. Hospice Program
2615 W. Washington St.
Waukegan, IL 60085
(312) 578-2220

Hospice for McHenry County
Box 835
Woodstock, IL 60098
(815) 338-5450

INDIANA
Lawrence County Area Hospice
1600 23rd St.
Bedford, IN 47421
(812) 275-3331

Hospice of Bloomington
PO Box 1149
Bloomington, IN 47402
(812) 336-5595

Parkview Hospice
2200 Randallia Drive
Fort Wayne, IN 46805
(219) 484-6636

St. Vincent Stress Center
8401 Harcourt
Indianapolis, IN 46260
(317) 875-4600

Ball Memorial Hospice
2401 University
Muncie, IN 47304
(317) 747-4274

Reid Hospice Home Care Program
Reid Hospital–1401 Chester Blvd.
Richmond, IN 47374
(317) 983-3000

IOWA
Green Valley Hospice
208 W. Montgomery
Creston, IA 50801
(515) 782-7876

Charter Community Hospital
1818-48th St.
Des Moines, IA 50310
(515) 271-6000

Hospice of Central Iowa
2116 Grand Ave.
Des Moines, IA 50312
(515) 243-4235

Holy Family Hospice
826 N. Eighth
Estherville, IA 51334
(712) 362-2631

North Central Hospice, Inc.
Box 42
Hampton, IA 50441
(515) 456-3209, 4100

Hospice of Siouxland
801 Fifth St.
Sioux City, IA 51106
(712) 279-2514

KANSAS
Hospice of the Plains, Inc.
507 Elm St.
Hays, KS 67601
(913) 625-1139

Harvey County Hospice
PO Box 632
Newton, KS 67114
(316) 283-4989

Hospice of Olathe Community Hospital
300 S. Rogers Rd.
Olathe, KS 66061
(913) 782-1451

Topeka Hospice
1522 W. Eighth St.
Topeka, KS 66606

Cowley County Hospice, Inc.
PO Box 344
Winfield, KS 67156
(316) 221-4495

KENTUCKY
Hospice of Bowling Green
PO Box 1157
Bowling Green, KY 42101
(502) 782-3402

St. Elizabeth Home Health Hospice
501 Madison Ave.
Covington, KY 41011
(606) 292-4256

St. Anthony's Hospice, Inc.
PO Box 351
Henderson, KY 42420
(502) 826-2326

Pennyroyal Hospice, Inc.
320 W. 18th St.
Hopkinsville, KY 42240
(502) 886-5221

Community Hospice of Lexington
1105 Nicholasville Rd.
Lexington, KY 40503
(606) 252-2308

Hospice of Louisville, Inc.
101 W. Chestnut St.
Louisville, KY 40202
(502) 584-4834

Hospice Association, Inc.
PO Box 1403
Owensboro, KY 42302
(502) 684-5326

Madison County Hospice, Inc.
Fifth St. Offices, Room 406
Richmond, KY 40475
(606) 623-3441

LOUISIANA
Capitol Home Health Hospice
PO Box 111
Hammond, LA 70401
(504) 345-1830

Home Health Services of Louisiana, Inc.
2001 Canal St., Suite 211
New Orleans, LA 70112
(504) 581-6768

MAINE
Bath Brunswick Hospice
PO Box 741
Brunswick, ME 04011
(207) 729-3602

Franklin Memorial Hospital
Wilton Rd.
Farmington, ME 04938
(207) 778-6031

Hospice of Maine
32 Thomas Court
Portland, ME 04102
(207) 774-4417

York County Health Services Hospice
Box 15A, Industrial Park Rd.
Saco, ME 04072
(207) 284-4566

Hospice of York
c/o York Hospital
15 Hospital Drive
York, ME 03909
(207) 363-4321

MARYLAND
Visiting Nurse Association
5 E. Read St.
Baltimore, MD 21202
(301) 539-3961

Talbot Hospice
PO Box 480
Easton, MD 21601
(301) 822-2422

Hospice of Frederick County, Inc.
PO Box 1604
Frederick, MD 21701
(301) 694-6444

Hospice of St. Mary's, Inc.
PO Box 625
Leonardtown, MD 20650
(301) 475-2023

Hospice of Prince George's County, Inc.
8001 Annapolis Rd.
New Carrollton, MD 20784
(301) 459-6104

Hospice of Garrett County, Inc.
253 N. Fourth St.
Oakland, MD 21550
(301) 334-8111

Coastal Hospice
PO Box 1733
Salisbury, MD 21801
(301) 742-8732

Arundel Hospice, Inc.
517 Benfield Rd., Suite 301
Severna Park, MD 21146
(301) 544-0656

Holy Cross Hospital Home Hospice Program
1500 Forest Glen Rd.
Silver Spring, MD 20910
(301) 565-1171

MASSACHUSETTS
Hospice Care, Inc.
39 Hospital Rd.
Arlington, MA 02174
(617) 646-3770

Hospice of Community Health Agency, Inc.
141 Park St.
Attleboro, MA 02703
(617) 222-0118

Hospice for Children
243 Forest St.
Fall River, MA 02721

VNA of South Middlesex Hospice
50 Lawrence St.
Framingham, MA 01701
(617) 875-3511

VNA of Haverhill Hospice, Inc.
Knipe School
Oxford Ave.
Haverhill, MA 01830
(617) 372-5484

Hospice Program of Greater Lawrence
451 Andover St.
North Andover, MA 01845
(617) 689-0383

Laboure Center VNS
371 W. Fourth St.
South Boston, MA 02127
(617) 268-9670

Visiting Nurse Hospice
12 Beacon St.
Stoneham, MA 02180
(617) 438-3770

MICHIGAN
Southwestern Michigan Health Care
960 Agard St.
Benton Harbor, MI 49022
(616) 927-5100

Hospice of Petoskey
706 Jackson, Box 2091
Boyne City, MI 49712
(616) 348-4253 or 347-9700

Barry Eaton District Health Department
Eaton Community Hospice
528 Beech St.
Charlotte, MI 48817
(517) 543-1050

Hospice of the Straits
748 S. Main St.
Cheboygan, MI 49721
(616) 627-5601

Hurley Home Care Hospice
1 Hurley Plaza
Flint, MI 48502
(313) 257-9000

Hospice of Greater Grand Rapids, Inc.
1901 Robinson Rd., S.E.
Grand Rapids, MI 49506
(616) 454-1426

Hospice of Jackson
437 Fern Ave.
Jackson, MI 49202
(313) 783-2648

Hospice of Greater Kalamazoo, Inc.
301 W. Cedar
Kalamazoo, MI 49007
(616) 345-0273

Hospice of Saginaw
3037 Davenport
Saginaw, MI 48602
(517) 754-1446

Hospice for Clinton County
805 S. Oakland St.
St. John's, MI 48879
(517) 224-6881

Hospice at Home, Inc.
Box 675
St. Joseph, MI 49085
(616) 983-0402

Grand Traverse Area Hospice
c/o Munson Medical Center
Traverse City, MI 49684
(616) 922-9000

MINNESOTA
Community Hospice of Crookston
323 S. Minnesota
Crookston, MN 56716
(218) 281-4682

Itasca Hospice Project, Inc.
PO Box 74
Grand Rapids, MN 55744
(218) 326-3401

Children's Hospital of St. Paul
345 N. Smith Ave.
St. Paul, MN 55102
(612) 298-8666

MISSOURI
Ozark Mountain Hospice
117 E. Main
Bronson, MO 65616
(417) 334-1222

St. Luke's Hospice Care Program
232 S. Woods Mill Rd.
Chesterfield, MO 63017
(314) 361-1212

Hospice of Care
1333 S. 63rd
Houston, MO 65483
(417) 967-3311

VNA of Greater Kansas City
527 W. 39th St.
Kansas City, MO 64111
(816) 531-1200

Community Hospice Care
2510 S. Brentwood
St. Louis, MO 63144
(314) 968-9115

VNA of Greater St. Louis
1129 Mackline
St. Louis, MO 63110
(314) 533-9680

MONTANA
Anaconda Pintler Hospice
PO Box 596
Anaconda, MT 59711
(406) 563-7070, 5422

Hospice of St. Peter's
2475 Broadway
Helena, MT 59601
(406) 442-2480, x6785

Hospice of Missoula
PO Box 8273
Missoula, MT 59807
(406) 549-7757

NEBRASKA
Hospice of Tabitha
4720 Randolph
Lincoln, NE 68510
(402) 483-7671

NEVADA
Nathan Adelson Hospice
4141 S. Swenson
Las Vegas, NV 89109
(702) 733-0320

NEW HAMPSHIRE
Seacoast Hospice
26 Prospect Ave.
Exeter, NH 03801
(603) 778-7391

Hospice of Cheshire County
83 Court
Keene, NH 03431
(603) 352-2253

Hospice of the Upper Valley
PO Box 225
Lebanon, NH 03766
(603) 448-5182

Hospice of the Kearsarge Valley
PO Box 1097
New London, NH 03257
(603) 526-6544

Hospice of Northern Carroll County
PO Box 401
North Conway, NH 03860
(603) 356-3320

Hospice of Southern Carroll County, Inc.
Box 1162
Wolfeboro, NH 03894
(603) 569-5190

NEW JERSEY
Englewood Hospital Hospice Program
350 Engle St.
Englewood, NJ 07670
(201) 894-3313

Hospice Program of Hackensack
385 Prospect Ave.
Hackensack, NJ 07601
(201) 441-2050

Monmouth Medical Center–Pediatric Oncology
    Clinic
300 Second Ave.
Long Branch, NJ 07747
(201) 222-5200

The Hospice Inc.
331 Claremont Ave.
Montclair, NJ 07042
(201) 783-7879

Children's Specialized Hospital
New Providence Rd.
Mountainside, NJ 07091
(201) 233-3720

Hospice-Jersey Shore Medical Center
1945 Corlies Ave.
Neptune, NJ 07753
(201) 775-5500

Children's Hospice of New Jersey
15 S. Ninth St.
Newark, NJ 07107
(201) 268-8000

Raritan Bay Medical Center Hospice
530 New Brunswick Ave.
Perth Amboy, NJ 08863
(201) 442-3700, x5173

Supportive Care Hospice Program
325 Witherspoon St.
Princeton, NJ 08540
(609) 734-4626

MCOSS Nursing Services, Inc.
141 Bodman Place
Red Bank, NJ 07701
(201) 747-1204

Overlook Hospital
193 Morris Ave.
Summit, NJ 07901
(201) 522-2846

Ocean County Health Department
CN2191 Sunset Ave.
Toms River, NJ 08754
(201) 349-8000, x307

Passaic Valley Hospice
50 Galesi Drive
Wayne, NJ 07470
(201) 256-4636

NEW MEXICO
Eastern New Mexico Hospice, Inc.
Box 1983
Clovis, NM 88101
(505) 762-0002

Mesilla Valley Hospice
PO Box 15146
Las Cruces, NM 88004
(505) 523-4700

Visiting Nurse Service Hospice
1316 Apache Ave.
Santa Fe, NM 87501
(505) 471-9201

NEW YORK
St. Peter's Hospice
315 S. Manning Blvd.
Albany, NY 12208
(518) 454-1688

Palliative Care Center–St. Mary's Hospital for
  Children
29-01 216 St.
Bayside, NY 11360
(718) 224-0400

The Brooklyn Hospice
4915 Tenth Ave.
Brooklyn, NY 11219
(718) 853-2800, x364

Nursing Sisters Home Visiting Service, Inc.
310 Prospect Park W.
Brooklyn, NY 11215
(718) 965-7350

Southern Tier Hospice Care
175 Grand Central Ave.
Elmira Heights, NY 14903
(607) 734-1570

Phelps Memorial Hospital Hospice Program
North Broadway
North Tarrytown, NY 10591
(914) 631-5100

NORTH CAROLINA
Mountain Area Hospice Inc.
PO Box 16
Asheville, NC 28802
(704) 255-0231

Hospice at Charlotte, Inc.
PO Box 22118
Charlotte, NC 28222
(704) 375-0100

Triangle Hospice
3605 Shannon Rd.
Durham, NC 27705
(919) 493-1491

Home Health Services Hospice Care
Cumberland County
PO Box 5334
Fayetteville, NC 28305
(919) 483-3489

Hospice at Greensboro
301 N. Eugene
PO Box 3508
Greensboro, NC 27402
(919) 274-4592

Hospice of East Carolina
1003 S. Clark St.
Box 7145
Greenville, NC 27834
(919) 758-5932

Hospice of Burke County, Inc.
PO Box 2107
Morganton, NC 28655
(704) 433-8842

Hospice of Wake County
619 Oberlin
Raleigh, NC 27605
(919) 833-0161

C.J. Harris Community Hospital H.H.A.
59 Hospital Rd.
Sylva, NC 28779
(704) 586-8941

NORTH DAKOTA
St. Joseph's Hospice
Seventh St., W.
Dickinson, ND 58601
(701) 225-7200

United Hospital Hospice
1200 S. Columbia Rd.
Grand Forks, ND 58201
(701) 780-5000

OHIO
Visiting Nurse Service, Inc.
1200 McArthur Drive
Akron, OH 44320
(216) 745-1601

Hospice of Dayton, Inc.
2181 Embury Park Rd.
Dayton, OH 45414
(513) 278-0060

Hospice of Hancock County
1815 S. Main St.
Findlay, OH 45840
(419) 424-0380

Hospice of Memorial Hospital
715 S. Taft Ave.
Fremont, OH 43420
(419) 332-7321

Hospice of Darke County
748 Chestnut St.
Greenville, OH 45331
(513) 548-4884

St. Rita's Medical Center Hospice
730 W. Market St.
Lima, OH 45801
(419) 227-3361

Madison County Home Health Hospice
210 N. Main
London, OH 43140
(614) 852-1372

St. Joseph Hospital
205 W. 20th St.
Lorain, OH 44052
(216) 245-6851

Hospice of Lake County, Inc.
5976 Heisley Rd.
Mentor, OH 44060
(216) 974-8516

Hospice of Middletown, Inc.
105 McKnight Drive
Middletown, OH 45044
(513) 424-2111, x951

Stein Hospice Service
516 Columbus Ave.
Sandusky, OH 44870
(419) 625-5269

Community Home Care–Hospice Services
2615 E. High St.
Springfield, OH 45501
(513) 325-0531, x1318

Community Hospice Care
PO Box 160
Tiffin, OH 44883
(419) 447-4040

Northwest Ohio Hospice Association
3350 Collingswood
Toledo, OH 43610
(419) 241-6609

Trumbull County VNA Hospice Program
219 N. River Rd.
Warren, OH 44483
(216) 394-8144

OKLAHOMA
Cross Timbers Hospice
PO Box 2514
Ardmore, OK 73401
(405) 223-3516

Hospice of Central Oklahoma, Inc.
4215 N.W. 23rd St., Suite 101
Oklahoma City, OK 73107
(405) 843-1269

OREGON
Hospice of Bend, Oregon
PO Box 1146
Bend, OR 97702
(503) 389-1430

Benton Hospice Service, Inc.
PO Box 100
Corvallis, OR 97330
(503) 757-9616

Visiting Nurse Association Hospice Program
3611 S.W. Hood
Portland, OR 97201
(503) 241-3477

Mid-Willamette Valley Hospice
PO Box 2292
Salem, OR 97308
(503) 588-5418

PENNSYLVANIA
Abington Memorial Hospital
1200 York Rd.
Abington, PA 19001
(215) 576-2009

Visiting Nurse Association
1421 Highland Ave.
Abington, PA 19001
(215) 884-0272

Centre County Home Health Service
221 Wittigh St.
Bellefonte, PA 16823
(814) 355-1557

Columbia Gontour Home Health Service
408 Central Rd.
Bloomsbury, PA 17815
(717) 784-1723

Hospice Services, Inc.
214 S. McKean
Butler, PA 16001
(412) 282-6806

Coatesville–Brandywine Home Health Agency
1219 E. Lincoln Hwy.
Coatesville, PA 19320
(215) 384-4200

Hospice Services of Erie
1305 Peach
Erie, PA 16501
(814) 454-2831

Susquehanna Nursing Service
3901 Derry St.
Harrisburg, PA 17111
(717) 564-9191

Wayne County Memorial Hospital
Park & West St.
Honesdale, PA 18431
(717) 253-5151

Good Samaritan Hospital Hospice
Fourth and Walnut Sts.
Lebanon, PA 17042
(717) 272-7611, x535

Hospice: The Bridge–Lewistown Hospital
Highland Ave.
Lewistown, PA 17044
(717) 248-5411

Hospice of St. Francis
S. Marcus & Phillips St.
New Castle, PA 16101
(412) 658-3511

Chandler Hall Hospice Home Health Agency
Buck Rd. & Reardon St.
Newtown, PA 18940
(215) 968-4786

Wissahickon Hospice
8835 Germantown Ave.
Philadelphia, PA 19119
(215) 247-0277

Bradford County Citizens Health Foundation
RD 2, Box 82 A-1
Towanda, PA 18848
(717) 265-3510

Hospice of Warren
108 Coyuga Ave.
Warren, PA 16365
(814) 726-1525

Hospice Care, Inc.
PO Box 168, 59 S. Washington
Waynesburg, PA 15370
(412) 627-8270

Hospice of York
218 E. Market St.
York, PA 17403
(717) 845-3608

RHODE ISLAND
Northwest Community Nursing Health Service
PO Box 234
Harmony, RI 02829-0234
(401) 949-3801

SOUTH CAROLINA
York County Hospice, Inc.
PO Box 2742 CRS
Rock Hill, SC 29731
(803) 329-4663

SOUTH DAKOTA
Prairie Hospice
Fifth & Foster
Mitchell, SD 57301
(605) 996-6531

TENNESSEE
Jackson Area Hospice
PO Box 2301
Jackson, TN 38302
(901) 427-7963

Holston Valley Hospice Home Health Agency
PO Box 238
Kingsport, TN 37662
(615) 246-3322

Memphis Hospice, Inc.
PO Box 17725
Memphis, TN 38187-0725
(901) 527-8361

TEXAS
St. Anthony's Hospice
PO Box 950
Amarillo, TX 79176-0001
(806) 376-4441, x5955

Hospice of Austin
4300 N. Lamar Blvd.
Austin, TX 78756
(512) 458-1041

Children's Medical Center
1935 Amelia St.
Dallas, TX 75235
(214) 920-2000

Visiting Nurse Association of Texas Home
  Hospice
8200 Brookriver Drive, Suite 200N
Dallas, TX 75247
(214) 689-0000

Hospice of El Paso
1900 N. Oregon
El Paso, TX 79902
(915) 532-5699

Galveston Hospice Group, Inc.
111-36th, Box 2448
Galveston, TX 77553
(713) 765-5548

Hospice of VNA
3100 Timmons, #200
Houston, TX 77027
(713) 840-7744

New Age Hospice of Houston, Inc.
7 Chelsea Place
Houston, TX 77006
(713) 528-2098

VNA, Inc.
3212-34th St.
Lubbock, TX 79410
(806) 793-9067

Hospice of Midland, Inc.
Box 2621
Midland, TX 79705
(915) 682-2855

The Southeast Texas Hospice
PO Box 2385
Orange, TX 77630
(713) 886-0622

Hospice of East Texas, Inc.
721 Clinic Drive
Tyler, TX 75701
(214) 593-2171

UTAH
Hospice of Utah County, Inc.
368 W. 1150 North
Provo, UT 84601
(801) 373-3191

Hospice of Salt Lake–Community Nursing
  Service
1370 S.W. Temple
Salt Lake City, UT 84115
(801) 486-3612

VERMONT
Central Vermont Hospice
MR #1
Barre, VT 05641
(802) 229-9121

Orleans and N. Essex Home Health Agency
3 Lakemont Rd.
Newport, VT 05855
(802) 334-7897

VIRGINIA
Riverside Hospital Hospice
500 J. Clyde Morris Blvd.
Newport News, VA 23601
(804) 599-2718

Roanoke Memorial Hospitals Hospice
PO Box 13367
Roanoke, VA 24033
(703) 981-7411

Edmarc, Inc.
410 N. Broad St.
PO Box 1684
Suffolk, VA 23434
(804) 539-2041

WASHINGTON
Hospice of Whatcon County
1111 Cornwall
Bellingham, WA 98225
(206) 734-9724

TriCities Chaplaincy Hospice
7514 W. Yellowstone
Kennewick, WA 99336-1101
(509) 783-2416

Community Home Health
1035 11th Ave.
Longview, WA 98632
(206) 425-8510

Hospice of Clallam County
PO Box 2014
Port Angeles, WA 98362
(206) 452-2956

Hospice of Seattle
7814 Greenwood Ave., N.
Seattle, WA 98103
(206) 784-9221

Transition Services Program
811 First Ave.
Seattle, WA 98104-1498
(206) 328-9700

Hospice of Yakima
St. Elizabeth Medical Center
110 S. Ninth Ave.
Yakima, WA 98902
(509) 575-5000

WEST VIRGINIA
Morgantown Hospice, Inc.
PO Box 4222-1000
Van Voorhis Rd.
Morgantown, WV 26505
(304) 293-4536

WISCONSIN
Lafayette County Hospice
800 Clay St.
Darlington, WI 53530
(608) 776-4006

Lifeline Community Hospice
825 S. Iowa St.
Dodgeville, WI 53533
(608) 935-2711

Bellin Hospice Program
PO Box 1700
Green Bay, WI 54301
(414) 468-3480

Hudson Memorial Hospital Hospice
400 Wisconsin St.
Box 361
Hudson, WI 54016
(715) 386-9321

Hospice Alliance
5159-Sixth Ave.
Kenosha, WI 53140
(414) 658-8344

LaCrosse Lutheran Hospital Pediatric
1910 S Ave.
LaCrosse, WI 54601
(608) 785-0530, x3025

Hospice Care, Inc.
303 Lathrop St.
Madison, WI 53705
(608) 255-0915

Milwaukee Children's Hospital-Hospice
    Program
1700 W. Wisconsin Ave.
PO Box 1997
Milwaukee, WI 53201
(414) 931-1010

Milwaukee Visiting Nurse Association
10045 W. Lishon Ave.
Milwaukee, WI 53222
(414) 276-2295

Rogers Memorial Hospital
34810 Pabst Rd.
Oconomowoc, WI 53066
(414) 567-5535

Mercy Hospice
631 Hazel St.
Oshkosh, WI 54901
(414) 236-2336

Hospice Program–Prairie du Chien Memorial
    Hospital
705 E. Taylor
Prairie du Chien, WI 53821
(608) 326-2431

Wausau Hospice Program
333 Pine Ridge Blvd.
Wausau, WI 54401
(415) 847-2121

WYOMING
Central Wyoming Cancer Center & Hospice
    Program
233 S. Jackson
Casper, WY 82601
(307) 577-4832

SOURCE: *Children's Hospice International.*

ORGANIZATIONS

Children's Hospice International
1800 Diagonal Rd., Suite 600
Alexandria, VA 22314
(703) 684-4464

National organization to promote the establishment of hospices for children. A source of information. Some publications, including a newsletter. Will provide the names of hospices that accept children and additional information upon request.

National Hospice Organization
1901 N. Fort Myer Drive
Suite 402
Arlington, VA 22209
(703) 243-5900

National membership organization for hospices of all types—community based, free standing, hospital based, those in nursing homes and those operated by home health agencies. Monthly newsletter monographs, and a hospice directory. Will answer questions from the public, and provide a list of hospices in a certain state upon request.

BOOKS

Dying at Home, **Harriet Copperman,** London-New York: Wiley, 1984.

Dying Dignified, **Thomas Andrew Gonda,** Menlo Park, CA: Addison-Wesley, 1984.

Graceful Dying: A Practical Approach to Terminal Care, **Thomas Andrew Gonda,** and **John Edward Ruark,** Menlo Park, CA: Addison-Wesley, 1983.

Home Health Care: Home Birthing to Hospice Care, **Allen D. Spiegel,** Owings Mills, MD: National Health Publishing, 1983.

The Hospice Alternative: A New Context for Death and Dying, **Anne Munley,** New York: Basic Books, 1983.

Hospice, U.S.A., **edited by Austin Kutscher, et al.** New York: Columbia University Press, 1983.

Living with Death and Dying, **Elisabeth Kubler-Ross,** New York: Macmillan, 1981.

Too Old to Cry . . . Too Young to Die, **Edith Pendleton,** Nashville: Thomas Nelson Publishers, 1980; written by teens for teens.

HUNTINGTON'S DISEASE

See also Rehabilitation, page 460, and Genetic Counseling, page 226.

Huntington's disease, also called Huntington's chorea, is an inherited degenerative disorder of the central nervous system, leading to loss of muscle control, dementia, and death. It leaves its victims with bizarre signs of mental deterioration—unintelligible speech, facial distortions, uncontrollable movements, depression, and paranoia. Unfortunately, these symptoms are often mistaken for signs of drunkenness or various forms of mental illness. The condition is relentlessly progressive and appears without warning in midlife.

Huntington's disease has been recognized for centuries. It was named for George Huntington, the physician who most fully described it in 1872. It is passed on through the genes from parent to child. All or none of the offspring of an afflicted parent could inherit the gene. It strikes males and females alike and usually does not show up until a person is 30 to 50 years old, although in some cases it does not appear until old age. One type of the disorder strikes children as young as two years old, although it is exceedingly rare.

If a child inherits the gene, the disease is sure to appear if the person lives long enough to develop symptoms. The chance of inheriting the gene is 50 percent for each child of a parent with Huntington's disease. If the gene is not inherited, there is no danger of being a silent carrier of the disease to future generations. About 20,000 Americans have Huntington's disease, and authorities estimate another 100,000 are at risk for developing it, making it one of the more common genetic disorders.

Cause: A faulty gene, present at birth. Apparently, a gene turns on Huntington's at a certain age, causing cells in certain parts of the brain to die, thus ending production of essential neurotransmitters (chemicals) that send messages throughout the brain.

Symptoms: The disease produces both physical and mental disturbances. Both the symptoms and the progression of the disease are variable. The early signs often are irritability, listlessness, apathy, poor judgment, memory loss, slurred speech, unsteady gait, tics, facial spasms, even severe depressions or hallucinations. Eventually, as the disease progresses, often over a decade or two, the whole body may be gripped by uncontrollable dancelike movements—thus the early name, chorea, from the Greek word for dance. There may be difficulty in swallowing, loss of bladder and bowel control, and incomprehensible speech. In some the abnormal movements may be mild; others may be confined to a wheelchair or bed. Death often comes from infections, or from heart failure, to which the Huntington's patient is especially vulnerable.

However, the progression of Huntington's disease may not be as incapacitating as once thought. Many people with Huntington's disease are quite able to remain independent and take care of themselves for many years after the onset of the disease. Others can remain at home with some assistance and thus avoid being institutionalized.

Diagnosis: Physicians diagnose Huntington's disease on the basis of a physical examination and a family history. There is no foolproof laboratory test for Huntington's disease, although brain scans, such as the CAT scan and the PETT scan, can often detect the abnormalities characteristic of Huntington's disease. Laboratory tests to rule out diseases with similar symptoms are often done.

Treatment: There is no cure, but drugs are often used to lessen abnormal movements and mood disturbances. Although a family physician might diagnose and oversee the treatment of Huntington's disease, care should be directed by a neurologist familiar with the disease. Individuals with Huntington's disease need exercise, and like others with physical disabilities, they may need special devices for the handicapped, such as special eating and communicating equipment.

A part of dealing with Huntington's disease is often psychological. Diagnosis often engenders fear, anger, guilt, shame, and denial in the patient and family. Genetic counseling is usually advised to explain the risk of Huntington's disease and its genetic pattern and to help family members decide whether to conceive children who may also inherit the Huntington's gene. Of course, quite often parents are unaware they have the disease until long after children are born. For years the gene has been so elusive that scientists could not develop a test to detect it. Now scientists have found a genetic "marker" for Huntington's disease, which will lead to new methods of diagnosing the disease and detecting it in the fetus.

WHERE TO FIND TREATMENT FOR HUNTINGTON'S DISEASE

Huntington's disease is treated by neurologists. *See* page 621, for a roster of leading neurologists who head departments of neurology at medical schools. They are a good source of treatment and/or medical referrals to other specialists.

For additional referrals to local medical specialists and health professionals experienced in managing Huntington's patients, you can also contact the Huntington's Disease Society of America, 140 W. 22nd St., New York, NY 10040.

RESEARCH ROSTER FOR HUNTINGTON'S DISEASE

To help speed up research that may lead to a cure for Huntington's disease, a national roster of Huntington's patients and families was established. The purpose is to find and engage those with Huntington's disease in national research projects of both a statistical and clinical nature. Here's how it works: A person with Huntington's disease signs up with the registry on a purely voluntary and confidential basis and provides information about himself or herself related to the disease. Researchers can then obtain information that does not involve names for statistical compilations that may uncover important patterns to the disease.

If a researcher wants to be put in contact with persons with Huntington's disease and their fam-

ilies, suitable individuals from the roster will be selected and told about the proposed research project. If they agree in writing, their names will be given to the researcher, who can then contact them to discuss the project further.

If you have a history of Huntington's disease in your family and want to be included in the roster, contact:

HD Roster
Department of Medical Genetics
Indiana University School of Medicine
1100 W. Michigan St.
Indianapolis, IN 46223
(317) 264-2241

BRAIN TISSUE BANKS

Huntington's patients and others with neurological and psychiatric disorders may want to donate their brain tissue for research after death. Others who do not have such diseases may also want to donate brain tissue for comparative research purposes.

The federal government helps fund centers that collect brain tissue for study. For more information contact:

W.W. Tourtellotte, M.D.
Director
Human Neurospecimen Bank
VA Wadsworth Hospital Center
Los Angeles, CA 90073
(213) 824-4307 (collect)
(213) 478-3711 (24 hours collect)

Edward D. Bird, M.D.
Director
The Brain Tissue Resource Center
McLean Hospital
Belmont, MA 02178
(617) 855-2400 (24 hours collect)

RESEARCH AND TREATMENT AT THE NATIONAL INSTITUTES OF HEALTH

Investigators at the NIH Clinical Center in Bethesda, Maryland, are conducting biochemical and experimental therapy studies with some selected Huntington's patients. Consideration for participation is by physician referral. For more information your physician can contact:

Office of the Director
The Clinical Center
Building 10, Room 2C-146
National Institutes of Health
Bethesda, MD 20892
(301) 496-4891

ORGANIZATIONS

Huntington's Disease Society of America
140 W. 22nd St.
New York, NY 10040
(212) 242-1968

A national voluntary health organization, providing support and services to Huntington's disease patients and their families. Local chapters nationwide. A source of information and publications. Will send material upon request.

National Huntington's Disease Association
1182 Broadway, Suite 402
New York, NY 10001
(212) 684-2781

National voluntary health organization for Huntington's disease patients and families. 59 chapters throughout the country. A source of information and mutual support. Maintains a network of social workers trained in dealing with the problems of Huntington's patients and families. Both national office and local chapters make referrals to medical specialists, centers, and nursing homes nationwide. Sponsors research. Will provide more information upon request.

BOOKS

Heirloom, **Dorothy Snyder,** Boulder, CO: Stonehenge Press, 1981; 381 Ponderosa Drive, Boulder, CO 80303.

Home Health Care, **Joann Friedman,** New York: W.W. Norton, 1986.

Living with Huntington's Disease: A Book for

Patients and Families, **Dennis Phillips, Ph.D.,** Milwaukee: University of Wisconsin Press, 1982.

The 36-Hour Day, **Nancy Mace** and **Peter Rabins, M.D.,** Baltimore: The Johns Hopkins University Press, 1981.

FREE MATERIALS

Single copies are free

Experiences of a Huntington's Disease Patient, 12 pages.

Caring for the HD Patient at Home, 8 pages.

Huntington's Disease, 6 pages.

Huntington's Disease Society of America
140 W. 22nd St., Sixth Floor
New York, NY 10111
(212) 757-0443

Clinical Care of the Huntington's Disease Patient and Family, brochure.

National Huntington's Disease Association
1182 Broadway, Suite 402
New York, NY 10001
(212) 684-2781

Huntington's Disease: Hope Through Research, 28 pages.

A Neurologist Speaks with Huntington's Disease Families, brochure.

National Institute of Neurological and Communicative Disorders and Stroke
9000 Rockville Pike
Bethesda, MD 20892

INFERTILITY AND CHILDBIRTH

Infertility is a growing problem for American couples. One in six, or about five million couples, are infertile, which is defined as the inability to conceive after a year of trying, or to carry a pregnancy to term and delivery. Previously, the blame was placed almost universally on the woman but it is now recognized that the male is equally responsible: The difficulty rests with the woman about 40 percent of the time and with the man, 40 percent. In other cases, both have reproductive deficiencies.

Some couples are reluctant to admit their reproductive problems and fail to seek help from a family physician or a fertility specialist. However, childless couples, unlike their counterparts of the past, do have many promising medical choices in addition to adoption. There are new drugs, devices, corrective surgical techniques, *in vitro* (better known as test-tube) fertilization, surrogate mothering, and embryo transplant available at centers around the country. The solutions to infertility are growing far more sophisticated. An estimated 70 percent of all couples can be helped.

Cause: There are several possible causes of infertility among women, including hormonal disturbances preventing ovulation (responsible for about one-fifth of female infertility); endometriosis, a disease in which tissue that normally lines the uterus grows in the abdominal cavity, around the reproductive organs and into the fallopian tubes, causing inflammation, scarring, and infertility, said by some experts to be the major cause of female infertility; and blocked or malformed fallopian tubes.

Men may suffer from defective semen (low sperm count, sluggish sperm movement, malfunctioning sperm, perhaps caused by an enzyme deficiency); a condition called varicocele (an enlarged vein in the testicle that interferes with sperm activity—the leading cause of male infertility according to one major study); and blockage of the duct between the testes and penis caused by a vasectomy or venereal disease.

Underlying contributors to these defects may be exposure to radiation, toxic chemicals, or heat; fetal damage during critical reproductive development (perhaps from chemicals or drugs, such as DES (diethylstilbestrol), a hormone prescribed for millions of pregnant women during the fifties and sixties). A number of pharmaceutical drugs, such as those used to treat cancer, arthritis, psoriasis, gout, epilepsy, and high blood pressure, may also contribute to impotency or infertility. Infertility can be temporary. Studies show that even some men exposed to high doses of radiation regained their fertility after three-and-a-half years.

Age may be a factor for both men and women. Studies show that infertility increases with age, and many couples are waiting longer to have children; thus, conception is more difficult at the time some couples desire it. This could be due to unknown internal biological changes or to the fact that sterilizing toxic chemicals and other influences in the environment have had longer to work.

Diagnosis: The difficulties can be determined by physical examinations and laboratory tests.

Most couples having difficulty conceiving should consult an infertility specialist.

Treatment: A common cause of male infertility, the varicocele, is easily corrected by a simple surgical procedure called a varicocelectomy. It is reportedly successful 70 percent of the time in men who have adequate sperm counts. The enlarged vein is simply tied off with sutures. The surgery is increasingly done at outpatient clinics, often with a local anesthetic. A new outpatient surgery technique for varicocele blocks off the vein with a small silicone balloon implant inserted by a catheter.

In some cases, surgery can also reverse a vasectomy, although reversal is not guaranteed, and a vasectomy should be regarded as permanent when undertaken. With new microsurgical techniques, however, success rates have been as high as 90 percent in restoring ejaculation of sperm and 75 percent in inducing pregnancy in certain cases. Such surgery requires a specially trained urologist. Success with older surgical techniques, still used by many doctors, is about 25 percent. Rates of success go down if the reversal operation is done more than 10 years after the vasectomy. In certain instances the reversal simply will not work. Reversing a vasectomy is major surgery. For the names of experts in reversing vasectomies, contact the American Fertility Society, 2131 Magnolia Ave., Birmingham, AL 35256; (205) 251-9764.

New surgical techniques also increase the chances of pregnancy for women. Endometriosis can be alleviated by surgery or drugs. Damaged tubes can be repaired by microsurgery in many cases. About half of the women who have hormonal problems preventing pregnancy are rendered fertile by a variety of pharmaceutical drugs. Some women who have been sterilized can regain fertility. There are other solutions as well, including the following:

Artificial insemination: Artificial insemination by a donor (AID) is a well-established alternative, used mainly when the male is infertile. Some couples also use it if there is a danger of passing on a genetic defect through the male sperm. AID is increasingly being used by single women who want to have a child but do not want to be married. As many as 20,000 infants born every year are conceived by AID. Either fresh or frozen sperm are inserted into the vagina at the proper time of the month. Though this procedure may have to be repeated many times, the overall success rates for AID are nearly 60 percent. One study showed that the success rate for AID ranged from 20 to 100 percent depending on the experience of the doctor; those who did the most procedures had the highest success rates. This demonstrates how important it is to choose a large, well-established, experienced clinic and physician.

Test-tube babies: *In vitro* fertilization clinics are springing up rapidly; many are affiliated with universities and hospitals. In this procedure, the eggs are removed from the woman during ovulation by a laparoscopy and put into a petri dish. The husband's sperm is then put into the dish with the egg, and the mixture is incubated. The fertilized egg—the embryo—is then inserted into the woman's uterus. There is then a waiting period to see whether the fertilized egg is implanted and whether pregnancy takes place. Studies show pregnancy occurs in about 10–20 percent of the cases, although the fetus may not survive, and the whole procedure may have to be repeated. This method was originally endorsed only for women with blocked or nonexistent tubes (a condition that accounts for at least 600,000 cases of infertility). But some clinics accept women for other reasons, including husbands with low sperm counts. Researchers believe the technique will spread and become more successful with time and experience.

GIFT (gamete intrafallopian transfer): This new technique can be used in cases of deficient sperm production or when the woman's reproductive tract is chemically destructive to sperm. The technique was developed by Dr. Ricardo Asch, University of Texas Health Science Center in San Antonio and has, he says, a 30 percent success rate.

Doctors use a laparoscope to extract ripe egg cells from the woman. These are then mixed with about 100,000 sperm from the man and reinserted into an oviduct from the ovary. Thus, this technique allows the embryo to be fertilized in a more natural fashion, within the mother's body.

Surrogate mothers: A growing and controversial solution to infertility is the use of another woman to bear the child. Surrogate mothering is done when the female is incapable of carrying a child. The couple designates a woman—the surrogate mother—to be artificially inseminated with the man's sperm (or with the sperm of another chosen man) and to carry the baby to delivery. Surrogate mothering has run into some medical and legal problems, but it is increasingly used and has been granted legal protection in some states. One advantage, experts and couples say, is that it is better than adoption because they can manipulate the process to have some biological connection to the child.

Embryo transfer: A more radical alternative to *in vitro* fertilization and the surrogate mother, this technique has long been used in the breeding of prize animals. The egg of a donor woman is fertilized through artificial insemination by the male partner's sperm; the fertilized egg is then transferred to the infertile woman who carries it to term and gives birth. This is appropriate for women without ovaries or with genetic disease.

EMBRYO TRANSFER PIONEERS

This procedure was pioneered at the University of California at Los Angeles. Although still experimental, it is being done at other infertility centers throughout the country. The procedure is part of a commercial enterprise organized by The Reproduction & Fertility Clinic in Chicago. For more information contact:

John Buster, M.D.
Harbor UCLA Medical Center
1000 W. Carson St.
Torrance, CA 90509
(213) 533-2101

Dr. Buster performed the first embryo transfers.

Randolph Seed, M.D.
The Reproduction & Fertility Clinic, Inc.
999 N. Lakeshore Drive
Chicago, IL 60611
(312) 280-8960

Infertility Center of New York
14 E. 60th St.
New York, NY 10022
(212) 371-0811

SOME LEADING *IN VITRO* FERTILIZATION CENTERS

The number of hospitals and centers doing *in vitro* fertilization is growing rapidly. The following centers have set up such services. Generally, you can also expect these centers to have leading specialists in all aspects of infertility. The new centers are almost always organized by those with a long-time interest in, and experience with, infertility. Some centers are headed by the country's most prestigious experts in infertility.

ALABAMA

University of Alabama–Birmingham Medical Center
Laboratory for IVF
547 Old Hillman Building, University Station
Birmingham, AL 35294
(205) 934-5631
Director: Benjamin Younger, M.D.

ARIZONA

Arizona Center for Fertility Studies
IVF Program
4614 E. Shea Blvd., D-260
Phoenix, AZ 85028
(602) 996-7896
Directors: Jay S. Nemiro, M.D., Robert McGaughey, Ph.D.

Phoenix Fertility Institute P.C.
Good Samaritan Hospital
1300 N. 12th St., Suite 522
Phoenix, AZ 85006
(602) 996-7896
Director: Tawfik H. Rizkallah, M.D.

Robert H. Tamis, M.D. & Associates (private)
2720 N. 20th St., #220
Phoenix, AZ 85006
(602) 279-2941
Director: Robert H. Tamis, M.D.

CALIFORNIA
Alta Bates Hospital
In Vitro Fertilization Program
3001 Colby St.
Berkeley, CA 94705
(415) 540-1416
Director: Ryszard J. Chetkowski, M.D.

Berkeley–East Bay Advanced Reproductive
    Services (private)
2999 Regent St., Suite 201
Berkeley, CA 94705
(415) 841-5510
Director: Ferdinand J. Beernink, M.D.

Central California IVF Program
Fresno Community Hospital
PO Box 1232
Fresno, CA 93715
(209) 439-1914
Director: Carlos E. Sueldo, M.D.

Fertility Institute of San Diego
Sharp/Children's Medical Center
9834 Genessee Ave., Suite 300
La Jolla, CA 92037
(619) 455-7520
Director: Joseph F. Kennedy, M.D.

Scripps Clinic and Research Foundation
    (private)
10666 N. Torrey Pines Rd.
La Jolla, CA 92037
(619) 457-8680
Director: Jeffrey Rakoff, M.D.

Century City Hospital
2070 Century Park E.
Los Angeles, CA 90067
(213) 201-6619
Director: Dianne Moore Smith, Ph.D.

Southern California Fertility Institute
California Institute for IVF Inc. (private)
"Right to Parenthood (RTP)" Program
12301 Wilshire Blvd., Suite 415
Los Angeles, CA 90025
Director: William Karow, M.D.

UCLA School of Medicine
Department of Ob/Gyn: IVF Program
Los Angeles, CA 90024
(213) 825-7755
Director: David R. Meldrum, M.D.

University of Southern California School of
    Medicine
IVF-Embryo Replacement Program
Hospital of the Good Samaritan
637 S. Lucas Ave.
Los Angeles, CA 90017
(213) 226-3421
Directors: Richard Marrs, M.D., Joyce
    Vargyas, M.D.

Robert M. Adams, M.D. (private)
966 Cass St., Suite 200
Monterey, CA 93940
(408) 649-1144
Director: Robert Adams, M.D.

Northridge Hospital Medical Center
IVF Program
18300 Roscoe Blvd.
Northridge, CA 91328
(818) 996-2289
Directors: Drs. Sheldon L. Schein, Paul M.
    Greenberg

Northern California Fertility Center (private)
87 Scripps Drive, Suite 202
Sacramento, CA 95825
(916) 929-3596
Director: Gary K. Stewart, M.D.

University of California, San Francisco
IVF Program
Department of Ob/Gyn & Reproductive
    Sciences
Room M 1480
San Francisco, CA 94143
(415) 666-1824
Directors: Drs. Robert H. Glass, Mary C.
    Martin

John Muir Memorial Hospital
Department of Ob/Gyn: IVF Program
1601 Ygnacio Valley Rd.
Walnut Creek, CA 94598
(415) 937-6166
Directors: Drs. Donald Galen, Arnold
    Jacobson, Elwood Kronick

Whittier Hospital Medical Center
The Genesis Program for In Vitro Fertilization
Center for Human Development
15151 Janine Drive
Whittier, CA 90605
(213) 945-3561, x549
Directors: Vellore Bhupathy, M.D., Robert A.
  Orlando, M.D.

COLORADO
Reproductive Genetics In Vitro PC (private)
455 S. Hudson St., Level Three
Denver, CO 80222
(303) 399-1464
Director: George Henry, M.D.

University of Colorado Health Sciences Center
IVF Program
4200 E. Ninth Ave., Box B198
Denver CO 80262
(303) 394-8365
Director: Bruce H. Albrecht, M.D.

CONNECTICUT
University of Connecticut Health Center
Division of Reproductive Endocrinology &
  Infertility
Farmington, CT 06790
(203) 674-2110
Directors: Donald Maier, M.D., Anthony
  Luciano, M.D.

Mount Sinai Hospital
Department of Ob/Gyn: Division of
  Reproductive Endocrinology and Infertility
675 Hartford Ave.
Hartford, CT 06112
(203) 242-6201
Director: Augusto P. Chong, M.D.

Yale University Medical School
Department of Ob/Gyn: IVF Program
333 Cedar St.
New Haven, CT 06510
(203) 785-4019, 4792
Director: Alan DeCherney, M.D.

DISTRICT OF COLUMBIA
Columbia Hospital for Women Medical Center
IVF Program
2425 L St., N.W.
Washington, DC 20037
(202) 293-6500
Director: Richard Falk, M.D.

George Washington University Medical Center
Department of Ob/Gyn: IVF Program
901 23rd St., N.W.
Washington, DC 20037
(202) 676-4614
Director: Robert J. Stillman, M.D.

FLORIDA
Memorial Medical Center of Jacksonville
In Vitro Fertilization Program
3343 University Blvd. S.
Jacksonville, FL 32216
(904) 391-1149
Director: Marwan M. Shaykh, M.D.

University of Miami
Department of Ob/Gyn: D-5
PO Box 016960
Miami, FL 33101
(305) 547-5818
Director: T. T. Hung, M.D., Ph.D.

Naples Life Program (private)
775 First Ave. N.
Naples, FL 33940
(813) 262-1653
Director: Donald W. Ketterhagen, M.D.

Humana Women's Hospital (USF)
3030 W. Buffalo Ave.
Tampa, FL 33607
(813) 872-2988
Directors: George B. Maroulis, M.D., Barry
  S. Verkauf, M.D.

GEORGIA
Atlanta Center for Fertility and Endocrinology
Northside Hospital
5675 Peachtree–Dunwoody Rd., N.E.
Atlanta, GA 30342
(404) 256-8000
Director: Camran Nezhat, M.D.

Atlanta Fertility Institute
Georgia Baptist Medical Center
300 Boulevard N.E.
Atlanta, GA 30312
(404) 659-5211
Director: Amir H. Ansari, M.D.

Reproductive Biology Associates (private)
993C Johnson Ferry Rd., Suite 315
Atlanta, GA 30342
(404) 843-3064
Directors: Benjamin Brackett, Ph.D., Hilton
  Kort, M.D., Joe Massey, M.D.

Augusta Reproductive Biology Associates
(private)
810–812 Chafee
Augusta, GA 30904
(404) 724-0228
Directors: Edouardo J. Servy, M.D., Jan
Sehdler, Ph.D.

Medical College of Georgia
Humana Hospital-IVF Section
Augusta, GA 30912
(404) 863-3232, x6646
Director: Paul McDonough, M.D.

HAWAII
Pacific In Vitro Fertilization Institute
Kapiolani Women's & Children's Hospital
1319 Punahou St., Suite 1040
Honolulu, HI 96826
(808) 946-2226
Directors: Drs. B. Chun, T. Huang, T.
Kosasa, P. McNamee, C. Morton, F. Terada

Kauai Medical Group, Inc.
University of Hawaii: G.N. Wilcox Memorial
Hospital
Department of Ob/Gyn
3420-B Kuhio Highway
Lihue, HI 96766
(808) 245-1119
Director: Frederick D. Sengstacke, II, M.D.

ILLINOIS
Michael Reese–University of Chicago
IVF-ET Program
31st St. at Lake Shore Drive
Chicago, IL 60616
(312) 791-4000
Director: Edward L. Marut, M.D.

Mount Sinai Hospital Medical Center
Department of Ob/Gyn: IVF Program
California Ave. at 15th St.
Chicago, IL 60608
(312) 650-6727
Directors: Norbert Gleicher, M.D., Jan
Friberg, M.D.

Rush Medical College
IVF Program: Department of Ob/Gyn
600 S. Paulina St.
Chicago, IL 60616
(312) 942-6609
Director: W. Paul Dmowski, M.D., Ph.D.

University of Illinois College of Medicine
Department of Ob/Gyn
840 S. Wood St.
Chicago, IL 60612
(312) 996-7430
Director: M. Yusoff Dawood, M.D.

INDIANA
Indiana University Medical Center
Department of Ob/Gyn: Section of
Reproductive Endocrinology
926 W. Michigan St., N 262
Indianapolis, IN 46223
(317) 264-4057
Director: Marguerite K. Shepard, M.D.

Pregnancy Initiation Center (Humana Women's
Hospital)
8091 Township Line Rd., Suite 110
Indianapolis, IN 46260
(317) 872-5103
Director: John C. Jarrett, II, M.D.

KANSAS
Kansas University Gynecological & Obstetrical
Foundation
University of Kansas College of Health
Sciences
39th and Rainbow Blvd.
Kansas City, KS 66103
(913) 588-6246
Director: William J. Cameron, M.D.

KENTUCKY
University of Kentucky
Department of Ob/Gyn
Kentucky Center for Reproductive Medicine
Lexington, KY 40536
(606) 233-5410
Director: Emery A. Wilson, M.D.

Norton Hospital
IVF Program
601 S. Floyd St., Room 304
Louisville, KY 40202
(502) 562-8154
Director: Marvin A. Yussman, M.D.

LOUISIANA
The Fertility Institute of New Orleans
Humana Women's Hospital, East Orleans
6020 Bullard Ave.
New Orleans, LA 70128
(504) 246-8971
Director: Richard Dickey, M.D.

Tulane Fertility Program
IVF Program
1415 Tulane Ave.
New Orleans, LA 70112
(504) 588-2341
Director: Ian H. Thorneycroft, M.D.

MARYLAND
Baltimore IVF Program (private)
2435 W. Belvedere Ave., #41
Baltimore, MD 21215
(301) 542-5115
Director: Moshe Salomy, M.D.

Greater Baltimore Medical Center (private)
IVF Program of the Women's Fertility Center
6701 N. Charles St.
Baltimore, MD 21204
(301) 828-2484
Director: Frederick Weinstein, M.D.

The Johns Hopkins Hospital
Division of Reproductive Endocrinology: IVF
  Program
600 N. Wolfe St.
Baltimore, MD 21205
(301) 955-8759
Director: John A. Rock, M.D.

Union Memorial Hospital
IVF Program: Department of Ob/Gyn
201 E. University Parkway
Baltimore, MD 21218
(301) 235-5255
Director: Rafael Haciski, M.D.

Genetic Consultants
Washington Adventist Hospital
5616 Shields Drive
Bethesda, MD 20817
(301) 530-6900
Directors: Drs. Mark Geier, John Young

MASSACHUSETTS
Beth Israel Hospital
Department of Ob/Gyn: IVF Program
330 Brookline Ave.
Boston, MA 02215
(617) 735-5923
Directors: Melvin Taymor, M.D., Machelle
  Seibel, M.D.

Brigham and Womens Hospital
IVF Program
75 Francis St.
Boston, MA 02115
(617) 732-4220
Director: Patricia M. McShane, M.D.

In Vitro Fertilization Center of Boston at
  Boston University Medical Center
75 E. Newton St.
Boston, MA 02118
(617) 247-5928
Director: Kenneth C. Edelin, M.D.

New England Medical Center Hospitals
Division of Reproductive Endocrinology
260 Tremont St.
Boston, MA 02111
(617) 956-6066
Director: R. Nuran Turksoy, M.D.

Greater Boston In Vitro Associates (private)
Newton-Wellesly Hospital
2000 Washington St., Suite 342
Newton, MA 02162
(617) 965-7270
Directors: John H. Derry, M.D., Peter M.
  Martin, M.D., Robert A. Newton, M.D.,
  Director of Andrology

MICHIGAN
University of Michigan Medical Center
L-2120 Women's Hospital
Department of Ob/Gyn
Ann Arbor, MI 48109
(313) 763-4323
Director: Jonathan Ayers, M.D.

Blodgett Memorial Medical Center
IVF Program
1900 Wealthy St., S.E., Suite 330
Grand Rapids, MI 49506
(616) 774-0700
Director: Robert D. Visscher, M.D.

Hutzel Hospital/Wayne State University
IVF Program
4707 St. Antoine
Detroit, MI 48201
(313) 494-7547
Director: David M. Magyar, D.O.

William Beaumont Hospital
In Vitro Fertilization Program
3601 W. 13 Mile Rd.
Royal Oak, MI 48072
(313) 288-2380
Director: S. Jan Behrman, M.D.

MINNESOTA
University of Minnesota VIP Program
Department of Ob/Gyn
Box 395, Mayo Memorial Building
420 Delaware St., S.E.
Minneapolis, MN 55455
(612) 373-8852
Director: George Tagatz, M.D.

Mayo Clinic
Department of Reproductive Endocrinology &
   Infertility
200 First St., S.W.
Rochester, MN 55905
(507) 284-3188

MISSISSIPPI
University of Mississippi Medical Center
IVF Program
Department of Ob/Gyn
Jackson, MS 39216
(601) 987-4662
Director: Bryan D. Cowan, M.D.

MISSOURI
Jewish Hospital
Department of Ob/Gyn: IVF Program
216 S. Kingshighway
St. Louis, MO 63110
(314) 454-7834
Director: Ronald Strickler, M.D.

Missouri Baptist Hospital
In Vitro Fertilization Program, Room 301
3015 N. Ballas Rd.
St. Louis, MO 63131
(314) 432-1212, x5295
Director: Romeo Perez, M.D.

NEBRASKA
University of Nebraska Medical Center
Department of Ob/Gyn
42nd and Dewey Ave.
Omaha, NE 68105
(402) 559-4212
Director: Raymond Schulte, M.D.

NEVADA
Northern Nevada Fertility Clinic (private)
350 W. Sixth St.
Reno, NV 89503
(702) 322-4521
Director: Geoffrey Sher, M.D.

NEW JERSEY
UMD: Rutgers Medical School
Department of Ob/Gyn: IVF Program
Academic Health Science Center, CN19
New Brunswick, NJ 08903
(201) 937-7635
Director: Ekkehard Kemmann, M.D.

University Hospital
Department of Ob/Gyn
100 Bergen St.
Newark, NJ 07103
(201) 456-6029
Director: Cecelia Schmidt, M.D.

NEW YORK
Children's Hospital of Buffalo
Reproductive Endocrinology and Infertility
   Unit
IVF-ET Program
140 Hodge Ave.
Buffalo, NY 14222
(716) 878-7232
Director: Abraham K. Munabi, M.D.

Westchester In Vitro Fertility Group (private)
88 Ashford Ave.
Dobbs Ferry, NY 10522
(914) 693-8820
Director: Andrew Y. Silverman, M.D.

North Shore University Hospital
Division of Human Reproduction: IVF
300 Community Drive
Manhasset, NY 11030
(516) 562-4470
Director: Richard Bronson, M.D.

Advanced Fertility Services, PC (private)
1625 Third Ave.
New York, NY 10028
(212) 369-8700
Director: Hugh D. Melnick, M.D.

Columbia–Presbyterian Medical Center
Presbyterian Hospital IVF-ET Program
622 W. 168th St.
New York, NY 10032
(212) 694-8013
Director: Georgianna Jagiello, M.D.

Cornell University Medical College
Program of In Vitro Fertilization
515 E. 71st St., 2nd Floor
New York, NY 10021
(212) 472-4693
Director: Alan S. Berkeley, M.D.

Mount Sinai Medical Center
In Vitro Fertilization Program
One Gustave Levy Place
Annenberg 20-60
New York, NY 10029
(212) 650-5927
Director: Jon W. Gordon, M.D., Ph.D.

St. Luke's–Roosevelt Hospital Center
IVF-ET Program
1111 Amsterdam Ave.
New York, NY 10025
(212) 870-6603
Director: Hussein K. Amin, M.D.

University of Rochester CARE Program
University of Rochester Medical Center
Rochester, NY 14642
(716) 275-4422
Director: Eberhard Muechler, M.D.

NORTH CAROLINA
Chapel Hill Fertility Services (private)
109 Conner Drive, Suite 2104
Chapel Hill, NC 27514
(919) 968-4656
Director: James Dingfeld, M.D.

Eastowne Ob/Gyn and Infertility (private)
700 Eastowne Drive
Chapel Hill, NC 27514
(919) 942-4100
Director: James Dingfelder, M.D.

North Carolina Memorial Hospital
Fertility Center: IVF Program
Chapel Hill, NC 27514
(919) 966-5438
Director: Luther M. Talbert, M.D.

Duke University Medical Center
Department of Ob/Gyn: IVF Program
Durham, NC 27710
(919) 684-5327
Director: Mark A. Bernhisel, M.D., PO Box
  3143, DUMC

OHIO
Akron City Hospital
IVF-ET Program
525 E. Market St.
Akron, OH 44309
(216) 375-3585
Director: Nicholas J. Spirtos, D.O.

Jewish Hospital of Cincinnati
Department of Ob/Gyn: IVF Program
3120 Burnet Ave., Suite 204
Cincinnati, OH 45229
(513) 221-3062 or 569-2150
Director: Sheldon Pelchovitz, M.D.

University of Cincinnati Medical Center
IVF Program
Division of Reproductive Endocrinology &
  Infertility
Department of Ob/Gyn
231 Bethesda Ave.
Cincinnati, OH 45267
(513) 872-6368
Director: O'dell M. Owens, M.D.

Cleveland Clinic Foundation
In Vitro Fertilization Program
9500 Euclid Ave.
Cleveland, OH 44106
(216) 444-2240
Director: Martin M. Quigley, M.D.

MacDonald Hospital for Women
IVF Program
2105 Adelbert Rd.
Cleveland, OH 44106
(216) 844-1514
Director: Cynthia M. Austin, M.D.

Mount Sinai Medical Center of Cleveland
LIFE Program
University Circle
Cleveland, OH 44106
(216) 421-5884
Director: Wulf H. Utian, M.D.

Infertility and Gynecology, Inc.
Grant Hospital
1450 Hawthorne Ave.
Columbus, OH 43203
(614) 253-8383
Director: Nichols Vorys, M.D.

University Reproductive Center
Ohio State University Hospitals
410 W. 10th Ave.
Columbus, OH 43210
(614) 421-8937, 8511
Director: Moon H. Kim, M.D.

Miami Valley Hospital
In Vitro Fertilization Program
1 Wyoming St.
Dayton, OH 45409
(513) 223-6192, x4066
Director: Robert C. Winslow, M.D.

OKLAHOMA
Oklahoma University Health Sciences Center
Section of Reproductive Endocrinology &
  Infertility
PO Box 26901, 4SP720
Oklahoma City, OK 73190
(405) 271-8700
Director: Ponjola Coney, M.D.

Hillcrest Infertility Center
1145 S. Utica, #1209
Tulsa, OK 74104
(918) 584-2870
Directors: J. Clark Bundron, M.D., J.W.
  Edward Wortham, Ph.D.

OREGON
Oregon Reproductive Research & Fertility
  Program
Oregon Health Science University School of
  Medicine
3181 S.W. Sam Jackson Park Rd.
Portland, OR 97201
(503) 225-8449
Director: Kenneth A. Burry, M.D.

PENNSYLVANIA
Rolling Hill Hospital
60 E. Township Line Rd.
Elkins Park, PA 19117
(215) 663-6728
Director: Michael Birnbaum, M.D.

Albert Einstein Medical Center
Department of Ob/Gyn
York and Tabor Rds.
Philadelphia, PA 19141
(215) 456-7990
Director: Martin Freedman, M.D.

Hospital of the University of Pennsylvania
Department of Ob/Gyn: IVF Program
3400 Spruce St., Suite 106
Philadelphia, PA 19104
(215) 662-2981
Directors: Luigi Mastroianni, Jr., M.D.,
  Celso-Ramon Garcia, M.D.

The Pennsylvania Hospital
In Vitro Fertilization–Embryo Transfer
  Program
Eighth & Spruce Sts.
Philadelphia, PA 19107
(215) 829-5095
Director: Esther Eisenberg, M.D.

Magee-Women's Hospital
IVF Program
Forbes Ave. & Halket St.
Pittsburgh, PA 15213
(412) 647-4000
Director: Carolyn B. Coulam, M.D.

SOUTH CAROLINA
Medical University of South Carolina
Department of Ob/Gyn: IVF Program
171 Ashley Ave.
Charleston, SC 29425
(803) 792-2861
Director: Charles C. Tsai, M.D.

The Southeastern Fertility Center
Roper Hospital
315 Calhoun St.
Charleston, SC 29401
(803) 722-3294
Directors: Grant Patton, M.D., John Black,
  Ph.D.

TENNESSEE
East Tennessee State University
Department of Ob/Gyn
PO Box 19570A
Johnson City, TN 37614
(615) 928-6426, x334
Directors: Drs. Melvin G. Dodson, Pickens A.
  Gantt

East Tennessee Baptist Hospital
Family Life Center
7A Office 715
Box 1788, Blount Ave.
Knoxville, TN 37901
(615) 632-5011
Director: I. Ray King, M.D.

University of Tennessee Memorial Research
    Center and Hospital
1924 Alcoa Highway
Knoxville, TN 37920
(615) 971-4958
Director: Robert A. Wild, M.D.
Coordinator: Michael R. Caudle, M.D.

Vanderbilt University
In Vitro Fertilization Program
D3200 Medical Center N.
Nashville, TN 37232
(615) 322-6576
Director: Anne Colston Wentz, M.D.

TEXAS
St. David's Community Hospital
In Vitro Fertilization–ET Program
PO Box 4039 (919 E. 32nd St.)
Austin, TX 78765
(512) 397-4107 or 476-7111
Director: Thomas Vaughn, M.D.

Trinity In Vitro/Embryo Transfer Program
Trinity Medical Center
4323 N. Josey Lane, Suite 206
Carrollton, TX 75007
(214) 394-0114
Director: W. F. "Dub" Howard, M.D.

Presbyterian Hospital of Dallas
PO Box 17 (8160 Walnut Hill Lane)
Dallas, TX 75231
(214) 891-2624
Director: James D. Madden, M.D.

The University of Texas–Southwestern Medical
    School
Department of Ob/Gyn: IVF Program
5323 Harry Hines Blvd.
Dallas, TX 75230
(214) 688-3111
Directors: David S. Guzick, M.D., Clare
    Edman, M.D.

Fort Worth Associates for Human
    Reproduction (private)
Harris Institute
1325 Pennsylvania Ave.
Fort Worth, TX 76104
(817) 335-0909, 334-6813
Director: Alan Johns, M.D.

University of Texas Medical Branch
Department of Ob/Gyn: IVF Program
Galveston, TX 77550
(409) 761-3985
Director: Manubai Nagamani, M.D.

Baylor College of Medicine
Department of Ob/Gyn: IVF Program
1 Baylor Plaza
Houston, TX 77030
(713) 797-0322 or 791-9861
Contact: Johnelle May, R.N., Coordinator

Texas Woman's Hospital
IVF Program
7600 Fannin
Houston, TX 77054
(713) 795-7257

University of Texas Health Science Center
Department of Ob/Gyn & Reproductive
    Science
6431 Fannin, Suite 3270
Houston, TX 77030
(713) 792-5360
Directors: Pedro Beauchamp, M.D., Donald P.
    Wolf, Ph.D.

The West Houston Fertility Center
Sam Houston Memorial Hospital
In Vitro Fertilization Center
1615 Hillendahl Blvd.
PO Box 55130
Houston, TX 77055
(713) 932-5600
Director: Dr. Ivor Safro

Texas Tech University Health Sciences Center
School of Medicine: Department of Ob/Gyn
PO Box 4569
Lubbock, TX 79430
(806) 743-2335
Director: Frank D. De Leon, M.D.

University of Texas Health Science Center
Department of Ob/Gyn: IVF Program
7703 Floyd Curl Drive
San Antonio, TX 78284
(512) 691-6181
Director: Ricardo Asch, M.D.

UTAH
University of Utah
Division of Reproductive Endocrinology
50 Medical Drive N.
Salt Lake City, UT 84132
(801) 581-4837
Director: William Keye, M.D.

VERMONT
University of Vermont
Department of Ob/Gyn: Division of
   Reproductive Endocrinology and Infertility
Given Building
Burlington, VT 05405
(802) 656-2272
Director: Mark Gibson, M.D.

VIRGINIA
Genetics and IVF Institute (Fairfax Hospital)
3020 Javier Rd.
Fairfax, VA 22031
(703) 698-7355
Director: Joseph D. Schulman, M.D.

Eastern Virginia Medical School
Jones Institute for Reproductive Medicine
825 Fairfax Ave., 6th Floor
Hoffheimer Hall
Norfolk, VA 23507
(804) 446-8935
Directors: Howard W. Jones, Jr., M.D.,
   Georgianna Seegar Jones, M.D.

Medical College of Virginia
IVF Program
Box 34-MCV Station
Richmond, VA 23298
(804) 786-9636
Director: Sanford M. Rosenberg, M.D.

WASHINGTON
Swedish Hospital Medical Center
Reproductive Genetics
747 Summit Ave.
Seattle, WA 98104
(206) 292-2483
Director: Laurence E. Karp, M.D.

University of Washington IVF Program
Department of Ob/Gyn: RH-20
Seattle, WA 98195
(206) 543-8483
Director: Michael Soules, M.D.

Infertility and Reproductive Associates
W. 104 Fifth Ave., Room 410
Spokane, WA 99204
(509) 455-8111
Director: George H. Rice, M.D.

WISCONSIN
University of Wisconsin Clinics
IVF Program
600 Highland Ave.
H4/630 CSC
Madison, WI 53792
(608) 263-1217
Director: Sander S. Shapiro, M.D.

University of Wisconsin–Milwaukee Clinical
   Campus
Department of Ob/Gyn
Mount Sinai Medical Center
950 N. 12th
PO Box 342
Milwaukee, WI 53201
(414) 289-8609
Director: Mark R. Neff, M.D.

Waukesha Memorial Hospital
IVF Program
725 American Ave.
Waukesha, WI 53186
(414) 544-2722
Director: K. Paul Katayama, M.D.

SOURCE: *American Fertility Society.*

SPERM BANKS

ARKANSAS
Frozen Semen Bank
Department of Anatomy
University of Arkansas for Medical Sciences
Little Rock, AR 72205
(501) 660-2098
J. K. Sherman, Ph.D.

CALIFORNIA
Valley Cryo Bank
17207 Ventura Blvd.
Encino, CA 91436
(213) 981-7822
Cyrus Milan, M.D.

Repository for Germinal Choice
450 S. Escondido Blvd.
Escondido, CA 92025
(619) 743-0772
Robert Graham, M.D.

Southern California Cryobank, Inc.
2080 Century Park E., #308
Los Angeles, CA 90067
(213) 553-9828
Cappy Rothman, M.D.
Charles Sims, M.D.

Tyler Medical Clinic
921 Westwood Blvd.
Los Angeles, CA 90049
(213) 477-6765
Stanley Friedman, M.D.

Sperm Bank of Northern California
2930 McClure St.
Oakland, CA 74609
(415) 444-2014
Barbara Reboy

COLORADO
Western Cryobank (Cryogenic Lab. branch)
10 N. Meade
Colorado Springs, CO 80909
(303) 578-9414
Charles Johnson, M.D.

Genetic Reserves
2005 E. 18th Ave.
Denver, CO 80206
(303) 321-4212
Edward A. Rhodes, M.D.

DISTRICT OF COLUMBIA
Washington Fertility Study Center
2600 Virginia Ave., N.W.
Washington, DC 20037
(202) 333-3100
Salvatore Leto, Ph.D.

GEORGIA
Xytex Corporation
1100 Emmit St.
Augusta, GA 30904
(404) 724-5615
Armand Karow, Ph.D.

ILLINOIS
Cryo Lab Facility
100 E. Ohio St.
Chicago, IL 60611
(312) 751-2632
Alfred Morris, M.S.

LOUISIANA
Louisiana Fertility Services
515 Westbank Expressway
Gretna, LA 70053
(504) 366-7233
Louis Levinson, M.D.

MASSACHUSETTS
Northwest Sperm Bank
2000 Washington St., Suite 322
Newton, MA 02162
(617) 332-1228
Robert A. Newton, M.D.

MICHIGAN
International Cryogenics, Inc.
189 Townsend St., Suite 203
Birmingham, MI 48011
(313) 644-5822
Willis H. Stephens, M.D.

MINNESOTA
Cyrogenic Laboratories
1935 W. County Rd. B-2
Roseville, MN 55113
(612) 636-3792
John H. Olson, M.S.

MISSOURI
Midwest Fertility Foundation & Laboratory,
    Inc.
2900 Baltimore, Suite 520
Kansas City, MO 64108
(816) 756-0040
Elwin Grimes, M.D.

NEBRASKA
Genetic Semen Bank
University of Nebraska Medical Center
42nd and Dewey Ave.
Omaha, NE 68105
(402) 559-5070
Warren G. Sanger, Ph.D.

NEW YORK
Erie Medical Center (Idant Branch)
50 High St.
Buffalo, NY 14203
(716) 883-2213

Idant Laboratory
645 Madison Ave.
New York, NY 10022
(212) 935-1430
Joseph Feldschuh, M.D.

OREGON
Infertility Laboratory
University of Oregon Health Science Center
3181 S.W. Sam Jackson Park Rd.
Portland, OR 97201
(503) 225-8261
Nancy J. Alexander, Ph.D.

PENNSYLVANIA
Semen Bank
Department of Obstetrics & Gynecology
Pennsylvania Hospital
8th & Spruce Sts.
Philadelphia, PA 19107
(215) 829-5018
William W. Beck, M.D.

WASHINGTON
Seattle Urological Associates
1221 Madison, Suite 1210
Seattle, WA 98104
(206) 292-6488
Wayne Weissman, M.D.

WYOMING
Rocky Mountain Cryobank
PO Box 3033
Jackson, WY 83001
(307) 733-4142
C.W. Ely, Jr., M.D.

SOURCE: *American Association of Tissue Banks.*

INFERTILITY ORGANIZATIONS

The American Fertility Society
Suite 201
2131 Magnolia Ave.
Birmingham, AL 35256
(205) 251-9764

A professional association of physicians, a primary source of information on all aspects of
fertility and infertility for the public. Pamphlets,
brochures, a monthly medical journal. Maintains
a master list of its members who are expert in
general fertility work-ups, vasectomy reversals,
artificial insemination by donor, microsurgery,
in vitro fertilization. Will provide a list of names
of physicians by specialty and by locality to anyone who writes or calls with a specific request.

Endometriosis Association
PO Box 92187
Milwaukee, WI 53202

A U.S.-Canadian self-help, education and research membership organization dealing with all
aspects of endometriosis, including infertility.
Pamphlets, information sheets, a newsletter.
Some local groups that make referrals for treatment. Will provide more information upon request.

RESOLVE, Inc.
PO Box 474
Belmont, MA 02178
(617) 484-2424

A national self-help, mutual support organization. Over 40 chapters throughout the country where men, women and couples meet to discuss their infertility problems with each other and a trained professional. A major source of information on infertility. The national office can refer you to infertility specialists, therapists, adoption services, *in vitro* clinics, artificial insemination specialists. Also offers telephone counseling during weekdays. Fact sheets, reprints, books, a monthly newsletter. Will provide more information upon request.

ALTERNATIVE CHILDBIRTH ORGANIZATIONS

Ordinarily the medical aspects of childbirth are between a woman and her physician, and no specialists of the type noted in this book are necessary. In recent years, however, a backlash has developed against the high technology of childbirth, and many American women are choosing to view pregnancy and childbirth as a normal event rather than as a medical crisis. Many now prefer more ''natural'' methods of childbirth and delivery at home or in freestanding birth centers with medical and hospital backup *only if needed*.

This section is for parents who want to know how to find information about *alternatives* to traditional methods of childbirth. Organizations have formed to help parents find such alternate facilities or resources. Some are listed below.

American Academy of Husband-Coached
   Childbirth
The Bradley Method®
PO Box 5224
Sherman Oaks, CA 91413
(800) 423-2397—Pregnancy Hotline (except
   California, Hawaii, and Alaska)
(818) 788-6362

A national organization to train instructors in the Bradley Method of natural childbirth. A source of information for the public. Makes referrals nationwide to Bradley teachers. Pamphlets, publications, including books and films, available through classes. Maintains a pregnancy hotline, which you can call to find local instructors. Will provide more information upon request.

American Society for Psychoprophylaxis in
   Obstetrics
Lamaze Method of Childbirth
1840 Wilson Blvd., Suite 204
Arlington, VA 22201
(703) 524-7802

Membership organization of physicians, nurses, nurse-midwives, teachers of the Lamaze method, parents, and others interested in the method. About 40 local chapters and 10 affiliates. A major source of information on the Lamaze method. Sponsors classes, trains and certifies Lamaze teachers, makes referrals to local chapters that conduct classes and support groups. Magazines, books, pamphlets. Will provide more information and the name of a local chapter in your area upon request.

C/SEC (Cesareans/Support, Education, and
   Concern)
22 Forest Rd.
Framingham, MA 01701
(617) 877-8266

National membership organization of professionals and parents interested in cesarean delivery. A major source of information and emotional support surrounding cesarean, especially education about cesarean prevention and vaginal birth after a cesarean. Support groups in many areas. Telephone, correspondence and person-to-person contact. Books, pamphlets, reading lists. Makes referrals to physicians who share the organization's concerns. Will provide more information upon request.

International Association of Parents and Professionals for Safe Alternatives in Childbirth (NAPSAC)
PO Box 429
Marble Hill, MO 63764
(314) 238-2010

National voluntary membership organization. Over 100 local chapters. A major source of information on childbirth education, nutrition in pregnancy, natural childbirth, midwifery, breast feeding, non-hospital births. Publications, including a *Directory of Alternative Birth Services*, listing about 4,500 home birth services, freestanding birth centers, midwives, and other alternatives. Holds seminars for parents coast to coast. Will send more information and the name of a local chapter in your area upon request.

International Childbirth Education Association
PO Box 20048
Minneapolis, MN 55420
(612) 854-8660

A nationwide, voluntary organization of consumers and health-care providers interested in informed "freedom of choice" in childbirth. Acts as a referral service for childbirth preparation classes, certifies childbirth educators, holds conferences. Has coordinators in every state and province in Canada who provide information locally. Publishes and sells numerous publications. Operates a mail-order bookstore.

National Association of Childbearing Centers
R.D. #1, Box 1
Perkiomenville, PA 18074
(215) 234-8068

National membership organization. A comprehensive resource for the public and professionals on freestanding birth centers. Promotes guidelines, standards, licensure, public information, and assistance to freestanding birth centers. Newsletter. Will send information to expectant mothers on birth centers, and the names of birth centers in your area upon request and receipt of a self-addressed, stamped envelope.

NURSE-MIDWIVES

Delivery by nurse-midwives, nurses with two years of special training in childbirth, is becoming more common. The number of babies delivered by nurse-midwives doubled between 1975 and 1980. At first, many obstetricians opposed delivery by midwives and restricted their presence in hospitals, but much of that opposition is now subsiding, and nurse-midwives often work in hospitals, sometimes as part of a team with an obstetrician. In fact, most midwife births are still in a hospital setting.

The nurse-midwife puts more emphasis on the normal delivery, without the use of high technology and drugs except when absolutely necessary. Nurse-midwives are now in all parts of the country. You can find one by contacting the following nurse-midwives association or one of the schools of nursing that train nurse-midwives, listed below.

American College of Nurse-Midwives
1522 K St., N.W.
Washington, DC 20005
(202) 347-5445

A national organization to promote the use of nurse-midwives. A major source of information to the public on nurse-midwives. Makes referrals to nurse-midwives throughout the country. Accredits nurse-midwive schools. Pamphlets. Will provide more information upon request.

SOME LEADING CENTERS FOR NURSE-MIDWIVES

The following universities do extensive training and education of nurse-midwives and can be sources of information and references in local communities about how to find midwives and use their services.

ARIZONA
College of Nursing
Nurse-Midwifery Program
University of Arizona
Tucson, AZ 85721
(602) 626-7481, 6154

CALIFORNIA
Family Nurse Practice
Nurse-Midwifery
University of California, San Diego, T-009
La Jolla, CA 92093
(619) 294-3685

Nurse-Midwifery Program
Women's Hospital, Room 8K5
University of Southern California
1240 N. Mission Rd.
Los Angeles, CA 90033
(213) 226-3386

Women's Health Care Training Project
Stanford University
703 Welch Rd., #F1
Palo Alto, CA 94304
(415) 723-7046

San Francisco General Hospital
University of California at San Francisco
Room 2127
1001 Potrero Ave.
San Francisco, CA 94110
(415) 821-5106 or 647-7828

COLORADO
School of Nursing Graduate Program
University of Colorado Health Sciences Center
Box C 288
4200 E. Ninth Ave.
Denver, CO 80262
(303) 394-8654

CONNECTICUT
Maternal Newborn (Nurse-Midwifery) Program
Yale University
855 Howard Ave.
Box 3333
New Haven, CT 06510
(203) 785-2423

DISTRICT OF COLUMBIA
Georgetown University School of Nursing
3700 Reservoir Rd., N.W.
Washington, DC 20007
(202) 625-6993

FLORIDA
School of Nursing
University of Miami
1540 Corniche
Coral Gables, FL 33124
(305) 284-3619

T. Hillis Miller Health Center College of
  Nursing
University of Florida at Gainesville
PO Box J-197
Gainesville, FL 32610
(904) 392-4214

GEORGIA
Neil Hodgson Woodruff School of Nursing
Emory University
Atlanta, GA 30322
(404) 727-6918

ILLINOIS
Rush-Presbyterian–St. Lukes' Medical Center
600 S. Paulina St.
Chicago, IL 60612
(312) 942-6604

College of Nursing
Department of Maternal-Child Nursing
Nurse-Midwifery Program
University of Illinois at Chicago, Health
  Sciences Center
PO Box 6998
Chicago, IL 60680
(312) 996-7937

KENTUCKY
College of Nursing
University of Kentucky
760 Rose St.
Lexington, KY 40536-0232
(606) 233-5406, 6620

Frontier School of Midwifery and Family
  Nursing
Frontier Nursing Service
Hyden, KY 41749
(606) 672-2312

MARYLAND
Nurse-Midwifery Program
Malcom Grow USAF Medical Center
United States Air Force
Andrews Air Force Base, MD 20331
(301) 981-6104

MINNESOTA
School of Nursing
University of Minnesota
6-101 Unit F
308 Harvard St.
Minneapolis, MN 55455
(612) 624-6494

NEW JERSEY
School of Allied Health Professions
Nurse-Midwifery Program
University of Medicine and Dentistry of New
    Jersey
100 Bergen St.
Newark, NJ 07103
(201) 456-4298

NEW YORK
Downstate Medical Center
College of Health Related Professions
Nurse-Midwifery Program, Box 93
State University of New York
450 Clarkson Ave.
Brooklyn, NY 11203
(212) 270-1359, 1360

Columbia University Graduate Program in
    Maternity Nursing and Nurse-Midwifery
Columbia Presbyterian Medical Center
630 W. 168th St.
New York, NY 10032
(212) 305-2808

OHIO
Frances Payne Boalton School of Nursing
Case Western Reserve
2121 Abington Rd.
Cleveland, OH 44106
(216) 368-2532

OREGON
School of Nursing
Department of Family Nursing
Nurse-Midwifery Program
Oregon Health Sciences University
3181 S.W. Sam Jackson Park Rd.
Portland, OR 97201
(503) 225-8382

PENNSYLVANIA
School of Nursing
Nursing Education Building
University of Pennsylvania
420 Service Drive, S2
Philadelphia, PA 19104
(215) 898-4335

SOUTH CAROLINA
Nurse-Midwifery Program
College of Nursing
Medical University of South Carolina
171 Ashley Ave.
Charleston, SC 29425
(803) 792-3066

TENNESSEE
Nurse-Midwifery Program
Department of Nursing Education
Meharry Medical College
10005 D.B. Todd Blvd., Box 61-A
Nashville, TN 37207
(615) 327-6494

TEXAS
Nurse-Midwifery Program
Baylor College of Medicine
1 Baylor Plaza
Houston, TX 77050
(713) 751-8257

UTAH
College of Nursing
Graduate Speciality in Nurse-Midwifery
University of Utah
25 S. Medical Drive
Salt Lake City, UT 84112
(801) 581-8274

SOURCE: *American College of Nurse-Midwives.*

BOOKS

Assertive Childbirth, **Susan McKay,**
Englewood Cliffs, NJ: Prentice Hall, 1983.

*The Baby Decision: How to Make the Most
Important Choice of Your Life,* **Merle
Bombardieri,** New York: Rawson Wade
Publishers, 1981.

Beating the Adoption Game, **Cynthia Martin,**
San Diego: Oaktree Publications, 1980.

*Birth Trap: The Legal Low-Down on High-
Tech Obstetrics,* **Y. Brackbill, J. Rice,** and
D. Young, St. Louis: Mosby Press, 1984.

*Childbirth With Love: A Complete Guide to
Fertility, Pregnancy, and Childbirth for
Caring Couples,* **Niels H. Lauersen,** New
York: Putnam's, 1983.

Conquering Infertility, **Dr. Stephen L.
Corson,** Norwalk, CT: Appleton-Century-
Crofts, 1983.

Coping with Infertility, **Judith A. Stigger,**
Minneapolis: Augsburg Publishing House,
1983.

The Fertility Handbook, **Aaron S. Lifchez,
M.D.,** and **Judith A. Fenton,** New York:
Clarkson N. Potter, 1980; One Park Ave.,
New York, NY 10016.

Getting Pregnant in the 1980s, **Robert H.
Glass** and **Ronald J. Ericsson,** Berkeley:
University of California Press, 1982.

A Good Birth, A Safe Birth, **Diana Korte** and
Roberta Scaer, New York: Bantam Books,
1984.

How to Get Pregnant, **Dr. Sherman J.
Silber,** New York: Charles Scribner's Sons,
1980.

Husband-Coached Childbirth, **Robert A.
Bradley, M.D.,** New York: Harper & Row,
1981.

Infertility: A Guide for the Childless Couple,
Barbara Eck Menning, Englewood Cliffs,
NJ: Prentice Hall, 1977. Menning is the
founder of RESOLVE, Inc.

*Making Babies: The New Science and Ethics of
Conception,* **Peter Singer** and **Deane Wells,**
New York: Charles Scribner's Sons, 1985.

*A Matter of Life: The Story of a Medical
Breakthrough,* **Robert Edwards** and
Patrick Steptoe, New York: William
Morris, 1980.

Natural Childbirth the Bradley Way, **Susan
McCutcheon-Rosegg,** New York: Dutton,
1984.

*New Conceptions: A Consumer's Guide to the
Newest Infertility Treatments,* **Lori B.
Andrews, J.D.,** New York: St. Martin's
Press, 1984.

New Hope for Problem Pregnancies, **Dianne
Hales** and **Robert K. Creasy,** New York:
Harper and Row, 1982.

Surviving Pregnancy Loss, **Rochelle
Friedman, M.D.,** and **Bonnie Gradstein,**
New York: Little Brown and Co., 1982.

What Every Pregnant Woman Should Know,
Gail Brewer and **Tom Brewer, M.D.,** New
York: Penguin Books, 1985.

*When Pregnancy Fails: Families Coping with
Miscarriage, Stillbirth and Infant Death,*
Susan Borg and **Judith Lasker,** Boston:
Beacon Press, 1981.

You Can *Have A Baby: Everything You Need
to Know About Fertility,* **Dr. Joseph H.
Bellina** and **Josleen Wilson,** New York:
Crown Publishers, 1985.

Your Search for Fertility, **Graham H.
Barker,** New York: Morrow, 1981.

MATERIALS FOR SALE

*How to Organize a Basic Study of the Infertile
Couple,* booklet detailing the kinds of tests
for infertility; though written for physicians,
it is instructive for couples.

*Report of the Ad Hoc Committee on Artificial
Insemination, 1980.*

Vasectomy: Facts About Male Sterilization

American Fertility Society
2131 Magnolia Ave.
Birmingham, AL 35256
(205) 251-9764

A Decade of Change in Cesarean Childbirth,
36 pages.

Education for Vaginal Birth After Cesarean, 4
  pages.
Frankly Speaking, 56 pages.
Planning for Birth, 6 pages.

C/SEC
22 Forest Rd.
Framingham, MA 01701
(617) 877-8266

The Directory of Alternative Birth Services and
  Consumer Guide

NAPSAC International
PO Box 429
Marble Hill, MO 63764

Fact sheets on:
Adoption
Artificial Insemination
Choosing a Specialist
Endometriosis
In Vitro Fertilization
Laparoscopy: What to Expect
Medical Evaluation of the Couple
Medical Management of Male Infertility
Miscarriage: Medical Facts
Semen Analysis
Surgical Techniques for Tubal Repair
Varicocele: Surgical and Medical Treatment

RESOLVE, Inc.
PO Box 474
Belmont, MA 02178
(617) 484-2424

KIDNEY DISEASES

Serious kidney and urinary tract diseases afflict more than 12 million Americans. About 10 out of every 100,000 Americans can expect to have kidney failure. It affects children and adults of all ages, even the newborn. Chronic kidney disease is on the rise; however, with dialysis and more recent successes with kidney transplants, kidney disease is becoming less often fatal, although it is rarely cured. Approximately 70,000 people are kept alive on dialysis therapy, and more than 6,000 have had successful kidney transplants. Dramatic advances in organ transplants promise life extension for more victims of kidney disease.

Cause: Since the kidneys have an important life-preserving function—they clean and filter the blood and help regulate blood pressure and blood content—they can be affected by any number of infections, toxins, other chronic diseases, and congenital defects. Infections of the kidneys, despite modern treatments, still kill about 8,000 persons a year and are the most common disorder of the kidneys and urinary tract. Up to 20 percent of all those who go on dialysis lose kidney function because of urinary tract infections.

Glomerulonephritis, usually called nephritis or Bright's disease, is an inflammation of the nephrons, the millions of small blood vessel filters that perform most of the kidneys' functions; the disease, often of unknown cause, can lead to kidney failure—requiring dialysis or transplantation. High blood pressure and the complications of diabetes are major causes of chronic kidney damage and degeneration. Obstructions, such as kidney stones, cysts, and genetic abnormalities, also can lead to much distress and serious damage. Poisonous chemicals and pharmaceutical drugs can suddenly or pro-gressively knock out kidney function, requiring lifesaving dialysis or other measures.

When the kidneys fail, they can no longer cleanse the blood; in cases of acute kidney failure, the person can be saved by short-term dialysis or other therapy in one out of two cases. When the damage is progressive and severe, it can result in what specialists call "end-stage renal disease": Without an artificial kidney (dialysis) or a kidney transplant, the person can be expected to die within a few months.

Symptoms: Increased frequency of urination; bloody urine; pain when urinating; gradual swelling, notably around the ankles; puffiness around the eyes (especially in children); lower back pain below the rib cage; high blood pressure (which can be a cause as well as a symptom of kidney disease).

Diagnosis: Most kidney diseases can be spotted by urine and blood tests, X-rays, and, if needed, kidney biopsy—removal and examination of kidney cells under a microscope.

Treatment: Drugs, surgery, radiation, and the full armament of modern medicine are used in treating various kinds of kidney diseases. Because of recent research, there is a new interest in specialized diets to prevent the progression of kidney disease. A restriction of high-protein and phosphate foods is believed to retard the loss of kidney function and is being intensively studied.

In end-stage disease there are two major life-saving therapies—dialysis and kidney transplant. Dialysis is more common; blood is purified periodically by techniques that mimic the kidneys'. Dialysis may be done at home, in a kidney dialysis center, or in a hospital. It can be done through the veins (hemodialysis) or through the abdominal cavity (peritoneal dialysis).

CONTINUOUS AMBULATORY PERITONEAL DIALYSIS (CAPD)

Recently, a simple technique—requiring no electricity, machinery, blood-thinning drugs, or technicians—was developed, which allows patients to perform their own dialysis without being tied down to a machine. The technique is called continuous ambulatory peritoneal dialysis (CAPD). A catheter is permanently inserted into the peritoneal cavity and attached to a small plastic bag that is empty most of the time and is worn under the patient's clothes. The patient drains used dialysis solution from the abdominal cavity into the bag three to five times a day and attaches a fresh bag of solution, which is transferred into the peritoneal cavity where it accomplishes the same kind of blood cleansing as the kidneys. This technique allows patients to walk around and perform normal activities while their blood is being cleansed. There have been some reports of complications. However, these are becoming less frequent and serious. It is expected that many patients now on conventional dialysis will use CAPD.

For more information on CAPD, contact:

Dr. Karl D. Nolph
Director, Division of Nephrology
Clinical Coordinating Center of the NIH
    CAPD Registry
Department of Medicine
University of Missouri Health Sciences Center
Columbia, MO 65212
(314) 882–7991

The center has published a *CAPD Travel Guide*, listing CAPD centers in the United States and foreign countries.

KIDNEY TRANSPLANTS

Of all the kidney treatments, kidney transplants are the most dramatic and, if successful, the most effective; they allow the person to proceed with life free of most of the complications of kidney disease. In recent years, transplants from relatives (a so-called "matched" kidney) have been successful in prolonging life for as long as five years in about 70 percent of the cases. That is compared with an in-center dialysis five-year survival rate of 36 percent.

The main hazard of kidney transplant is rejection: The patient's immune system mobilizes to destroy the foreign tissue. New drugs, such as cyclosporine, are often successful in controlling the patient's immune system, allowing the transplanted organ to survive. Some predict that new selective immune-suppressing drugs will make kidney transplants about 90 percent successful in the near future. Preservation of the kidneys prior to transplant can be a problem, and kidneys for transplant are in short supply. Thousands of people who could benefit from kidney transplants have died because there are not enough organs to go around.

How to donate your kidneys

To donate your kidneys after your death, contact the National Kidney Foundation for a donor card.

National Kidney Foundation
2 Park Ave.
New York, NY 10016
(212) 889–2210

SOME LEADING KIDNEY TRANSPLANT SPECIALISTS AND CENTERS

The following centers, according to federal government records, have generally done about 50 or more kidney transplants a year, designating them as leaders and pioneers in the field. Although you may not need a transplant, you may still benefit from knowing which centers are performing the most kidney transplants. These centers are usually staffed with experts in all kinds of kidney diseases.

ALABAMA
Nephrology Research and Training Center
University of Alabama School of Medicine
University Station
Birmingham, AL 35294
(205) 934-3653
Robert G. Luke, M.D.

ARIZONA
Good Samaritan Medical Center
1033 E. McDowell Rd.
Phoenix, AZ 85006
(602) 239-4336
Ben A. Vander Werf, M.D., Phoenix
   Transplant Center

CALIFORNIA
St. Vincent's Medical Center
2131 W. Third St.
Los Angeles, CA 90057
(213) 483-7707
Robert Mendez, M.D., Chairman, Renal
   Transplantation

UCLA Center for Health Sciences
10833 LeConte Ave.
Los Angeles, CA 90024
(213) 825-3430
Leon G. Fine, M.D., Division of Nephrology

University Hospital
UCSD Medical Center
225 Dickinson St.
San Diego, CA 92103
(619) 294-6628
Nicholas Halasz, M.D.

Presbyterian Hospital
Pacific Medical Center
2333 Buchanan St.
San Francisco, CA 94115
(415) 563-4321, x2915
Barry Levin, M.D., Medical Director
Derek Sampson, M.D., Geoffrey Collins,
   M.D., Surgeons

Department of Medicine
University of California—San Francisco
San Francisco, CA 94143
(415) 666-2172
Floyd C. Rector, M.D.

COLORADO
Department of Medicine
University of Colorado Medical Center
4200 E. Ninth Ave.
Denver, CO 80220
(303) 394-7203
Robert W. Schrier, M.D.

DISTRICT OF COLUMBIA
Department of Medicine
Georgetown University Hospital
3800 Reservoir Rd., N.W.
Washington, DC 20007
(202) 625-7257
George E. Schreiner, M.D.

Washington Hospital Center
110 Irving St., N.W.
Washington D.C. 20010
(202) 541-6058
Jimmy Light, M.D.

FLORIDA
Department of Medicine
Shands Hospital
Gainesville, FL 32610
(904) 392-3756
C. Craig Tisher, M.D., Adult Nephrology
George A. Richard, M.D., Pediatric
   Nephrology
Jackson Memorial Hospital
1611 N.W. 12th Ave.
Miami, FL 33136
(305) 547-6315
Les Orson, M.D.

Tampa General Hospital
Davis Islands
Tampa, FL 33606
(813) 253-0711
John R. Ackerman, M.D.

GEORGIA
Department of Medicine—Nephrology
Emory University School of Medicine
69 Butler St., S.E.
Atlanta, GA 30303
(404) 588-4700
Edmund Bourke, M.D.

ILLINOIS

Section of Nephrology
Department of Medicine
The University of Chicago
950 East 59th St.
Chicago, IL 60637
(312) 962-1051
Fredric L. Coe, M.D.
Adrian I. Katz, M.D.

University of Illinois Hospital
1740 W. Taylor St.,
Chicago, IL 60612
(312) 996-6771
Martin Mozes, M.D.

INDIANA

Renal Division
Department of Medicine
Indiana University Medical Center
1100 W. Michigan St.
Indianapolis, IN 46223
(317) 264-7453
Stuart A. Kleit, M.D.

IOWA

Department of Medicine
University Hospitals
University of Iowa College of Medicine
Iowa City, IA 52242
(319) 356-4409
John B. Stokes, III, M.D.

KANSAS

St. Francis Hospital
929 N. St. Francis Ave.
Wichita, KS 67214
(316) 268-5890
Charles Shield, M.D.

KENTUCKY

Renal Division
Department of Medicine
University of Kentucky Medical Center
Lexington, KY 40506
(606) 233-6677
Bruce Lucas, M.D., Renal Transplant Program

LOUISIANA

Tulane Medical Center Hospital
1415 Tulane Ave.
New Orleans, LA 70112
(504) 588-5303
Edward Etheredge, M.D.

MARYLAND

Johns Hopkins Hospital
600 N. Wolfe St.
Baltimore, MD 21205
(301) 955-5165
G. Melville Williams, M.D.

MASSACHUSETTS

Renal Unit
Department of Medicine
Massachusetts General Hospital
Boston, MA 02114
(617) 726-3772
Dennis A. Ausiello, M.D.

Department of Medicine
Peter Brent Brigham Hospital
721 Huntington Ave.
Boston, MA 02115
(617) 732-5850
Barry M. Brenner, M.D.

MICHIGAN

Department of Internal Medicine (Renal Unit)
University of Michigan Medical Center
1405 E. Ann St.
Ann Arbor, MI 48109
(313) 764-4160
Richard L. Tannen, M.D.

Division of Nephrology
Department of Medicine
Henry Ford Hospital
2799 W. Grand Blvd.
Detroit, MI 48202
(313) 876-2600
Nathan W. Levin, M.D.

MINNESOTA

Regional Kidney Disease Program
701 Park Ave.
Minneapolis, MN 55415
(612) 347-5800
Robert Christian Andersen, M.D.

University of Minnesota Hospital
Minneapolis, MN 55455
(612) 373-7652
Robert L. Vernier, M.D.
Alfred F. Michael, M.D.

Rochester Methodist Hospital
201 W. Center St.
Rochester, MN 55902
(507) 284-2511
Sylvester Sterioff, M.D.

NEW JERSEY
Department of Medicine
College of Medicine & Dentistry of New
   Jersey
100 Bergen St.
Newark, NJ 07107
(201) 456-4100
Norman Lasker, M.D.

Newark Beth Israel Medical Center
201 Lyons Ave.
Newark, NJ 07112
(201) 926-7555
Hossein Eslami, M.D.

NEW YORK
Department of Medicine
Albany Medical College
Albany, NY 12208
(518) 445-5176
M. Donald McGoldrick, M.D.

Department of Medicine
Montefiore Medical Center
111 E. 210 St.
Bronx, NY 10467
(212) 920-5442
Norman Bank, M.D.

The Brooklyn Hospital
121 DeKalb Ave.
Brooklyn, NY 11205
(718) 403-8160
Mary DelMonte, M.D.

Department of Pediatrics
New York Hospital
Cornell Medical Center
525 E. 68th St.
New York, NY 10021
(212) 472-5400
Matthew R. Kaplan, M.D.

Presbyterian Hospital
622 W. 168th St.
New York, NY 10032
(212) 305-6469
Mark Hardy, M.D.

NORTH CAROLINA
Division of Nephrology
Department of Medicine
Duke University Medical Center
Durham, NC 27710
(919) 684-2116
Vincent W. Dennis, M.D.

OHIO
University Hospital
234 Goodman St.
Cincinnati, OH 45267
(513) 872-4156
J. Wesley Alexander, M.D.

Department of Hypertension and Nephrology
Cleveland Clinic Foundation
9500 Euclid Avenue
Cleveland, OH 44106
(216) 444-6764
Ray W. Gifford, Jr., M.D.

University Hospitals of Cleveland
2074 Abington Rd.
Cleveland, OH 44106
(216) 844-3689
James Schulak, M.D.

Division of Nephrology
Department of Medicine
The Ohio State University Hospital
410 W. 10th Ave.
Columbus, OH 43210
(614) 421-4997
Lee A. Hebert, M.D.

OREGON
Department of Medicine
University of Oregon
Health Sciences Center
Portland, OR 97201
(503) 225-8490
William M. Bennett, M.D.

PENNSYLVANIA
Albert Einstein Medical Center
York & Tabor Rds.
Philadelphia, PA 19141
(215) 457-4444
Aaron D. Bannett, M.D.

Department of Medicine
Hospital of the University of Pennsylvania
3600 Spruce St.
Philadelphia, PA 19104
(215) 662-3601
Zaiman S. Agus, M.D.

Thomas Jefferson University Hospital
11th & Walnut St.
Philadelphia, PA 19107
(215) 928-8813
Bruce Jarrell, M.D.

Presbyterian-University Hospital
39th & Market Sts.
Pittsburgh, PA 15213
(412) 624-2682
Thomas R. Hakala, M.D.

TENNESSEE
University of Tennessee
Center for the Health Sciences
951 Court Ave.
Memphis, TN 38103
(901) 528-5764
Fred E. Hatch, Jr., M.D.

Department of Medicine
Division of Nephrology
Vanderbilt University Hospital
Nashville, TN 37232
(615) 322-4794
Richard L. Gibson, M.D.

TEXAS
Methodist Central Hospital
301 W. Colorado Blvd.
Dallas, TX 75265
(214) 944-8181
Pedro Vergne-Marini, M.D.

Parkland Memorial Hospital
5201 Harry Hines Blvd.
Dallas, TX 75235
(214) 688-2754
J. Harold Helderman, M.D.

Department of Pediatrics
University of Texas
Health Sciences Center
Southwestern Medical School
5323 Harry Hines Blvd.
Dallas, TX 75235
(214) 688-3438
Ronald J. Hogg, M.D.

Department of Medicine
University of Texas Medical Branch
Galveston, TX 77550
(409) 761-1811
H. E. Sarles, M.D.
A. R. Remmers, Jr., M.D.

Texas Kidney Institute
Hermann Hospital
1203 Ross Sterling Ave.
Houston, TX 77030
(713) 797-4991
Barry Kahan, M.D.

Department of Medicine
University of Texas Health Science Center at
    San Antonio
7703 Floyd Curl Drive
San Antonio, TX 78284
(512) 691-6338
Jay Stein, M.D.

UTAH
LDS Hospital Transplant Center
325 Eighth Ave.
Salt Lake City, UT 84143
(801) 321-1234
Lawrence E. Stevens, M.D.

University of Utah Medical Center
50 N. Medical Drive
Salt Lake City, UT 84132
(801) 581-2634
Ed Nelson, M.D., Surgeon
Wayne Border, M.D., Nephrologist

VIRGINIA
Norfolk General Hospital
600 Gresham Drive
Norfolk, VA 23507
(804) 628-3906
Chris Silliman, M.D.

WISCONSIN
Nephrology Program
University Hospital H4514
600 Highland Ave.
Madison, WI 53792
(608) 263-3315
David P. Simpson, M.D.

Kurtis Froedtert Memorial Lutheran Hospitals
9200 Wisconsin Ave.
Milwaukee, WI 53226
(414) 259-3070
H.M. Kauffman, M.D.

SOURCE: *Author's compilation based on figures from the
Health Care Financing Administration.*

KIDNEY STONES

Kidney stones are one of our oldest and most painful maladies, and there is some evidence that they are on the rise. Two to 4 percent of the population can expect to have kidney stones at some time; more than one million Americans are hospitalized every year for treatment of kidney and urinary tract stones. About 95 percent of these stones occur in the kidneys; the other 5 percent occur in the bladder.

The stones are hard build ups, usually of calcium and oxalate. These stones can grow so large they cannot be passed out through the drainage tubes of the kidney and may obstruct the flow of urine, causing pain, infection, and kidney damage. Smaller stones may become lodged in the passageways from the kidneys; others may pass through, often with severe pain. Kidney stones can range in size from that of a grain of salt to a golf ball. The incidence of kidney stones varies with geographic location; they are particularly prevalent in the southeastern United States, commonly call the "stone belt." Three times more men get kidney stones than women.

Cause: The causes are complex and multiple and include diet, drinking too little fluid, climate, and heredity. The stones may be formed because of metabolic abnormalities, infections, or misuse of medications.

Symptoms: Sudden, severe pain is the most common symptom, often in the back, side, and groin. There may be blood in the urine and soreness and tenderness in the abdomen; if urinary tract infection is present, there may also be fever, vomiting, nausea, loss of appetite, and chills.

Diagnosis: The physician can confirm the presence and position of the stone by X-ray and/or ultrasound.

Treatment: The first line of treatment is to try to flush out the stone by having the patient drink large amounts of fluid. In 90 percent of the cases the stone finally passes through, but the rest of the time a physician must remove or destroy the stones. There is the possibility of recurrence. Research shows that if there is just one stone, chances are only one in five that the person will develop another stone in five years. If there is more than one stone, the risk of developing additional stones within five years rises to 80 percent. Part of the treatment for kidney stones is trying to prevent further formation through a change in diet or with drugs.

As a last resort, surgery to remove kidney stones is still performed, but other procedures are becoming increasingly common. Some experts predict that surgical removal may become a thing of the past. Urologists are now using needles and tubes instead of a scalpel to get small stones out, and they are destroying larger ones with shock waves. Many American medical centers are using a method developed in West Germany to break up kidney stones. The patient sits in a bath of water, and a powerful shock wave is administered to the precise position of the kidney stone, pulverizing it. The rest of the body is unharmed.

SPECIALISTS IN SHOCK-WAVE THERAPY

The equipment needed to pulverize the kidney stones is called a lithotripter. The following hospitals and medical centers have lithotripters and are pioneering the use of this new treatment for kidney stones.

ALABAMA
Dr. Derrill Crowe
Brookwood Medical Center
2010 Brookwood Drive
Birmingham, AL 35209
(205) 877-2714

Dr. William Cooner
Springhill Memorial Hospital
3719 Dauphin St.
Mobile, AL 36608
(205) 344-9630, x1884

ARIZONA
Dr. William W. Bohnert
St. Joseph's Hospital & Medical Center
Urology Department
PO Box 2071
Phoenix, AZ 85001-2071
(602) 264-4431

ARKANSAS
Dr. Tony Barnett
St. Vincent Infirmary
No. 2
St. Vincent Circle
Little Rock, AR 72205
(501) 664-1762

CALIFORNIA
Dr. Robert Roth
Lahey Clinic Medical Center
41 Mall Rd.
Burbank, CA 91505
(617) 273-8420

Dr. Peter Fugelso
St. Joseph Medical Center
Buena Vista & Alameda
Burbank, CA 91505
(818) 840-7945

Dr. Darrell W. Lange
Medical Director
Glendale Adventist Hospital
Kidney Stone Center of Southern California
1509 Wilson Terrace
Glendale, CA 91206
(818) 240-8000, x7922

Dr. David Coleman
Memorial Medical Center of Long Beach
2801 Atlantic Ave.
Long Beach, CA 90801-1428
(213) 595-3454

Professor Christian G. Chaussy, M.D.
UCLA Medical Center
School for Medicine
Division of Urology
10833 Le Conte Ave.
Los Angeles, CA 90024
(213) 825-1172

Dr. Dominique Manzoni
Los Gatos Community Rehabilitation Center
Los Gatos Community Hospital
815 Pollard Rd.
Los Gatos, CA 95030
(408) 378-6131, x 4045

Dr. Robert R. Dale
Los Gatos Surgical Center
15195 National Ave.
Los Gatos, CA 95030
(408) 356-6177

Dr. Joaquin Thuroff
UCSF—H.C. Moffitt Hospital
M418 Moffitt Hospital
505 Parnassus Ave.
San Francisco, CA 94143
(415) 476-8273

Dr. Robert Saffian
Medical Center of Tarzana (AMI-2)
Lithotripter Facility
18321 Clark St.
Tarzana, CA 91356
(818) 708-5444

FLORIDA
Dr. Martin Madonsky
North Broward Hospital
1625 S.E. Third Ave.
Fort Lauderdale, FL 33316
(800) 821-4224

Dr. Birdwell Finlayson
The University of Florida
1600 S.W. Archer Rd.
Gainesville, FL 32610
(904) 392-2501

Dr. James Porterfield
Florida Medical Plaza
2501 N. Orange Ave.
Orlando, FL 32804
(305) 897-1818

GEORGIA
Dr. Kenneth Walton
Emory University School of Medicine
Department of Urology
1365 Clifton Rd., N.E.
Atlanta, GA 30322
(404) 321-0111

Dr. Thomas Schoborg
Georgia Baptist Medical Center
Department of Urology
300 Boulevard, N.E.
Atlanta, GA 30312
(404) 524-5082

Dr. Ralph Newton
Coliseum Park Hospital
350 Hospital Drive
Macon, GA 31213
(912) 745-9461, x4877

Dr. Samuel Torres
Head Urologist
Memorial Medical Center
4700 Waters Ave.
Savannah, GA 31403
(912) 356-8000, x3341

ILLINOIS
Dr. C. McKiel, Jr.
Rush Presbyterian/St. Luke Medical Center
1753 W. Congress Parkway
Chicago, IL 60612
(312) 942-6447

Dr. John B. Graham
University of Chicago
Northwest Memorial Hospital
Passavant Pavilion
Chicago, IL 60611
(312) 962-3080

Dr. Robert Flinn
St. Francis Medical Center
530 N.E. Glen Oak Ave.
Peoria, IL 61637
(309) 673-1900

INDIANA
Dr. Daniel M. Newman
Methodist Hospital of Indiana
1604 N. Capital Ave.
Indianapolis, IN 46202
(317) 929-3692

IOWA
Dr. Stefan A. Loening
University of Iowa
Hospitals and Clinics
Department of Urology
Newton Rd.
Iowa City, IA 52242
(319) 356-2226, 1616

KENTUCKY
Dr. John Hubbard
Head Urologist
Humana Hospital
4001 Dutchmans Lane
Louisville, KY 40207
(502) 893-1180

LOUISIANA
Dr. Raju Thomas
Louisiana Lithotripter, Inc.
Tulane University
1415 Tulane Ave., 3rd Floor
New Orleans, LA 70112
(504) 587-7666

Dr. William Brannan
Oschner Clinic
1514 Jefferson Highway
New Orleans, LA 70121
(504) 838-4083

MASSACHUSETTS
Dr. Stephen Dretler
Massachusetts General
Ambulatory Care Center
Fruit St.
Boston, MA 02114
(617) 726-3512

Dr. Robert Roth
Lahey Clinic Medical Center
41 Mall Rd.
Burlington, MA 01803
(617) 273-8420

MICHIGAN
Dr. Edward McGuire
University of Michigan
A. Alfred Taubman Medical Health Center
1500 E. Medical Center Drive
Box 0330
Ann Arbor, MI 48109
(313) 936-5765

Dr. Ray Littleton
Henry Ford Hospital
2799 W. Grand Blvd.
Detroit, MI 48202
(313) 876-2062

MINNESOTA
Dr. John Hulberg
University of Minnesota Hospital
Mayo Memorial Building
420 Delaware St., S.E.
Minneapolis, MN 54455
(612) 373-8780

Dr. Joseph W. Segura
The Mayo Clinic/St. Mary's Hospital
Department of Urology
100 First St., S.W.
Rochester, MN 55905
(507) 286-2511

MISSOURI
Dr. Ralph Clayman
Barnes Hospital
Barnes Hospital Plaza
St. Louis, MO 63110
(314) 362-8209

NEW JERSEY
Dr. Louis Keeler
Mid-Atlantic Kidney Stone Center
Garden State Community Medical Center
1 Brick Rd.
Marlton, NJ 08053
(609) 983-7337

NEW YORK
Dr. William R. Fair
The New York Hospital
525 E. 68th St.
New York, NY 10023
(212) 472-2272

NORTH CAROLINA
Dr. J. Weinerth
Duke University Medical Center
Box 3343
Durham, NC 27710
(919) 684-4157

Dr. William Jordan
Highsmith-Rainey Hospital
150 Roberson St.
Fayetteville, NC 28301
(919) 485-8871

Dr. Frederick Howell
President
Hawthorne Medical Mall
1901 S. Hawthorne Rd.
Winston-Salem, NC 27103
(919) 768-8821

Dr. David McCullough
North Carolina Baptist Hospital
300 S. Hawthorne Rd.
Winston-Salem, NC 27103
(919) 748-4131

OHIO
Dr. Inayat Malik
Bethesda Oak Hospital
619 Oak St.
Cincinnati, OH 45206
(513) 569-6050

Dr. Steven Streem
Dr. Martin Resnick
Dr. Jerard DeOreo
Calcilex Corporation
10605 Carnegie Ave.
Cleveland, OH 44106
(216) 444-2420

Dr. Henry A. Wise, II
Ohio Kidney Stone Management, Inc.
Ohio Kidney Stone Center
3525 Olentangy River Rd.
Columbus, OH 43214
(614) 462-2216

Dr. Richard Tapper
Genito-Urinary Surgeons
Toledo Hospital
3939 Monroe St.
Toledo, OH 43606
(419) 473-2651

PENNSYLVANIA
Dr. Alan J. Wein
University of Pennsylvania
School of Medicine
5 Silverstein
2400 Spruce St.
Philadelphia, PA 19104
(215) 662-2891

TENNESSEE
Dr. Aubra D. Branson
HCA–Park West Hospital
Park West Professional Building
9320 Park West Blvd.
Knoxville, TN 37923
(615) 690-5152

Dr. Robert McLellan
Baptist Hospital
2000 Church St.
Nashville, TN 37236
(615) 329-7300

TEXAS
Dr. James Cochran
Presbyterian Hospital
Lithotripter Center S.W., Inc.
8220 Walnut Hill Lane
ESWL Suite 214
Dallas, TX 75231
(214) 691-1902

Dr. Donald P. Griffith
The Baylor College
Methodist Hospital
One Baylor Plaza
Houston, TX 77030
(713) 799-4001

VIRGINIA
Dr. Jay Gillenwater
University of Virginia
School of Medicine
Jefferson Park Ave.
Charlottesville, VA 22908
(804) 924-2224

WASHINGTON
Dr. Robert Gibbons
VA Mason Kidney Stone Center
PO Box 900
Seattle, WA 98111-0900
(206) 624-1144

CANADA
V.A. Rowley, M.D.
Vancouver General Hospital
Centennial Pavilion
855 W. 12th Ave.
Vancouver, B.C. V5Z 1M9
Canada

SOURCE: *National Kidney Foundation.*

GOVERNMENT-SPONSORED KIDNEY STONE RESEARCH CENTERS

The National Institutes of Health supports three centers specializing in kidney stone research.

University of Chicago
Michael Reese Medical Centers
2929 S. Ellis Ave.
Chicago, IL 60616
Frederic Coe, M.D.
(312) 791-2000

University of Florida
Gainesville, FL 32610
Birdwell Finlayson, M.D.
(904) 392-2501

University of Texas Health Science Center
5323 Harry Hines Blvd.
Dallas, TX 75235
Charles Pak, M.D.
(214) 688-3111

ORGANIZATIONS

American Kidney Fund
7315 Wisconsin Ave.
Bethesda, MD 20814-3266
(301) 986-1444
(800) 638-8299
(800) 492-8361 (in Maryland)

A national nonprofit voluntary organization offering educational materials and financial assis-

tance to kidney patients who demonstrate need. Will provide information upon request.

National Association of Patients on
  Hemodialysis and Transplantation, Inc.
150 Nassau St.
New York, NY 10038
(212) 619-2727

A national voluntary membership organization for patients with kidney disease. A number of local chapters throughout the country, formed to give mutual support. Source of information for patients, their families, other interested persons. Pamphlets, a monthly news magazine. Special services: sponsors a children's camp for those on dialysis: maintains an up-to-date list of dialysis centers worldwide which accept transient patients. Will provide more information upon request.

The National Kidney Foundation
2 Park Ave.
New York, NY 10016
(212) 889-2210

A national organization for kidney patients, health professionals and others interested in kidney diseases, 54 local affiliates that conduct patient service programs and make referrals. Numerous brochures, quarterly newsletter, medical journals. Conducts an organ donor program. Will provide more information upon request.

BOOKS

Gary Coleman: Medical Miracle, **The Coleman Family** and **Bill Davidson,** New York: Coward, McCann & Geohegan, 1983.

The Gourmet Renal Nutrition Cookbook, **edited by Meredith C. Greene, R.D.,** New York: Lenox Hill Hospital, 1983; Lenox Hill Hospital, Dialysis Unit, 100 E. 77th St., New York, NY 10021.

Just What the Doctor Ordered: Gourmet Recipes Developed with Boston's Beth Israel Hospital for Low-Calorie, Diabetic, Low-Fat, Low-Cholesterol, Low-Sodium, Bland, High-Fiber and Renal Diets, **Harriet Wilinsky Goodman** and **Barbara Morse,** New York: Holt, Rinehart and Winston, 1983.

A Patient's Guide to Dialysis and

Transplantation, **Roger Gabriel, M.D.,** Hingham, MA: Kluwer Boston, 1983; Kluwer Boston, Inc., 190 Old Derby St., Hingham, MA 02043.

Understanding Your New Life With Dialysis: A Patient's Guide for Physical and Psychological Adjustment, **Edith T. Oberley** and **Terry D. Oberley,** Springfield, IL: Charles C. Thomas, 1983.

When Your Kidneys Fail: A Handbook for Patients and Their Families, **Mickie Hall Faris,** Los Angeles: National Kidney Foundation, 1982; a comprehensive guide; National Kidney Foundation of Southern California, 6820 La Tijero Blvd. Suite 111, Los Angeles, CA 90045.

MATERIALS, FREE AND FOR SALE

Free (single copies)

Children and Kidney Disease, 22 pages.
Diabetes and the Kidneys, 12 pages.
Dialysis Patient, 7 pages.
Facts About Kidney Diseases and Their Treatment, 18 pages
Facts About Kidney Stones, 6 pages.
Give A Kidney, leaflet.
High Blood Pressure and Its Effects on the Kidneys, 6 pages.
''The Kid,'' 16 pages (for children).

American Kidney Fund
7315 Wisconsin Ave.
Bethesda, MD 20814-3266

Prevention and Treatment of Kidney Stones, 16 pages.
Understanding Urinary Tract Infections, 12 pages.

National Institute of Diabetes and Digestive and Kidney Diseases
9000 Rockville Pike, Building 31, Room 9A04
Bethesda, MD 20892
(301) 496-3583

About Kidney Stones, 6 pages.
Dialysis, 6 pages.
How Can Urinary Tract Obstructions Affect You?, 6 pages.
If You Needed a Kidney or Other Vital Organ

to Live, Would You Be Able To Get One?, 6
  pages.
Questions Parents Ask About Nephrosis, 10
  pages.
Transplantation, 6 pages.
What Everyone Should Know About Kidneys,
  16 pages.
*Working with Kidney Failure: Rehabilitation
  and Employment*, 10 pages.

National Kidney Foundation
2 Park Ave.
New York, NY 10016
(212) 889-2210

For sale

NA-K, Sodium-Potassium Counter, 11 pages; a
  food reference for the dialysis patient.
Living With Renal Failure, 6 pages.
Renal Failure and Diabetes, 6 pages.

National Association of Patients on
  Hemodialysis and Transplantation, Inc.
150 Nassau St., Suite 1305
New York, NY 10038
(212) 619-2727

LEPROSY

Leprosy (Hansen's disease) is an infectious disease that afflicts about 12 million people around the world, notably in Asia and Africa, and is of increasing concern in the United States. An unprecedented number of new cases of leprosy were reported in the United States in 1982, mainly due to the immigration of persons from areas where leprosy is prevalent. Most of the new cases originate in those entering the country from Central and South America, the Philippines, and Asia. Most of the American victims contracted the disease overseas. Currently, about 5,000 persons in the United States are being treated for leprosy.

Cause: Bacteria *(Mycobacterium leprae)* attack the skin and peripheral nerves. Despite its reputation for being highly contagious, leprosy rarely afflicts more than 1 percent of any population; the overwhelming majority of any population is not susceptible to the infection. For susceptible individuals, leprosy can spread readily by airborne droplets and perhaps by skin-to-skin contact. The infectious agent has an incubation period of a few months to perhaps 20 years; the average is three to five years.

Symptoms: Nerve damage with loss of sensation; paralysis; skin lesions; deformities of face, hands and feet; and blindness. If treated promptly and properly there is no disfigurement, and the disease is rarely fatal.

Diagnosis: The disease is diagnosed by a pattern of symptoms, skin smears, and biopsies of the skin and nerve lesions. In the past, diagnosis was often delayed, allowing the disease to get a damaging hold on the patient. Diagnosis today is made, on the average, within six months.

Treatment: Unquestionably, leprosy is not the scourge it was in ancient times, although in many countries the infection is still inadequately treated. Modern drugs have done wonders to defeat leprosy but not to eradicate it. Experts say that with the combination of several drugs used in the United States, even the most severe leprosy infections can be cured. Surgery is sometimes performed to repair damage in severe cases.

WHERE TO FIND TREATMENT FOR LEPROSY

There is a single major treatment, research, and educational center for leprosy. It is operated by the federal government and is located in Louisiana. All cases are reported to this center, and those who need hospitalization and extensive treatment, such as rehabilitative surgery, or who do not respond to other treatments are often referred to this center by their physicians.

National Hansen's Disease Center
Carville, LA 70721
(504) 642-7771
(800) 642-2477 (physicians and patients)

In recent years the center has set up satellite regional centers around the country that also treat leprosy, and people who require only outpatient care are usually treated at these centers.

REGIONAL LEPROSY CENTERS

ARIZONA
Maricopa County Health Department
1825–1845 E. Roosevelt
Phoenix, AZ 85006
Douglas Campos-Outcalt, M.D.
(602) 258-6381

CALIFORNIA
Seton Medical Center
1900 Sullivan Ave.
Daley City, CA 94015
Robert Gelber, M.D.
(415) 991-6652

County of Los Angeles
Department of Health Services
1175 N. Cummings St.
Los Angeles, CA 90033
Thomas Rea, M.D.
(213) 226-5261

North San Diego Health Center
2440 Grand Ave.
San Diego, CA 92109
Antonia Lopez, M.D.
(619) 274-1223

FLORIDA
University of Miami
Department of Dermatology
1611 N.W. 12th Ave.
Miami, FL 33136
Francisco Ramos-Caro, M.D.
(305) 547-5958

HAWAII
State of Hawaii
Department of Health
3650 Maunalei Ave.
Honolulu, HI 96816
Ron Metler, M.D.
(808) 735-2473

ILLINOIS
University of Illinois
College of Medicine
840 S. Wood St.
Chicago, IL 60612
Sophie Worobec, M.D.
(312) 996-0193

LOUISIANA
New Orleans Home and Rehabilitation Center
612 Henry Clay Ave.
New Orleans, LA 70118
Robert Jacobson, M.D.
(504) 895-4833

MASSACHUSETTS
Brighton Marine Public Health Center
77 Warren St.
Brighton, MA 02135
Donald Lucas, M.D.
(617) 782-3400

NEW YORK
Bayley Seton Hospital
Bay and Vanderbilt Sts.
Staten Island, NY 10304
William Levis, M.D.
(718) 390-5757

PUERTO RICO
University of Puerto Rico
Department of Dermatology
GPO Box 5067
San Juan, PR 00936
Pablo Almodovar, M.D.
(809) 765-7950

TEXAS
Texas Department of Health
1100 W. 49th
Austin, TX 78756
Luis Escobedo, M.D.
(512) 458-7455

WASHINGTON
Pacific Medical Center
1200 12th Ave. S.
Seattle, WA 98144
James P. Harnisch, M.D.
(206) 326-4142

OTHER PUBLIC AND PRIVATE TREATMENT CENTERS

University of South Florida
Medical Center
12901 N. 30th St.
Box 19
Tampa, FL 33612
Bienvenido Yangco, M.D.
(813) 974-4096

Cook County Hospital
Division of Dermatology
1835 W. Harrison St.
Chicago, IL 60612
Sidney Barsky, M.D.
(312) 633-6000

Bellevue Hospital
Department of Dermatology
Tropical Medicine/HD Clinic
First Ave. & 28th St.
New York, NY 10016
Miguel Sanchez, M.D.
(212) 340-5245

Hansen's Disease Clinic
Department of Dermatology
Oregon Health Sciences Unit
3181 S.W. Sam Jackson Drive
Park Road
Portland, OR 97201
Frank Parker, M.D., William Marriott, M.D.
(503) 225-8597

SOURCE: *National Hansen's Disease Center.*

ORGANIZATION

American Leprosy Missions
1 Broadway
Elmwood Park, NJ 07407
(201) 794-8650

A nonprofit international donor-supported organization, dedicated to finding people with leprosy and helping them get treatment and rehabilitation. Works extensively overseas. Provides medical reprints and audiovisual materials. More information upon request.

MATERIALS FOR SALE

So You Have Hansen's Disease, 44-minute videotape (Beta or VHS). *The Star,* bimonthly magazine covering the medical questions.

National Hansen's Disease Center
Carville, LA 70721

LUNG DISEASES

See also Asthma and Allergies, page 84, Cancer, page 124, Smoking, page 506.

More than nine million Americans have a frightening disease in which they literally cannot breathe. They cannot get enough air into or out of their lungs: Insufficient amounts of oxygen circulate in the bloodstream, starving tissues. The general term for this condition is chronic obstructive pulmonary disease (COPD) or chronic obstructive lung disease (COLD). Because of increased smoking, air pollution, and exposure to environmental and occupational chemicals, such pulmonary damage is the fastest growing cause of death and disability in this century. The diseases, including emphysema and chronic bronchitis, account for about 66,000 deaths a year, making them the fifth leading cause of death. The number of deaths has jumped by 60 percent since 1968.

Typical victims are men (about 80 percent), but the death rate for women with these diseases has taken an alarming jump recently, due to increased cigarette smoking. The progressive lung destruction takes a long time to show up; symptoms usually don't become apparent or troublesome before age 50 or 60. However, by that time much of the lung damage is irreversible.

EMPHYSEMA AND BRONCHITIS

The causes of chronic bronchitis and emphysema are essentially the same. The mechanisms and the symptoms of the two diseases are slightly different. In chronic bronchitis, the major breathing apparatus—the tubes leading into the lungs—are inflamed, swollen, and blocked by thick secretions. The persistent cough, the well-known "smoker's hack," is a warning sign that damage is occurring. In emphysema, the smaller internal tissues, the airways and air sacs, are damaged or destroyed. The air sacs can be destroyed without warning signs, and the destruction is irreversible. Further destruction can be prevented by stopping smoking or avoiding other harmful chemical exposures.

Cause: It is generally agreed that cigarette smoking is primarily at fault. Physicians say it is almost unheard of for a lifetime *nonsmoker* to develop such lung damage. Stopping smoking slows the progression of the disease. Air pollutants—sulfur dioxide, nitrous oxide, cotton dust, aerosols, and other gases and chemicals—are thought to bring on or aggravate COPD. People who smoke and also inhale such pollutants are at added risk. Certain people, for genetic reasons, also have a deficiency of an enzyme inhibitor, alpha-1-antitrypsin, which makes them extraordinarily susceptible to such lung diseases. Some lung tissue destruction occurs in all smokers. It is not known why the disease is progressive and fatal in some, and not others.

Symptoms: Since the lung damage develops gradually over several decades, the symptoms may be ignored until the lung destruction is permanent. The main symptom of emphysema is shortness of breath with special difficulty in exhaling. Because of the destruction of tissue in the small airways where gases are exchanged, air is often trapped in the lungs, leading to the typical barrel chest of sufferers of emphysema. The major symptom of chronic bronchitis is the persistent coughing up of a thick, yellow-greenish sputum over a three-month period for two successive years. Death usually results from infections or complications, such as a heart attack, possibly brought on by electrolyte or blood-gas imbalances. Survival time depends on the impairment of lung function. If lung function is one-third of normal, about two out of three patients under age 65 will probably survive five years. And those who survive five years have a 50/50 chance of living another five years.

Diagnosis: Unfortunately, most serious obstructive lung disease is discovered after damage is extensive. Chest X-rays will not detect emphysema or chronic bronchitis in the early stages. Usually doctors depend on a medical history and pulmonary function tests, particularly spirometry (which measures how rapidly and how much air flows out of the lungs) for diagnosis. No tests detect the disease before from 40 to 60 percent of the damage is done.

Treatment: There is no cure; treatment is aimed at relieving the symptoms and trying to retard progress of the disease. Drugs are used, notably theophylline, which can dramatically alleviate symptoms in some patients but has little or no effect on many others. Several new experimental drugs are being developed including some that may help block the biochemical imbalance leading to the destruction of lung tissue in emphysema.

Additionally, there are promising experiments in replacing the critical alpha-1-antitrypsin in those who are genetically deficient.

Better techniques for managing the disease are appearing. Many people with chronic obstructive pulmonary disease can now be mobile, thanks to a new system developed by Dr. Henry Heimlich, a surgeon and inventor of the "Heimlich Maneuver," a lifesaving procedure for choking victims. With the new system called the Heimlich Micro-Trach (HMT), patients ordinarily housebound to large oxygen tanks can go out and stay out for several hours by carrying a portable oxygen supply in a six-pound shoulder bag. The system improves and usually extends the patient's life.

For more information on the HMT oxygen delivery system and physicians who are outfitting patients with the system, send a self-addressed stamped enveloped to:

Dr. Henry Heimlich
Heimlich Institute
Xavier University
PO Box 8858
Cincinnati, OH 45208
(513) 531-1053

For many with chronic obstructive pulmonary disease, expert, comprehensive care from a team of professionals equipped to handle what is called "pulmonary rehabilitation" may make the difference between whether a person is bedridden or able to function at maximum, even if limited, ability.

Many medical centers have pulmonary rehabilitation teams to deal with the problem, either in a hospital or on an outpatient basis. The large centers often have a multidisciplinary team that includes not only an expert clinician but also such specialists as a professional nurse, respiratory therapist, physical therapist, occupational therapist, dietitian, social worker and cardiopulmonary technologist as well.

The purpose of such care is to restore functioning as much as possible, and to ward off infections. The care includes instruction in hygiene of the bronchial tubes and proper methods of breathing. Drugs are administered if necessary, notably antibiotics to fight infections, and steroids. Patients learn how to use respiratory equipment, including bronchodilators to help open breathing passages. Exercises often improve breathing, and dramatically increase a patient's ability to walk and climb stairs. Whether such a care program increases survivability is controversial, but it can greatly improve the quality of life during the illness.

OCCUPATIONAL LUNG DISEASES

A number of serious lung diseases are associated with various occupations. Workers' lungs are scarred after years of inhaling tiny particles of foreign substances. These diseases are categorized as pneumoconioses and have similar symptoms and treatments, although the inhaled substances are different.

Asbestosis: A progressive lung disease caused by breathing particles of asbestos into the lungs over a period of years. About 11 million American workers have been exposed to asbestos. It may take 15 to 20 years after exposure for the symptoms to appear. It is most common in workers exposed to asbestos from jobs in mining, milling, construction, or repair of brake linings. Cigarette smokers are especially susceptible. Symptoms usually appear before the disease can be spotted by X-rays. The first symptom is shortness of breath after exertion, followed by a dry cough, chest pain, recurring respiratory infections, and heart failure due to an enlarged heart. Asbestos particles in the lungs may also cause mesothelioma, an incurable cancer of the lining of the lung.

Silicosis: A progressive lung disease caused by inhaling silica dust (mostly from quartz) for many years (usually 10 or more years), silicosis is frequently found in foundry workers, boiler scalers, and stonecutters. The tiny particles cannot be processed by the lungs and destroy lung tissue. Early symptoms are shortness of breath, especially after exercising and a dry cough (notably in the morning). Later, there may be central nervous system changes, such as confusion and lethargy, and disturbed sleep. Diagnosis is usually made by chest X-rays, revealing nodules in the lungs, and pulmonary function tests. The disease is incurable. It is treated by trying to relieve symptoms and prevent infections. Sufferers from silicosis are susceptible to tuberculosis.

Black lung disease (coal worker's pneumoconiosis): This progressive lung disease is caused by breathing coal dust particles, usually over a period of 15 or more years. The disease may be present without symptoms for some time. Later, victims may cough up an inky black, coal-flecked, or gray sputum and be plagued by shortness of breath, wheezing, and development of a barrel chest. Complications include heart failure, tuberculosis, and, in cigarette smokers, possible emphysema and chronic bronchitis. Diagnosis is made by X-rays and pulmonary function studies. Treatment tries to relieve respiratory symptoms through bronchodilator therapy, drugs, and physical therapy techniques. Therapy is also aimed at controlling infections.

WHERE TO FIND TREATMENT FOR LUNG DISEASES

For some leading sources of treatment and medical referrals for respiratory diseases, *see* page 639. The physicians listed are heads of pulmonary disease departments or divisions at leading medical schools. They can be expected to be knowledgeable about the latest therapies, and can also be good referral sources.

Lung disease specialists treat and manage all kinds of respiratory problems, including emphysema, COPD, asthma, tuberculosis, nonoperable and postoperable lung cancer, histoplasmosis, sarcoidosis, pneumonia, silicosis, asbestosis, and black lung disease.

GOVERNMENT RESPIRATORY DISEASE CENTERS

The National Heart, Lung, and Blood Institute sponsors 21 centers that conduct both basic (laboratory) and clinical (patient) research on certain lung diseases. These centers do not accept patients primarily for treatment, but they have directors who are eminent authorities on lung diseases and staffs who are knowledgeable about the latest therapies.

These specialized centers of research can be considered leading reservoirs of knowledge and referral on treatment, especially experimental treatments, of certain lung diseases.

ARIZONA
Benjamin Burrows, M.D.
Arizona Health Sciences Center
1501 Campbell Ave.
Tucson, AZ 85724
(602) 626-6387
Chronic airways diseases

CALIFORNIA
Kenneth M. Moser, M.D.
University of California Medical Center San
  Diego
225 W. Dickinson St.
San Diego, CA 92103
(619) 294-5970
Adult respiratory failure

John F. Murray, M.D.
San Francisco General Hospital
1001 Potrero Ave.
San Francisco, CA 94110
(415) 821-8313
Pulmonary vascular disease

William H. Tooley, M.D.
Cardiovascular Research Institute
University of California
696 Moffitt Hospital
San Francisco, CA 94143
(415) 666-1910
Pediatric pulmonary diseases

COLORADO
Robert Mason, M.D.
National Jewish Hospital & Research Center
National Jewish Center for Immunology and
  Respiratory Medicine
1400 Jackson St.
Denver, CO 80206
(303) 398-1302
Fibrotic & immunologic interstitial lung
  diseases

LOUISIANA
Hans Weill, M.D.
Tulane University School of Medicine
1700 Perdido St.
New Orleans, LA 70112
(504) 588-5265
Fibrotic & immunologic interstitial lung
  diseases

MASSACHUSETTS
Mary E. Avery, M.D.
Children's Hospital Corporation
300 Longwood Ave.
Boston, MA 02115
(617) 735-8330
Pediatric pulmonary diseases

Lynne M. Reid, M.D.
Children's Hospital Medical Center
300 Longwood Ave.
Boston, MA 02115
(617) 735-7440
Pulmonary vascular diseases

Warren M. Zapol, M.D.
Harvard Medical School
Massachusetts General Hospital
Department of Anesthesia
Boston, MA 02114
(617) 726-3030
Adult respiratory failure

MINNESOTA
Warren J. Warwick. M.D.
University of Minnesota Medical School
420 Del St., S.E.
PO Box 184 Mayo
Minneapolis, MN 55455
(612)373-8886
Pediatric pulmonary diseases

MISSOURI
Thomas M. Hyers, M.D.
Director, Division Pulmonary Diseases
St. Louis University School of Medicine
1402 S. Grand Blvd.
St. Louis, MO 63104
(314) 577-8857
Adult respiratory failure

NEW YORK
L. Stanley James, M.D.
Columbia University
College of Physicians and Surgeons
630 W. 168th St.
New York, NY 10032
(212) 694-6527
Pediatric pulmonary diseases

NORTH CAROLINA
Wallace A. Clyde, Jr., M.D.
University of North Carolina
535 Burnet, Womack Building, 229H
Chapel Hill, NC 27514
(919) 966-2331
Pediatric pulmonary diseases

TENNESSEE
Kenneth L. Brigham, M.D.
Vanderbilt University
Pulmonary Circulation Center
Medical Center North
Nashville, TN 37232
(615) 322-2386
Pulmonary vascular diseases

Mildred T. Stahlman, M.D.
Vanderbilt University Medical Center
S-4307 Division of Neonatology
Nashville, TN 37232
(615) 322-3475
Pediatric pulmonary diseases

TEXAS
Waldemar G. Johanson, Jr., M.D.
University of Texas
7703 Floyd Curl Drive
San Antonio, TX 78284
(512) 691-6011
Adult respiratory failure

WASHINGTON
Leonard D. Hudson, M.D.
Harborview Medical Center
325 Ninth Ave.
Seattle, WA 98104
(206) 223-3356
Adult respiratory failure

William A. Hodson, M.S.
University of Washington
Department of Pediatrics, RD-20
Seattle, WA 98195
(206) 543-1060
Pediatric pulmonary diseases

WISCONSIN
Philip M. Farrell, M.D.
University of Wisconsin Center for Health
  Sciences
600 Highland Ave.
Madison, WI 73792
(608) 263-8555
Pediatric pulmonary diseases

SOURCE: *National Heart, Lung, and Blood Institute.*

LUNG DISEASE RESEARCH AND TREATMENT AT THE NATIONAL INSTITUTES OF HEALTH

Several long-term studies are ongoing at the NIH Clinical Center in Bethesda, Maryland, involving those with certain lung diseases. Included are patients with mild to moderate emphysema but without chronic bronchitis, patients with hereditary emphysema (alpha-1-antitrypsin deficiency), and patients with "interstitial lung diseases," such as pulmonary fibrosis and the pneumoconioses (or occupational lung diseases). Consideration for participation is by physician referral only. For more information, your physician can contact:

Office of the Director
The Clinical Center
Building 10, Room 2C-146
National Institutes of Health
Bethesda, MD 20892
(301) 496-4891

or:

Ronald Crystal, M.D.
(301) 496-1597

HOTLINE

(800) 222-LUNG
(303) 398-1477—Colorado

A specially trained nurse is available Monday through Friday from 8:30 A.M. to 5:00 P.M. Rocky Mountain Time to answer questions about lung diseases. In addition, the caller can receive information about the National Jewish Hospital—National Asthma Center, which operates the hotline and is a well-recognized center for treating a variety of lung diseases. The Center will also provide the names of local physicians who were trained at the Center to manage lung diseases, or who practice in the caller's area.

ORGANIZATIONS

American Lung Association, National
  Headquarters
1740 Broadway
New York, NY 10019
(212) 315-8700

The major voluntary health association concerned with lung diseases. State and local affiliates throughout the country. A major source of information. Publishes numerous pamphlets, booklets, journals and other materials on lung diseases. Supports research on lung diseases. Sponsors prevention and educational programs. Will provide more information upon request. For the name of an American Lung Association affiliate in your area, consult your local telephone directory white pages or contact the national headquarters.

National Heart, Lung, and Blood Institute
National Institutes of Health
9000 Rockville Pike
Building 31, 4A21
Bethesda, MD 20892
(301) 496-4236

This is the Institute within the National Institutes of Health most concerned with lung diseases. Supports research on all kinds of lung diseases. Helps set national policy on lung disease-related issues. Publishes booklets, fact sheets and reports. Will provide more information upon request.

BOOKS

Enjoying Life With Emphysema, **Dr. Thomas L. Petty,** Philadelphia: Lea & Febiger, 1984.

Lung Diseases of Children: an Introduction, New York: American Lung Association, 1986.

MATERIALS

Single copies are free

Chronic Obstructive Pulmonary Disease, 14 pages.
The Lungs: Medicine for the Layman, 24 pages.

National Heart, Lung, and Blood Institute
9000 Rockville Pike
Building 31, 4A21
Bethesda, MD 20892
(301) 496-4236

Free or for a small donation

About Lungs and Lung Diseases
As you Live . . . You Breathe
Asbestos: Lung Hazards on the Job
Byssinosis: Lung Hazards on the Job
Chronic Bronchitis Facts
Chronic Cough Facts
Did you Know That There is a Lung Disease Which Affects Primarily Farmers?
Dust Diseases Facts

Emphysema: Answers to Your Questions
Emphysema Facts
Facts in Brief About Lung Disease
Health Hazards in the Arts
Help Yourself to Better Breathing
Histo Facts
In Defense of the Lung
Lung Hazards in the Workplace
Pills, Pills, Pills

Shortness of Breath Facts
Silicosis: Lung Hazards on the Job
TB Outside the Lungs
Tuberculosis? A Handbook for TB Patients
Tuberculosis Facts

Local American Lung Associations listed in
   the white pages of your telephone directory.

MENTAL RETARDATION AND DEVELOPMENTAL AND LEARNING DISABILITIES

See also Autism, page 105, Cerebral Palsy, page 148, Epilepsy, page 211, Speech and Language Problems, page 510.

About 9 million Americans are mentally retarded or have developmental disabilities, an umbrella term for some major or minor brain dysfunction that prevents normal development. This category can include disabilities such as cerebral palsy, epilepsy, autism, and learning disorders. The handicaps range in degree from mild to very severe. Quite often those affected need a complement of medical and rehabilitative services to help them live up to their potential. The same facilities often serve this entire population, and medical research on various disabilities is often lumped together. Since all of these disabilities originate in some form of brain damage, the disorders may overlap; for example a child with autism is often mentally retarded. At one time there were few places where parents could find help for children with these types of disabilities—today there are many. Here are descriptions and some of the help available.

MENTAL RETARDATION

Mental retardation is the general term applied to those who have sub-average intelligence (an IQ of 70 or lower), have difficulties adapting to the world and whose deficiencies show up during childhood (usually before age 5). When most people think of mental retardation they think of Down syndrome, with its distinctive characteristics. Actually, nearly 90 percent of all mental retardation is mild, not physically apparent, and has no known cause. Mild mental retardation is defined as an IQ between 50 and 70; moderate, between 35 and 50; severe, between 20 and 35; profound, below 20.

Cause: Unknown in the vast majority of cases. It is thought to be a combination of environmental and biological factors. For example, a disproportionately high number of people with mild mental retardation come from the ranks of the disadvantaged, which may point to environmental factors.

On the other hand, there is no socioeconomic distinction among the more severely retarded minority who have biologically identifiable abnormalities, such as chromosomal and metabolic defects. Within this group, the leading cause of mental retardation is Down syndrome, a genetic disorder usually characterized by an extra chromosome. Other causes are "fragile-X syndrome," a chromosomal defect affecting males only, hydrocephalus (water on the brain), and prenatal infections, such as rubella or German measles.

The chances of having a mentally retarded child increase with the age of the parents. Women under age 30 have less than one chance in a thousand of bearing a child with Down—compared with one chance in 400 for women age 35, one chance in 100 for women age 40, and one chance in 12 for women age 48. The age of the father, too, may be critical, especially if he is over 55. From 25 to 30 percent of the extra chromosomes responsible for Down syndrome come from the father.

Diagnosis: Many mentally retarded youngsters are not identified as such until they reach school and their inability to learn normally is noticed. However, Down syndrome is almost always spotted at birth by its distinctive symptoms: slanting eyes, slightly protruding tongue, short hands, feet, and trunk. Children with frag-

ile-X syndrome typically have big heads, protruding ears, and large testicles.

Children with Down syndrome generally have low IQ's and are slow in developing physically. They may also have heart defects and be susceptible to respiratory infections. The life expectancy of Down youngsters is now about 70—close to that of the general population.

The prenatal test amniocentesis can detect Down syndrome during pregnancy. If the test proves positive, a woman may choose to have an abortion. Since the risk of Down syndrome increases with age, the test is recommended especially for women over age 35.

Treatment: Mental retardation is not curable or reversible although some foreign studies have found improvement in children with fragile-X syndrome after the administration of certain vitamins and drugs. A study using vitamins and minerals on children with Down syndrome in this country found preliminary evidence of benefit, but the results were not confirmed by subsequent studies. However, it is well known that proper management of the mentally retarded, especially early in life, can do wonders in helping them reach their potential: Many can become partially or nearly totally independent.

LEARNING DISABILITIES

There is a large group of Americans who are not mentally retarded—in fact, many have high intelligence—but who have difficulty learning in the traditional way. Many scientists believe these people have a minimal kind of brain dysfunction that puts them out of the mainstream and constitutes a kind of handicap. These are youngsters who do not perceive language in the usual sense, who may have trouble reading, writing, and doing math; some cannot sustain attention or concentration. They may be hyperactive and be a discipline problem in school. Some suffer from dyslexia, a disorder that makes mastery of language very difficult. Dyslexics commonly have great difficulty spelling, confusing "p" with "b" and "was" with "saw".

Some estimates put the number of youngsters with learning disabilities due to slight irregularities of brain function at 15 percent of the popula-

tion. The causes are generally unknown and are undoubtedly multiple. Some disabilities could result from injuries to the nervous system before, during, or soon after birth. There is growing evidence of genetic influences, notably in dyslexia. Ferreting out the biological causes is a subject of intense scientific interest. Regardless of cause, it is agreed that youngsters with minor or major learning disabilities should be identified as early as possible, so they can receive special attention to help them succeed.

To deal with the general problem, researchers, physicians, psychologists, social workers, rehabilitation specialists, and other health professionals have adopted the term developmental disabilities, which is a catch-all term for those with any kind of brain dysfunction, minor or major, that distinguishes them from the mainstream and often requires special medical, social, and educational help. It also includes those with cerebral palsy (page 148) autism (page 105), and epilepsy (page 211). *See also* Speech and Language Problems, page 510.

WHERE TO FIND HELP

In the past two decades the recognition of a need for special facilities to detect, evaluate, treat, and manage youngsters with developmental disabilities has grown enormously. There is now a network of facilities designed to assist them.

Many excellent rehabilitation facilities include developmental disabilities for infants and preschool children as a part of their program. Recently, the Commission on Accreditation of Rehabilitation Facilities (a well-recognized accrediting body) has started accrediting rehabilitation programs that specialize in infant and early childhood programs. A list of recently accredited places follows. For more information, contact:

Director of Developmental Disabilities
    Program
The Commission on Accreditation of
    Rehabilitation Facilities
2500 N. Pantano Rd.
Tucson, AZ 85715
(602) 886-8575

REHABILITATION CENTERS THAT SPECIALIZE IN INFANT AND EARLY CHILDHOOD DEVELOPMENTAL PROGRAMS

ARIZONA
Institute for Human Development
Northern Arizona University
C.U. Box 5630
Flagstaff, AZ 86011
(602) 774-2181
Richard W. Carroll, Director

Marc Center
924 N. Country Club Drive
Mesa, AZ 85201
(602) 969-3800
Randall L. Gray, Executive Director

TCH, Inc.
Tempe Center for the Handicapped, Inc.
250 W. First St.
Tempe, AZ 85281
(602) 894-2355
David B. Cutty, Executive Director

ARKANSAS
Easter Seal Rehabilitation Center
PO Box 5148
Little Rock, AR 72225
(501) 663-8331
James E. Butler, Executive Director

CALIFORNIA
Contra Costa Association for Retarded Citizens
2280 Diamond Blvd., Suite 365
Concord, CA 94520
(415) 827-4495
Rhea Nilon, Executive Director

Redwoods United, Inc.
PO Box 1400
Eureka, CA 95502-1400
(707) 443-0811
Raymond E. Rozales, Executive Director

Lemon Grove Infant Development Program
    Association for Retarded Citizens—San
    Diego
2770 Glebe Rd.
Lemon Grove, CA 92045
(619) 574-7575
Dr. Richard B. Farmer, Executive Director

Rehabilitation Institute of Southern California
1800 E. LaVeta Ave.
Orange, CA 92666
(714) 633-7400
Praim S. Singh, Executive Director

Foundation for the Retarded of the Desert
PO Box 1183
Palm Desert, CA 92261
(714) 346-0591
Keith Rhodes, Executive Director

Community Association for Retarded, Inc.
3864 Middlefield Rd.
Palo Alto, CA 94303
(415) 494-0550
Ralph M. Scheer, Executive Director

Infant Center
Contra Costa Association for Retarded Citizens
950 El Pueblo Drive
Pittsburgh, CA 94565
(415) 827-4495
Rhea Nilon, Executive Director

Casa Colina Hospital for Rehabilitative
  Medicine
255 E. Bonita Ave.
Pomona, CA 91767
(714) 593-7521
Dale E. Eazell, Chief Operating Officer

Indian Wells Valley Association for Retarded
  Citizens
216 N. Gold Canyon Drive
Ridgecrest, CA 93555
(619) 375-9787
Dr. Suzanne Hard, Executive Director

Indian Wells Valley Work Activity Center
Indian Wells Valley Association for Retarded
  Citizens
318 Arondo
Ridgecrest, CA 93555
(619) 375-9787
Dr. Suzanne Hard, Executive Director

Association for Retarded Citizens–San Diego
5384 Linda Vista Rd., Suite 100
San Diego, CA 92110
(619) 574-7575
Dr. Richard B. Farmer, Executive Director

Poplar Center
515 E. Poplar Ave.
San Mateo, CA 94401
(415) 342-3558
Elsie B. Vickery, Executive Director

Gateway Projects, Inc.
240 Garden Highway
Yuba City, CA 95991
(916) 673-2125
Stephen V. Thomas, Executive Director

COLORADO
Rehabilitation Center
Boulder Memorial Hospital
311 Mapleton Ave.
Boulder, CO 80302
(303) 443-0230
Warren Clark, President

Developmental Preschool Developmental
  Training Services, Inc.
1720 Brookside
Canon City, CO 81212
(303) 275-0550
Paulette L. Bolton, Deputy Director

Developmental Training Services, Inc.
PO Box 1249
Canon City, CO 81212
(303) 275-1616
Roger G. Jensen, President

Rocky Mountain Rehabilitation Center
2501 East Yampa St.
Colorado Springs, CO 80909
(303) 473-3475
William F. Montfort, President

HOPE CENTER for the Developmentally
  Disabled, Inc.
3601 Martin L. King Blvd.
Denver, CO 80205
(303) 388-4801
George E. Brantley, Executive Director

United Cerebral Palsy Association of Denver,
  Inc.
2727 Columbine St.
Denver, CO 80205
(303) 355-7337
David Heartman, Executive Director

Hilltop Special Services Division
1331 Hermosa Ave.
Grand Junction, CO 81506
(303) 244-6191
William Wright, Administrator

CONNECTICUT
Easter Seal Rehabilitation Center of Eastern
  Fairfield County, Inc.
26 Mill Hill Ave.
Bridgeport, CT 06610
(203) 366-7551
Edmund S. McLaughlin, President

Easter Seal Goodwill Industries Rehabilitation
  Center, Inc.
20 Brookside Ave.
New Haven, CT 06515-9985
(203) 389-4561
Malcolm H. Gill, President

Easter Seal Rehabilitation Center of Greater
  Waterbury, Inc.
22 Tompkins St.
Waterbury, CT 06708
(203) 754-5141
George A. Mango, Executive Director

DELAWARE
Delaware Curative Workshop, Inc.
1600 Washington St.
Wilmington, DE 19802
(302) 656-2521
Mae D. Hightower-Vandamm, Executive
  Director

FLORIDA
Upper Pinellas Association for Retarded
  Citizens, Inc.
2199 Calumet St.
Clearwater, FL 33575
(813) 441-2854
James E. Leach, Executive Director

Easter Seal Society of Volusia and Flagler
  Counties, Inc.
PO Box 9117
Daytona Beach, FL 32020
(904) 255-4568
David M. Timko, Executive Director

Easter Seal Society of Dade County, Inc.
1475 N.W. 14th Ave.
Miami, FL 33125
(305) 325-0470
Albert P. Calli, Executive Director

Easter Seal Society of De Soto, Manatee, and
  Sarasota Counties, Inc.
401 Braden Ave.
Sarasota, FL 33580
(813) 355-7637
Donald L. Wise, Executive Director

Pinellas Association for Retarded Children
3100 75th St. N.
St. Petersburg, FL 33710
(813) 345-9111
Bert Muller, President

Tri-County Rehabilitation Center, Inc.
PO Box 597
Stuart, FL 33495
(305) 287-7600
Suzanne Hutcheson, Executive Director

GEORGIA
Easter Seal Children's Center
3161 Maple Drive, N.E.
Atlanta, GA 30305
(404) 261-6262
Susan E. Woodhall, Director

ILLINOIS
Association for Individual Development
309 New Indian Trail Court
Aurora, IL 60506
(312) 896-0707
E. Duane Thompson, Executive Director

Infant Program
Association for Individual Development
309 W. New Indian Trail Court
Aurora, IL 60506
(312) 844-5040
E. Duane Thompson, Executive Director

Clinton County Rehabilitation Center, Inc.
Route 50 W. Box 3B
Breese, IL 62230
(618) 594-3689
John J. Sedivy, Executive Director

Pulaski-Alexander Mental Health Association,
  Inc.
218 10th St.
Cairo, IL 62914
(618) 734-2665
Roger W. Hannan, Executive Director

Developmental Services Center
1304 W. Bradley Ave.
Champaign, IL 61821
(217) 356-7294
William Gingold, Executive Director

Birth Thru Three Program
Coles County Association for the Retarded
825 18th St.
Charleston, IL 61920
(217) 348-0127
Janice Grewell, Executive Director

Coles County Association for the Retarded
PO Box 487
Charleston, IL 61920
(217) 345-7058
Janice Grewell, Executive Director

Helping Hand Rehabilitation Center
9649 W. 55th St.
Countryside, IL 60525
(312) 352-3580
E. Evans Ronshausen, Executive Director

Kreider Services, Inc.
PO Box 366
Dixon, IL 61021
(815) 288-6691
Arlan L. McClain, Executive Director

Naron Wood Center for Children
Association for Retarded Citizens–Effingham
   County
2502 S. Veterans Drive
Effingham, IL 62401
(217) 857-3186
Michael W. Fortner, Executive Director

Jayne Shover Easter Seal Rehabilitation
   Center, Inc.
799 S. McLean Blvd.
Elgin, IL 60120
(312) 742-3264
Peggy Muetterties, Executive Director

Career Development Center
Rural Route #5, Box 357
Fairfield, IL 62837
(618) 842-2691
Donald C. Knight, Executive Director

Mental Health Services of Franklin and
   Williamson Counties, Inc.
PO Box 401
Herrin, IL 62948
(618) 942-7378
Floyd E. Cunningham, Administrator

Proviso Association for Retarded Citizens
4100 Litt Drive
Hillside, IL 60162
(312) 547-3560
Jan Suchala, Executive Director

Easter Seal Rehabilitation Center of Will-
   Grundy Counties, Inc.
257 Springfield Ave.
Joliet, IL 60435
(815) 727-5457
Debra K. Gagliardo-Condotti, Executive
   Director

McDonough County Rehabilitation Center
900 S. Deer Rd.
Macomb, IL 61455
(309) 837-4876
James H. Starnes, Executive Director

Warren Achievement Center, Inc.
1314 S. Main St.
Monmouth, IL 61462
(309) 734-8331
Joan McVey, President

Jefferson County Comprehensive Services, Inc.
PO Box 428
Mount Vernon, IL 62864
(618) 242-7300
John J. Hansen, Executive Director

Opportunity Center of Southeastern Illinois,
   Inc.
PO Box 519
Olney, IL 62450
(618) 395-2418
Larry Maxwell, President

LaSalle County Easter Seal Society
1013 Adams St.
Ottawa, IL 61350
(815) 434-0857
Deborah Bernardini, Executive Director

Allied Agency Peoria Association for Retarded
   Citizens
320 E. Armstrong Ave.
Peoria, IL 61603
(309) 672-6308
Ronald B. Wisecarver, Executive Director

Easter Seal Center, Inc.
320 E. Armstrong
Peoria, IL 61603
(309) 672-6330
John Pavek, Executive Director

Easter Seal Foundation Serving Rock Island
and Mercer Counties
3808 Eighth Ave.
Rock Island, IL 61201
(309) 786-2434
George McDoniel, Executive Director

Coleman Tri-County Services
PO Box 689
Shawneetown, IL 62984-9998
(618) 269-4211
Roger W. Mahan, Executive Director

Rock River Valley Self Help Enterprises, Inc.
2300 W. LeFevre Rd.
Sterling, IL 61081
(815) 626-3115
John L. Stern, Executive Director

Association for Retarded Citizens/Effingham
County
618 W. Main St.
Teutopolis, IL 62467
(217) 857-3186
Michael W. Fortner, Executive Director

Children's Services
Developmental Services Center
1409 W. Park St.
Urbana, IL 61801
(217) 356-9176
Dr. William Gingold, Executive Director

Proviso Early Intervention Program
810 Newcastle
Westchester, IL 60153
(312) 547-3550
Jan Suchala, Executive Director

INDIANA
Allen County Society for Crippled Children
and Adults, Inc.
3320 N. Clinton St.
Fort Wayne, IN 46805
(219) 745-0566
Percy Talati, Executive Director

Allen County Society for Crippled Children
and Adults, Inc., Children's Center
2323 Fairfield Ave.
Fort Wayne, IN 46807
(219) 745-0566
Percy Talati, Executive Director

Crossroads Rehabilitation Center, Inc.
3242 Sutherland Ave.
Indianapolis, IN 46205
(317) 924-3251
James J. Vento, President

Bona Vista Programs, Inc.
PO Box 2496
Kokomo, IN 46902
(317) 457-8273
Paul F. Wagner, President

KANSAS
Children's Services Offices
Developmental Services of Northwest Kansas,
Inc.
PO Box 451
Colby, KS 67701
(913) 625-5678
James Blume, President

Arrowhead West
PO Box 1353
Dodge City, KS 67801
(316) 227-8803
Donald J. Pendergast, President

Children's Center
Arrowhead West, Inc.
1100 E. Wyatt Earp Blvd.
Dodge City, KS 67801
(316) 227-8803
Donald J. Pendergast, President

Developmental Services of Northwest Kansas,
Inc.
PO Box 1016
Hays, KS 67601
(913) 625-5678
James W. Blume, President

Training and Evaluation Center of Hutchinson,
Inc. (T.E.C.H.)
1228 N. Halstead
Hutchinson, KS 67501
(316) 663-1596
Maurice F. Cummings, President

Big Lakes Developmental Center, Inc.
1500 Hayes Drive
Manhattan, KS 66502
(913) 776-9201
James K. Shaver, Executive Director

Service Development Office
Developmental Services of Northwest Kansas,
   Inc.
517 Main
Stockton, KS 67669
(913) 625-5678
James Blume, President

Starkey Developmental Center, Inc.
144 S. Young
Wichita, KS 67209
(316) 942-4221
John C. Frye, Executive Director

KENTUCKY
J.U. Kevil Mental Retardation/Mental Health
   Center
10th St., Extended
Mayfield, KY 42066
(502) 247-5396
Larry G. Knight, Executive Director

West Kentucky Easter Seal Center
2229 Mildred St.
Paducah, KY 42001
(502) 444-9687
Richard B. Brown, Executive Director

MARYLAND
Mt. Washington Pediatric Hospital, Inc.
1708 W. Rogers Ave.
Baltimore, MD 21209
(301) 578-8600
Francis A. Pommett, President

MASSACHUSETTS
Youville Rehabilitation and Chronic Disease
   Hospital
1575 Cambridge Street
Cambridge, MA 02238
(617) 876-4344
Sister Annette Caron, Executive Director

Lakeville Hospital Rehabilitation Center
Main St.
Lakeville, MA 02346
(617) 947-1231
John R. Pratt, Executive Director

The Children's Developmental Disabilities
   Center
Massachusetts Cerebral Palsy Association of
   the South Shore Area, Inc.
105 Adams St.
Quincy, MA 02169
(617) 479-7443
Arthur Ciampa, Executive Director

Valley Infant Development Services
31 Park St.
Springfield, MA 01103
(413) 739-3954
Ellen Berger, Director

MICHIGAN
Beekman Center Workshop, Inc.
2901 Wabash Rd.
Lansing, MI 48910
(517) 374-4900
John M. Breaugh, Administrator

MINNESOTA
Polinsky Medical Rehabilitation Center, Inc.
530 E. Second St.
Duluth, MN 55805
(218) 727-5083
David B. Jordahl, Executive Director

Mankato Rehabilitation Center, Inc.
PO Box 328
Mankato, MN 56001
(507) 345-4507
Arne J. Berg, Executive Director

Cerebral Palsy Center, Inc.
360 Hoover St., N.E.
Minneapolis, MN 55413
(612) 331-5958
Regis H. Barber, Executive Director

Courage Center
3915 Golden Valley Rd.
Minneapolis, MN 55422
(612) 588-0811
David Phillips, Executive Director

Saint Paul Rehabilitation Center, Inc.
319 Eagle St.
St. Paul, MN 55102
(612) 227-8471
Ronald E. Anderson, President

MISSOURI
Exceptional Ones, Inc.
PO Box 46
Mapaville, MO 63065
(314) 464-2060
Dr. Anthony A. Casey, Executive Director

United Cerebral Palsy of Buchanan County
1025 N. 22nd St.
St. Joseph, MO 64506
(816) 364-3836
Barbara Wilkerson, Executive Director

Canterbury Center
United Cerebral Palsy Association of Greater
St. Louis
8645 Old Bonhomme Rd.
University City, MO 63132
(314) 994-1600
David A. Young, Executive Vice President

NEW HAMPSHIRE
Easter Seal Society/Goodwill Industries of
New Hampshire, Inc.
555 Auburn St.
Manchester, NH 03103
(603) 623-8863
Paul S. Boynton, Vice President of
Rehabilitation

Early Intervention Program
Nashua Memorial Hospital
PO Box 2014
Nashua, NH 03601
(603) 883-5521
Joan Izen, Coordinator

NEW JERSEY
Lourdes Regional Rehabilitation Center
1600 Haddon Ave.
Camden, NJ 08103
(609) 757-3500
James B. Makos, President and CEO

Robert Wood Johnson, Jr. Rehabilitation
Institute
John F. Kennedy Medical Center
Edison, NJ 08818
(201) 321-7050
Gerald Feldman, Administrator

Morris County Society for Crippled Children
and Adults
260 Tabor Rd.
Morris Plains, NJ 07950
(201) 539-5636
Margery Oppenheimer, Executive Director

Children's Specialized Hospital
150 New Providence Rd.
Mountainside, NJ 07091
(201) 233-3720
Richard B. Ahlfeld, Executive Director

NEW YORK
Bergholz School
United Cerebral Palsy Association of Niagara
County, Inc.
6700 Schultz Rd.
Bergholz, NY 14304
(716) 285-5761
Joseph O. Mineo, Executive Director

Rehabilitation Services, Inc.
PO Box 310
Binghamton, NY 13902
(607) 722-2364
Dr. George W. Sandiford, President–Medical
Director

Children's Center
United Cerebral Palsy Association of Western
New York, Inc.
31 Rossler Ave.
Buffalo, NY 14206
(716) 894-0130
Duane Schielke, Executive Director

United Cerebral Palsy Association of Western
New York, Inc.
7 Community Drive
Buffalo, NY 14225
(716) 833-3231
Duane Schielke, Executive Director

Circle Hill School
United Cerebral Palsy Association of Greater
Suffolk, Inc.
Scholar Lane
Commack, NY 11725
(516) 543-5100
Ira E. Jacobs, Executive Director

Smiths Lane School
United Cerebral Palsy Association of Greater
    Suffolk, Inc.
Azalea Lane
Commack, NY 11725
(516) 543-5100
Ira E. Jacobs, Executive Director

United Cerebral Palsy Association of Greater
    Suffolk
159 Indian Head Rd.
Commack, NY 11725
(516) 543-5100
Ira E. Jacobs, Executive Director

Rockland County Center for the Physically
    Handicapped, Inc.
260 Little Tor Rd. N.
New City, NY 10956
(914) 634-4648
Goodwin D. Katzen, Executive Director

Educational and Treatment Center
United Cerebral Palsy Association of Niagara
    County, Inc.
245 30th St.
Niagara Falls, NY 14303
(716) 285-5761
Joseph O. Mineo, Executive Director

United Cerebral Palsy Association of Niagara
    County, Inc.
2103 Mackenna Ave.
Niagara Falls, NY 14303
(716) 285-5761
Joseph O. Mineo, Executive Director

United Cerebral Palsy Association of Nassau
    County, Inc.
380 Washington Ave.
Roosevelt, NY 11575
(516) 378-2000
Salvatore Gullo, Executive Director

Helen Hayes Hospital
Route 9W
West Haverstraw, NY 10993
(914) 947-3000
Robert Lindsay, Chief Executive Officer

NORTH CAROLINA
Southeastern Speech and Hearing Services of
    North Carolina, Inc.
PO Box 53415
Fayetteville, NC 28305
(919) 485-5145
L. Brooks Gore, Executive Director

OHIO
The Cleveland Society for the Blind
PO Box 1988
Cleveland, OH 44106
(216) 791-8118
James E. Goodwin, Executive Director

Easter Seal Rehabilitation Center of Central
    Ohio, Inc.
565 Children's Drive W.
Columbus, OH 43205
(614) 228-5523
John R. Murphy, Executive Director

Rehabilitation Service of North Central Ohio,
    Inc.
270 Sterkel Blvd.
Mansfield, OH 44907
(419) 756-1133
Robert C. Linstrom, Executive Director

Betty Jane Memorial Rehabilitation Center
65 St. Francis Ave.
Tiffin, OH 44883
(419) 447-9811
M. Eugene Winters, Executive Director

Children's Rehabilitation Center
855 Howland-Wilson Rd., N.E.
Warren, OH 44484
(216) 856-2107
Barbara Anderson, Executive Director

Easter Seal Society of Mahoning, Trumbull,
    and Columbiana Counties
299 Edwards St.
Youngstown, OH 44502
(216) 743-1168
Andrew Douglas, Executive Director

PENNSYLVANIA
Erie County Crippled Children's Society, Inc.
101 E. Sixth St.
Erie, PA 16507
(814) 459-2755
Frank J. Chiz, Executive Director

Easter Seal Society of Allegheny County
110 Seventh St.
Pittsburgh, PA 15222
(412) 281-7244
Andrew J. Wasko, Executive Director

D.T. Watson Rehabilitation Hospital
Camp Meeting Rd.
Sewickley, PA 15143
(412) 741-9500
Steven J. Mozolak, Executive Director

Hope Enterprises, Inc.
PO Box 1837
Williamsport, Pa 17703-1837
(717) 326-3745
Merle S. Arnold, President

RHODE ISLAND
Sargent Rehabilitation Center
229 Waterman St.
Providence, RI 02906
(401) 751-3113
Marilyn F. Serra, President

SOUTH CAROLINA
Charles Lea Center
Charles Lea Center for Rehabilitation and
   Special Education, Inc.
195 Burdette St.
Spartanburg, SC 29302
(803) 585-0322
Glenn A. Brumfield, Executive Director

TENNESSEE
Les Passees Rehabilitation Center
49 N. Dunlop Memphis, TN 38103
(901) 529-0233
Gloria D. McDaniel, Administrator

TEXAS
West Texas Rehabilitation Center/Abilene
4601 Hartford
Abilene, TX 79605
(915) 692-1633
Shelley V. Smith, President

Brazos Valley Rehabilitation Center
1318 Memorial Drive
Bryan, TX 77802
(713) 822-0193
Jim Thompson, Executive Director

Easter Seal Society for Children
5701 Maple Ave.
Dallas, TX 75235
(214) 358-5261
Jack E. Andrews, Executive Director

Permian Basin Rehabilitation Center
620 N. Alleghaney
Odessa, TX 79761
(915) 332-8244
John W. Clarke, Executive Director

West Texas Rehabilitation Center/San Angelo
West Texas Rehabilitation Center/Abilene
3001 S. Jackson
San Angelo, TX 76904
(915) 692-1633
Shelley V. Smith, President

Easter Seal Rehabilitation Center, Inc.
2203 Babcock Rd.
San Antonio, TX 78229
(512) 699-3911
Mr. Randel W. Aaron, Executive Director

Bell County Rehabilitation Center
2000 Marland Wood Rd.
Temple, TX 76502
(817) 778-6785
Richard Schaub, Executive Director

Temple Memorial Treatment Center/Easter
   Seal Society
PO Box 147
Texarkana, TX 75501
(214) 794-2705
Janet Hoag, Executive Director

North Texas Easter Seal Rehabilitation Center,
   Inc.
516 Denver St.
Wichita Falls, TX 76301
(817) 322-0771
Nils Richardson, Executive Director

VERMONT
Rutland Mental Health Service, Inc.
PO Box 222
Rutland, VT 05701
(802) 775-2381
Gilbert D. Aliber, Executive Director

WASHINGTON
Hearing, Speech, & Deafness Center
1620 18th Avenue
Seattle, WA 98122
(206) 323-5770
Julia S. Winn, Director

Northwest Center Early Childhood
  Development Program
Northwest Center for the Retarded
2919 First Ave. W.
Seattle, WA 98119
(206) 281-9222
Linda Gil, Director

Northwest Center for the Retarded
1600 W. Armory Way
Seattle, WA 98119
(206) 282-3547
James N. McClurg, Executive Director

WEST VIRGINIA
Easter Seal Rehabilitation Center
1305 National Rd.
Wheeling, WV 26003
(304) 242-1390
Rosemary M. Front, Executive Director

WISCONSIN
Black River Industries, Inc.
PO Box 341
Medford, WI 54451
(715) 743-2950
Ronald D. Alexander, General Manager

Rehabilitation Center of Sheboygan, Inc.
PO Box 685
Sheboygan, WI 53082-0685
(414) 458-8262
Ronald L. Van Rooyen, President

Curative Rehabilitation Center
9001 Watertown Plank Rd.
Wauwatosa, WI 53226
(414) 259-1414
Eugene M. Cox, President

SOURCE: *Commission on Accreditation of Rehabilitation Facilities*

UNIVERSITY-AFFILIATED LEARNING DISABILITIES CENTERS AND SPECIALISTS (UAFs)

There is a national network of 50 centers, partly supported by the federal government and affiliated with major universities or medical schools, that diagnose, treat, and manage mental retardation and developmental disabilities, as well as conduct research. They are often referred to as University-Affiliated Facilities (UAFs) or University-Affiliated Programs (UAPs). Some of the centers have various specialties, but the focus is on multidisciplinary teams that can deal with the full scope of problems—including physical, medical, nutritional, speech, hearing, visual, educational, psychological, social, dental, and vocational.

Many of the centers, often geared to infants and young children, also see adolescents and adults. The centers are considered a central referral diagnostic source, especially for difficult cases. You can contact the centers directly, although they generally receive their clients through physician or health professional referrals.

For more information about the programs of any of the centers, you can contact:

American Association of University-Affiliated
  Programs
8605 Cameron St.
Suite 406
Silver Spring, MD 20910
(301) 588-8252

ALABAMA
Sparks Center for Developmental and Learning
  Disorders
University of Alabama—Birmingham
1720 Seventh Ave. S.
Birmingham, AL 35233
Director: Gary J. Myers, M.D.
(205) 934-5471

ARIZONA
Dine Center for Human Development
Navajo Community College
Tsaile, AZ 86556
Director: Loren Sekayumptewa
(602) 724-3351

CALIFORNIA
Division of Clinical Genetics and
  Developmental Disabilities
Department of Pediatrics
College of Medicine
University of California—Irving
Irvine, CA 92717
Director: Kenneth W. Dumars, M.D.
(714) 634-5791

University-Affiliated Training Program
Center for Child Development and
  Developmental Disorders
Children's Hospital of Los Angeles
4650 Sunset Blvd.
Los Angeles, CA 90027
Director: Wylda Hammon, M.D.
(213) 669-2151

University-Affiliated Facility
Mental Retardation Program
University of California—Los Angeles
760 Westwood Plaza
Los Angeles, CA 90024
Director: James Q. Simmons, M.D.
(213) 825-0395

COLORADO
Rocky Mountain Child Development Center
University of Colorado Health Sciences Center
Box C234
4200 E. Ninth Ave.
Denver, CO 80262
Director: William K. Frankenburg, M.D.
(303) 394-7224

DISTRICT OF COLUMBIA
Georgetown University Child Development
  Center
CG-52 Bles Building
3800 Reservoir Rd. N.W.
Washington, DC 20007
Director: Phyllis R. Magrab, Ph.D.
(202) 625-7675

FLORIDA
Mailman Center for Child Development
University of Miami School of Medicine
PO Box 016820, Miami, FL 33101
Director: Robert S. Stempfel, M.D.
(305) 547-6635

GEORGIA
University-Affiliated Program of Georgia
University of Georgia
850 College Station Rd.
Athens, GA 30610
Director: Richard Talbott, Ph.D.
(404) 542-1685

ILLINOIS
Illinois Institute for Developmental Disabilities
1640 W. Roosevelt Rd.
Chicago, IL 60608
Director: Kenneth R. Swiatek, Ph.D.
(312) 996-1590

INDIANA
Developmental Training Center
Indiana University
2853 E. 10th St.
Bloomington, IN 47405
Director: Henry J. Schroeder, Ed.D.
(812) 335-6508

Riley Child Development Program
Riley Hospital for Children
702 Barnhill Drive
Indianapolis, IN 46223
Director: Ernest E. Smith, M.D.
(317) 264-2051

IOWA
University Hospital School
The University of Iowa
Division of Developmental Disabilities
Iowa City, IA 52242
Director: Alfred Healy, M.D.
(319) 353-5972

KANSAS
Kansas University-Affiliated Facility—Kansas
  City, Children's Rehabilitation Unit
Kansas University Medical Center
39th & Rainbow Blvd.
Kansas City, KS 66103
Director: Joseph Hollowell, M.D., M.P.H.
(913) 588-5900

Kansas University-Affiliated Facility—Central
   Office
Bureau of Child Research
223 Haworth Hall
University of Kansas
Lawrence, KS 66045
Director: Richard L. Schiefelbusch, Ph.D.
(913) 864-4295

Kansas University-Affiliated Facility—Parsons
2601 Gabriel
Parsons, KS 67357
Director: Joseph E. Spradlin, Ph.D.
(316) 421-6550, x254

KENTUCKY
University of Kentucky Human Development
   Program
114 Porter Building
730 S. Limestone
Lexington, KY 40506-0205
Director: Melton C. Martinson, Ph.D.
(606) 257-1715

LOUISIANA
Human Development Center
Louisiana State University Medical Center
Building 138
1100 Florida Ave.
New Orleans, LA 70119
Director: Robert E. Crow
(504) 568-8397

Children's Center
Louisiana State University Medical Center
3730 Blair
Shreveport, LA 71103
Director: Clydie K. Mitchell
(318) 227-5108

MAINE
University-Affiliated Handicapped Children's
   Program
Eastern Maine Medical Center
489 State St.
Bangor, ME 04401
Director: Paul H. LaMarche, M.D.
(207) 947-3711

MARYLAND
The Kennedy Institute for Handicapped
   Children
707 N. Broadway
Baltimore, MD 21205
Director: Hugo Moser, M.D.
(301) 522-5405

MASSACHUSETTS
Developmental Evaluation Clinic
Children's Hospital Medical Center
300 Longwood Ave.
Boston, MA 02115
Director: Allen C. Crocker, M.D.
(617) 735-6509

Eunice Kennedy Shriver Center for Mental
   Retardation
Walter E. Fernald State School
200 Trapelo Rd.
Waltham, MA 02254
Director: Eileen M. Ouellette, M.D.
(617) 642-0230

MINNESOTA
Gillette Developmental Disabilities Program
Gillette Children's Hospital
200 E. University Ave.
St. Paul, MN 55113
Director: Robert Bruininks, Ph.D.
(612) 373-8383

MISSISSIPPI
University-Affiliated Program of Mississippi
Southern Station, Box 5163
University of Southern Mississippi
Hattiesburg, MS 39401
Director: Robert Campbell, Ed.D.
(601) 268-7309

MISSOURI
University-Affiliated Facility for
   Developmental Disabilities
University of Missouri—Kansas City
2220 Holmes St.
Kansas City, MO 64108
Director: Carl F. Calkins, Ph.D.
(816) 276-1770

MONTANA
Montana University-Affiliated Program
University of Montana
Missoula, MT 59812
Director: Richard B. Offner, Ph.D.
(406) 243-5467

NEBRASKA
Meyer Children's Rehabilitation Institute
University of Nebraska Medical Center
444 S. 44th St.
Omaha, NE 68131
Director: Bruce Buehler, M.D.
(402) 559-5233

NEW JERSEY
University-Affiliated Facility
University of Medicine & Dentistry of New
  Jersey
Rutgers Medical School
Box 101
Piscataway, NJ 08854
Director: Larry Taft, M.D.
(201) 937-7888

NEW YORK
Rose F. Kennedy Center
Albert Einstein College of Medicine
Yeshiva University
1410 Pelham Parkway S.
Bronx, NY 10461
Director: Herbert J. Cohen, M.D.
(212) 430-2440

Developmental Disabilities Center
St. Lukes—Roosevelt Hospital
428 W. 59th St.
New York, NY 10019
Director: Louis Z. Cooper, M.D.
(212) 870-6844

University-Affiliated Program for
  Developmental Disabilities
University of Rochester Medical Center
PO Box 671
601 Elmwood Ave.
Rochester, NY 14642
Director: Philip W. Davidson, Ph.D.
(716) 275-2986

Mental Retardation Institute
Westchester County Medical Center
Valhalla, NY 10595
Director: Ansley Bacon-Prue, Ph.D.
(914) 347-4545

NORTH CAROLINA
Division for Disorders of Development and
  Learning
Biological Sciences Research Center 220H
University of North Carolina
Chapel Hill, NC 27514
Director: Melvin D. Levine, M.D.
(919) 966-5171

OHIO
University-Affiliated Cincinnati Center for
  Developmental Disabilities
Pavilion Building
Elland & Bethesda Aves.
Cincinnati, OH 45229
Director: Jack H. Rubinstein, M.D.
(513) 559-4621

The Nisonger Center
The Ohio State University
McCampbell Hall
1580 Cannon Drive
Columbus, OH 43210
Director: Michael J. Guralnick, Ph.D.
(614) 422-8365

OREGON
Center on Human Development
University of Oregon
901 E. 18th St.
Eugene, OR 97403
Director: Hill Walker, Ph.D.
(503) 686-3591

Child Development & Rehabilitation Center
Crippled Children's Division
Oregon Health Sciences University
PO Box 574
Portland, OR 97207
Acting Director: Gerald Smith, Ed.D.
(503) 225-8364

PENNSYLVANIA
Developmental Disabilities Program
Temple University, Ritter Annex
13th St. & Columbia Ave.
Philadelphia, PA 19122
Director: Edward Newman, Ph.D.
(215) 787-1356

RHODE ISLAND
Child Development Center
Rhode Island Hospital
593 Eddy St.
Providence, RI 02902
Director: Siegfried M. Pueschel, M.D., Ph.D.
(401) 277-5071

SOUTH CAROLINA
UAF Program of South Carolina—USC
Center for Developmental Disabilities
Benson Building, Pickens St.
University of South Carolina
Columbia, SC 29208
Director: Richard R. Ferrante, Ph.D.
(803) 777-4839

SOUTH DAKOTA
Center for the Developmentally Disabled
Julian Hall
University of South Dakota
Vermillion, SD 57069
Director: Charles A. Anderson, Ed.D.
(605) 677-5311

TENNESSEE
Child Development Center
University of Tennessee
711 Jefferson Ave.
Memphis, TN 38105
Director: Gerald Golden, M.D.
(901) 528-6512

TEXAS
University-Affiliated Center
Suite 748
6011 Harry Hines Blvd.
Dallas, TX 75235
Director: Doman K. Keele, M.D.
(214) 688-2883

UTAH
Developmental Center for Handicapped
  Persons
UMC 68
Utah State University
Logan, UT 84322
Director: Marvin Fifield, Ed.D.
(801) 750-1982

VIRGINIA
Virginia Institute for Developmental
  Disabilities
1015 W. Main Street
Richmond, VA 23284
Director: Howard Garner
(804) 257-8485

WASHINGTON
Child Development and Mental Retardation
  Center
University of Washington
Seattle, WA 98195
Director: Donald F. Farrell, M.D.
(206) 543-3224

WEST VIRGINIA
University-Affiliated Center for Developmental
  Disabilities
509 Allen Hall/PO Box 6122
West Virginia University
Morgantown, WV 26506-6122
Director: Ashok S. Dey
(304) 293-4692

West Virginia Genetics Evaluation and
  Counseling Center
West Virginia University School of Medicine
Morgantown, WV 26506
Director: Stephen R. Amato, M.D., Ph.D.
(304) 293-7331

WISCONSIN
Clinical Services Unit, Waisman Center
University of Wisconsin
1500 Highland Ave.
Madison, WI 53705-2280
Director: Terrence R. Dolan, Ph.D.
(608) 263-5940

SOURCE: *American Association of University-Affiliated Programs.*

GOVERNMENT-SUPPORTED RESEARCH IN MENTAL RETARDATION

The National Institute of Child Health and Human Development supports several centers around the country that investigate the biological and behavioral aspects of mental retardation and other developmental disabilities and new ways of dealing with the disorders. The patients used in this research are selected by the investigators.

Patients are usually referred to the centers by their own physicians, so you generally cannot volunteer for such research. However, most, but not all, of the centers have screening, diagnostic evaluation, treatment, and referral programs. A few maintain special schools.

MENTAL RETARDATION RESEARCH CENTERS

CALIFORNIA
Mental Retardation Research Center
Neuropsychiatric Institute
Center for the Health Sciences
University of California at Los Angeles
760 Westwood Plaza
Los Angeles, CA 90024
Dr. Nathaniel A. Buchwald, Director
(213) 825-0313

COLORADO
The John F. Kennedy Child Development
  Center
University of Colorado Health Sciences
  Center
4200 E. Ninth Ave.
Denver, CO 80220
Stephen Goodman, M.D., Director
(303) 394-7940

ILLINOIS
Joseph P. Kennedy Jr. Mental Retardation
  Research Center
Department of Pediatrics, Box 413
Wyler Children's Hospital–University of
  Chicago
5841 Maryland Ave.
Chicago, IL 60637
Dr. Glyn Dawson, Director
(312) 962-6430

KANSAS
Center for Research in Human Development
University of Kansas
New Haworth Hall, Room 223
Lawrence, KS 66045
Dr. Richard L. Schiefelbusch, Director
(913) 864-4295

MASSACHUSETTS
Mental Retardation Research Center
Boston Children's Hospital Medical Center
300 Longwood Ave.
Boston, MA 02115
Dr. Charles F. Barlow, Director
(617) 735-6385

Research in Mental Retardation
E. K. Shriver Center for Mental Retardation,
  Inc.
200 Trapelo Rd.
Waltham, MA 02154
Edwin H. Kolodny, M.D., Director
(617) 893-3500

NEW YORK
Rose F. Kennedy Center in Research in Mental
  Retardation and Human Development
Albert Einstein College of Medicine
1410 Pelham Parkway, S.
Bronx, New York 10461
Dr. Herbert G. Vaughan, Jr., Director
(212) 430-2468

NORTH CAROLINA
Child Development Research Center
Highway 54 Bypass W. 071-A
University of North Carolina
Chapel Hill, NC 27514
Dr. James Gallagher, Director
(919) 966-4121

OHIO
Institute of Developmental Research
The Children's Hospital Research Foundation
Elland Ave. & Bethesda
Cincinnati, OH 45229
Peter Dignan, M.D., Director
(513) 559-4471

TENNESSEE
The John F. Kennedy Center for Research on
  Education and Human Development
PO Box 40
Peabody College of Vanderbilt University
Nashville, TN 37203
Dr. Alfred Baumeister, Director
(615) 322-8242

WASHINGTON
Child Development and Mental Retardation
  Research Center
University of Washington
WJ-10
Seattle, WA 98195
Donald F. Farrell, M.D., Acting Director
(206) 543-3224

WISCONSIN
Harry A. Waisman Center on Mental
  Retardation and Human Development
Waismen Center
University of Wisconsin, Room 247
1500 Highland Ave.
Madison, WI 53706
Dr. Terrence R. Dolan, Director
(608) 263-5940

SOURCE: *National Institute of Child Health and Human Development.*

SOME SPECIAL SCHOOLS FOR CHILDREN WITH DYSLEXIA

Some parents with youngsters who have dyslexia may find it advisable to send them to special schools with programs of instruction geared to this disability. Some of these schools claim excellent results. There is no comprehensive list of such schools, but the Orton Dyslexia Society has had so many requests for such information that it has compiled the following list of schools. The Society emphasizes that it is not an accrediting body, does not endorse or recommend the following schools, and advises any parent interested in any educational facility with dyslexia programs to thoroughly check the school out and satisfy themselves that it meets their youngster's needs. The Society has a checklist of questions available for parents to ask about a school.

CALIFORNIA
Dunn School
PO Box 98
Los Olivos, CA 93441
(805) 688-6471
Grades 8–12, coed, boarding

COLORADO
The Denver Academy
1125 S. Race St.
Denver, CO 80210
(303) 777-5870
Grades 1–12, coed, boarding & day

CONNECTICUT
The Forman School
Norfolk Rd.
Litchfield, CT 06759
(203) 567-8712
Ages 13–19, coed, boarding

Grove School, Inc.
175 Copse Rd.
PO Box 646
Madison, CT 06443
(203) 245-2778
Ages 11–18, boys, boarding

Salisbury Summer School
Salisbury, CT 06068
(203) 435-2931
Grades 9–12, boys, boarding

FLORIDA
The Vanguard School
PO Box 928
Lake Wales, FL 33853
(813) 676-6091
Ages 6–16, coed, boarding & day

GEORGIA
Brandon Hall School
1701 Brandon Hall Drive
Atlanta, GA 30338
(404) 394-8177
Ages 11–19, coed, day; boys, boarding

ILLINOIS
The Brehm Preparatory School
1245 E. Grand
Carbondale, IL 62901
(618) 457-0371
Ages 12–21, coed, boarding

MASSACHUSETTS
Valleyhead School
PO Box 714
Lenox, MA 01240
(413) 637-3635
Girls

Leland Hall
Leland Rd.
Norfolk, MA 02056
(617) 528-0882
Ages 7–18, coed, boarding & day

Linden Hill School
S. Mountain Rd.
Northfield, MA 01360
(413) 498-2167
Ages 10–14, boys, boarding

Landmark School
412 Hale St.
Prides Crossing, MA 01965
(617) 927-4440
Ages 8–18, coed, boarding

The HighCroft School
Gale Rd.
Williamstown, MA 01267
(413) 458-8136
Ages 8–19, coed, boarding

NEW JERSEY
The Hun School of Princeton
Edgerstoune Rd.
PO Box 271
Princeton, NJ 08540
(609) 921-7600
Grades 7–12, coed, boarding & day

NEW YORK
The Kildonan School
Perry Corners Rd.
Amenia, NY 12501
(914) 373-8111
Ages 9–20, boys, boarding

Darrow School
PO Box 260
Shaker Rd.
New Lebanon, NY 12125
(518) 794-7700
Ages 13–19, coed, boarding & day

Trinity-Pawling School
Pawling, NY 12564
(914) 855-3100
Grades 9–12, boys, boarding; girls, day

The Knox School
Saint James, NY 11780
(516) 584-5500
Ages 12–18, coed, boarding & day

The Gow School
Emery Rd.
South Wales, NY 14139
(716) 652-3450
Grades 7–12, boys, boarding

NORTH CAROLINA
Patterson School
Route 5, Box 170
Lenoir, NC 28645
(704) 758-2374
Grades 7–12, coed, boarding

PENNSYLVANIA
The Phelps School
Malvern, PA 19355
(215) 644-1754
Ages 12–18

SOUTH CAROLINA
Trident Academy
PO Box 804
Mount Pleasant, SC 29464
(803) 884-7046
Grades K–12, coed, boarding locally

TEXAS
Dallas Academy
950 Tiffany Way
Dallas, TX 75218
(214) 324-1481
Ages 13–19, coed, 80 percent day

VERMONT
Bennington School
19 Fairview St.
Bennington, VT 15201
(802) 447-0773
Girls

Greenwood School
Box 58-A, RFD 2
Putney, VT 05346
(802) 387-4545
Ages 8–14, boys, boarding

Pine Ridge School
PO Box 138
Williston, VT 05495
(802) 434-2161
Ages 12–19, coed, boarding

VIRGINIA
Oakland School
Oakland Farm
Boyd Tavern, VA 22947
(804) 293-9059
Ages 8–16, coed, boarding & day

SOURCE: *Orton Dyslexia Society.*

SERVICES DIRECTORY FOR THE LEARNING DISABLED

This directory lists about 500 facilities and services throughout the United States for those with learning disabilities. It includes educational facilities, residential schools, day schools, speech-language training, career counseling, summer-camp programs, mental health services, and psychological counseling. There is a nominal mailing fee for a single copy.

Association for Children With Learning
  Diabilities
4156 Library Rd.
Pittsburgh, PA 15234

ORGANIZATIONS AND AGENCIES

Association for Children and Adults with
  Learning Disabilities
4156 Library Rd.
Pittsburgh, PA 15234
(412) 341-8077

National membership organization for professionals, parents and others concerned with learning disabilities. Fifty state affiliates, more than 775 local chapters. Pamphlets, research updates, bimonthly newsletter, booklets, audiovisual materials, a national directory of facilities and services for the learning disabled. Answers questions from the public. Will send more information upon request.

Association for Retarded Citizens of the United
  States
2501 Ave. J
Arlington, TX 76006
(817) 640-0204

A national voluntary, nonprofit, membership organization for those interested in improving the welfare of persons with mental retardation. 1300 state and local chapters around the country. A source of information and local services. Pamphlets, brochures, books, audiovisual materials, and a newspaper. Will provide more information and name of an affiliate near you upon request.

National Easter Seal Society, Inc.
2023 W. Ogden Ave.
Chicago, IL 60612
(312) 243-8400/Voice
(312) 243-8880/TDD

A national organization with state and local societies formed to give services to people with disabilities from any cause, including epilepsy, cerebral palsy, stroke, speech and hearing disorders, geriatric problems, fractures, arthritis, learning and developmental disorders, heart disease, spina bifida, accidents, multiple sclerosis. Maintains about 200 rehabilitation centers nationwide, with various services, depending on the local unit. A major source of information and self-help. Publishes pamphlets and booklets. Referrals to services are made through local Easter Seal affiliates listed in local phone directories. Will provide more information and the location of an Easter Seal affiliate near you upon request.

National Information Center for Handicapped
  Children and Youth
1555 Wilson Blvd.
Rosslyn, VA 22209
(703) 528-8480

A national government-supported service that answers questions from the public on all kinds of disabilities. A major source of computer-based information and referrals. Parents, for example, who want to know services in their community geared to the child with learning disabilities can call toll-free or write and receive a computerized printout of that information. Includes parent and child support groups, treatment centers, government agencies, rehabilitation facilities, legal rights, etc. Extensive publications, fact sheets on all disabilities, a newsletter, reading lists, and bibliographies.

The Orton Dyslexia Society
724 York Rd.
Baltimore, MD 21204
(301) 296-0232
(800) ABC-D123

Nonprofit, membership organization of professionals and the public. Local branches in many parts of the country. Information source for individuals, families, other interested persons on dyslexia. Supports medical research. Booklets, pamphlets, fact sheets, audiocassette tapes, a quarterly newsletter, *Perspectives*. Answers questions from the public, maintains lists of facilities specializing in dyslexia. Will send more information and name of a local branch in your area upon request.

BOOKS

Angel Unaware, **Dale Evans Rogers,** Old Tappan, NJ: Revell Co., 1984 (Down Syndrome).

The Complete Handbook of Children's Reading Disorders, **Hilde L. Mosse,** New York: Human Sciences Press, 1982.

Dyslexia and Your Child, **Rudolph F. Wagner,** New York: Harper & Row, 1979.

The Hidden Handicap, **Dr. Judith Ehre Kranes,** New York: Simon & Schuster, 1980 (learning disabilities).

Hope for the Families: New Directions for Parents of Persons With Retardation or Other Disabilities, **R. Perske,** Nashville: Abingdon Press, 1981.

A Little Time, **Anne Norris Baldwin,** New York: Viking Press, 1978 (Down Syndrome).

Me and Einstein, **Rose Blue,** New York: Human Sciences Press, 1979.

Our Special Child, **Bette M. Ross,** New York: Walker, 1981 (Down Syndrome).

Overcoming Dyslexia, **Beve Hornsby,** New York: Arco Publishers, 1984.

Secret Places of the Stairs, **Susan Sallis,** New York: Harper & Row, 1984 (Down Syndrome).

Teaching Your Down's Syndrome Infant: A Guide for Parents, **Marci Hanson,** Baltimore: University Park Press, 1977.

An Uncommon Gift, **James S. Evans,** Philadelphia: Westminster Press, 1983 (dyslexia).

Yes They Can: A Handbook for Effectively Parenting the Handicapped, Irvine, CA: Reality Productions Publications, 1981; Reality Productions Publications, PO Box 18452, Irvine, CA 92713.

The Young Child With Down's Syndrome, **S. M. Pueschel,** New York: Human Sciences Press, 1983.

MATERIALS, FREE AND FOR SALE

Free (single copies)

Learning Disabilities due to Minimal Brain Dysfunction: Hope Through Research, 22 pages.

National Institute of Neurological and Communicative Disorders and Stroke
9000 Rockville Pike
Bethesda, MD 20892

The Problem of Dyslexia, pamphlet.
What is Dyslexia? Pamphlet.

The Orton Dyslexia Society
724 York Rd.
Baltimore, MD 21204
(301) 296-0232

Developmental Dyslexia and Related Reading Disorders, brochure.
Facts About Down Syndrome for Women Over 35, 16 pages.

National Institute of Child Health and Human Development
9000 Rockville Pike
Bethesda, MD 20205

Dehumanization vs. Dignity, 12 pages.
Dignity of Risk and the Mentally Retarded, 11 pages.
How to Provide for Their Future, 52 pages.
Make the Most of Your Baby, 23 pages.
Primer for Parents of a Mentally Retarded Child, 18 pages.
Toilet Training Your Retarded Child, 8 pages.

Association for Retarded Citizens of the United States
2501 Ave. J
Arlington, TX 76006
(817) 640-0204

For sale

Annals of Dyslexia 1985
Sex Differences in Dyslexia
Readings for Parents, packet of materials.
Guidelines for Seeking Help for Dyslexic Students, pamphlet.
Parents' Guidelines to the Evaluation Process
Checklist for Schools, Camps

The Orton Dyslexia Society
724 York Rd.
Baltimore, MD 21204

Audiocassette tapes

Numerous audiocassettes on specific aspects of dyslexia, delivered by speakers at the Orton Dyslexia Society's annual conferences. Some topics are technical, but may be valuable to a sophisticated person who wants more knowledge. Some subjects: Biological Perspectives in Dyslexia, The Brain of the Learning Disabled Individual, Pediatric Aspects of Dyslexia, the Legal Rights of Dyslexics, A Pediatric Neurologist Looks at Dyslexia, An Uncommon Gift.

The Orton Dyslexia Society
724 York Rd.
Baltimore, MD 21204
(301) 296-0232

MULTIPLE SCLEROSIS

See also Rehabilitation, page 460.

Multiple sclerosis (MS) is a neurological disease that primarily strikes young adults; the median onset age is 30. An estimated 135,000 Americans have MS, according to federal health statistics. Some estimates put the figure as high as 250,000. The disease destroys the outside coating around the message-carrying nerve fibers in the brain and spinal cord. Plaque, or scar tissue, appears where the coating, or myelin, has been damaged or destroyed. Consequently, messages throughout the nervous system cannot be transmitted properly. MS most often strikes women, rarely strikes children or people older than 50, and most frequently affects whites and those who live in colder climates. MS is highly unpredictable. Although it can cause grave disability, in some persons it is so mild it is overlooked; it does not significantly shorten the life span.

Cause: Unknown. It is believed that there is a genetic susceptibility to the disease. Some speculate it is caused by a virus or a malfunction of the immune system.

Symptoms: The symptoms vary greatly and depend on which areas of the central nervous system are damaged. In most cases, the disease is also characterized by dramatic remissions and flare-ups, which appear to be tied to emotional stress in the view of some experts. Common indications of the disease include vision disorders (double vision, temporary blindness), muscle weakness, loss of coordination, "pins and needles" prickling, foot dragging, hand tremors, and dizziness. Partial or complete paralysis, loss of bladder and bowel control, and speech problems may develop. Periods of remission may last for months or even years. About 10–20 percent of patients simply become progressively worse.

Diagnosis: There is no single laboratory test to detect MS, and its unpredictable course and varied symptoms make diagnosis difficult. Confusion with many other neurological disorders is common. Certain procedures often point doctors toward a diagnosis: spinal fluid analysis, CAT scans, standard physical and neurological tests, and magnetic resonance imaging (MRI). It is common to diagnose MS only after a person has had several attacks or a pattern of attacks.

Treatment: There is no cure for MS, although current research is investigating new ways of treating the symptoms and helping patients better cope with the disease. Some of the research is promising. Powerful immunosuppressant drugs, and other techniques to modify the damaging effects of the autoimmune reactions are being extensively investigated.

MS patients may need physical therapy to keep muscles functioning and to minimize crippling. Special drugs are sometimes used to prevent spasms. If the disease becomes advanced, special aids, such as support railings, specially designed furniture, and wheelchairs, may be necessary to help patients cope with their incapacities and maintain independence.

WHERE TO FIND TREATMENT FOR MS

MS is generally diagnosed, evaluated, and treated by neurologists; patients may need special physical therapy at rehabilitation centers as the disease progresses. Centers around the country specialize in the diagnosis and care of MS. Most of them are in the neurology departments of leading medical centers. All of the centers on the following list are affiliated with chapters of the Multiple Sclerosis Society. You are well advised to take advantage of the patient services provided by the Society. The local chapters of the Society offer information, counseling and referrals to other agencies for special assistance, as well as rehabilitation, recreational, and equipment loan programs.

For a list of the heads of departments of neurology at leading medical schools, *see* page 621. These physicians also are excellent sources for treatment or medical referrals for multiple sclerosis, as well as for other neurological diseases.

MULTIPLE SCLEROSIS CLINICS

All of the listed clinics are affiliated with a local chapter of the National Multiple Sclerosis Society. The clinic is listed first, followed by the name and phone number of the affiliated chapter.

ALABAMA

Multiple Sclerosis Evaluation Clinic
University of Alabama
Birmingham, AL 35233
(205) 852-1592

Central Alabama Chapter
(205) 822-1592

ARIZONA

Multiple Sclerosis Clinic
Barrow Neurological Institute
St. Joseph's Hospital and Medical Center
Phoenix, AZ 85013
(602) 241-3000

Central Arizona Chapter
(602) 968-2488

CALIFORNIA

University of California, Irvine
Medical Center MS Clinic
Orange, CA 92668
(714) 634-5678

Orange County Chapter
(714) 633-9391

Rancho Los Amigos Hospital
Multiple Sclerosis Clinic
Downey, CA 90242
(213) 922-7022

Loma Linda University Medical Center
Multiple Sclerosis Clinic
Loma Linda University
Loma Linda, CA 92354
(714) 796-7311

UCLA Reed Neurological Center
Multiple Sclerosis Clinic
The Center for Health Sciences
Los Angeles, CA 90024
(213) 825-9111

Harbor UCLA Medical Center
Multiple Sclerosis Clinic
Torrance, CA 90509
(213) 825-9111

Huntington Memorial Hospital
Multiple Sclerosis Clinic
Pasadena, CA 91105
(213) 440-5000

Multiple Sclerosis Clinic
Valley Hospital Medical Center
Van Nuys, CA 91405
(818) 908-8735

Multiple Sclerosis Clinic
Wadsworth VA Medical Center
West Los Angeles, CA 90073
(213) 824-3223

Southern California Chapter
(213) 247-1175

COLORADO
Boulder Memorial Hospital
Multiple Sclerosis Clinic
Boulder, CO 80302
(303) 443-0230

Porter Memorial Hospital
Multiple Sclerosis Clinic
Denver, CO 80210
(303) 778-1955

Western Slope MS Clinic
St. Mary's Hospital
Grand Junction, CO 81502
(303) 243-1331

Central Colorado Chapter
(303) 691-2956

CONNECTICUT
MS Clinical Center
University of Connecticut Health Center
Farmington, CT 06115
(203) 674-3494

Greater Connecticut Chapter
(203) 236-3229

DELAWARE
Multiple Sclerosis Clinic
Wilmington Medical Center
Medical Center of Delaware
Wilmington, DE 19899
(302) 428-3274

Delaware Chapter
(302) 571-9956

GEORGIA
Multiple Sclerosis Clinic
Medical College of Georgia
Augusta, GA 30910
(404) 828-4531

Georgia Chapter
(404) 874-9797 or
(800) 822-3379

ILLINOIS
Multiple Sclerosis Clinic
Northwestern Medical Faculty Foundation
Chicago, IL 60611
(312) 649-6980

Rush-Presbyterian-St. Luke's
MS Center
Chicago, IL 60612
(312) 942-5000

University of Chicago
Outpatient Neurology Clinic
MS Center
Chicago, IL 60637
(312) 947-1000

MS Center
Loyola University
Medical Center
Maywood, IL 60153
(312) 531-3000

Nesset Health Center
Parkside Human Services Foundation
Lutheran General Hospital
Park Ridge, IL 60068
(312) 696-5059

Chicago-Northern Illinois Chapter
(312) 922-8000

Stretch Miller Memorial MS Clinic
St. Francis Hospital
Peoria, IL 61637
(309) 672-2000

Greater Illinois Chapter
(309) 688-1778

INDIANA
MS Outpatient Clinic
Robert Long Hospital
Indiana University Medical Center
Indianapolis, IN 46223
(317) 635-8431

Indiana State Chapter
(317) 634-8796

IOWA
MS Re-evaluative Clinic
Iowa Methodist Medical Center
Des Moines, IA 50303
(515) 283-6212

Western Iowa Chapter
(515) 223-8121

KANSAS
MS Clinic
Menorah Medical Center
Kansas City, KS 66102
(816) 276-3926

Mid-America Chapter
(913) 432-3926

MS Rehabilitation Clinic
St. Joseph Medical Center
Wichita, KS 67218
(316) 685-1111

South Central and Western Kansas Chapter
(316) 264-5425

KENTUCKY
Multiple Sclerosis Clinic
University of Kentucky
Lexington, KY 40536
(606) 233-6719

Kentucky Chapter
(502) 636-1700

LOUISIANA
Multiple Sclerosis Rehabilitation Clinic
F. Edward Hebert Hospital
New Orleans, LA 70114
(504) 362-1822

Louisiana Chapter
(504) 821-5821

MAINE
Multiple Sclerosis and Neurological Diseases
   Clinic
Maine Medical Center
Portland, ME 04102
(207) 871-0111

Maine Chapter
(207) 761-5815

MARYLAND
Johns Hopkins University Hospital
Multiple Sclerosis Comprehensive Care Clinic
Baltimore, MD 21205
(301) 955-5000

Multiple Sclerosis Rehabilitation Clinic
Union Memorial Hospital
Baltimore, MD 21218
(301) 554-2344

Multiple Sclerosis Center
University of Maryland Hospital
Baltimore, MD 21201
(301) 528-5605

Maryland Chapter
(301) 821-8626

MASSACHUSETTS
Beverly Hospital
Multiple Sclerosis Clinic, OPD
Beverly, MA 01915
(617) 922-3000

Brigham & Women's Hospital
Multiple Sclerosis Clinical and Research
   Center
Boston, MA 02115
(617) 732-7601

Tufts New England Medical Center
MS Clinic
Boston, MA 02111
(617) 956-5000

Framingham Union Hospital MS Clinic
Framingham, MA 01701
(617) 890-4990

University of Massachusetts
Medical Center MS Clinic
Department of Neurology
Worcester, MA 01605
(617) 856-0011

Massachusetts Chapter
(617) 890-4990

MICHIGAN
Multiple Sclerosis Clinic
University Health Center
Detroit, MI 48201
(313) 494-5050

MS Clinic, Mary Free Bed Hospital and
   Rehabilitation Center
Grand Rapids, MI 49503
(616) 242-0300

Midland Multiple Sclerosis Clinic
Midland Hospital Center
Midland, MI 48640
(517) 839-3000

Michigan Chapter
(313) 967-2211

MINNESOTA
Multiple Sclerosis Clinic
Fairview Community Hospital
Minneapolis, MN 55404
(612) 721-9100

Minnesota North Star Chapter
(612) 870-1500

MISSOURI
St. Francis Medical Center
MS Clinic
Cape Girardeau, MO 63701
(314) 335-1251

Washington University
Multiple Sclerosis Clinic
St. Louis, MO 63130
(314) 362-5000

Gateway Area Chapter
(314) 241-8285

NEVADA
MS Clinic, Department of Neurology
University of Nevada Medical School
Reno, NV 89520
(702) 784-6001

Northern Nevada Chapter
(702) 329-7180

NEW JERSEY
Bernard W. Gimbel Multiple Sclerosis
  Comprehensive Care Center at Holy Name
  Hospital
Teaneck, NJ 07666
(201) 837-0727

Bergen-Passaic Counties Chapter
(201) 837-0515

MS Diagnostic & Treatment Center
University Hospital
University of Medicine and Dentistry of New
  Jersey
Newark, NJ 07103
(201) 456-4300

Northern New Jersey Chapter
(201) 783-6442

NEW MEXICO
Multiple Sclerosis Clinic
University of New Mexico Hospital
Albuquerque, NM 87106
(505) 843-2111

New Mexico Central Chapter
(505) 888-4418

NEW YORK
Albany Medical Center
MS Neurology Clinic
Albany, NY 12208
(518) 445-3125

Sunnyview Multiple Sclerosis Clinic
Sunnyview Hospital & Rehabilitation Center
Schenectady, NY 12308
(518) 382-4500

Capital District Chapter
(518) 459-1631

Rehabilitation Services, Inc.
MS Clinic
Binghamton, NY 13905
(607) 722-5308

Greater Broome County Chapter
(607) 724-5464

South Nassau Community Hospital
MS Clinic
Oceanside, NY 11572
(516) 536-1600

Nassau County Chapter
(516) 579-9120

Medical Rehabilitation Research and Training
  Center for Multiple Sclerosis
Albert Einstein College of Medicine
Bronx, NY
(212) 921-9199

Multiple Sclerosis Care Center
Maimonides Medical Center
Brooklyn, NY
(212) 921-9199

Columbia-Presbyterian Multiple Sclerosis Care
  Center
Columbia-Presbyterian Medical Center
New York, NY
(212) 921-9199

New York City Chapter
Multiple Sclerosis Society
55 West 44th St.
New York, NY 10036
(212) 921-9199

Rochester Area Multiple Sclerosis Inc.
Strong Memorial Hospital
Rochester, NY 14620
(716) 271-0801

Rochester Area Chapter
(716) 271-0801

Brunswick Physical Medicine and
    Rehabilitation Hospital
MS Clinic
Amityville, NY 11701
(516) 264-5000

MS Medical Rehabilitation Center
St. Charles Hospital
Port Jefferson, NY 11794
(516) 473-2800

Suffolk County Chapter
(516) 421-3857

Multiple Sclerosis Clinic
Westchester County Medical Center
Valhalla, NY 10595
(914) 946-4024

Westchester County Chapter
(914) 694-3800

NORTH CAROLINA
Asheville Multiple Sclerosis Physical Therapy
    Clinic
Jean M. Harkey & Associates Facility
Asheville, NC 28813
(704) 253-6759

MS Clinic
Charlotte Rehabilitation Hospital
Charlotte, NC 28203
(704) 333-6634

Greater Carolinas Chapter
(704) 372-2955

NORTH DAKOTA
North Dakota Multiple Sclerosis Clinic and
    Treatment Group
St. Luke's Hospital
Fargo, ND 58107
(701) 235-5354 (Dr. Goodkin)

Dakota Chapter
(701) 235-2678

OHIO
MS Clinic
Ohio State University Hospitals
Columbus, OH 43210
(614) 421-8931

Mid-Ohio Chapter
(614) 291-2442

Multiple Sclerosis Diagnostic and Evaluation
    Clinic
Medical College of Ohio in Toledo
Toledo, OH 43699
(419) 385-4661

Northwest Ohio Chapter
(419) 531-1671

Multiple Sclerosis Comprehensive Clinical
    Center
St. Elizabeth Hospital Medical Center
Youngstown, OH 44512
(216) 788-2427

Northeast Ohio Chapter
(216) 434-3411

MS Clinic
St. Elizabeth Medical Center
Dayton, OH 45408
(513) 229-6000

Western Ohio Chapter
(513) 461-5232

OREGON
Multiple Sclerosis Clinic
University of Oregon Health Sciences Center
Portland, OR 97201
(503) 225-7967

Oregon Chapter
(503) 223-9511

PENNSYLVANIA
MS Diagnostic and Evaluation Center
Milton S. Hershey Medical Center
Pennsylvania State University
Hershey, PA 17033
(717) 534-8521

Central Pennsylvania Chapter
(717) 652-2108

MS Clinic
Good Shepherd Rehabilitation Hospital
Allentown, PA 18103
(215) 821-2121

Multiple Sclerosis Clinical Center
Thomas Jefferson University Hospital
Philadelphia, PA 19107
(215) 928-7365

Multiple Sclerosis Clinic of the Hospital of the
University of Pennsylvania
Department of Neurology, G-1
Philadelphia, PA 19104
(215) 662-4000

Greater Delaware Valley Chapter
(215) 963-0100

MS Clinic
Franklin Regional Medical Center
Franklin, PA 16323
(814) 437-7000

Northwestern Pennsylvania Chapter
(814) 838-4744

SOUTH CAROLINA
Multiple Sclerosis Clinic
Lexington County Hospital
Columbia, SC 29169
(803) 799-7848

South Carolina Chapter
(803) 799-7848

TENNESSEE
MS Physical Therapy Clinic
Patricia Neal Rehabilitation Center
Ft. Sanders Presbyterian Hospital
Knoxville, TN 37920
(615) 546-2811

MS Physical Therapy Clinic
Erlanger Medical Plaza
Chattanooga, TN 37403
(615) 778-7000

Setenga Chapter
(615) 624-2064

TEXAS
Multiple Sclerosis Clinic
Methodist Hospital
Physical Therapy Section
Lubbock, TX 79410
(806) 792-1011

Permian Basin Chapter
(915) 699-4944

UTAH
MS Clinic
University of Utah
Department of Neurology
Salt Lake City, UT 84132
(801) 581-2121

Utah State Chapter
(801) 575-8500

VIRGINIA
Multiple Sclerosis Clinic
Medical College of Virginia
Richmond, VA 23298
(804) 786-9718

Central Virginia Chapter
(804) 282-2358

WASHINGTON
Multiple Sclerosis Clinical Center
University Hospital
Seattle, WA 98195
(206) 543-3300

Puget Sound Chapter
(206) 624-3025

SOURCE: *National Multiple Sclerosis Society.*

GOVERNMENT MS RESEARCH CENTERS

The National Institute of Neurological and
Communicative Disorders and Stroke supports
centers for the study of the causes and most
effective treatments of MS. Some of these centers accept patients for experimental treatment
programs or rehabilitation. The personnel at the
centers are among the nation's top authorities
on MS.

CALIFORNIA
Scripps Clinic & Research Foundation
10666 N. Torrey Pines Rd.
La Jolla, CA 92037
Michael Oldstone, M.D.
(619) 455-8054

University of California at Los Angeles
Reed Neurological Research Center
710 Westwood Plaza
Los Angeles, CA 90024
George Ellison, M.D.
(213) 825-7313

University of California at San Francisco
Department of Neurology
San Francisco, CA 94143
Stanley Prusiner, M.D.
(415) 476-4483

MARYLAND
Johns Hopkins University
School of Medicine
720 Rutland Ave.
Baltimore, MD 21205
Guy McKhann, M.D.
(301) 955-5000

NEW YORK
Albert Einstein College of Medicine of
    Yeshiva University
1300 Morris Park Ave.
Bronx, NY 10461
Murray B. Bornstein, M.D.
(212) 430-2508

PENNSYLVANIA
Hospital of the University of Pennsylvania
3400 Spruce St.
Philadelphia, PA 19104
Donald H. Silberberg, M.D.
(215) 662-3386

Wistar Institute
3601 Spruce St.
Philadelphia, PA 19104
Hilary Koprowski, M.D.
(215) 898-3700

SOURCE: *National Institute of Neurological and Communicative Disorders and Stroke.*

RESEARCH AND TREATMENT AT THE NATIONAL INSTITUTES OF HEALTH

Selected patients with MS are being studied at the Clinical Center of the National Institutes of Health in Bethesda, Maryland. Of primary interest are families or twins with MS for genetic studies. Participation is by physician referral. For more information your physician can contact:

Office of the Director
The Clinical Center
Building 10, Room 2C-146
National Institutes of Health
Bethesda, MD 20892
(301) 496-4891

ORGANIZATION

National Multiple Sclerosis Society
205 E. 42nd St.
New York, NY 10017
(212) 986-3240

A voluntary membership organization for those with multiple sclerosis, their families and other interested persons. With about 140 chapters and branch chapters throughout the country, it is a major source of information and self-help. Offers brochures, booklets, a quarterly magazine. Some chapters are affiliated with MS clinics. Chapters provide numerous patient services, including referral services to clinics and community services, loans of medical equipment, a home care course for families and friends who care for an MS person, psychological counseling, swimming programs, vocational rehabilitation. Will provide more information upon request.

BOOKS

The Multiple Sclerosis Diet Book, **Ray Laver Swank,** New York: Doubleday, 1977.

Multiple Sclerosis: The Facts, **Walter Bryan Matthews,** London: Oxford University Press, 1980.

Multiple Sclerosis: A Guide for Patients and Families, **Labe C. Scheinberg, M.D.,** New York: Raven Press, 1983.

The Multiple Sclerosis Handbook for Patients, Family and Physicians, **Dr. Jack H. Petajan,** Utah Chapter, National Multiple Sclerosis Society, 1980.

Multiple Sclerosis: A Personal View, **Cynthia Birrer,** New York: Thomas, 1979.

The Pursuit of Hope, **Miriam Ottenberg,** New York: Rawson-Wade, 1978.

Research on Multiple Sclerosis; a loose leaf book that contains current information on all major research aspects of multiple sclerosis. New York: National Multiple Sclerosis Society, 1983.

FREE MATERIALS

Multiple Sclerosis: Hope Through Research, 18 pages; Multiple Sclerosis: NINCDS Research Program.

National Institute of Neurological and Communicative Disorders and Stroke
Building 31, Room 8A06
Bethesda, MD 20892

About Multiple Sclerosis: What Everyone Should Know, 16 pages.

Emotional Aspects of MS, 12 pages

MS: The Enemy of Young Adults, 6 pages.

A Practical Guide: Living With MS, 16 pages.

Someone You Know Has Multiple Sclerosis: A Book for Families, 28 pages.

Who Says Multiple Sclerosis Patients Can't Work?, 10 pages.

National Multiple Sclerosis Society
205 E. 42nd St.
New York, NY 10017
(212) 986-3240

MUSCULAR DYSTROPHY AND RELATED NEUROMUSCULAR DISEASES

See also Rehabilitation, page 460.

Muscular dystrophy is but one of more than 40 different disorders that strike the functioning of the body's neuromuscular system. Although all neuromuscular diseases involve deterioration of the muscle and cause similar disabilities, they may strike different parts of the body and have different characteristics. For example, ALS, amyotrophic lateral sclerosis, affects the motor nerve cells of the spinal cord; other neuromuscular diseases affect the peripheral nerves of the extremities, the junctions of nerve and muscle, and so forth. Some involve enzyme deficiencies, inflammation of the muscles, or abnormal functioning of the endocrine system. About half are clearly inherited; others are not known to be.

All of these disorders are grouped together here not only because of their underlying similarity, but because they are often treated by the same specialists. They also fall under the diagnosis and treatment network developed by the Muscular Dystrophy Association, which offers considerable assistance to those suffering from such diseases (*see* page 390). Thus, it is a convenience to medical consumers to view them as a single group of similar neuromuscular disorders, even though their causes, treatment, and management may vary.

MUSCULAR DYSTROPHY

There are several types of muscular dystrophy, but the most common form, recognized more than 100 years ago, is Duchenne muscular dystrophy. Named after the French physician who described it in 1861, Duchenne muscular dystrophy is the disease most people mean when they refer to muscular dystrophy. Like other neuromuscular diseases, it is characterized by a wasting away or degeneration of the muscles. Duchenne muscular dystrophy is a genetic and fatal disorder that strikes boys almost exclusively; an estimated 20–30 out of every 100,000 males born will suffer from the disease. It can be passed on through the mother if she carries the defective gene. About one-third of cases, however, have no previous family history.

Cause: The disease is transmitted genetically through females to their offspring. Each male child born to a carrier (the mother has no symptoms of the disease) has a 50 percent chance of inheriting the disease, and each female offspring has a 50 percent chance of passing the disease along to her own children. Researchers believe that at least one-third of the cases come from "spontaneous mutations" in which there is no family history of the disease. Sophisticated genetic tests can detect carriers with greater than 90 percent accuracy.

Symptoms: Duchenne muscular dystrophy usually does not become apparent until the child is about two years old. Even then, it may not be noticed for months or even years. Early development, such as sitting up and raising the head, may seem normal, but symptoms show up when the child begins to walk. Early symptoms include frequent falls, a slightly waddling walk, difficulty in rising from the floor, and a clumsy gait. These symptoms are sometimes diagnosed as an orthopedic problem. Later there is difficulty climbing stairs, a rolling movement to the hips while walking, and pains in the calves. The disease is progressive, leading to the use of a wheelchair and ending in death in early adulthood.

Diagnosis: Most muscular dystrophy, including Duchenne can be quickly and accurately diagnosed at a competent center on the basis of a physical examination and laboratory tests. Common tests are an electromyogram, which measures the electrical activity of the muscle, and serum enzyme tests that measure the amounts of muscle proteins in the blood. High amounts of circulating muscle proteins in the blood are a sure sign of damaged muscle. In the case of Duchenne muscular dystrophy, the critical test is the creatine phosphokinase (CPK) level in the blood serum.

Some forms of muscular dystrophy are diagnosed by urine tests and, in some cases, muscle biopsy is also required. Confirmation of Duchenne muscular dystrophy is followed by further tests to determine female carriers of the disease and by genetic counseling. Doctors are increasingly using CAT scans to monitor the condition of muscles both as a diagnostic tool and to trace the progression of neuromuscular diseases.

Treatment: The disease is incurable. Identification of the specific gene that causes Duchenne muscular dystrophy is the subject of extensive research and would dramatically aid the search for a cure. A variety of drugs have been tested, but none has altered the progression of the muscular dystrophies. Treatment of the disease consists of appropriate management, preferably by a team of experts in different specialties, such as neurologists, orthopedic surgeons, physiatrists, physical and occupational therapists and social workers. If the diagnosis is made early enough, much can be done to help the child lead a productive and comfortable life. The quicker the diagnosis is made, the more quickly the patient and family will have access to a competent facility for both physical and psychological care. Neurologists are the specialists who treat muscular dystrophy. (*See* page 621).

AMYOTROPHIC LATERAL SCLEROSIS (ALS OR LOU GEHRIG'S DISEASE)

ALS is one of the cruelest human illnesses. It is a progressive neuromuscular disorder that generally strikes adults between the ages of 35 and 70, with average age about 50; it is fatal. Two-thirds of the victims of ALS are men. The disease usually leads to total paralysis, caused by a gradual disintegration of certain nerves of the spinal cord and brain that control motor activity. The muscle cells controlled by these nerves then shrink or atrophy. The disease has been recognized and studied for more than a century. Between 3,000 and 5,000 new cases are diagnosed every year.

Cause: Unknown. Scientists still have few clues about the cause of the disease, although research has become more intense in recent years. Some theories: ALS is caused by a slow-acting virus, a toxic factor in the blood, premature aging, malfunction of male hormones, or a genetic deficiency in enzymes affecting motor nerve cells. To what extent, if any, ALS is genetically controlled is not known.

Symptoms: Typical early symptoms are weakness, nonresponsiveness, or twitching in one or both hands. As the small muscles of the hands progressively atrophy, it becomes difficult to manipulate small objects. Victims may also begin to notice a limpness in the arms, shoulder, and at the back of the neck, and weakness, stiffness and cramps in the legs.

In almost one-third of the victims. the disease strikes the respiratory muscles, causing a progressive slurring of speech and difficulty in swallowing and breathing. The disease progresses at varying rates, depending on the location of the nerve cells originally attacked. The progression is unpredictable and may be rapid or slow. Ultimately, virtually all voluntary muscles, except eye and sphincter muscles, waste away. Most patients live at least three to five years, and a few as long as 20 years, after diagnosis.

Diagnosis: ALS can be readily diagnosed by a neurologist, usually by laboratory tests, such as a spinal tap or electromyography (EMG), which detects changes in the electrical activity of motor nerve cells. Sometimes muscle biopsies are performed.

Treatment: There is currently no cure for ALS. However, some of the symptoms can be relieved. For example, certain drugs may reduce muscle cramping; exercise may strengthen some muscles; and support devices can help weak arms and legs. Recent research gives hope that drugs may be developed to cure the disease. A hormonal drug, TRH (thyrotropin-releasing hormone), provided the first evidence that drugs might help strengthen some muscles of ALS patients, although it does not halt progression of the disease. Several drugs are being tested in efforts to find a cure.

MYASTHENIA GRAVIS

Myasthenia gravis is a chronic muscle disease causing weakness and fatigue. It is considered an autoimmune disease—a disease in which the body's defense system goes awry and attacks its own tissues. Myasthenia gravis strikes people of all ages, but is likely to affect women two times more than men.

Cause: The trigger is an autoimmune response that appears to destroy certain receptor sites on muscle cell membranes for the neurotransmitter acetylcholine. Without this critical chemical, the ordinary transmission of signals from nerves to muscles is interrupted; muscles do not contract properly; and weakness and severe fatigue result. Scientists do not know why the immune system malfunctions in this manner; they believe it is related to abnormalities in the thymus gland, a gland behind the heart that regulates immune functions. Sufferers of this disease frequently have enlarged thymus glands or tumors on the gland.

Symptoms: The disease can attack swiftly but usually early symptoms are subtle. The first and classic sign is a weakness of the eye muscles. Eyelids may droop and the muscles that control the eyeballs may weaken. The disease may halt there or progress to double vision, weakness in the arms, hands, and fingers, and difficulty swallowing, breathing, and walking. Such muscular weakness may stabilize or worsen, and varies greatly among patients. The disease is rarely fatal, although a person who develops difficulty breathing may have to be hospitalized on a respirator in an emergency.

Diagnosis: It is often diagnosed easily by physical examination and history. Electrical nerve-muscle stimulation and drug injection tests help confirm the diagnosis. X-rays may show an enlargement of the thymus gland.

Treatment: There is no cure for the basic deficiency, but myasthenia gravis is quite successfully treated by drugs and surgery, or both. In severe cases a procedure called plasmapheresis (blood-plasma exchange) has produced dramatic temporary recovery. Drugs that suppress the immune system or correct the acetylcholine deficiency sometimes work to a limited degree in improving neuromuscular transmission. The removal of the thymus gland is common and reportedly causes striking improvement half of the time, especially in younger persons.

Plasmapheresis is the latest treatment for severe cases that do not respond to other treatments and are near paralysis. The procedure lowers the amounts of circulating antibodies that interfere with nerve transmissions to the muscles. Although the technique is dramatically effective in patients previously considered hopeless, it is time consuming, risky in some patients, and expensive. It is considered a reasonable therapy only for those who have severe cases or do not respond to other treatments. It is no longer experimental. It has also been tested on other autoimmune diseases, such as multiple sclerosis, rheumatoid arthritis, and ALS, with limited success.

TREATMENT THROUGH THE MUSCULAR DYSTROPHY ASSOCIATION

About 240 clinics nationwide are affiliated with the Muscular Dystrophy Association and its staff of local "field offices." The clinics are all part of leading medical centers and you can go to them as a private patient on your own; however, there are some advantages to going through the Muscular Dystrophy Association. You become eligible for a number of services, including a definitive diagnosis (it is MDA's policy to pay for authorized medical services *not* covered by private or public insurance plans or other community resources), possible participation in research supported by MDA, group support, psychological counseling, information about orthopedic aids, wheelchairs, and so forth.

Patients who make arrangements for appointments through the Muscular Dystrophy Association local offices are admitted for diagnostic examination only on the written recommendation of a physician who suspects a neuromuscular disease. The cost of the clinic services and laboratory tests for the establishment of an initial diagnosis is covered by MDA, even if the disease does not turn out to be one covered by the Association's program.

Note: Patients not referred by MDA field staff may be billed as private patients and therefore not eligible for MDA financial help. Here is a list of forms of muscular dystrophy and neuromuscular diseases covered by medical services of and clinics affiliated with the Muscular Dystrophy Association.

Muscular Dystrophies
Duchenne Muscular Dystrophy
(Pseudohypertrophic)
Becker Muscular Dystrophy
Emery-Dreifuss Muscular Dystrophy
Limb-Girdle Muscular Dystrophy
Juvenile Dystrophy of Erb
Facioscapulohumeral Muscular Dystrophy
(Landouzy-Dejerine)
Myotonic Dystrophy (Steinert's Disease)
Oculopharyngeal Dystrophy
Ocular Dystrophy
Distal Muscular Dystrophy
Congenital Muscular Dystrophy
Muscular Dystrophy of Late Onset

Motor Neuron Diseases
Amyotrophic Lateral Sclerosis (ALS)
Infantile Progressive Spinal Muscular Atrophy
(Type 1, Werdnig-Hoffmann Disease)
Intermediate Spinal Muscular Atrophy (Type 2)
Juvenile Spinal Muscular Atrophy (Type 3,
Kugelberg-Welander Disease)
Adult Spinal Muscular Atrophy (Aran-Duchenne
Type)

Inflammatory Myopathies
Polymyositis
Dermatomyositis
Myositis Ossificans

Diseases of Neuromuscular Junction
Myasthenia Gravis
Eaton-Lambert (Myasthenic) Syndrome

Diseases of Peripheral Nerve
Peroneal Muscular Atrophy (Charcot-Marie-Tooth
disease)
Friedreich's Ataxia
Dejerine-Sottas Disease

Myotonias
Myotonia Congenita (Thomsen's Disease)
Paramyotonia Congenita

Metabolic Diseases of Muscle
Phosphorylase Deficiency (McArdle's Disease)
Acid Maltase Deficiency (Pompe's Disease)
Phosphofructokinase Deficiency (Tarui's Disease)
Debrancher Enzyme Deficiency (Cori's or
Forbes' Disease)
Carnitine Palmityltransferase Deficiency
Periodic Paralysis

Myopathies Due to Endocrine Abnormalities
Hyperthyroid Myopathy
Hyperthyroid Myopathy

Less Common Myopathies
Central Core Disease
Nemaline Myopathy
Mitochondrial Disease
Myotubular Myopathy

MUSCULAR DYSTROPHY ASSOCIATION CLINICS

Here is a list of the clinics that treat neuromuscular diseases. To make an appointment at one of the clinics through the Muscular Dystrophy Association, see the white pages of your local phone directory for the number of your local MDA office.

For a list of the heads of departments of neurology at leading medical colleges, *see* page 621. These physicians are also excellent sources of treatment and/or medical referrals to specialists who treat muscular dystrophy.

ALABAMA
The Children's Hospital
Birmingham, AL 35233
John W. Benton, M.D., James W. Coker, Jr.,
  M.D., Codirectors
(205) 250-9100

University of Alabama Hospital
Birmingham, AL 35233
Shin J. Oh, M.D., Director
(205) 934-5314

The Clinic for Neurology
Huntsville, AL 35801
Lynn B. Boyer, M.D., George C. Morgan,
  M.D., Ph.D., Codirectors
(205) 533-8020

Providence Hospital
Mobile, AL 36604
Elias Chalhub, M.D., Robert L. Green, M.D.,
  Codirectors
(205) 438-7611

Baptist Medical Center
Montgomery, AL 36198
Richard V. Colan, M.D., W. Joseph
  Leuschke, M.D., Codirectors
(205) 288-2100

ARIZONA
Phoenix Children's Hospital
Phoenix, AZ 85008
Mark T. Felmus, M.D., Ronald O. Hadden,
  M.D., Codirectors
(602) 239-2400

The Mucio F. Delgado Clinic for
  Neuromuscular Disorders
University of Arizona Health Sciences Center
Tucson, AZ 85724
Lawrence Z. Stern, M.D., Director
(602) 626-0111

ARKANSAS
Sparks Regional Medical Center
Fort Smith, AR 72901
James H. Buic, M.D., Director
(501) 441-4000

Arkansas Children's Hospital
Little Rock, AR 72202
Fereydoun Dehkharghani, M.D., Director
(501) 370-1100

CALIFORNIA
Rancho Los Amigos Hospital
Downey, CA 90242
Irene S. Gilgoff, M.D., John D. Hsu, M.D.,
  Codirectors
(213) 922-7022

Valley Children's Hospital
Fresno, CA 93703
Joseph T. Capell, M.D., H. T. Hutchison,
  M.D., Codirectors
(209) 225-3000

Loma Linda University Medical Center
Loma Linda, CA 92354
Stephen Ashwal, M.D., James E. Shook,
  M.D., Codirectors
(714) 796-7311

Orthopaedic Hospital
Los Angeles, CA 90007
John D. Hsu, M.D., Director
(213) 742-1000

The Carl M. Pearson MDA Clinic for
  Neuromuscular Disorders
University of California, Los Angeles
Los Angeles, CA 90024
Thomas L. Anderson, M.D., John C. Keesey,
  M.D., Codirectors

University of Southern California Medical
  Center
Los Angeles, CA 90033
Valerie Askanas, M.D., W. King Engel,
  M.D., Codirectors
(213) 226-6501

Children's Hospital of Orange Country
Orange, CA 92668
Richard D. Dauben, M.D., Brain A. Ewald,
  M.D., Codirectors
(714) 997-3000

Stanford Medical Center
Children's Hospital at Stanford
Palo Alto, CA 94304
Larry Steinman, M.D., Director
(415) 327-4800

Stanford University Medical Center
Palo Alto, CA 94305
Leslie Dorfman, M.D., Director
(415) 497-2300

Casa Colina Hospital for Rehabilitative
  Medicine
Pomona, CA 91767
Julia Botvin-Madorsky, M.D., David Rice,
  M.D., Codirectors
(714) 593-7521

University of California, Davis—Sacramento
  Medical Center
Sacramento, CA 95817
William M. Fowler, M.D., Robert G. Taylor,
  M.D., Codirectors
(916) 453-3096

Children's Hospital
San Diego, CA 92123
Paul Schultz, M.D., Director
(619) 576-1700

Children's Hospital of San Francisco
San Francisco, CA 94119
Robert G. Miller, M.D., Director
(415) 668-3704

Santa Clara Valley Medical Center
San Jose, CA 95128
Herbert Goodman, M.D., Director
(408) 279-6827

Sansum Medical Clinic, Inc.
317 W. Pueblo Street
Santa Barbara, CA 93102
Richard M. Lowenthal, M.D., Donald E.
  Webb, M.D., Codirectors
(805) 682-2621

COLORADO
University of Colorado Health Science Center
Denver, CO 80262
Hans E. Neville, M.D., Steven P. Ringel,
  M.D., Codirectors
(303) 394-8446

CONNECTICUT
University of Connecticut Health Sciences
  Center
Farmington, CT 06032
Keshav, Ram Rao, M.D., Director
(203) 674-3540

Newington Children's Hospital
Newington, CT 06111
Barry S. Russman, M.D., Director
(203) 666-2461

DELAWARE
Alfred I. DuPont Institute
Wilmington, DE 19899
J. Richard Bowen, M.D., Harold Marks,
  M.D., Codirectors
(302) 651-4000

DISTRICT OF COLUMBIA
Children's Hospital National Medical Center
Washington, DC 20010
Gloria D. Eng, M.D., Director
(202) 745-5000

Georgetown University Hospital
Washington, DC 20007
Bennett Lavenstein, M.D., Desmond S.
  O'Doherty, M.D., Codirectors
(202) 625-0100

FLORIDA
Mease Hospital & Clinic
Dunedin, FL 33528
Jeffrey M. Karp, M.D., Director
(813) 733-1111

Broward General Medical Center
Fort Lauderdale, FL 33316
Harish D. Thaker, M.D., Director
(305) 463-3131

Lee Memorial Hospital
Fort Myers, FL 33902
Harris L. Bonnette, M.D., Director
(813) 332-1111

Nemours Children's Hospital
Jacksonville, FL 32207
Andrew K. Hodson, M.D., Louis S. Russo,
   Jr., M.D., Codirectors
(904) 721-4200

University Hospital
Jacksonville, Fl 32209
Louis S. Russo, Jr., M.D., Director
(904) 350-6899

Miami Children's Hospital
(Formerly Variety Children's Hospital)
Miami, FL 33155
Danilo Duenas, M.D., Director
(305) 666-6511

Mt. Sinai Medical Center
Miami Beach, FL 33140
Michael Goodson, M.D., Director
(305) 674-2121

Florida Hospital
Orlando, Fl 32803
Susan M. Mott, M.D., Joseph R. O'Connor,
   M.D., Codirectors
(305) 896-6611

Gulf Coast Community Hospital
Panama City, FL 32405
Michael L. Walker, M.D., Director
(904) 769-8341

Sacred Heart Hospital
Pensacola, FL 32504
John Axley, M.D., Director
(904) 476-7851

Memorial Hospital
Sarasota, FL 33579
Donald R. Vande Polder, M.D., Director
(813) 955-1111

Tallahassee Memorial Regional Medical Center
Tallahassee, FL 32303
William C. Kohler, M.D., Frederick Q.
   Vroom, M.D., Codirectors
(904) 681-1155

University of South Florida
Tampa, FL 33612
Raymond J. Fernandez, M.D., Maria Gieron-
   Korthals, M.D., Codirectors
(813) 974-2196

St. Mary's Hospital
West Palm Beach, FL 33407
Richard A. Chidsey, M.D., Walter C.
   Martinez, M.D., Codirectors
(305) 844-6300

GEORGIA
Phoebe Putney Memorial Hospital
Albany, GA 31703
John Baker M.D., Director
(912) 883-1800

Emory University Center for Rehabilitative
   Medicine
Atlanta, GA 30322
Donal Costigan, M.D., Director
(404) 329-7021

Medical College of Georgia
Augusta, GA 30912
Patricia L. Hartlage, M.D., Thomas R. Swift,
   M.D., Codirectors
(404) 828-0211

Medical Center of Central Georgia
Macon, GA 31208
Thomas Hope, M.D., Director
(912) 744-1000

St. Joseph's Hospital
Savannah, GA 31406
Herbert F. Sanders, M.D., Director
(912) 925-4100

Roosevelt Institute for Rehabilitation
Warm Springs, GA 31830
William J. Bailey, M.D., Director
(404) 655-3321

HAWAII
Capt. Yasumori H. Tomi MDA Clinic at
   Rehabilitation Hospital of the Pacific
Honolulu, HI 96817
Dennis M. Crowley, M.D., Director
(808) 531-3511

IDAHO

Saint Alphonsus Hospital
Boise, ID 83706
Thomas E. Henson, M.D., Richard W.
 Wilson, M.D., Codirectors
(208) 378-2121

ILLINOIS

Louis A. Weiss Memorial Hospital
Chicago, IL 60640
Irwin M. Siegel, M.D., Director
(312) 878-8700

Michael Reese Medical Center
Chicago, IL 60616
Morris Fisher, M.D., Peter Heydeman, M.D.,
 Codirectors
(312) 791-2000

Rush-Presbyterian-St. Luke's Hospital
Chicago, Illinois 60612
Irwin M. Siegel, M.D., Russell Hugh Glantz,
 M.D., Codirectors
(312) 942-5129

University of Illinois Hospital
Chicago, IL 60612
Irwin M. Siegel, M.D., Director
(312) 996-6803

Evanston Hospital
Evanston, IL 60201
Lawrence P. Bernstein, M.D., Director
(312) 492-2000

Hinsdale Sanitarium and Hospital
Hinsdale, IL 60521
Wilton H. Bunch, M.D., Kamal N. Ibrahim,
 M.D., Thomas D. Sullivan, M.D.,
 Codirectors
(312) 887-2400

Good Samaritan Hospital
Mount Vernon, IL 62864
Alan Froehling, M.D., Director
(618) 242-4600

Peoria School of Medicine
Peoria, IL 61656
Krishna Kalyana Raman, M.D., Director
(309) 671-3000

Proctor Hospital
Peoria, IL 61614
Xuan T. Truong, M.D., Director
(309) 691-4702

Franciscan Hospital Rehabilitation Center
Rock Island, IL 61201
Robert J. Chesser, M.D., Director
(309) 793-2121

Rockford Memorial Hospital
Rockford, IL 61103
Raymond F. Doyle, M.D., Director
(815) 968-6861

Memorial Medical Center
Springfield, IL 62781
James Russell Couch, M.D., Director
(217) 788-3000

Mercy Hospital
Urbana, IL 61801
John Gapfis, M.D., Director
(217) 337-2233

Marianjoy Rehabilitation Hospital
Wheaton, IL 60189
Vinod Sahgal, M.D., Director
(312) 653-7600

INDIANA

Elkhart General Hospital
Elkhart, IN 46515
Thomas R. Vidic, M.D., Director
(219) 294-2621

Lutheran Hospital
Fort Wayne, IN 46807
Jerry L. Mackel, M.D., C. J. Ottinger, M.D.,
 Codirectors
(219) 458-2001

Methodist Hospital of Indiana
Indianapolis, IN 46206
John Ellis, M.D., Bradford R. Hale, M.D.,
 Codirectors
(317) 924-6411

IOWA

Younker Memorial Rehabilitation Center
Des Moines, IA 50308
William D. deGravelles, Jr., M.D., Director
(515) 283-6212

University of Iowa Hospitals and Clinics
Iowa City, IA 52242
Victor Ionasescu, M.D., Director
(319) 356-1616
Children

University of Iowa Hospitals and Clinics
Iowa City, IA 52242
E. Peter Bosch, M.D., Director
(319) 356-1616
Adults

KANSAS
University of Kansas Medical Center
Kansas City, KS 66103
John B. Redford, M.D., Dewey K. Ziegler,
  M.D., Codirectors
(913) 588-5000

St. Francis Regional Medical Center
Wichita, KS 67201
Ely Bartal, M.D., Director
(318) 268-5000

St. Joseph Medical Center
Wichita, KS 67218
Dilawer Abbas, M.D., Albert R. Siegel,
  M.D., Codirectors
(316) 685-1111

KENTUCKY
University of Kentucky Medical Center
Lexington, KY 40536
Robert J. Baumann, M.D., Director
(606) 233-5000

St. Anthony Hospital
Louisville, KY 40204
Gregory L. Pittman, M.D., Director
(502) 587-1161

LOUISIANA
Baton Rouge General Medical Center
Baton Rouge, LA 70821
Carlos A. Garcia, M.D., Director
(504) 387-7767

Our Lady of Lourdes Hospital
Lafayette, LA 70501
Carlos A. Garcia, M.D., Director
(318) 234-7381

St. Francis Medical Center
Monroe, LA 71201
Michael E. Boykin, M.D., Director
(318) 362-4143

Louisiana State University School of Medicine
New Orleans, LA 70112-2822
Carlos A. Garcia, M.D., Director
(504) 568-4000

Louisiana State University Medical Center
Shreveport, LA 71130
Gwendolyn Hogan, M.D., Ju-Sung Wu,
  M.D., Codirectors
(318) 674-5000

MAINE
Eastern Maine Medical Center
Bangor, ME 04401
Paul H. LaMarche, M.D., Director
(207) 947-3711

Maine Medical Center
Portland, ME 04102
B. Cairbre McCann, M.D., Director
(207) 871-0111

MARYLAND
Johns Hopkins Hospital
Baltimore, MD 21205
Daniel B. Drachman, M.D., Director
(301) 955-5000

Maryland General Hospital
Baltimore, MD 21201
Salvatore R. Donohue, M.D., Michael
  Sellman, M.D., Codirectors
(301) 728-7900

MASSACHUSETTS
Boston University Medical Center
Boston, MA 02118
Robert G. Feldman, M.D., Edgar
  Oppenheimer, M.D., Codirectors
(617) 247-5000

Children's Hospital Corp.
Boston, MA 02115
Michael J. Bresnan, M.D., Fred Shapiro,
  M.D., Codirectors
(617) 735-6000

Massachusetts General Hospital
Boston, MA 02114
Dennis M. D. Landis, M.D., Director
(617) 726-2000

Tufts-New England Medical Center
Boston, MA 02111
Agatha Colbert, M.D., Theodore Munsat,
  M.D., Codirectors
(617) 956-5000

Lakeville Hospital
Lakeville, MA 02346
Leo R. Sullivan, M.D., Director
(617) 947-1231

Berkshire Medical Center
Pittsfield, MA 01201
Jay M. Ellis, M.D., Director
(413) 499-4161

Baystate Medical Center
Springfield, MA 01107
Joseph H. Donnelly, M.D., Robert S. Gerstle,
  M.D., Codirectors
(413) 787-3200

St. Vincent Hospital
Worcester, MA 01604
Norman E. Beisaw, M.D., Director
(617) 798-1234

MICHIGAN
Children's Hospital of Michigan
Detroit, MI 48201
Michael A. Nigro, D.O., Director
(313) 494-5301

Michigan State University Clinical Center
East Lansing, MI 48824
George E. Ristow, D.O., Director
(517) 353-1730

Hurley Medical Center
Flint, MI 48502
Devender Bhrany, M.D., Director
(313) 257-9000

Blodgett Memorial Medical Center
Grand Rapids, MI 49506
John F. Butzer, M.D., Robert H. Puite, M.D.,
  David H. Van Dyke, M.D., Codirectors
(616) 774-7444

Borgess Hospital
Kalamazoo, MI 49001
Jerald T. Finnegan, M.D., David G. Flagler,
  M.D., Dale E. Rowe, M.D., Codirectors
(616) 383-7000

Oakland General Hospital
Madison Heights, MI 48071
Michael A. Nigro, D.O. Director
(313) 967-7000

Midland Hospital Association
Midland, MI 48640
Kamal Sadjadpour, M.D., Director
(517) 839-3000

MINNESOTA
Miller-Dwan Hospital
Duluth, MN 55805
Steven K. Goff, M.D., Wolcott S. Holt,
  M.D., Codirectors
(218) 727-8762

Fairview Hospital
Minneapolis, MN 55435
Lowell D. Lutter, M.D., V. Richard Zarling,
  M.D., Codirectors
(612) 924-5000

University of Minnesota Hospitals
Minneapolis, MN 55455
Dennis Matthews, M.D., Robert I. Roelofs,
  M.D., Stephen Smith, M.D., Codirectors
(612) 373-8484

Mayo Clinic
Rochester, MN 55905
Andrew G. Engel, M.D., Manuel R. Gomez,
  M.D., Codirectors
(507) 284-3671

MISSISSIPPI
Gulf Coast Community Hospital
Biloxi, MS 39531
Shri K. Mishra, M.D., Director
(601) 388-6711

University of Mississippi Medical Center
Jackson, MS 39216
Shri K. Mishra, M.D., Director
(601) 984-5500

MISSOURI
St. Francis Medical Center
Cape Girardeau, MO 63701
Michael H. Brooke, M.D., Director
(314) 335-1251

University of Missouri Medical Center
Columbia, MO 65212
James M. Pickens, M.D., Director
(314) 882-3984

St. Louis University Medical Center
St. Louis, MO 63104
John D. McGarry, M.D., Director
(314) 771-7600

Washington University School of Medicine
St. Louis, MO 63110
Michael H. Brooke, M.D., Director
(314) 454-2000

Lester E. Cox Medical Center
Springfield, MO 65802
George Klinkerfuss, M.D., Michael Luzecky,
    M.D., Codirectors
(417) 836-3000

MONTANA
St. Vincent's Hospital
Billings, MT 59101
Lewis Robinson, M.D., Director
(406) 657-7000

Montana Deaconess Medical Center
Great Falls, MT 59405
William H. Labunetz, M.D., Bill J. Tacke,
    M.D., Codirectors
(406) 761-1200

NEBRASKA
University of Nebraska Medical Center
Omaha, NE 68105
Erich W. Streib, M.D., Sallie F. Sun, M.D.,
    Codirectors
(402) 559-7400

NEVADA
Southern Nevada Memorial Hospital
Las Vegas, NV 89102
R. Kirby Reed, M.D., Director
(702) 383-2000

Saint Mary's Hospital
Reno, NV 89502
William C. Torch, M.D., Director
(702) 323-2041

NEW HAMPSHIRE
Mary Hitchcock Memorial Hospital
Hanover, NH 03756
Colin Allen, M.D., Richard E. Nordren,
    M.D., Codirectors
(603) 646-5000

NEW JERSEY
Children's Seashore House
Atlantic City, NJ 08404
Wilma C. Kellerman, M.D., Director
(609) 345-5191

John F. Kennedy Medical Center
Edison, NJ 08818
Bernard Sandler, M.D., Director
(201) 321-7000

Englewood Hospital
Englewood, NJ 07631
Michael L. Gruber, M.D., Peter Kornfeld,
    M.D., Stanley J. Myers, M.D., Codirectors
(201) 894-3000

Monmouth Medical Center
Long Branch, NJ 07740
Christos P. Anayiotos, M.D., Judith F.
    Topilow, M.D., Codirectors
(201) 222-5200

United Hospitals Orthopedic Center
Newark, NJ 07107
Arnold Feldman, M.D., Director
(201) 268-8000

University Hospital
Newark, NJ 07103
Marvin Ruderman, M.D., Director
(201) 456-4300

Kennedy Memorial Hospitals
University Medical Center
Stratford, NJ 08084
Donald A. Barone, D.O., Director
(609) 784-4000

NEW MEXICO
University of New Mexico Hospital
Albuquerque, NM 87106
Russell D. Snyder, M.D., Director
(505) 843-2111

NEW YORK
Albany Medical Center
Albany, NY 12208
Ronald Bailey, M.D., Reynaldo Lazaro,
    M.D., Codirectors
(518) 445-3125

Hospital of the Albert Einstein College of
    Medicine
Bronx, NY 10461
Alfred J. Spiro, M.D., Director
(212) 430-2000

State University of New York Downstate
    Medical Center
Brooklyn, NY 11203
Roger W. Kula, M.D., Director
(718) 270-2401

Erie County Medical Center
Buffalo, NY 14215
Jerry G. Chutkow, M.D.
(716) 898-3707

Nassau County Medical Center
East Meadow, NY 11554
Joel Delfiner, M.D., Director
(516) 542-0123

Twin Tiers Rehabilitation Center
St. Joseph's Hospital
Elmira, NY 14902
Jonathan Cooper, M.D., Director
(607) 733-6541

Women's Christian Association Hospital
Jamestown, NY 14701
Jerry G. Chutkow, M.D., Director
(716) 487-0141

United Hospital Service, Inc.
Wilson Hospital
Johnson City, NY 13790
Robert R. Taylor, Jr., M.D., Director
(607) 773-6000

Long Island Jewish–Hillside Medical Center
New Hyde Park, NY 11042
Steven H. Horowitz, M.D., Director
(212) 470-2000

Hospital for Joint Diseases and Medical Center
New York, NY 10003
Alfred D. Grant, M.D., Director
(212) 598-6000

Hospital for Special Surgery
New York, NY 10021
Peter Tsairis, M.D., Director
(212) 598-6000

Jerry Lewis Neuromuscular Disease Center
Institute of Rehabilitation Medicine
New York University Medical Center
New York, NY 10016
Joseph Goodgold, M.D., Leon Greenspan,
   M.D., Codirectors
(212) 340-6200

Mount Sinai Hospital and Medical Center
New York, NY 10029
Adam N. Bender, M.D., Director
(212) 650-6500

Presbyterian Hospital
Columbia Presbyterian Medical Center
New York, NY 10032
Robert E. Lovelace, M.D., Joseph Willner,
   M.D., Codirectors
(212) 694-2500

St. Vincent's Hospital and Medical Center
New York, NY 10011
Harry Bartfeld, M.D., Hyman Donnenfeld,
   M.D., Codirectors
(212) 790-7000

University of Rochester School of Medicine
   and Dentistry and Strong Memorial Hospital
Rochester, NY 14642
David Goldblatt, M.D., Robert C. Griggs,
   M.D., Richard T. Moxley, M.D.,
   Codirectors
(716) 275-2644

State University of New York at Stony Brook
   University Hospital
Stony Brook, NY 11794
John J. Halperin, M.D., Robert Y. Moore,
   M.D., Codirectors
(516) 444-2701

State University of New York Upstate Medical
   Center
Syracuse, NY 13210
Carl J. Crosley, M.D., Director
(315) 473-5540

Children's Hospital and Rehabilitation Center
Utica, NY 13502
Carl J. Crosley, M.D., Director
(315) 724-5101

Westchester County Medical Center
Valhalla, NY 10595
Stanley B. Holstein, M.D., Director
(914) 347-7000

Mercy Hospital of Watertown
Watertown, NY 13601
David O. Van Eenenaam, M.D., Director
(315) 782-7400

White Plains Hospital Medical Center
White Plains, NY 10601
Sheldon Alter, M.D., Director
(914) 681-1200

NORTH CAROLINA
Memorial Mission Hospital
Asheville, NC 28801
Dennis L. Martin, M.D., Director
(704) 255-4000

University of North Carolina at Chapel Hill
Chapel Hill, NC 27514
Colin D. Hall, M.D., Ch.B., James F.
   Howard, Jr., M.D., Codirectors
(919) 966-4161

Charlotte Rehabilitation Hospital
Charlotte, NC 28203
Ronald C. Demas, M.D., Philip Lesser, M.D.,
  Codirectors
(704) 333-6634

Duke University Medical Center
Durham, NC 27710
Allen D. Roses, M.D., Director
(919) 684-5587

Humana Hospital
Greensboro, NC 27408
Martin A. Hatcher, M.D., Director
(919) 373-8555

Forsyth Memorial Hospital
Winston-Salem, NC 27103
Carlo P. Yuson, M.D., Director
(919) 773-3000

NORTH DAKOTA
Dakota Hospital
Fargo, ND 58103
Donald Eliot Goodkin, M.D., Director
(701) 280-4100

OHIO
University of Cincinnati Medical Center
Cincinnati, OH 45267
Paul Barkhaus, M.D., Henry G. Grinvalsky,
  M.D., Susan T. Innaconne, M.D., Frederick
  J. Samaha, M.D., Codirectors
(513) 872-4628

Cleveland Metropolitan General Hospital
Cleveland, OH 44109
Maurice Victor, M.D., Director
(216) 398-6000

Ohio State University Hospital
Columbus, OH 43210
Ernest W. Johnson, M.D., Director
(614) 421-8000

St. Elizabeth Medical Center
Dayton, OH 45408
Samuel E. Pitner, M.D., Margaret Turk,
  M.D., Codirectors
(513) 229-6000

The Toledo Hospital
Toledo, OH 43606
Ronald R. Wade, M.D., Edward J. Orecchio,
  M.D., Codirectors
(419) 473-4218

St. Elizabeth Hospital
Youngstown, OH 44501
Robert L. Gilliland, M.D., Steven M.
  Kalavsky, M.D., Codirectors
(216) 746-7211

OKLAHOMA
Baptist Medical Center
Oklahoma City, OK 73112
John D. Bodensteiner, M.D., Sherman B.
  Lawton, M.D., Codirectors
(405) 949-3011

Children's Medical Center
Tulsa, OK 74135
David H. Barber, M.D., Director
(918) 664-6600

Oklahoma Osteopathic Hospital
Tulsa, OK 74127
John D. DeWitt, D.O., Director
(918) 587-2561

OREGON
Sacred Heart Hospital
Eugene, OR 97440
Paul W. Jones, M.D., Director
(503) 686-7300

Rogue Valley Memorial Hospital
Medford, OR 97501
Kevin J. Sullivan, M.D., Director
(503) 773-6281

Good Samaritan Hospital
Portland, OR 97210
John H. Kennedy, M.D., Jacob H. Wilson,
  M.D., Codirectors
(503) 229-7711

PENNSYLVANIA
Good Shepherd Rehabilitation Hospital
Allentown, PA 18103
Terry Heiman-Patterson, M.D., Director
(215) 821-2121

Geisinger Medical Center
Danville, PA 17822
Paul R. Spilsbury, M.D., Director
(717) 271-6211

Elizabethtown Hospital & Rehabilitation
  Center of the Pennsylvania State University
Elizabethtown, PA 17022
Edward P. Schwentker, M.D., Director
(717) 367-1161

Hamot Medical Center
Erie, PA 16550
Karl F. Frankovitch, M.D., Director
(814) 455-6711

Lee Hospital
Johnstown, PA 15901
John J. Seeber, M.D., Paul R. Hyman, M.D.,
  Codirectors
(814) 535-7541

Children's Hospital of Philadelphia
Philadelphia, PA 19104
Peter H. Berman, M.D., Director
(215) 596-9100

Henry M. Watts, Jr. Neuromuscular Disease
  Research Center
Hospital of the University of Pennsylvania
Philadelphia, PA 19104
William J. Bank, M.D., Donald L. Schotland,
  M.D., Codirectors
(215) 662-4000

Children's Hospital of Pittsburgh
Pittsburgh, PA 15213
Michael A. Alexander, M.D., Henry B.
  Wessel, M.D., Codirectors
(412) 647-2345

Shadyside Hospital
Pittsburgh, PA 15232
T. S. Danowski, M.D., Director
(412) 622-2121

University Health Center of Pittsburgh
Pittsburgh, PA 15213
Oscar M. Reinmuth, M.D., Director
(412) 647-2345

Wilkes-Barre General Hospital
Wilkes-Barre, PA 18764
Abdol H. R. Samii, M.D., Director
(717) 829-8111

Williamsport Hospital
Williamsport, PA 17701
Young W. Park, M.D., Director
(717) 322-7861

PUERTO RICO
Hospital Santo Asilo de Damas
Ponce, PR 00731
Wilma Lluberas, M.D., Director
(809) 843-5151

Metropolitan Hospital
Rio Piedras, PR 00922
Arturo F. Lluberas, M.D., Director
(809) 783-6200

RHODE ISLAND
Child Development Center
Rhode Island Hospital
Providence, RI 02902
Siegfried Pueschel, M.D., Thomas Wachtel,
  M.D., Codirectors
(401) 277-4000

SOUTH CAROLINA
Anderson Memorial Hospital
Anderson, SC 29621
J. David deHoll, M.D., Michael B. Fry,
  M.D., Codirectors
(803) 261-1000

Medical University of South Carolina
Charleston, SC 29425
Edward L. Hogan, M.D., John Gross, M.D.,
  Codirectors
(803) 792-3131

Richland Memorial Hospital
Columbia, SC 29203
D. Nelson Gunter, M.D., Joseph W. Taber,
  Jr., M.D., Codirectors
(803) 765-7011

SOUTH DAKOTA
Rapid City Rehabilitation Hospital, Inc.
Rapid City, SD 57701
K. Alan Kelts, M.D., Director
(605) 343-8500

McKennan Hospital
Sioux Falls, SD 57101
K. G. Koob, M.D., Director
(605) 339-8000

TENNESSEE
Siskin Memorial Foundation
Chattanooga, TN 37404
Robert C. Coddington, M.D., Joseph V.
  LaVecchia, M.D, Codirectors
(615) 265-3491

Johnson City Medical Center
Johnson City, TN 37601
Jude Smith, M.D., Stephen M. Kimbrough,
  M.D., G. Dean Wilson, Jr., M.D.,
  Codirectors
(615) 461-6111

East Tennessee Children's Hospital
Knoxville, TN 37916
John H. Bell, M.D., Director
(615) 546-7711

University of Tennessee College of Medicine/
  Baptist Memorial Hospital
Memphis, TN 38146
Tulio Bertorini, M.D., Robert P. Christopher,
  M.D., Codirectors
(901) 522-5252

Vanderbilt University Medical Center
Nashville, TN 37232
Owen B. Evans, M.D., Gerald M. Fenichel,
  M.D., Codirectors
(615) 322-7311

TEXAS
St. Anthony's Hospital
Amarillo, TX 79107
Michael G. Ryan, M.D., Rush A. Snyder, Jr.,
  M.D., Codirectors
(803) 376-4411

Brackenridge Hospital
Austin, TX 78701
Rodney Simonsen, M.D., Jerry Tindel, M.D.,
  Codirectors
(512) 476-6461

Ada Wilson Hospital
Corpus Christi, TX 78411
Ernesto H. Guido, M.D., John D. McKeever,
  M.D., Codirectors
(512) 853-9977

Southwestern Medical School University of
  Texas Health Science Center
Dallas, TX 75235
Howard Feit, M.D., Ronald G. Haller, M.D.,
  Codirectors
(214) 688-3111

Texas Neurological Institute
Dallas, TX 75230
Allan L. Naarden, M.D., Director
(214) 661-7000

Providence Memorial Hospital
El Paso, TX 79902
A. B. Bakr, M.D., Directors
(915) 542-6011

Fort Worth Children's Hospital
Fort Worth, TX 76104
Robert E. McMichael, M.D., Director
(817) 336-9861

University of Texas Medical Branch
Galveston, TX 77550
John R. Calverly, M.D., Gerald S. Golden,
  M.D., Codirectors
(713) 765-1011

Neurosensory Center of Baylor College of
  Medicine
Houston, TX 77080
Stanley H. Appel, M.D., Director
(713) 799-4951

Texas Institute for Rehabilitation and Research
Houston, TX 77225
Barry L. Bowser, M.D., Director
(713) 797-1440

University of Texas Health Sciences Center
Houston, TX 77225
Ian J. Butler, M.D., Director
(713) 792-2121

Methodist Hospital
Lubbock, TX 79410
Donald R. Craig, M.D., William H. Gordon,
  M.D., Codirectors
(806) 792-1011

McAllen General Hospital
McAllen, TX 78501
Frank E. McDonald, M.D., Juan Trevenio,
  M.D., Codirectors
(512) 687-7611

Medical Center Hospital
Odessa, TX 79760
Sam Reuben Lehman, M.D., Director
(915) 333-7111

Santa Rosa Medical Center
San Antonio, TX 78207
Joel Y. Rutman, M.D., Saul B. Wilen, M.D.,
  Kaye E. Wilkins, M.D., Codirectors
(512) 228-2011

University of Texas Health Science Center
San Antonio, TX 78284
Allen B. Gruber, M.D., Director
(512) 691-6011

Wilson N. Jones Memorial Hospital
Sherman, TX 75090
Fred L. Snipes, M.D., Director
(214) 893-4611

Scott and White Clinic
Temple, TX 76508
Darrell Crisp, M.D., Rich Lenchan, M.D.
(817) 774-2111

University of Texas Health Center at Tyler
Tyler, TX 75710
Preston Harrison, Jr., M.D., Richard F.
  Ulrich, M.D., Codirectors
(214) 877-3451

Wichita Falls Clinic
Wichita Falls, TX 76302
Stephen Farmer, D.O., Director
(817) 766-3551

UTAH
University of Utah Medical Center
Salt Lake City, UT 84132
Fred A. Ziter, M.D., Director
(801) 581-2680

VERMONT
Medical Center Hospital of Vermont
Burlington, VT 05401
Walter G. Bradley, M.D., Edward S. Emery
  III, M.D., James B. McQuillen, M.D.,
  Codirectors
(802) 656-2345

VIRGINIA
Handicapped Children's Clinic/Children's
  Rehabilitation Center
University of Virginia Medical Center
Charlottesville, VA 22901
Peter Blasco, M.D., Michael D. Sussman,
  M.D., Codirectors
(804) 924-5161

University of Virginia Jerry Lewis
  Neuromuscular Center
University of Virginia Hospital
Charlottesville, VA 22908
T. R. Johns, M.D., Director
(804) 924-0211

Norfolk General Hospital
Norfolk, VA 23507
Albert B. Finch, M.D., Director
(804) 628-3361

Crippled Children's Hospital
Richmond, VA 23220
Robert T. Leshner, M.D., Director
(804) 321-7474

Medical College of Virginia Hospitals
Richmond, VA 23298
William Campbell, M.D., Robert T. Leshner,
  M.D.
(804) 786-0932

Roanoke Neurological Associates
Roanoke, VA 24014
Michael A. Sisk, M.D., Director
(703) 342-0211

WASHINGTON
Children's Orthopedic Hospital
Seattle, WA 98105
Kenneth Jaffee, M.D., Jerrold M. Milstein,
  M.D., Codirectors
(206) 634-5000

University of Washington Hospital
Seattle, WA 98195
George H. Kraft, M.D., S. Mark Sumi, M.D.,
  Codirectors
(206) 543-3300

Deaconess Hospital
Spokane, WA 99210
William R. Bozarth, M.D., John V. Stephens,
  M.D., Codirectors
(509) 458-5800

Mary Bridge Children's Health Center
Tacoma, WA 98405
Marcel Malden, M.D., Director
(206) 272-1281

St. Mary Community Hospital
Walla Walla, WA 99362
Herbert H. Hendricks, M.D., Toomas Eisler,
  M.D., Codirector
(509) 525-3320

Yakima Valley Memorial Hospital
Yakima, WA 98902
Barbara J. DeLateur, M.D., Director
(509) 575-8000

WEST VIRGINIA
St. Francis Hospital
Charleston, WV 24322
Lee H. Pratt, M.D., Director
(304) 348-8500

West Virginia University Hospital
Morgantown, WV 26506
Alexander V. Fakadej, M.D., Ludwig
  Gutmann, M.D., Codirectors
(304) 293-4632

Ohio Valley Medical Center
Wheeling, WV 26003
Srini Govindan, M.D., Director
(304) 234-0123

WISCONSIN
Bellin Memorial Hospital
Green Bay, WI 54301
W. David Jones, M.D., Director
(414) 433-3500

University of Wisconsin Hospitals and Clinics
Madison, WI 53792
Benjamin R. Brooks, M.D., Henry A. Peters,
  M.D., Robert L. Sufit, M.D., Codirectors
(608) 263-6400

Marshfield Clinic
Marshfield, WI 54449
David B. Frens, M.D., Director
(715) 387-5511

Froedtert Memorial Lutheran/Medical College
  of Wisconsin
Milwaukee, WI 53226
Michael McQuillen, M.D., Director
(414) 344-8800

Milwaukee Children's Hospital
Milwaukee, WI 53233
Herbert M. Swick, M.D., Director
(414) 931-1010

SOURCE: *Muscular Dystrophy Association.*

ALS ASSOCIATION CENTERS

The ALS Association supports patient services at the following institutions. Each center has a multidisciplinary team dedicated to quality care of the ALS patient and consists of clinical neurologists, social workers, occupational therapists, physical therapists, nurse specialists, speech therapists, and psychotherapists.

University of Miami School of Medicine
Department of Neurology
1501 N.W. Ninth Ave., D4-5
Miami, FL 33136
Robert T. Shebert, M.D.
Director, ALS Clinical Services
(305) 547-6731

University of Chicago Medical Center
Department of Neurology
Pritzker School of Medicine
950 E. 59th St.
Chicago, IL 60637
Jack P. Antel, M.D.
Director, ALS Clinical Services
(312) 962-6221

Mt. Sinai Medical Center
Department of Neurology
Fifth Ave. and 100th St.
New York, NY 10029
James T. Caroscio, M.D.
Director, ALS Clinical Services
(212) 650-8168

Hahnemann University Hospital
Department of Neurology
Broad and Vine Sts.
Philadelphia, PA 19102
Elliott L. Mancall, M.D.
Director, ALS Clinic
(215) 448-8036

The neuromuscular diseases clinics sponsored by the Muscular Dystrophy Association, also have expertise in treating ALS.

GOVERNMENT-SUPPORTED ALS CENTERS

The following centers are supported by the National Institute of Neurological and Communicative Disorders and Stroke.

Dr. Michael Oldstone
Scripps Clinic & Research Foundation
10666 N. Torrey Pines Rd.
La Jolla, CA 92307
(714) 455-9100

Dr. Guy McKhann
Johns Hopkins Hospital
Department of Neurology
Blalock 1415
600 N. Wolfe St.
Baltimore, MD 21205
(301) 955-3282

NEUROMUSCULAR DISEASES RESEARCH AND TREATMENT AT THE NATIONAL INSTITUTES OF HEALTH

Research projects are being conducted at the Clinical Center of the National Institutes of Health in Bethesda, Maryland, on myasthenia gravis, ALS, and some of the inflammatory myopathies, especially in regard to the immune system. You can receive treatment at NIH and participate in their research only if you meet certain criteria and are referred by a physician. For more information your physician can contact:

Office of the Director
The Clinical Center
Building 10, Room 2C-146
National Institutes of Health
Bethesda, MD 20892

Patient Referral Service
(301) 496-4891

ORGANIZATIONS

The ALS Association
185 Madison Ave.
New York, NY 10016
(212) 679-4016

15300 Ventura Blvd.
Suite 315
Sherman Oaks, CA 91403
(818) 990-2151

A nonprofit voluntary health agency to fight ALS. Raises funds to support research into the cause and cure of ALS, acts as a clearinghouse for information on ALS, provides counseling and medical referrals for patients and families. Local and regional chapters. A newsletter and other materials. Will provide more information upon request.

Friedreich's Ataxia Group in America, Inc.
PO Box 11116
Oakland, CA 94611
(415) 655-0833

An international nonprofit organization for those with Friedreich's Ataxia. Chapters in many parts of the country. Supports research, offers mutual self-help through chapters, helps educate the public and medical profession about the disorder, provides a newsletter. Will give more information upon request.

Muscular Dystrophy Association
810 Seventh Ave.
New York, NY 10019
(212) 586-0808

A voluntary organization with about 175 local chapters. Conducts research into the causes and cures for muscular dystrophy and related neuro-muscular diseases. Supports university-based clinical research centers and more than 240 out-patient muscular dystrophy clinics throughout the country, where the diseases are diagnosed and treated. The care at the clinics is provided at no direct cost to families, if it is not reim-bursed by health insurance. Also sponsors out-door camps for young people ages 6 to 21 and works with community groups, school officials, and legislative groups in support of programs for the handicapped. To find an MDA chapter near you, write the national headquarters, or con-sult your local telephone directory.

Myasthenia Gravis Foundation
7-11 S. Broadway
White Plains, NY 10601
(914) 328-1717

A national membership organization for patients, physicians, nurses and others concerned about

myasthenia gravis with 52 chapters and branches nationwide. A major source of information. Sup-ports research. Helps support clinics and treat-ment centers for the disease. Has "drug banks" in many local areas through which patients can get myasthenia gravis medications at reduced rates. Manuals for patients and professionals. Will provide more information upon request.

National Ataxia Foundation
600 Twelve Oaks Center
15500 Wayzata Blvd.
Wayzata, MN 55391
(612) 473-7666

A national nonprofit organization to combat all types of hereditary ataxia (lack of muscular coor-dination). Chapters in some parts of the country. A source of information. Makes referrals to neurologists who have a special interest and expertise in ataxias. Brochures, quarterly news-letter, a manual on speech and swallowing problems. Will provide more information upon request.

BOOKS

Under the Shadow, **Anne Knowles,** New York: Harper & Row, 1983; muscular dystrophy.

Hereditary Ataxia: A Guidebook for Managing Speech and Swallowing Problems, Wayzata, MN: National Ataxia Foundation.

MATERIALS, FREE AND FOR SALE

Free (single copies)

Home Care for the Patient with Amyotrophic Lateral Sclerosis, 18 pages.
Managing ALS: Finding Help What is ALS? Some Questions and Answers, leaflet.

The ALS Association
185 Madison Ave.
New York, NY 10016

ALS: Amyotrophic Lateral Sclerosis, 10 pages.
Charcot—Marie—Tooth Disease, 6 pages.
The CPK Test for Detection of Female Carriers of Duchenne Muscular Dystrophy, 8 pages.

Duchenne Muscular Dystrophy, 15 pages.
Learning to Live With Neuromuscular Disease: A Message for Parents of Children with a Neuromuscular Disease, 10 pages.
Living with Progressive Childhood Illness: Parental Management of Neuromuscular Disease, 22 pages.
Muscular Dystrophy Fact Sheet, 10 pages.
Myasthenia Gravis, 6 pages.
Myotonic Dystrophy, 6 pages.
101 Questions & Answers About Muscular Dystrophy, 21 pages.
Plasmapheresis, 8 pages; for treatment of myasthenia gravis.

Polymyositis/Dermatomyositis, 6 pages.
Spinal Muscular Atrophy, 8 pages.
*Who Is At Risk? The Genetics of Duchenne
    Muscular Dystrophy,* 12 pages.

Muscular Dystrophy Association
810 Seventh Ave.
New York, NY 10019
(212) 586-0808

Facts About MG for Patients and Families,
    booklet.
*Myasthenia Gravis—The Disease and a Case
    History,* booklet.

The Myasthenia Gravis Foundation
7-11 S. Broadway
White Plains, NY 10601

Hereditary Ataxia, 8 pages.

National Ataxia Foundation
600 Twelve Oaks Center
15500 Wayzata Blvd.
Wayzata, MN 55391
(612) 473-7666

*ALS: Lou Gehrig's Disease: Hope Through
    Research*
Myasthenia Gravis: Hope Through Research

National Institute of Neurological and
    Communicative Disorders and Stroke
Building 31, Room 8A06
Bethesda, MD 20892

For sale

*Managing ALS: Managing Muscular
    Weakness,* 270 pages.

The ALS Association
15300 Ventura Blvd., Suite 315
Sherman Oaks, CA 91403

NEUROFIBROMATOSIS

See also Genetic Counseling, page 226.

Neurofibromatosis (NF), also known as "Elephant Man Disease," is a genetic disorder that can be inherited or can result from a spontaneous mutation. An estimated 100,000 Americans have neurofibromatosis; it shows up in about one in every 3,000 births. It is a rare disorder, but common among the genetic diseases.

Cause: Genetic. A child with an affected parent has a 50/50 chance of having the disease. It cannot be detected through prenatal screening of an unborn child.

Symptoms: The disorder is characterized by many small or large tumors or nodules just under the skin. There may also be curvature of the spine, enlargement and deformation of bones, deafness, blindness in one or both eyes, and tumors on the brain or spinal cord. It is important to note that severe disfigurement, of the type popularized in the book, play, and movie, *The Elephant Man,* is exceedingly rare. Although some people with the disorder suffer some deformities, others have merely a few brown spots or skin lumps that are virtually unnoticeable.

The course of neurofibromatosis is unpredictable. In a small percentage of cases the tumors become malignant.

Diagnosis: The disorder can sometimes be spotted in infants at birth by the presence of six or more light brown spots on the skin. However, the spots may appear up to a year after birth and increase in number and size during the first 10 years of life. Tumors may show up in childhood, but usually not until adolescence; they have developed as late as age 50.

Treatment: Neurofibromatosis is incurable, but there are a number of treatments available to lessen the severity of the disease, including surgery to correct curvature of the spine, neurosurgery to remove tumors, and plastic surgery to remove skin tumors and, if necessary, to correct facial deformities.

People with the disease and their families often need psychological counseling and support and genetic counseling. If the condition is suspected, you can contact a genetics department at a nearby university medical center, or one of the centers or agencies dedicated to genetic counseling (*see* page 227).

SOME LEADING SPECIALISTS AND TREATMENT CENTERS FOR NEUROFIBROMATOSIS

The following clinics specialize in the diagnosis and treatment of NF:

Neurofibromatosis Clinic
Children's Hospital National Medical Center
Washington, DC 20010
Director: Dr. Kenneth Rosenbaum
(202) 745-2187

Neurofibromatosis Clinic
Massachusetts General Hospital
Boston, MA 02114
Director: Dr. Robert Martuza
(617) 726-3776

Neurofibromatosis Clinic
Mt. Sinai School of Medicine
New York, NY 10029
Director: Dr. Allan Rubenstein
(212) 650-7875

Neurofibromatosis Clinic
Children's Hospital
Philadelphia, PA 19104
Director: Dr. Anna Meadows
(215) 596-9644

Dr. Linton A. Whitaker, chief of plastic surgery at the Philadelphia Children's Hospital, is widely recognized for craniofacial surgery to correct deformities from this disorder.

Neurofibromatosis Clinic
Baylor School of Medicine
Houston, TX 77030
Director: Dr. Vincent Riccardi
(713) 790-6103

SOURCE: *National Neurofibromatosis Foundation.*

RESEARCH AND TREATMENT AT THE NATIONAL INSTITUTES OF HEALTH

Selected patients with neurofibromatosis are admitted at the National Institutes of Health's Neurofibromatosis Clinic in Bethesda, Maryland. The purpose is early diagnosis and treatment evaluation. Patients are admitted by physician referral only. For more information, your physician can contact:

Office of Director
The Clinical Center
Building 10, Room 2C-146
National Institutes of Health
Bethesda, MD 20892
(301) 496-4891

ORGANIZATION

National Neurofibromatosis Foundation, Inc.
141 Fifth Ave., Suite 7-S
New York, NY 10010
(212) 460-8980

A nonprofit, voluntary health organization. Provides information and guidance to families with neurofibromatosis. Offers pamphlets and a quarterly newsletter. Sponsors research. Answers questions from the public. Has local chapters in many parts of the country. Contact for more information and location of nearest chapter.

BOOKS

The Elephant Man, **Bernard Pomerance,** New York: Grove Press, 1979.
The Elephant Man, **Ashley Montague,** New York: E. P. Dutton, 1979
Neurofibromatosis, **edited by Vincent M. Riccardi** and **John J. Mulvihill,** New York: Raven Press, 1981.
The True History of the Elephant Man, **Michael Howell,** New York: Penguin Books, 1980.

FREE MATERIALS

Neurofibromatosis, fact sheet.
*Neurofibromatosis: Information for Patients
and Families,* 20 page booklet.

National Institute of Neurological and
  Communicative Disorders and Stroke
Bethesda, MD 20892

OSTEOPATHIC MEDICINE

Most physicians in the United States have an M.D. (doctor of medicine) degree, but there is another type of physician, called an osteopath, who receives a D.O. (doctor of osteopathic medicine). Like M.D.'s, D.O.'s can practice all branches of medicine and surgery and can prescribe drugs. The main difference is that D.O.'s graduate from colleges of osteopathic medicine and emphasize manipulative procedures of the musculoskeletal system—muscles, bones, and joints—to diagnose and help cure all kinds of diseases.

D.O.'s also have a long tradition of treating patients "holistically"—treating the whole entity instead of the diseased part—and many are interested in nutrition. Thus, osteopathic physicians insist they offer an alternative to conventional drug-surgery therapy. The overwhelming majority, more than 85 percent of the osteopaths in the United States, do primary care and are more apt to be located in smaller towns and cities. But, like M.D.'s, osteopaths specialize as allergists, anesthesiologists, cardiologists, obstetricians, pathologists, pediatricians, etc.

Because their tradition differs from that of M.D.'s, osteopaths are often mistakenly not considered "real" doctors, and in the past have been opposed by the general medical establishment. But much of the opposition has diminished, and D.O.'s and M.D.'s sometimes practice together. Also, D.O.'s are often confused in the public's mind with chiropractors. Chiropractors offer *only* physical manipulation and are not licensed to give full-range medical services, such as drugs and surgery; osteopaths are. In most states, D.O.'s take the same license exams as M.D.'s and are recognized by all states as fully accredited professionals.

PROFESSIONAL ORGANIZATION

The osteopathic medical profession has set up its own network of hospitals and medical schools and its own medical association.

American Osteopathic Association
212 E. Ohio St.
Chicago, IL 60611
(312) 280-5882

Serves as the main body for standards of osteopathic medicine, as the American Medical Association does for M.D.'s. Comprised of osteopathic physicians, surgeons, graduates of approved schools of osteopathic medicine, and affiliate members, such as hospitals. Accredits colleges and hospitals. Sponsors research. Offers several publications, including a monthly journal.

OSTEOPATHIC PHYSICIANS AND HOSPITALS

The American Osteopathic Association publishes an annual national directory of osteopathic physicians and will refer you to an osteopath in your locality if you contact them.

There are many osteopathic hospitals that are staffed mostly by osteopathic physicians, some specializing in various medical fields. If you prefer care by osteopaths either as an inpatient or outpatient, these hospitals are a good point of reference.

Here is a list of osteopathic hospitals according to a survey by the American Osteopathic Association. Asterisks (*) indicate accreditation from the American Osteopathic Association.

ARIZONA
*Mesa General Hospital Medical Center
515 N. Mesa Drive
Mesa, AZ 85210
(601) 969-9111

*Parker Community Hospital
PO Box 1149
Parker, AZ 85283
(602) 669-9201

*Community Hospital Medical Center
6501 N. 19th Ave.
Phoenix. AZ 85015
(602) 249-3434

*Phoenix General Hospital
1950 W. Indian School Rd.
PO Box 21331
Phoenix, AZ 85036
(601) 279-4411

*Scottsdale Community Hospital
8435 E. McDowell Rd.
Scottsdale, AZ 85257
(602) 945-7600

*Tucson General Hospital, Inc.
3838 N. Campbell Ave.
Tucson, AZ 85719
(602) 327-5431

CALIFORNIA
Burbank Community Hospital
466 E. Olive Ave.
Burbank, CA 91501
(818) 953-6500

Rio Hondo Memorial Hospital
8300 E. Telegraph Rd.
Downey, CA 90240
(213) 806-1821

*Pacific Hospital of Long Beach
2776 Pacific Ave.
PO Box 1268
Long Beach, CA 90801
(213) 595-1911

Doctors Hospital of Montclair
5000 San Bernardino St.
Montclair, CA 91763
(714) 625-5411

*Ontario Community Hospital
550 N. Monterey Ave.
Ontario, CA 91764
(714) 984-2201

*Hillside Hospital
1940 El Cajon Blvd.
San Diego, CA 92104
(619) 297-2251

Simi Valley Community Hospital
1575 Erringer Rd.
Simi Valley, CA 93065
(805) 527-9383

COLORADO
*Eisenhower Medical Center
33 Barnes Ave.
PO Box 15700
Colorado Springs, CO 80909
(303) 475-2111

*Rocky Mountain Hospital
4701 E. Ninth Ave.
Denver, CO 80220
(303) 393-5701

Community Hospital
1065 Walnut Ave.
Grand Junction, CO 81501
(303) 242-0920

*Memorial Hospital
928 Twelfth St.
Greeley, CO 80631
(303) 352-3123

DELAWARE
*Riverside Osteopathic Hospital
700 Lea Blvd.
PO Box 845
Wilmington, DE 19802
(302) 764-6120

FLORIDA

*Daytona Beach General Hospital, Inc.
1340 Ridgewood Ave.
Holly Hill, FL 32017
(904) 677-5100

*Humana Hospital of South Broward
5100 W. Hallandale Blvd.
Hollywood, FL 33023
(305) 966-8100

*Jacksonville Medical Center
4901 Richard St.
PO Box 10398
Jacksonville, FL 32207
(904) 737-3120

*Sun Coast Hospital
2025 Indian Rocks Rd.
PO Box 2025
Largo, FL 34294-2025
(813) 581-9474

*Westchester General Hospital
2500 S.W. 75th Ave.
Miami, FL 33155
(305) 264-5252

*Southeastern Medical Center
1750 N.E. 167 St.
North Miami Beach, FL 33162
(305) 945-5400

*Orlando General Hospital, Inc.
7727 Lake Underhill Drive
Orlando, FL 32822
(305) 277-8110

Peninsula Medical Center
264 S. Atlantic Ave.
Ormond Beach, FL 32074
(904) 672-4161

*Metropolitan General Hospital, Inc.
7950 66th St., N.
Pinellas Park, FL 33565
(813) 546-9871

*Doctors General Hospital
6701 W. Sunrise Blvd.
Plantation, FL 33313
(305) 581-7800

*Harborside Hospital
401 15th St., N.
St. Petersburg, FL 33705
(813) 821-2021

*University General Hospital
10200 Seminole Blvd.
Seminole, FL 33544
(813) 397-5511

*Carrollwood Community Hospital
7171 N. Dale Mabry Highway
Tampa, FL 33614
(813) 935-1191

Wellington Regional Medical Center
10101 Forest Hill Blvd.
West Palm Beach, FL 33414
(305) 798-4440

GEORGIA

*Doctors Hospital
2160 Idlewood Rd.
Tucker, GA 30084
(404) 496-6700

ILLINOIS

*Chicago Osteopathic Medical Center
5200 S. Ellis Ave.
Chicago, IL 60615
(312) 947-3000

*Olympia Fields Osteopathic Medical Center
20201 Crawford Ave.
Olympia Fields, IL 60461
(312) 747-4000

INDIANA

*Westview Hospital
3630 Guion Rd.
Indianapolis, IN 46222
(317) 924-6661

*Wirth Osteopathic Hospital
Highway 64 W.
Oakland City, IN 47660
(812) 749-6111

*Michiana Community Hospital
2515 E. Jefferson Blvd.
South Bend, IN 46615
(219) 288-8311

IOWA

*Davenport Medical Center
1111 W. Kimberly Rd.
Davenport, IA 52806
(319) 391-2020

*Des Moines General Hospital
603 E. 12th St.
Des Moines, IA 50307
(515) 263-4200

Manning General Hospital
410 Main St.
Manning, IA 51455
(712) 653-2072

KANSAS
Wellington Hospital
924 S. Washington Ave.
Wellington, KS 67152
(316) 326-3353

*Riverside Hospital
2622 W. Central Ave.
Wichita, KS 67203
(316) 945-9161

MAINE
*Taylor Hospital
268 Stillwater Ave.
Bangor, ME 04401
(207) 942-5286

*Osteopathic Hospital of Maine, Inc.
335 Brighton Ave.
Portland, ME 04102
(207) 774-3921

*Waterville Osteopathic Hospital
200 Kennedy Memorial Drive
Waterville, ME 04901
(207) 873-0731

MASSACHUSETTS
*Massachusetts Osteopathic Hospital &
   Medical Center
222 S. Hungtington Ave.
Boston, MA 02130
(617) 522-4300

MICHIGAN
*Bay Osteopathic Hospital
3250 E. Midland Rd.
Bay City, MI 48706
(517) 686-2920

*Belding Community Hospital, Inc.
1534 W. State St.
Belding, MI 48809
(616) 794-0400

*Visitors Hospital
1301 Main St.
Buchanan, MI 49107
(616) 695-3851

*Carson City Osteopathic Hospital
406 E. Elm
Carson City, MI 48811
(517) 584-3131

*Clare Osteopathic Hospital, Inc.
104 W. 6th St.
Clare, MI 48617
(517) 386-9951

*Aurora Hospital Osteopathic
3737 Humboldt
Detroit, MI 48208
(313) 361-8000

MOMC
Adult Mental Health Hospital
5435 Woodward Ave.
Detroit, MI 48202
(313) 494-0400

*MOMC Acute Care Hospital
2700 Martin Luther King, Jr. Blvd.
Detroit, MI 48208
(313) 361-8000

*Northwest General Hospital
8741 W. Chicago Blvd.
Detroit, MI 48204
(313) 934-3030

Northwest General Hospital, Mental Health
   Services Department
8741 W. Chicago
Detroit, MI 48204
(313) 934-3030

*Botsford General Hospital
28050 Grand River Ave.
Farmington Hills, MI 48024
(313) 471-8000

*Flint Osteopathic Hospital
3921 Beecher Rd.
Flint, MI 48502
(313) 762-4600

*Garden City Osteopathic Hospital
6245 N. Inkster Rd.
Garden City, MI 48135
(313) 421-3300

Metropolitan Hospital
1919 Boston St., S.E.
Grand Rapids, MI 49506
(616) 247-7200

*Detroit Osteopathic Hospital
12523 Third Ave.
Highland Park, MI 48203
(313) 252-4000

*Jackson Osteopathic Hospital
110 N. Elm Ave.
Jackson, MI 49202
(517) 787-1440

*Lansing General Hospital, Osteopathic
2727 S. Pennsylvania
Lansing, MI 48910
(517) 372-8220

*Saint Lawrence Hospital
1210 W. Saginaw
Lansing, MI 48915
(517) 372-3610

*Oakland General Hospital
27251 Dequindre Rd.
Madison Heights, MI 48071
(313) 967-7000

*Harrison Community Hospital
26755 Ballard Rd.
Mount Clemens, MI 48035
(313) 465-5501

*Mount Clemens General Hospital
1000 Harrington Blvd.
Mount Clemens, MI 48043
(313) 466-8000

*Muskegon General Hospital
1700 Oak Ave.
Muskegon, MI 49442
(616) 773-3311

Heritage Hospital
3020 Peck St.
Muskegon Heights, MI 49444
(616) 739-7141

Memorial Hospital of Manistee County
Rogers Memorial Drive
Onekama, MI 49675
(616) 889-4294

*Pontiac Osteopathic Hospital
50 N. Perry Ave.
Pontiac, MI 48058
(313) 338-5000

*Saginaw Osteopathic Hospital
515 N. Michigan Ave.
Saginaw, MI 48602
(517) 771-5100

*Sheridan Community Hospital (Osteopathic)
301 N. Main St.
Sheridan, MI 48884
(517) 291-3261

*Southfield Rehabilitation Center
22401 Foster Winter Drive
Southfield, MI 48075
(313) 569-1500

*Mecosta Memorial Hospital
18087 Pierce Rd.
Stanwood, MI 49346
(616) 823-2071

*Traverse City Osteopathic Hospital
550 Munson Ave.
Traverse City, MI 49684
(616) 922-8400

*Riverside Osteopathic Hospital
150 Traux St.
Trenton, MI 48183
(313) 676-4200

*Bi-Country Community Hospital
13355 E. Ten Mile Rd.
Warren, MI 48089
(313) 756-1000

MISSOURI
Cameron Community Hospital
1015 W. Fourth St.
Cameron, MO 64429
(816) 632-2101

South Barry County Memorial District Hospital
87 Gravel St.
Cassville, MO 65625
(417) 847-4115

Chaffee General Hospital
537 W. Yoakum Ave.
Drawer C
Chaffee, MO 63740
(314) 887-3573

Golden Valley Memorial Hospital
Junction Highways 7 & 13 N
Clinton, MO 64735
(816) 885-5511

Reynolds County Memorial Hospital
PO Box 250
Ellington, MO 63638
(314) 663-2511

*Mineral Area Osteopathic Hospital
1212 Weber Rd.
Farmington, MO 63640-3398
(314) 756-4581

Hermann Area District Hospital
Rt. 1, Box 30
Hermann, MO 65041
(314) 486-2191

*Charles E. Still Osteopathic Hospital
1125 S. Madison St.
PO Box 1128
Jefferson City, MO 65102
(314) 635-7141

*Oak Hill Hospital
932 E. 34th St.
Joplin, MO 64801
(417) 623-4640

*Lakeside Hospital
8701 Troost Ave.
Kansas City, MO 64131
(816) 995-2000

*Park Lane Medical Center
5151 Raytown Rd.
Kansas City, MO 64133
(816) 358-8000

*The University of Health Sciences University
  Hospital
2105 Independence Blvd.
Kansas City, MO 64124
(816) 283-2000

Grim-Smith Hospital & Clinic
112 E. Patterson Ave.
Kirksville, MO 63501
(816) 665-7241

*Kirksville Osteopathic Health Center
800 W. Jefferson
Kirksville, MO 63501
(816) 626-2226

*Scotland County Memorial Hospital
Rte. 1, Box 53
Memphis, MO 63555
(816) 465-8511

Moberly Regional Medical Center
1515 Union Ave.
PO Box 3000
Moberly, MO 65270
(816) 263-8400

*Phelps County Regional Medical Center
1000 W. 10th St.
Rolla, MO 65401
(314) 364-3100

*Normandy Osteopathic Hospital—North
7840 Natural Bridge Rd.
St. Louis, MO 63121
(314) 389-0015

*Normandy Osteopathic Hospital—South
530 Des Peres Rd.
St. Louis, MO 63131
(314) 821-5850

*Springfield General Hospital
2828 N. National Ave.
PO Box 783
Springfield, MO 65801
(417) 869-5571

Pulaski County Memorial Hospital
Hospital Rd.
Waynesvile, MO 65583
(314) 774-6461

NEW JERSEY
*Kennedy Memorial Hospital University
  Medical Center, Cherry Hill Division
Chapel Ave. & Cooper Landing Rd.
Cherry Hill, NJ 08034
(609) 665-2000

*West Essex General Hospital
204 Hillside Ave.
Livingston, NJ 07039
(201) 992-6550

*Kennedy Memorial Hospital at Saddle Brook
300 Market St.
Saddle Brook, NJ 07662
(201) 368-6000

*Kennedy Memorial Hospital University
  Medical Center, Stratford Division
18 E. Laurel Rd.
Stratford, NJ 08084
(609) 784-4000

*Kennedy Memorial Hospital University
  Medical Center, Washington Township
  Division
Hurffville-Cross Keys Rds.
Turnersville, NJ 08012
(609) 589-3300

*Memorial General Hospital
1000 Galloping Hill Rd.
Union, NJ 07083
(201) 687-1900

NEW MEXICO
*Heights General Hospital
4701 Montgomery Blvd., N.E.
Albuquerque, NM 87109
(505) 888-7800

NEW YORK
*Baptist Medical Center of New York
2749 Linden Blvd.
Brooklyn, NY 11208
(718) 277-5100

*Coney Island Hospital
2601 Ocean Parkway
Brooklyn, NY 11235
(718) 615-4000

*St. Joseph's Hospital, Division of the
  Catholic Medical Center of Brooklyn and
  Queens
158-40 79th Ave.
Flushing, NY 11366
(718) 591-1000

*Massapequa General Hospital
750 Hicksville Rd.
PO Box 20
Seaford, NY 11783-0020
(516) 454-3498

OHIO
*O'Bleness Memorial Hospital
Hospital Drive
Athens, OH 45701
(614) 593-5551

*Otto C. Epp Memorial Hospital
8000 Kenwood Rd.
Cincinnati, OH 45236
(513) 745-2200

*Doctors Hospital North & West
1087 Dennison Ave.
Columbus, OH 43201
(614) 297-4000

*Cuyahoga Falls General Hospital
1900 23rd St.
Cuyahoga Falls, OH 44223
(216) 929-2911

*Grandview Hospital
405 Grand Ave.
Dayton, OH 45405
(513) 226-3200

Southview Hospital & Family Health Center
1997 Miamisburg & Centerville Rd.
Dayton, OH 45459
(513) 439-6000

*Northeastern Ohio General Hospital
2041 Hubbard Rd.
Madison, OH 44057
(216) 428-2121

*Selby General Hospital
1106 Colegate Drive
Marietta, OH 45750
(614) 373-0582

*Doctors Hospital, Inc. of Stark County
400 Austin Ave., N.W.
Massillon, OH 44646
(216) 837-7200

*Doctors Hospital of Nelsonville
W. Franklin St.
Nelsonville, OH 45764
(614) 753-1931

Fisher-Titus Memorial Hospital
272 Benedict Ave.
Norwalk, OH 44857
(419) 668-8101

Wayne General Hospital
230 S. Crown Hill Rd.
Orrville, OH 44667
(216) 682-6015

*Richmond Heights General Hospital
27100 Chardon Rd.
Richmond Heights, OH 44143
(216) 585-6500

*Firelands Community Hospital
1101 Decatur St.
Sandusky, OH 44870
(419) 626-7400

*Sandusky Memorial Hospital
2020 Hayes Ave.
Sandusky, OH 44870
(419) 627-5000

*Parkview Hospital—Osteopathic
1920 Parkwood Ave.
Toledo, OH 43624
(419) 242-8471

*Warren General Hospital
667 Eastland Ave., S.E.
Warren, OH 44484
(216) 373-9000

*Brentwood Hospital
4110 Warrensville Center Rd.
Warrensville Heights, OH 44122
(216) 283-2900

*St. John and West Shore Hospital
2900 Center Ridge Rd.
Westlake, OH 44145
(216) 835-8000

*Youngstown Osteopathic Hospital
1319 Florencedale Ave.
Youngstown, OH 44505
(216) 744-9200

OKLAHOMA

Afton Memorial Hospital
Drawer L
134 S. Main St.
Afton, OK 74331
(918) 257-8322

*Memorial Hospital Company, Inc.
523 N. 22nd St.
Collinsville, OK 74021
(918) 371-2591

*Enid Memorial Hospital
402 S. Fourth St.
PO Box 3467
Enid, OK 73701
(405) 234-3371

*Hillcrest Osteopathic Hospital
2129 S.W. 59th St.
Oklahoma City, OK 73119
(405) 685-6671

Moots Osteopathic Hospital, Inc.
8 N. Rowe
PO Box 188
Pryor, OK 74361
(918) 825-2155

*Oklahoma Osteopathic Hospital
Ninth & Jackson Sts.
Tulsa, OK 74127
(918) 587-2561

OREGON

Forest Glen Hospital, Inc.
495 S.W. First St.
PO Box 198
Canyonville, OR 97417
(503) 839-4213

*Eastmoreland General Hospital
2900 S.E. Steele St.
Portland, OR 97202
(503) 234-0411

PENNSYLVANIA

*Allentown Osteopathic Medical Center
1736 Hamilton St.
Allentown, PA 18104
(215) 770-8300

*Clarion Osteopathic Community Hospital
One Hospital Drive
Clarion, PA 16214
(814) 226-9500

*Metro Health Center
252 W. 11th St.
Erie, PA 16501
(814) 455-3961

*Millcreek Community Hospital
5515 Peach St.
Erie, PA 16509
(814) 864-4031

*Shenango Valley Osteopathic Hospital
2200 Memorial Drive
Farrell, PA 16121
(412) 981-3500

*United Community Hospital
RD No. 5, Box 5005
Cranberry Rd.
Grove City, PA 16127
(412) 458-5442

*Community General Osteopathic Hospital
PO Box 3000
4300 Londonderry Rd.
Harrisburg, PA 17105
(717) 632-3000

*Lancaster Osteopathic Hospital
PO Box 3002
1175 Clark St.
Lancaster, PA 17604
(717) 397-3711

*Delaware Valley Medical Center
200 Oxford Valley Rd.
Langhorne, PA 19047
(215) 750-3000

*Suburban General Hospital
2701 DeKalb Pike
Norristown, PA 19401
(215) 278-2000

*West Allegheny Hospital
777 Steubenville Pike
Oakdale, PA 15071
(412) 788-4900

*Metropolitan Hospital—Central Division
201 N. Eighth St.
Philadelphia, PA 19106
(215) 238-2000

*Metropolitan Hospital—Parkview Division
1331 E. Wyoming Ave.
Philadelphia, PA 19124
(215) 537-7400

*Osteopathic Medical Center of Philadelphia
4150 City Ave.
Philadelphia, PA 19131
(215) 581-6262

*Metropolitan Hospital—Springfield Division
Sproul & Thomson Rds.
Springfield, PA 19064
(215) 328-9200

*Troy Community Hospital
100 John St.
Troy, PA 16947
(717) 297-2121

*Memorial Hospital
325 Belmont St.
PO Box M-118
York, PA 17405
(717) 843-8623

RHODE ISLAND
*Cranston General Hospital, Osteopathic
1763 Broad St.
Cranston, RI 02905
(401) 781-9200

SOUTH DAKOTA
Community Memorial Hospital Association
2100 Davenport St.
Sturgis, SD 57785
(605) 347-2536

TENNESSEE
Northwest General Hospital
5310 Western Ave.
Knoxville, TN 37921-3299
(615) 584-9191

Coffee Medical Center
1001 McArthur Drive
Manchester, TN 37355
(615) 728-3586

Medical Center of Manchester
Rt. 6, Box 6015
Interstate Drive
Manchester, TN 37355
(615) 728-6354

Memorial Hospital
Highway 45 By-Pass
Trenton, TN 38382
(901) 855-4500

TEXAS
*Southwest Osteopathic Hospital
2828 W. 27th St.
PO Box 7408
Amarillo, TX 79109
(806) 358-3131

*Northeast Community Hospital
1301 Airport Freeway
Bedford, TX 76021
(817) 282-9211

Fannin County Hospital
504 Lipscomb
Bonham, TX 75418
(214) 583-8585

Comanche Community Hospital
211 S. Austin
Comanche, TX 76442
(915) 356-2012

Citizens Hospital of Commerce
2900 Sterling Hart Drive
Commerce, TX 75428
(214) 886-3161

*Corpus Christi Osteopathic Hospital
1502 Tarlton St.
PO Box 7807
Corpus Christi, TX 78415
(512) 886-2300

City Oaks Hospital
728 S. Corinth St.
Dallas, TX 75203
(214) 946-4000

*Dallas Family Hospital
2929 S. Hampton Rd.
Dallas, TX 75224
(214) 330-4611

*Dallas Memorial Hospital
5003 Ross Ave.
Dallas, TX 75206
(214) 824-3071

*Metropolitan Hospital
7525 Scyene Rd.
Dallas, TX 75227
(214) 381-7171

Concho County Hospital
Drawer L
Eden, TX 76837
(915) 869-5911

*Tigua General Hospital
7722 N. Loop Rd.
El Paso, TX 79915
(915) 779-2424

*Fort Worth Osteopathic Medical Center
1000 Montgomery St.
Fort Worth, TX 76107
(817) 731-4311

White Settlement Hospital
701 S. Cherry Lane
Fort Worth, TX 76108
(817) 246-2491

*Dallas/Fort Worth Medical Center—Grand
   Prairie
2709 Hospital Blvd.
Grand Prairie, TX 75051
(214) 641-5000

*Doctors Hospital, Inc.
5500 39th St.
Groves, TX 77619
(409) 962-5733

Doctors Hospital, Ltd.
5815 Airline Drive
Houston, TX 77076
(713) 695-6041

Eastway General Hospital
9339 N. Loop E.
Houston, TX 77029
(713) 675-3241

Omni Hospital & Medical Center
8214 Homestead Rd.
Houston, TX 77028
(713) 631-1550

*Community Hospital of Lubbock
5301 University Ave.
Lubbock, TX 79413
(806) 795-9301

Menard Hospital
PO Box 608
Menard, TX 76859
(915) 396-4515

Mesquite Physicians Hospital
1527 N. Galloway
Mesquite, TX 75149
(214) 285-6391

Mineola General Hospital, Inc.
807 Mimosa
Mineola, TX 75773
(214) 569-3821

Martin County Hospital District
R610 N. St. Peter Sts.
Stanton, TX 79782
(915) 756-3345

Doctors Memorial Hospital
1400 W. Southwest Loop 323
Tyler, TX 75701
(214) 561-3771

WASHINGTON
*Shorewood Osteopathic Hospital
12845 Ambaum Blvd., S.W.
Seattle, WA 98146
(206) 243-1455

*Waldo General Hospital
10560 Fifth Ave., N.E.
Seattle, WA 98125
(206) 364-2050

*Sunnyside Community Hospital
10th & Tacoma Ave.
PO Box 719
Sunnyside, WA 98944
(509) 837-2101

New Valley Osteopathic Hospital
3003 Tieton Drive
Yakima, WA 98902
(509) 453-6561

WEST VIRGINIA
*South Charleston Community Hospital
30 McCorkle Ave.
South Charleston, WV 25303
(304) 744-5311

Weirton Osteopathic Hospital, Inc.
3045 Pennsylvania Ave.
PO Box 2458
Weirton, WV 26062
(304) 723-1200

WISCONSIN
*Lakeview Hospital
10010 W. Bluemound Rd.
Milwaukee, WI 53226
(414) 771-5200

*Northwest General Hospital
5310 W. Capitol Drive
Milwaukee, WI 53216
(414) 447-8543

*New Berlin Memorial Hospital
13750 W. National Ave.
New Berlin, WI 53151
(414) 782-2700

SOURCE: *American Osteopathic Hospital Association.*

BOOKS

*Osteopathic Medicine: An American
   Reformation,* **George W. Northup, D.O.,**

Chicago: American Osteopathic Association,
1979.

FREE MATERIALS

Single copies are free

An Introduction to Osteopathic Medicine, fact
   sheet.
Osteopathic Medicine, 6 pages.
What Is a D.O.? What Is an M.D.? 6 pages.

*You're the Patient: Your Rights and
   Responsibilities,* 6 pages.

American Osteopathic Association
212 E. Ohio St.
Chicago, IL 60611
(312) 280-5882

PAGET'S DISEASE

Paget's disease (osteitis deformans) is a progressive and potentially crippling disorder of the bones in which the normal metabolic processes that control the constant resorption and regrowth of bone cells go awry. The bones become soft and then deformed as new bone is laid down rapidly and in disorderly fashion. About three million Americans have Paget's disease, many without knowing it. The disease almost always strikes after age 40, and is most common between ages 50 and 70. It is slightly more common in men. Some patients have no symptoms and do not need treatment. However, the disease can be devastating and disabling. Paget's disease tends to show up in people of Western European heritage and is most common in those from Great Britain, France and Germany.

Cause: Unknown. It is thought to have a genetic factor and appears to run in families. From 15 to 30 percent of those stricken have a family history of the disease. It has also been suggested that a slow-acting virus may trigger the onset of Paget's disease in susceptible individuals.

Symptoms: Pain is usually the first complaint, often in the back or hip. This may be due to associated arthritis or nerve damage. There is occasionally bone pain. Affected limbs may become bowed. If the skull is involved, as it frequently is, symptoms are headache, tinnitus (ringing in the ears), hearing loss, dizziness, other neurological disturbances, and sometimes an enlargement of the head.

Diagnosis: The main diagnosis is through X-ray, confirmed by biochemical tests of the blood and urine. Bone biopsy is rarely needed, although a bone scan may also be done. Diagnosis is usually made by a specialist. Diagnosis in some cases may be difficult and confusing, especially if the person also has arthritis, for the symptoms are often the same. Sometimes doctors make a differential diagnosis by injecting an antiarthritic drug into the joint; if there is instant relief, the assumption is the pain was caused by arthritis. Conversely, it is sometimes necessary to begin treatment for Paget's before the diagnosis is definitive.

Treatment: The disease cannot be cured, but it can be treated rather effectively by drugs that relieve the pain and discomfort and block progression of the disease. In rare cases surgery is necessary to repair the damage. Because the treatment of Paget's is rather new and the diagnosis often difficult, many people who need treatment do not get it. The disorder usually requires a specialist; general practitioners rarely have the experience to treat it.

Physicians who treat Paget's disease are endocrinologists, rheumatologists, and orthopedic surgeons. For the heads of departments in those medical specialties at leading medical colleges, *see* pages 594, 569, and 630 respectively. The physicians listed there can be sources of treatment and/or referrals to others specializing in the treatment of bone diseases.

Additionally, here is a list of physicians who have a special expertise and interest in treating Paget's disease.

SOME PAGET'S TREATMENT SPECIALISTS

ARIZONA

Eric P. Gall, M.D.
Professor, Chief Rheumatology Section
University of Arizona
Health Sciences Center
Tucson, AZ 85724
(602) 626-6041

Richard A. Silver, M.D.
Tucson Orthopaedic and Fracture Surgery
  Associates, Ltd.
PO Box 50187
Tucson, AZ 85703
(602) 884-9242

CALIFORNIA

David Baylink, M.D.
Professor of Medicine
Loma Linda University
Chief, Mineral Metabolism
Jerry L. Pettis Veterans' Hospital
11201 Benton St.
Loma Linda, CA 92357
(714) 825-7084, x2815

Gerald Finerman, M.D.
Division of Orthopaedic Surgery
UCLA School of Medicine
The Center for the Health Sciences
Los Angeles, CA 90024
(213) 825-6019

Theodore J. Hahn, M.D.
Professor of Medicine, UCLA
Endocrine Section (691/111D)
Wadsworth Medical Center (VA)
Wilshire and Sawtelle Blvds.
Los Angeles, CA 90073
(213) 824-4442 (for veterans)
(213) 825-7591 (outpatient appointments)

Frederick R. Singer, M.D.
Professor of Medicine
Department of Medicine
Section of Endocrinology
Clinical Research Center
University of Southern California
2025 Zonal Ave.
Los Angeles, CA 90033
(213) 226-4632

Neil E. Romanoff, M.D.
Wright #308
Eisenhower Medical Center
39000 Bob Hope Drive
Rancho Mirage, CA 92270
(714) 346-5639

William G. Cushard, Jr., M.D.
Endocrine Associates of Sacramento
77 Scripps Drive, Suite 100
Sacramento, CA 95825
(916) 929-3381

Paul H. Broadley, M.D.
770 Washington St.
San Diego, CA 92103
(714) 291-2723 (for orthopedic surgery)

Leonard J. Deftos, M.D.
Associate Professor of Medicine
Chief, Endocrine Section
VA Hospital
3350 La Jolla Village Drive
San Diego, CA 92161
(619) 453-7500, x3715

Marvin H. Meyers, M.D.
Clinical Professor
Orthopedic Surgery & Rehabilitation
University of California Medical Center
225 Dickinson St.
San Diego, CA 92103
(619) 453-7500, x3841

Claude D. Arnaud, M.D.
Daniel Bickle, M.D.
Gordon J. Strewler, M.D.
VA Medical Center
4150 Clement St., 111N
San Francisco, CA 94121
(415) 221-4810

Paul A. Fitzgerald, M.D.
Assistant Clinical Professor of Medicine
University of California, San Francisco
350 Parnassus Ave., Suite 710
San Francisco, CA 94117
(415) 665-1136

Felix O. Kolb, M.D.
3580 California St.
San Francisco, CA 94118
(415) 922-1330
(Referral only by patient's physician)

COLORADO
Mervyn L. Lifschitz, M.D.
Rose Medical Plaza
4545 E. Ninth Ave.
Denver, CO 80220
(303) 388-4673

CONNECTICUT
Lawrence Raisz, M.D.
Professor of Medicine
University of Connecticut
School of Medicine
Health Center
Farmington, CT 06032
(203) 674-2129

Robert Lang, M.D.
Associate Professor of Medicine
Department of Medicine
Room 2074 LMP
Yale University
School of Medicine
333 Cedar St.
New Haven, CT 06510
(203) 785-4181

FLORIDA
Stanley Wallach, M.D.
Chief, Medical Service
VA Medical Center
Bay Pines, FL 33504
(813) 398-9372
(Takes private patients at University of South
    Florida Clinics)

Irvin Stein, M.D.
2267 Silver Palm Rd., E.
Boca Raton, FL 33432
(305) 392-6161

Roy D. Altman, M.D.
Professor of Medicine
University of Miami School of Medicine
Chief, Arthritis Division
Miami VA Medical Center
PO Box 016960
Miami, FL 33101
(305) 547-5735 or 324-3188

Eric Reiss, M.D.
Department of Medicine (D4-10)
University of Miami School of Medicine
PO Box 016960
Miami, FL 33101
(305) 547-5735 or 324-3188

Adelina Flores, M.D.
Internal Medicine
Endocrinology & Metabolism
2400 Harbor Blvd., N.E.
Suite 12
Port Charlotte, FL 33952
(813) 629-4422

Louis R. Ricca, M.D.
763 Sixth Ave., S.
St. Petersburg, FL 33701
(813) 822-3525

John T. Garland, M.D.
Palm Beach Endocrine Associates
1000 45th St., Suite 2
West Palm Beach, FL 33407
(305) 845-6001

GEORGIA
Robert S. Weinstein, M.D.
Associate Professor of Medicine
Director, Metabolic Bone Disease Laboratory
Section of Metabolic and Endocrine Disease
Medical College of Georgia
Augusta, GA 30912
(404) 828-2131

HAWAII
Se Mo Suh, M.D., Ph.D.
Director, Bone-Mineral Research Laboratory
Shriners Hospitals
Honolulu Unit
1310 Punahou St.
Honolulu, HI 96826
(808) 955-7755

ILLINOIS
Murray J. Favus, M.D.
Associate Professor of Medicine
University of Chicago
Clinical Research Center
5841 S. Maryland St., Box 28
Chicago, IL 60637
(312) 962-6227

James W. Milgram, M.D.
Suite 922E
Water Tower Place
845 N. Michigan Ave.
Chicago, IL 60611
(312) 943-5550

W.G. Ryan, M.D.
Consultants in Endocrinology
1753 W. Congress Parkway
Chicago, IL 60612
(312) 942-6163

INDIANA
C. Conrad Johnston, Jr., M.D.
Professor of Medicine
Indiana University
School of Medicine
Director, Division of Endocrinology and
  Metabolism
Indiana University Medical Center
1100 W. Michigan St.
Indianapolis, IN 46223
(317) 264-8554

IOWA
Joseph A. Buckwalter, M.D.
University of Iowa Hospitals
Department of Orthopedics
1201 RCP
Iowa City, IA 52242
(319) 356-2223

MARYLAND
Giraud V. Foster, M.D.
Department of Gynecology and Obstetrics
Johns Hopkins Hospital
600 N. Broadway
Baltimore, MD 21205
(301) 955-3399

MASSACHUSETTS
Samuel H. Doppelt, M.D.
Massachusetts General Hospital
CRP-E
Boston, MA 02114
(617) 726-8534
(Orthopedic surgeon)

Robert G. Feldman, M.D.
Professor and Chairman
Department of Neurology
Boston University
Medical Center
School of Medicine
80 E. Concord St.
Boston, MA 02118
(617) 274-5136
(Sees only patients with neurological problems)

Stephen M. Krane, M.D.
Professor of Medicine
Harvard Medical School
Chief, The Arthritis Unit
Massachusetts General Hospital
Bulfinch 1
Boston, MA 02114
(617) 726-2871

Robert M. Neer, M.D.
John T. Potts, Jr., M.D.
David M. Slovik, M.D.
Massachusetts General Hospital
Endocrine Associates
ACC-6
Boston, MA 02114
(617) 726-8720

Michael F. Holick, Ph.D, M.D.
MIT–Department of Nutrition, 56-217
77 Massachusetts Ave.
Cambridge, MA 02139
(617) 723-8720

MICHIGAN
Boy Frame, M.D.
Michael Kleerekoper, M.D.
A. Michael Parfitt, M.D.
Sudhaker Rao, M.D., and fellows
Bone and Mineral Division
Henry Ford Hospital
2799 W. Grand Blvd.
Detroit, MI 48202
(313) 876-2377, 2363
(313) 876-2361 (for Dr. Parfitt)

MINNESOTA
Hunter Heath III, M.D.
Mayo Clinic and Mayo Medical School
5-164 W. Joseph Building
Rochester, MN 55905
(507) 284-2511

Stephen Hodgson, M.D.
David Hoffman, M.D.
Edward G. Lufkin, M.D.
Donald A. Scholz, M.D.
Mayo Clinic
Rochester, MN 55905
(507) 284-2511

B. Lawrence Riggs, M.D.
Chairman, Division of Endocrinology and
    Metabolism
Mayo Clinic
Rochester, MN 55905
(507) 284-2511

MISSOURI
Louis Avioli, M.D.
Stanley Birge, M.D.
William A. Peck, M.D.
Michael Whyte, M.D.
Department of Medicine
Division of Bone and Mineral Metabolism
The Jewish Hospital of St. Louis
216 S. Kingshighway
Washington University School of Medicine
St. Louis, MO 63110
(314) 454-7765
(314) 454-7766 (for Dr. Whyte)

NEBRASKA
J.C. Gallagher, M.D.
Professor of Medicine
St. Joseph's Hospital
601 N. 30th St.
Omaha, NE 68131
(402) 280-4516

NEW JERSEY
Mark Wiesen, M.D.
1100 Clifton Ave.
Clifton, NJ 07013
(201) 471-2692

George Schneider, M.D.
Chief of Endocrinology
Newark Beth Israel
Medical Center
201 Lyons Ave.
Newark, NJ 07112
(201) 228-2047

NEW YORK
Robert Busch, M.D.
1 Executive Park Drive
Albany, NY 12203
(518) 489-4704

Uriel S. Barzel, M.D.
Professor of Medicine
Albert Einstein College of Medicine
Montefiore Medical Group
3444 Kossuth Ave.
Bronx, NY 10467
(212) 920-5291

Joseph J. DeRose, M.D.
Associate Professor of Clinical Family Practice
Downstate Medical Center
State University of New York
450 Clarkson Ave.
Brooklyn, NY 11203
(718) 270-1801

Florence Shai, M.D.
VA Medical Center (111)
Endocrinology
800 Poly Place
Brooklyn, NY 11209
(718) 836-6600, x312
(Veterans only)

John F. Aloi, M.D.
Professor of Medicine
Nassau Hospital
164 Commack Rd.
Commack, NY 11725
(516) 499-0796
or:
222 Station Place, N.
Mineola, NY 11501
(516) 248-1217

Italo Zanzi, M.D.
Associate Professor of Medicine
Cornell University Medical College
Department of Medicine
North Shore University Hospital
Manhasset, NY 11030
(516) 562-4400
(By referral from patient's physician only)

Asher Haymovits, M.D.
500A E. 87th St.
New York, NY 10028
(212) 988-4800

Melvin Horwith, M.D.
Professor, Clinical Medicine
Division of Endocrinology
New York Hospital
Cornell Medical Center
517 E. 71st St.
New York, NY 10021
(212) 472-5652
(By referral from patient's physician only)

Thomas Jacobs, M.D.
Columbia-Presbyterian Hospital
161 Fort Washington Ave.
New York, NY 10032
(212) 305-5578

Joseph M. Lane, M.D.
Hospital for Special Surgery
535 E. 70th St.
New York, NY 10021
(212) 606-1172

Ethel S. Siris, M.D.
Associate Professor of Medicine
Columbia-Presbyterian Medical Center
630 W. 168th St.
New York, NY 10032
(212) 305-2529

Antonio Culebras, M.D.
Associate Professor
Department of Neurology
SUNY, Upstate Medical Center
Chief, Neurology Service
VA Medical Center
800 Irving Ave.
Syracuse, NY 13210
(315) 473-4627, 7461
(Sees only patients with neurological problems)

Robert Lindsay, M.D.
Director of Research
Helen Hayes Hospital
Route 9W
West Haverstraw, NY 10993
(914) 947-3000

NORTH CAROLINA
Stephen A. Grubb, M.D.
Chapel Hill Orthopedic Clinic and Spine
  Center, P.A.
110 S. Estes Drive
Chapel Hill, NC 27514
(919) 929–7796

OKLAHOMA
John A. Mohr, M.D.
Assistant Chief, Medical Service (111)
VA Medical Center
921 N.E. 13th St.
Oklahoma City, OK 73104
(405) 272-9876, x3250 or 270-5149

OREGON
Michael R. McClung, M.D.
Associate Professor of Medicine
Director, Bone and Mineral Clinic
Oregon Health Sciences University
3181 S.W. Sam Jackson Park Rd.
Portland, OR 97201
(503) 225-7360

PENNSYLVANIA
Maurice Attie, M.D.
John G. Haddad, M.D.
Department of Medicine
Endocrine Section
531 Johnson Pavilion G2
University of Pennsylvania
Philadelphia, PA 19104
(215) 898-6521

Leslie I. Rose, M.D.
Hahnemann University
Division of Endocrinology and Metabolism
230 N. Broad St.–MS 426
Philadelphia, PA 19102
(215) 448-8114

SOUTH CAROLINA
Norman H. Bell, M.D.
Professor of Medicine and Pharmacology
VA Medical Center
109 Bee St.
Charleston, SC 29403
(803) 577-5011 x350

TENNESSEE
Genaro M.A. Palmieri, M.D.
Professor of Medicine
UTCHS–College of Medicine
Coleman Building, Box 3B
956 Court Ave., Room 3C17
Memphis, TN 38163
(901) 528-5743

TEXAS
Robert F. Gagel, M.D.
Division of Endocrinology
Baylor College of Medicine
1921 Lauderdale Ave.
Houston, TX 77030
(713) 795-7484

Lawrence Mallette, M.D.
Medical Service–VA Hospital
2002 Holcombe Blvd.
Houston, TX 77221
(713) 795-7484

V. Schneider, M.D.
University of Texas Health Science Center at
    Houston
Division of Endocrinology
Houston, TX 77025
(713) 792-4838

Gregory Mundy, M.D.
Division of Endocrinology
Department of Medicine
University of Texas Health Science Center
San Antonio, TX 78284
(512) 691-6524

Lt. Col. Thomas J. Taylor, M.C.
Brooke Army Medical Center (HSHE-MDE)
San Antonio, TX 78234
(512) 221-4715

WASHINGTON
Charles Chestnut, M.D.
Department of Medicine/Radiology
University of Washington Hospitals
Seattle, WA 98105
(206) 543-3538

SOURCE: *Paget's Disease Foundation.*

ORGANIZATION

Paget's Disease Foundation
PO Box 2772
Brooklyn, NY 11202
(718) 596-1043

This national nonprofit membership organization is a source of information for the public and physicians on Paget's disease. Questions from the public are answered and referrals are made to specialists. Conferences and programs are sponsored. Brochures, scientific reprints, and a semiannual newsletter are published. Special services include listing sources for discounted prescription drugs. More information will be provided upon request.

FREE MATERIALS

Understanding Paget's Disease, 10 pages.

National Institute of Arthritis and
    Musculoskeletal and Skin Diseases
Building 31, Room 9A04
Bethesda, MD 20892

PAIN

See also Headaches, page 246, Cancer, page 124.

Chronic pain is America's number-one medical complaint. It is the most common reason for seeing a doctor and for taking medication. Experts estimate that about 86 million Americans—one-third of the population—live with some kind of recurring pain. Of those, one-half to two-thirds are partially or totally disabled for periods of days, weeks, or months, and sometimes permanently. Yet, until recently, very little attention has been given to the medical treatment of pain. Consequently, there are large gaps in the understanding of pain. Nobody has precisely defined the physiological mechanism that produces pain, although there is a growing understanding of the role of prostaglandins, endorphins, and other chemicals that are involved in the transmission of pain to the brain.

Current research is turning up more knowledge about pain—with promises of new treatments. The field is moving fast; experts say they are much more sophisticated about the nature of pain and relieving it than they were just five years ago. Some experts say science has learned more about pain in the last 10 years than in the previous 100.

Chronic pain comes in all dimensions and stems from numerous conditions and diseases. By far the most common is back pain, especially lower back pain, a puzzling ailment so widespread that it keeps as many as seven million Americans away from work periodically or permanently. Chronic pain also occurs with arthritis, headaches, and neurological dysfunctions, such as sciatica. One of the most dreaded sources of chronic pain is terminal cancer.

Often, doctors are unable to find a specific organic reason for pain; it frequently has a strong psychological basis; for example, flaring up, during emotional stress. Sometimes, the pain persists even though the organic cause has been treated and considered corrected. For that reason among others, pain is one of the most frustrating and perplexing maladies to treat.

Fortunately, some pioneering doctors realized the importance of pain therapy. In 1960, Dr. John Bonica, one of the nation's most highly respected pain specialists, established the first comprehensive pain clinic at the University of Washington School of Medicine in Seattle. This clinic became the model of treatment for chronic pain. Since then, numerous pain clinics have sprung up nationwide. Many of the best ones are affiliated with university medical centers and hospitals. These are generally multidisciplinary pain centers, staffed by a broad variety of specialists, including physiatrists (doctors who specialize in rehabilitation), orthopedists, physical therapists, neurologists, psychiatrists, and occupational therapists. Such clinics are highly rated by pain experts because they offer comprehensive diagnosis and many different treatments.

Additionally, there are hundreds of pain centers around the country that specialize in a single type of pain treatment, for example, surgery. Many experts fear that such clinics deny patients the full range of options and may cause them to run from one specialist to another seeking help when one form of treatment fails. It is common for back-pain sufferers to be treated by several doctors without relief.

427

TYPES OF TREATMENTS

Therapies change as researchers learn more about pain. Treatment for all kinds of pain, notably back pain, is growing more conservative.

Surgery: Nerve surgery for chronic back pain, once common, is not performed as often today. Although less radical types of spinal and nerve surgery are evolving, some pain clinic specialists say surgery should be performed only in extreme and limited circumstances and is unnecessary in most cases of chronic pain. Specialists have found that surgery may give temporary relief, but it sometimes does not work permanently and often leaves sufferers "low-back cripples." In some cases, specialists report, victims who have had as many as 10 operations still have recurring back pain. If a surgeon recommends back surgery, it is important to get a second opinion.

Exercise: There is new emphasis on specific exercises to relieve pain; rest used to be the traditional remedy. Doctors realize now that prescribed inactivity actually promotes pain by leading to a deterioration of certain muscles and suppressing the production of endorphins, natural opiate pain killers stimulated by exercise. Arthritics are now encouraged to walk, stretch, and do specific joint exercises to relieve pain. Back-pain victims often dramatically improve through specific exercises to strengthen back and abdominal muscles and to improve their postures. Some centers offer extensive exercise programs with back calisthenics and aerobic dancing for people who have had or are contemplating having back surgery.

Little-known specialists called physiatrists are emerging as probably the most successful physicians for dealing with back pain. Physiatrists are physicians who specialize in rehabilitating the disabled. Although physiatrists may use medicines, they concentrate on exercises and physical therapy, instead of drugs and surgery. However, they can spot the need for surgery and recommend it if necessary. Pain and physical rehabilitation centers routinely include physiatrists on their staffs.

One survey of 500 patients with back pain showed that they found the greatest relief from physiatrists. According to the same survey, physical therapists were second best in relieving back pain. Least successful in alleviating chronic pain, according to the patients surveyed, were neurologists who tended to rely heavily on drugs.

For more information and the names of physiatrists in your area, contact:

American Academy of Physical Medicine and
  Rehabilitation
30 N. Michigan Ave.
Chicago, IL 60602

Drugs: The use of powerful drugs, mainly narcotics, to combat chronic pain is on the downswing, although they are still the treatment of choice for terminal cancer patients. Antidepressants are used effectively to relieve both depression and pain; the analgesic (pain-killing) mechanism is not known. Anticonvulsants also relieve some specific types of pain from neurological conditions or from spinal cord injuries. Injections of the drug chymopapain, an enzyme that dissolves the troublesome part of herniated discs, are sometimes given, although this therapy is not recommended in many cases.

Some physicians rely on drugs to treat pain, leaving the underlying cause unrecognized and unaltered. One study at the Mayo Clinic found that 65 percent of 144 patients with nonmalignant pain were addicted to some type of drug. Such patients were also less likely to respond to other pain-relief therapies.

The number-one choice against much chronic pain is aspirin and aspirin substitutes like acetaminophen. Aspirin is still one of the most remarkable pain killers and anti-inflammatory agents of all time.

Nerve stimulation: An electric aspirin, as it is often called, is one of the fastest growing therapies for chronic pain. Brief jolts of electricity are transmitted through the skin to nerve endings. Doctors are not sure how it works—it may block pain signals from getting to the brain, or it may trigger production of pain-relieving endorphins. The most common technique is TENS (transcutaneous electrical nerve stimulation): Electrodes are taped to the skin and electrical impulses administered by a small generator about the size of a deck of cards. TENS has reportedly been most effective in treating the pain of cancer, certain types of neuralgia, low back pain, and headaches. Some studies show TENS has a 40 percent success rate for chronic pain; others show a lower success over a long period of time. Patients may develop a tolerance to the effects. Some researchers are conducting experiments using a new type of laser to stimulate nerves and combat pain; it is a so-called cold laser and directs a low-powered beam onto the skin and nerves.

Psychological component: More practitioners are recognizing that pain often depends on emotional makeup and responses. In fact, they suspect that many treatments work at least partially because of a placebo effect. Behavior modification has proved quite successful in relieving emotionally induced chronic pain.

Other treatments: Some pain specialists successfully use hypnosis, self-hypnosis, biofeedback, acupuncture, relaxation exercises, and family therapy.

WHERE TO FIND TREATMENT

Experts advise anyone with recurring pain that lasts more than two months to contact a comprehensive pain clinic where you will receive a thorough evaluation in efforts to relieve the pain and get at the cause. There is no question that pain specialists with a broad perspective on pain are more likely to give appropriate treatment.

Despite this recommendation, only about 3 percent of Americans suffering chronic pain consult these specialists. Early treatment at a pain clinic often prevents an acute problem from developing into a long-term chronic one, according to experts.

SOME LEADING PAIN CLINICS

ALABAMA
University of Alabama at Birmingham
Pain Management Center
1920 Seventh Ave., S.
Birmingham, AL 35294
Director: Joel Haber, Ph.D.
(205) 934-6174

Pain Rehabilitation Center
1717 Sixth Ave., S.
Birmingham, AL 35233
(205) 934-4011

CALIFORNIA
New Hope Pain Center & Pain Research
  Foundation
100 S. Raymond Ave.
Alhambra, CA 91801
Director: Benjamin L. Crue, M.D.
(213) 570-1607

*St. Jude Hospital and Rehabilitation Center
101 E. Valencia Mesa Drive
Fullerton, CA 92632
(714) 871-3280

*Rehabilitation Institute
Glendale Adventist Medical Center
1509 Wilson Terrace
Glendale, CA 91206
Director: David R. Igler
(213) 240-8000, x896

*Center for Diagnostic and Rehabilitation
  Medicine
Daniel Freeman Hospital Medical Center
333 N. Prairie Ave.
Inglewood, CA 90301
Director: Norman S. Namerow, M.D.
(213) 674-7050, x3465

*New Directions Rehabilitation Center
Centinela Hospital Medical Center
PO Box 720
Inglewood, CA 90307
(213) 673-4660

University of California, Irvine
California College of Medicine
Irvine, CA 92717
Director, Hypnotherapy and Pain Evaluation:
   Donald W. Schafer, M.D. (Psychiatry)
(714) 634-5921

University of California, Irvine
California College of Medicine
Irvine, CA 92717
Chief, Physical Medicine and Rehabilitation:
   Jen Yu, M.D. (pain management program)
(714) 634-6504

UCLA Pain Management Center
10833 Le Conte Ave.
Los Angeles, CA 90024
Director: Dr. Richard Kroening
(213) 825-4292, 3229

*Center for Rehabilitation Medicine—Pain
   Program
Northridge Hospital Medical Center
18300 Roscoe Blvd.
Northridge, CA 91328
Director: Ronald Rozanski, Coordinator of
   Pain Program
Medical Director of Pain Program: Thomas
   Hedge, M.D.
(213) 885-5338

*Casa Colina Hospital for Rehabilitative
   Medicine
255 E. Bonita Ave.
Pomona, CA 91767
(714) 593-7521

University of California
San Diego Medical Center
Pain Treatment Program
225 Dickinson St., H-614
San Diego, CA 92103
Medical Director: J. Hampton Atkinson, M.D.
Program Director: Edwin Kremer, Ph.D.
(619) 294-5592

Stanford University Medical Center
Pain Clinic
Department of Anesthesia
Stanford, CA 94305
Clinic Chief: L. Eltherington, M.D.
Department Chairman: Barrie Fairley, M.D.
(415) 723-6238

*Center for Rehabilitation Medicine
Valley Hospital Medical Center
14500 Sherman Circle
Van Nuys, CA 91405
(213) 997-0101

COLORADO
*Rehabilitation Center
Boulder Memorial Hospital
311 Mapleton Ave.
Boulder, CO 80302
(303) 443-0230

*Spalding Rehabilitation Hospital
1919 Ogden St.
Denver, CO 80218
(303) 861-0504

University of Colorado Health Sciences Center
Pain Clinic
Physical Medicine and Rehabilitation
4200 E. Ninth Ave.
Denver, CO 80202
Director: F.P. Maloney, M.D.
(303) 394-7102, 7078

*Hilltop Rehabilitation Hospital
1100 Patterson Rd.
Grand Junction, CO 81506
(303) 244-6007

CONNECTICUT
Yale University School of Medicine
Yale Behavioral Medicine Clinic
25 Park St.
New Haven, CT 06519
Director: Hoyle Leigh, M.D.
(203) 785-2112, 2617

DISTRICT OF COLUMBIA
Georgetown University Hospital
Department of Anesthesiology
Pain Clinic
3800 Reservoir Rd., N.W.
Washington, DC 20007
Director: Shin S. Kang, M.D.
Codirectors: Russell T. Wall, M.D.
Petra Movotny-Joseph, M.D.
(202) 625-7163

George Washington University Medical Center
Pain Program
2150 Pennsylvania Ave., N.W.
Washington, DC 20037
Director: Marc Hertzman, M.D.
(202) 676-3355

Washington Pain Center
2026 R St., N.W.
Washington, DC 20009
Director: Lorenz Ng, M.D.
(202) 387-4735

FLORIDA

University of Florida Health Center
Pain and Stress Management Laboratory
Box J-165, JHMHC
Department of Clinical Psychology
Gainesville, FL 32610
Director: Michael Feuerstein, M.D.
(904) 392-4551, 2944

Mount Sinai Medical Center
Pain Center—Anesthesiology
4300 Alton Rd.
Miami Beach, FL 33140
Director: Frank Moya, M.D.
(305) 674-2070

University of Miami School of Medicine
University of Miami Comprehensive Pain
  Center
South Shore Hospital
600 Alton Rd., Suite 505
Miami Beach, FL 33139
Director: Hubert L. Rosomoff, M.D.
(305) 672-2100

*Rehabilitation Institute of West Florida
PO Box 18900
Pensacola, FL 32523-8900
(904) 474-5358

Pain Management Program
Tampa General Hospital
University of South Florida
College of Medicine
12901 N. 30th St., Box 55
Tampa, FL 33612
Director: Shashidhar H. Kori, M.D.
(813) 972-2000, x6873

GEORGIA

Emory University—Woodruff Health Sciences
  Center
Emory Pain Control Center
Center for Rehabilitation Medicine
1441 Clifton Rd., N.E.
Atlanta, GA 30322
Director: Steven Brena, M.D.
(404) 329-5492

ILLINOIS

Rehabilitation Institute of Chicago
The Center for Pain Studies
345 E. Superior St.
Chicago, IL 60611
Director: Robert G. Addison, M.D.
(312) 649-6011

Rush-Presbyterian-St. Luke's Medical Center
Rush Pain Center
1753 W. Congress Parkway
Chicago, IL 60612
Director: Anthony D. Ivankovich, M.D.
(312) 942-6631

University of Chicago Medical Center
Chronic Pain Program
5841 S. Maryland Ave.
Chicago, IL 60637
Director: Frederick Brown, M.D.
(312) 947-1000

University of Illinois
Temporomandibular Joint and Facial Pain
  Research Center
PO Box 6998
Chicago, IL 60680
Federal government-supported center.

University of Illinois at Chicago
Pain Clinic
University of Illinois Hospital
1740 W. Taylor St.
Chicago, IL 60612
Director: Alon P. Winnie, M.D.
(312) 996-6803

IOWA

University of Iowa Hospitals and Clinics
Pain Clinic—Anesthesia Department
Iowa City, IA 52242
Director: Edward S. Wegrzynowski, M.D.
(319) 356-2320

Mercy Pain Center
Mercy Hospital Medical Center
6th & University
Des Moines, IA 50314
Director: James Blessman, M.D.
(515) 247-4430

KANSAS
University of Kansas Medical Center
Pain Clinic
Department of Anesthesiology
39th & Rainbow Blvd.
Kansas City, KS 66103
Director: Kasumi Arakawa, M.D.
(913) 588-3315

KENTUCKY
Chronic Pain Clinic
Ambulatory Care Building
University of Louisville School of Medicine
Louisville, KY 40292
Director: William Conwill, M.D.

LOUISIANA
Pain Program
Tulane University School of Medicine
1430 Tulane Ave.
New Orleans, LA 70112
Director: Alan W. Grogono, M.D.
(504) 588-5067

*Physical Medicine and Rehabilitation Center
Physicians & Surgeons Hospital
PO Box 4466
Shreveport, LA 71104
(318) 227-3950

MARYLAND
Johns Hopkins University
Pain Treatment Program
600 N. Wolfe St.
Baltimore, MD 21205
Directors: Donlin Long, M.D.,
Godfrey Pearlson, M.D.
(301) 955-3270

University of Maryland Medical System Pain
   Clinic
Baltimore, MD 21201
Director: Walter F. Baile, M.D.,
Arthur V. Milholland, M.D.
(301) 528-6846

MASSACHUSETTS
Beth Israel Hospital
Pain Management Unit
330 Brookline Ave.
Boston, MA 02215
Director: Carol Warfield, M.D.
(617) 735-3334

Brigham and Women's Hospital
Pain Treatment Service
75 Francis St.
Boston, MA 02115
Director: Angelo G. Rocco, M.D.
(617)732-6708

Massachusetts General Hospital
Neurological Pain Service
Ambulatory Care Building
15 Parkman
Boston, MA 02114
Directors: Raymond J. Maciewicz, M.D.,
   Charles E. Poletti, M.D.
(617) 726-2777

Massachusetts Rehabilitation Hospital
Boston Pain Unit
125 Nashua St.
Boston, MA 02114
Director: Gerald Aronoff, M.D.
(617) 720-6510

New England Deaconess Hospital
William P. Arnold Center for Research &
   Treatment of Pain
185 Pilgrim Rd.
Boston, MA 02215
Director: Melvin J. Krant, M.D.
(617) 732-9727

*Spaulding Rehabilitation Hospital
125 Nashua St.
Boston, MA 02114
(617) 720-6400

Tufts University School of Medicine
Pain Clinic
New England Medical Center
171 Harrison Ave.
Boston, MA 02111
Director: Parminder Phull, M.D.
(617) 956-5634

New England Rehabilitation Hospital
One Rehabilitation Way
Woburn, MA 01801
(617) 935-5050

University of Massachusetts Medial Center
Pain Control Center
55 Lake Ave., N.
Worcester, MA 01609
Director: W. Thomas Edwards, M.D., Ph.D.
(617) 856-2640, 3763

MICHIGAN
University of Michigan Medical Center
Pain Clinic
3203 Upjohn Center
Ann Arbor, MI 48109
Director: A Michael deRosayro, M.D.
(313) 763-5459

MINNESOTA
Pain Treatment Program
University of Minnesota Hospital and Clinic
Box 297 UMHC
Minneapolis, MN 55455
Director: Glenn Gullickson, M.D.
(612) 626-5740

Mayo Clinic
Pain Clinic
200 First St., S.W.
Rochester, MN 55905
Director: Josef Wang, M.D.
(507) 284-8311

MISSOURI
Howard A. Rusk Rehabilitation Center
University of Missouri Hospital and Clinics
One Hospital Drive
Columbia, MO 65212
Directors: Robert Willard, M.D., Robert
  Frank, Ph.D.
(314) 882-1071

St. Louis University School of Medicine
Pain Management–Division of Behavioral
  Medicine
1221 S. Grand Blvd.
St. Louis, MO 63104
Directors: Raymond Tait, Ph.D. (clinical),
  Ronald Margolis (division)
(314) 577-8700

NEBRASKA
University of Nebraska Medical Center
Pain Management Center
S.S.P. Building, 4th Floor
42nd & Dewey Ave.
Omaha, NE 68105
Director: Charles J. Golden, Ph.D.
(402) 559-4364

NEW JERSEY
Betty Bacharach Rehabilitation Hospital
Jim Leeds Rd.
Pomona, NJ 08240
(609) 652-7000

NEW MEXICO
University of New Mexico Hospital
Chronic Pelvic Pain Clinic
2211 Lomas, N.E.
Albuquerque, NM 87131
Director: John Slocumb, M.D.
(505) 277-4051

NEW YORK
Pain Management Center
SUNY at Buffalo School of Medicine
Buffalo General Hospital
100 High St.
Buffalo, NY 14203
Director: Marc Viguera, M.D.
(716) 845-2226

Columbia—Presbyterian Medical Center
Anesthesiology—Pain Treatment Service
622 W. 168th St.
New York, NY 10032
Directors: Leonard Brand, M.D., David
  Richlin, M.D.
(212) 694-7114

Memorial Sloan-Kettering Cancer Center
Pain Clinic
1275 York Ave.
New York, NY 10021
Director: Kathleen Foley, M.D.
(212) 794-7050
Cancer pain

Pain Treatment Center
Montefiore Medical Center
111 E. 210th St.
New York, NY 10467
Director: Edith R. Kepes, M.D.
(212) 920-4440

New York University Medical Center
Pain Consultation Service
530 First Ave.
New York, NY 10016
Director: Levon Capan, M.D.
(212) 340-7316

New York University Medical Center
Comprehensive Pain Center
530 First Ave.
New York, NY 10016
Director: B. Berthold Wolf, M.D.
(212) 340-6620

Pain Center
Department of Psychiatry
University Hospital
SUNY at Stony Brook Health Sciences Center
Level 5, Room 434
Stony Brook, NY 11794
Director: Charles Godwin, M.D.
(516) 444-2570

Pain Clinic
SUNY Health Science Center at Syracuse
750 E. Adams St.
Syracuse, NY 13210
Director: P. Sebastian Thomas, M.D.
(315) 473-5540

NORTH CAROLINA
Pain Clinic
PO Box 3060
Durham, NC 27706
Codirectors: Blain Nashhold, M.D., Bruno J.
  Urban, M.D.
(919) 684-6542, 3511

Bowman Gray School of Medicine
Pain Clinic
Department of Psychiatry and Behavioral
  Medicine
300 S. Hawthorne
Winston-Salem, NC 27103
Director: Laurence A. Bradley, M.D.
(919) 748-4238

OHIO
University of Cincinnati Medical Center
Pain Control Center
231 Bethesda Ave.
Cincinnati, OH 45267
Director: P. Prithvi Raj, M.D.
(513) 872-5963

Case Western Reserve University School of
  Medicine
The Pain Center
University Hospitals of Cleveland
Department of Neurology
2074 Abington Rd.
Cleveland, OH 44106
Director: Jennifer S. Kiregler, M.D.
(216) 844-4857

Ohio State University Hospitals
Pain Management Program
2148 Dodd Hall
472 W. Eighth Ave.
Columbus, OH 43210
Director: W. Brian O'Malley, M.D.
(614) 421-3830

*Good Samaritan Medical Center and
  Rehabilitation Center
800 Forest Ave.
Zanesville, OH 43701
(614) 454-5469

OREGON
*The Portland Pain Center
Emanuel Rehabilitation Center
3001 N. Gantenbein
Portland, OR 97227
Directors: Douglas F. Renholds, M.D.,
  Gregory T. Smith, Ph.D.
(503) 280-4400

Northwest Pain Center
10615 S.E. Cherry Blossom Drive, Suite 170
Portland, OR 97216
Director: Joel Seres, M.D.
(503) 256-1930

PENNSYLVANIA
Pain Management Service
The Milton S. Hershey Medical Center
The Pennsylvania State University
Hershey, PA 17033
Director: Wayne K. Marshall, M.D.
(717) 531-8521

Pain Treatment Unit
Center for Behavioral Medicine
Hospital of the University of Pennsylvania
3400 Spruce St.
Philadelphia, PA 19104
Directors: Michael J. Pertschuk, M.D., Martin
  D. Cheatle, M.D.
(215) 662-3507

Pain Center
Jefferson Medical College of Thomas Jefferson
   University
11th & Walnut Sts.
Philadelphia, PA 19107
Chief: Robert Woo, M.D.
(215) 928-6161

Magee Rehabilitation Hospital
Six Franklin Plaza
Philadelphia, PA 19102
(215) 864-7100

Temple University Health Services Center
Temple University Pain Control Center
3401 N. Broad St.
Philadelphia, PA 19140
Director: Edward Resnick, M.D.
(215) 221-2100

Center for Pain Evaluation and Treatment
University of Pittsburgh
School of Medicine
Room 701, Eye & Ear Hospital
230 Lothrop St.
Pittsburgh, PA 15213
Director: Dennis Turk, Ph.D., Professor of
   Psychiatry and Anesthesiology
(412) 647-2096

University Health Center of Pittsburgh
Presbyterian University Hospital Pain Control
   Clinic
Pittsburgh, PA 15213
Director: Ruben Tenicela, M.D.
(412) 647-3680

SOUTH CAROLINA
*Pain Treatment
Greenville General Hospital
701 Grove Rd.
Greenville, SC 29605
Director: David Tollison, M.D.
(803) 242-8088

TENNESSEE
*Baptist Memorial Hospital
Regional Rehabilitation Center
1025 E.H. Crump Blvd.
Memphis, TN 38104
(901) 522-6550

University of Tennessee
Memphis College of Medicine
Pain Center
1025 E.H. Crump
Memphis, TN 38104
Director: William North, M.D.
(901) 528-5800

Vanderbilt University Medical Center
Pain Control Center
1161 21st Ave., S.
Nashville, TN 37232
Director: Winston C.V. Parris, M.D.
(615) 322-6683

TEXAS
University of Texas Health Science Center—
   Dallas
Department of Anesthesiology
Dallas, TX 75235
Directors: Adolph Giesecke, M.D., James
   Lipton, Ph.D.
(214) 688-2679

University of Texas Health Science Center—
   Dallas
Chronic Back Pain—Division of Orthopedic
   Surgery
Dallas, TX 75235
Director: Vert Mooney, M.D.
(214) 688-3524

Baylor College of Medicine
Pain Control and Biofeedback Clinic
6560 Fannin, Suite 900
Houston, TX 77030
Director: H. Martin Blacker, M.D.
(713) 799-5796

University of Texas Health Science Center at
   Houston
Pain Rehabilitation Program
6410 Fannin, Suite 600
Houston, TX 77030
Director: James Kelley, M.D.
(713) 792-4847

North Texas Back Institute
3801 W. 15th St.
Plano, TX 75075
Clinical Director: Alan Morris
(214) 867-2720

University of Texas Health Science Center at
  San Antonio
Anesthesiology Pain Clinic
7703 Floyd Curl Drive
San Antonio, TX 78284
Director: Somayaji Ramamurthy, M.D.
(512) 694-2600 or 291-6664

UTAH
Pain Clinic
University of Utah School of Medicine
50 N. Medical Drive
Salt Lake City, UT 84132
Director: Scot Russell, Ph.D.
(801) 581-8076

VIRGINIA
Medical College of Virginia
Pain Management Clinic
MCV Station, Box 516
Richmond, VA 23298
Director: Amir Rafii, M.D.
(804) 786-9162

WASHINGTON
University of Washington School of Medicine,
  RC-76
Pain Clinic
Seattle, WA 98195
Director: John D. Loeser, M.D.
(206) 543-3574

*Rehabilitation Department
St. Joseph Hospital and Health Care Center
PO Box 2197
Tacoma, WA 98405
(206) 627-4101

WISCONSIN
University of Wisconsin–Madison
Pain Clinic
Clinical Sciences Center
600 Highland Ave.
Madison, WI 53792
Director: Carl Getto, M.D.
(608) 263-8094

Medical College of Wisconsin
Pain Clinic
8700 W. Wisconsin Ave.
Milwaukee, WI 53226
Director: Steven Abrams, M.D.
(414) 257-6259

Curative Rehabilitation Center
1000 N. 92nd St.
Wauwatosa, WI 53226
Director: Eugene Cox
(414) 259-1414

SOURCE: *Commission for Accreditation of Rehabilitation Facilities and author's survey of leading medical schools.*

*Accredited by Commission on Accreditation of Rehabilitation Facilities (CARF).

PAIN RESEARCH AT THE NATIONAL INSTITUTES OF HEALTH

In a multidisciplinary center devoted entirely to research on pain, investigators at the National Institutes of Health (National Institute of Dental Research) in Bethesda, Maryland, study the basic mechanisms of pain and test out the effectiveness of new and standard chronic pain treatments. Selected patients with severe oral-facial or other types of chronic pain are accepted for treatment and research. Participation in the studies is by physician referral only. For more information your physician can contact:

Office of the Director
The Clinical Center
Building 10, Room 2C-146
National Institutes of Health
Bethesda, MD 20892
(301) 496-4891

ORGANIZATIONS

National Chronic Pain Outreach Association,
  Inc.
8222 Wycliffe Court
Manassas, VA 22110
(703) 368-7357

A national voluntary mutual support organization for pain sufferers and their families. About 30 chapters around the country. The chapters meet, usually twice a month, for "care and share" and information sessions. A quarterly newsletter.

A source of information on pain. Will answer questions and send information upon request with a self-addressed, stamped, legal-size envelope.

National Committee on the Treatment of
    Intractable Pain
PO Box 9553, Friendship Station
Washington, DC 20016
(301) 983-1710

An advocacy, educational membership organization, favoring more effective methods of controlling pain, including legalization of heroin for

terminal cancer patients and extensive use of hospices.

National YMCA Headquarters
110 N. Wacker Drive
Chicago, IL 60606
(312) 977-0031

The YMCA offers a six-week "Healthy Back" program in many chapters throughout the country. For more information contact a local YMCA chapter.

BOOKS

The American Medical Association Guide to Back Care, **Marion Steinmann,** New York: Random House, 1984.

Back School and Other Conservative Approaches to Low Back Pain, **Arthur H. White,** St. Louis: Mosby, 1983.

Backache: Its Evolution and Conservative Treatment, **David P. Evans,** Baltimore: University Park Press, 1982.

Backache Relief, **Dava Sobel** and **Arthur C. Klein,** New York: Times Books, 1985.

Bonnie Prudden's Guide to Pain Free Living, **Bonnie Prudden,** New York: Dial Press, 1984.

Chronic Pain, **Joseph A. Kotarba,** Beverly Hills, CA: Sage Publications, 1983.

Chronic Pain: America's Hidden Epidemic, **Steven Brena, M.D.,** New York: Atheneum, 1978.

Free Yourself from Neck Pain and Headache, **David F. Fardon,** Englewood Cliffs, NJ: Prentice-Hall, 1983.

Listen To Your Pain, **Ben E. Benjamin,** New York: Viking Press, 1984.

The Pain Book, **Frederick W. Kerr,** Englewood Cliffs, NJ: Prentice-Hall, 1981.

Pain Control: The Bethesda Program, **Bruce Smoller** and **Brian Schulman,** New York: Doubleday, 1982.

Understanding Back Pain: A Patient Handbook, **R. W. Porter,** New York: Churchill Livingstone, 1983.

Your Aching Back: A Doctor's Guide to Relief, **Augustus A. White, III, M.D.,** New York: Bantam Books, 1983.

MATERIALS, FREE AND FOR SALE

Free (single copies)

Pain Control, 44 pages.

American Cancer Society
777 Third Ave.
New York, NY 10017

Chronic Pain, Hope Through Research, 28 pages.

National Institute of Neurological and
    Communicative Disorders and Stroke
Building 31, Room 8A06
Bethesda, MD 20892

For sale

Low Back Pain: What It is, What Can Be Done, **Irvin Block.**

Public Affairs Pamphlets
381 Park Ave. S.
New York, NY 10016

Be Good To Your Back, **Charles Burton,
   M.D.,** and **Gail Nida, R.N.,** 57 pages,
   book-size format.
*The Sister Kenny Institute Gravity Lumbar
   Therapy Program,* **Charles Burton, M.D.,**
   and **Gail Nida, R.N.,** 1982; 48 pages,

book-size format; how to control low back
and or leg pain from herniated intervertebral
lumbar disc.
*A Patient's Guide to Wellness: Coping With
   Chronic Pain,* **David Florence, M.D.,** 26
   pages, book-size format.

Sister Kenny Institute
800 E. 28th St.
Minneapolis, MN 55407

PARKINSON'S DISEASE

See also Rehabilitation, page 460.

Parkinson's disease, once called "the shaking palsy," strikes the central nervous system, usually causing tremors and slowed movements of the arms, legs, and trunk. It affects about half a million Americans, although the figures are not firm. According to one major survey, 40 percent of Parkinson's cases had not been diagnosed. Parkinson's disease rarely appears before age 30, and it is more common in men. Although not considered genetic, it does occasionally run in families. The risk of developing Parkinson's disease increases as you age.

Cause: Unknown, but doctors do know the disease causes degenerative changes in certain cells in the brain. This leads to a deficiency of a brain chemical called dopamine; without sufficient amounts of this chemical, brain messages cannot be transmitted smoothly, and the symptoms of Parkinson's disease appear.

Symptoms: Stiffness of the muscles, slowness of muscle activity, and often, but not always, tremors. The disease usually shows up first on one side of the body and slowly worsens. Later symptoms may be stooped posture, loss of facial expression, difficulty walking and talking, and impaired handwriting and balance. Tremors, if they appear, are usually in the fingers or wrist, but can involve other parts of the body. In the late stages, patients may develop a "Parkinson's dementia," similar to that found in Alzheimer's disease. However, it is not certain whether this incidence is higher than would be expected in people of their ages.

Diagnosis: Parkinson's disease can be difficult to diagnose because there is no biological test that confirms it. Diagnosis is usually made through medical history, pattern of symptoms, and differential diagnosis—the ruling out of any other cause, such as brain tumor or other neurological disorders.

Treatment: The development of a drug in the 1960s to correct dopamine deficiency means that Parkinson's disease is by no means the "hopeless" disease it was 25 years ago. In most patients, the symptoms can be partially or completely relieved for a time, even though the underlying disease progresses. The breakthrough treatment for Parkinson's disease is a drug called levodopa (L-dopa), which increases brain levels of dopamine. The most common drug is Sinemet, a combination of L-dopa and carbidopa, which has fewer side effects and more potency than L-dopa alone. Doctors now have several formulations of Sinemet, which they can adjust individually to patients.

Still, researchers are not entirely satisfied with the drug treatment. Authorities are increasingly concerned about the long-term adverse effects of L-dopa. New evidence shows that not only dopamine but other brain chemicals may be in short supply in the brains of Parkinson's sufferers. Therefore, new alternative drugs to treat Parkinson's disease are coming on the market. Further, current L-dopa–type drugs are sometimes not prescribed for persons with mild symptoms because the effects tend to wear off, giving the drugs a limited span of effectiveness. There is also no evidence that the early use of such drugs alters the course of the underlying disease. Because the drugs are so potent and the side effects often severe, and because the choice of drugs is changing, it is important that a neurologist supervise the treatment.

WHERE TO FIND TREATMENT FOR PARKINSON'S DISEASE

The following are leading authorities on Parkinson's disease. Most are also doing clinical research on the disease and may be available for consultation of treatment of certain cases, or can refer you or your primary physician to other specialists in Parkinson's disease.

For a list of heads of departments of neurology at leading medical colleges, *see* page 621. These physicians can be excellent sources of treatment and/or referrals to others who specialize in the treatment of Parkinson's disease.

Sufferers of Parkinson's disease will also need proper exercise and physical therapy (*see* Rehabilitation Centers, page 460). If possible, have a physiatrist—a physician specializing in rehabilitation medicine—design an exercise program for a disabled Parkinson's patient.

SOME LEADING SPECIALISTS

CALIFORNIA
Charles H. Markham, M.D.
Department of Neurology, RNRC
UCLA School of Medicine
Los Angeles, CA 90024
(213) 825-6578

COLORADO
Dr. Margaret M. Hoehn
3535 Cherry Creek N. Drive
Suite 407-A
Denver, CO 80209
(303) 393-6287

ILLINOIS
Harold L. Klawans, M.D.
Associate Chairman and Professor
Department of Neurological Sciences
Rush-Presbyterian-St. Lukes Medical Center
1753 W. Congress Parkway
Chicago, IL 60612
(312) 942-5938

MICHIGAN
Dr. John B. Penney, Jr.
Department of Neurology
University of Michigan
1405 E. Ann St.
Ann Arbor, MI 48109
(313) 763-4778

Peter A. LeWitt, M.D.
Lafayette Clinic
951 E. Lafayette St.
Detroit, MI 48207
(313) 256-9350

MINNESOTA
Manfred D. Muenter, M.D.
Associate Professor of Neurology
Department of Neurology
Mayo Clinic
200 First St., S.W.
Rochester, MN 55901
(507) 284-2833

NEW JERSEY
Roger C. Duvoisin, M.D.
Department of Neurology
Rutgers Medical College
PO Box 101
Piscataway, NJ 08854
(201) 463-4545

NEW YORK
Stanley Fahn, M.D.
Room 02-0201
Neurological Institute
710 W. 168th St.
New York, NY 10032
(212) 694-5277
Dr. Fahn is director of the Parkinson's Clinic at the Columbia University Medical Center.

Abraham N. Lieberman, M.D.
New York University Medical Center
530 First Ave.
New York, NY 10016
(212) 340-6351

Ira Shoulson, M.D.
University of Rochester Medical Center
Department of Neurology
601 Elmwood Ave.
Rochester, NY 14642
(716) 275-5130

OHIO
Dr. Harold Mars
3609 Park E.
Beechwood, OH 44122
(216) 831-6085

Dr. George Paulson
Chairman, Department of Neurology
Ohio State University
452 Means Hall
1655 Upham Drive
Columbus, OH 43210
(614) 421-4973

OREGON
Dr. John G. Nutt
Department of Neurology
Oregon Health Sciences University
3181 S.W. San Jackson Park Road
Portland, OR 97201
(503) 225-7772

TEXAS
Joseph Jankovic, M.D.
Department of Neurology
Baylor College of Medicine
Texas Medical Center
Houston, TX 77030
(713) 799-5971

VIRGINIA
Dr. Frederick Wooten
Department of Neurology, Box 394
University of Virginia Medical Center
Charlottesville, VA 22908
(804) 924-8369

SOURCE: *Parkinson's Disease Foundation and United Parkinson Foundation.*

BRAIN TISSUE BANKS

Since the cause of Parkinson's disease is obscure, the study of brain tissue is invaluable in research. The Parkinson's Disease Foundation and Columbia University have established the first brain bank specifically for the study of the brains of Parkinson's victims. For more information on donating brain tissue after death, write to:

The Parkinson's Disease Foundation
Columbia University Medical Center
650 168th St.
New York, NY 10032

Additionally, the federal government's National Institute of Neurological and Communicative Diseases and Stroke supports two brain-tissue specimen banks. For information write or call:

Dr. Wallace W. Tourtellotte, Director
Human Neurospecimen Bank
VA Wadsworth Hospital Center
Los Angeles, CA 90037
(213) 824-4307 or 478-3711
(24 hours, collect)

Dr. Edward D. Bird, Director
Brain Tissue Resource Center
McLean Hospital
115 Mill St.
Belmont, MA 02178
(617) 855-2400
(24 hours, collect)

ORGANIZATIONS

American Parkinson Disease Association
116 John St.
New York, NY 10038
(212)732-9550

A privately funded voluntary health organization, dedicated to research on and treatment of Parkinson's disease. Funds 31 referral systems around the country connected with neurological clinics in hospitals. Funds research into Parkinson's. Also helps set up local support groups. Provides free evaluations in 31 clinics nationwide for people who suspect they may have Parkinson's. Publishes booklets and newsletters. Makes medical referrals. Will provide more information upon request.

Parkinson's Disease Foundation
Columbia University Medical Center
650 W. 168th St.
New York, NY 10032
(212) 923-4700

A nonprofit, endowed organization, dedicated to the study of Parkinson's disease and related disorders, including cerebral palsy, Alzheimer's disease, Huntington's disease, dystonia, familial tremor, and tardive dyskinesia. The Foundation mainly sponsors research into the cause, prevention and treatment of these diseases. It also acts as a source of information for patients and physicians on all aspects of such diseases and supports patient service activities at a Parkinson's Clinic at the Columbia University Medical Center, which is one of the leading centers in the country for research on and treatment of Parkinson's. The Foundation publishes a newsletter and self-help booklets for patients with Parkinson's and related diseases, as well as the proceedings of symposia sponsored by the Foundation. The Foundation keeps a list of more than 300 self-help groups nationwide, and upon request will supply the names of self-help groups in your area.

Parkinson's Educational Program USA
1800 Park Newport, Suite 302
Newport Beach, CA 92660
(714) 640-0218
(800) 344-7872 (outside California)

A nonprofit organization dedicated to disseminating information on Parkinson's. Sponsors conferences, workshops, publishes a newsletter, sells a number of publications, audio- and home videotapes and other items geared to Parkinson's patients. Assists in establishing local support groups throughout the country. Maintains a speakers' bureau. Will send a list of local support groups and publications and product price list upon request.

United Parkinson Foundation
360 W. Superior St.
Chicago, IL 60610
(312) 664-2344

A membership organization for patients, family members, medical personnel and other interested persons. Purpose: to disseminate reliable information about symptoms, medication and therapy on Parkinson's; to foster, promote and support scientific research on the disease; to assist patients and families in finding proper medical treatment. Publishes a quarterly newsletter, distributes exercise booklets and sponsors nationwide seminars on Parkinson's. Makes medical referrals and referrals to self-help groups. Will provide more information upon request.

BOOKS

Parkinson's Disease: A Guide for Patient and Family, **Roger C. Duvoisin, M.D.,** New York: Raven Press, 1983.

Parkinson's Disease: The Facts, **Gerald Stern** and **Andrew Lees,** New York: Oxford University Press, 1982.

Parkinson's Disease: The Patient's View, **Sidney Dorros,** Cabin John, MD: Seven Locks Press, 1982; Seven Locks Press, Inc., PO Box 72, Cabin John, MD 20818; also

recorded as a Talking Book, available from many public libraries, for those who cannot hold a book or turn the pages.

Portrait of Myself, **Margaret Bourke-White,** New York: Simon and Schuster, 1963; the famous photographer's battle with Parkinson's disease.

We Are Not Alone: Learning to Live with Chronic Illness, **Sefra Kobrin Pitzele,** Minneapolis: Thompson & Co., 1985.

MATERIALS, FREE AND FOR SALE

Free

Aids, Equipment and Suggestions to Help the Patients with Parkinson's Disease in the Activities of Daily Living, 22 pages.
Home Exercises for Patients with Parkinson's Disease, 16 pages.
A Manual for Patients with Parkinson's Disease, 37 pages.
Speech Problems and Swallowing Problems in Parkinson's Disease, 16 pages.

American Parkinson Disease Association
116 John St.
New York, NY 10038
(212) 732-9950

Parkinson's Disease, Hope Through Research, 26 pages.

National Institute of Neurological and Communicative Diseases and Stoke
Bethesda, MD 20892
(301) 496-5751

Exercises for the Parkinson Patient with Hints for Daily Living, illustrated. *The Parkinson Patient At Home,* 16 pages.

Parkinson's Disease Foundation
Columbia University Medical Center
650 W. 168th St.
New York, NY 10032
(212) 923-4700

All About Parkinson's Drugs Progress, Promise and Hope, 12 pages.
You Are Not Alone, 32-page booklet.

Parkinson's Educational Program
1800 Park Newport, Suite 302
Newport Beach, CA 92660

One Step At A Time; exercise booklet.

United Parkinson's Foundation
360 W. Superior St.
Chicago, IL 60610

Audio- and videotapes for sale

Exercise With Beverly Steward, audio- and videotape.
Exercise With Us, videotape.
Fitness Exercises for Parkinsonians, audiotape with booklet.
Range of Motion Exercises, audiotape.

More than 50 videotapes (VHS and beta) and numerous audiotapes on various aspects of Parkinson's disease, including treatment and research. Catalog available on request.

Parkinson's Educational Program–USA
1800 Park Newport, Suite 302
Newport Beach, CA 92660

The Exercise Program: an illustrated booklet with two audiocassettes.

United Parkinson's Foundation
360 W. Superior St.
Chicago, IL 60610

PHOBIAS

Phobias—irrational debilitating fears often accompanied by panic attacks—are a major, but amazingly treatable mental disorder. As many as 13 million American adults, about 8 percent of the population, suffer from anxiety disorders, including phobias, according to a government study. Experts estimate that in more than 90 percent of the cases the phobia can be brought under control in a relatively short time with proper treatment.

Anything that produces anxiety so severe as to cause panic or abnormal physical reactions can be considered a phobia—such as fear of animals, insects, thunderstorms, dark places, blood, dentists, injections by needle, riding in cars, planes, crossing bridges, heights, speaking in public and so forth. Because people tend to avoid any situation in which they might possibly confront the object of fear or with which they associate a panic attack, phobias seriously curtail activities and alter a person's ability to function in society. Phobias can be psychologically debilitating.

"Simple" phobias in which people fear a specific object are the most common. But the phobia for which people most frequently seek treatment is agoraphobia, the Greek work for "fear of the marketplace." Agoraphobia is a complex and often devastating disorder of multiple fears accompanied by intense panic attacks that make a person afraid to leave a safe person or place. Agoraphobia accounts for about 70 percent of all treated phobias, and an estimated three out of four victims are women.

Agoraphobia almost always starts with panic attacks. The first panic attack usually occurs between the late teens and early thirties; the average age of sufferers is 24. It is often followed by more panic attacks and increased fears of being in public; eventually, the person may be afraid to leave the house. These panic attacks unless somehow prevented lead to full-blown agoraphobia in 85 percent of the cases, especially in women.

Although sometimes there may be a rational or partially rational reason for a phobia, the degree of intensity of the fear extends far beyond the rational reason.

Cause: The precise cause is unknown, but recent research shows that agoraphobia is a biological, possibly a hereditary disorder: It tends to run in families. That does not mean, however, that every susceptible person develops a phobia. Research suggests that something must trigger the panic attacks in biologically susceptible people. The trigger may be stress. Recent studies indicate that about 80 percent of the initial panic attacks associated with agoraphobia occur within six months to one year after a major life crisis, such as a divorce, job change, death in the family or severe illness.

Recent studies also show that caffeine can stimulate panic attacks. High doses of caffeine—about seven cups of coffee in a day—can trigger phobic panic attacks in normal people who have never had a panic attack. As few as two cups of coffee can produce panic attacks in certain phobics, indicating they are more sensitive to caffeine. Experts note that for some phobics simply avoiding caffeine will lessen the panic attacks.

Symptoms: A phobic reaction carries with it what experts call a "sensation storm" of physical reactions. Generally, the heart beats faster, in what may be characterized as a panic attack; when it happens the first time, some people think they are having a heart attack, dying, or going crazy. Other symptoms include a cold sweat, shortness of breath, dizziness, "noodle legs," even diarrhea.

Treatment: Phobias are one of the most consistently successfully treated of all mental problems, and it is tragically unnecessary for most persons to suffer from phobias. Before the 1950s phobias, like many other mental complaints, were treated almost exclusively by psychoanalysis and conventional talk therapy with overwhelming failure. In some cases, antipsychotic drugs and even electroconvulsive shock treatments have been used in futile efforts to cure phobias. The current treatment is a highly successful short-term therapy based on "systematic desensitization," generally by gradual exposure to the fear itself.

During such therapy, the phobic confronts the fear surrounding the dreaded object, and by doing so experiences and learns to cope with the resultant anxiety, eventually mastering the fear. It is a gradual, well-defined, step-by-step approach to the fear, done under the supervision of a specialist, sometimes a psychiatrist. Gradually, the fear lessens as the person becomes "desensitized."

Some phobia experts, such as Dr. Joseph Wolpe, a professor of psychiatry at the Medical College of Pennsylvania, claim that the desensitization can sometimes be done in the mind; for example, imagining seeing a spider, approaching it, etc. Thus, "simple phobias" can be treated mostly in the imagination.

Most therapists, however, insist that recovery is much faster and more successful if the phobic is exposed to the real fear itself in the same systematic fashion, usually with the support of a therapist or a "phobia aide" who is a recovered phobic. This type of treatment is called "exposure therapy": Therapists go with the victims to the scene of the fear and help them endure the ensuing panic and conquer the fear. Such therapy apparently works for all kinds of phobias, and advocates claim success in from 80 to more than 90 percent of the instances. Failures result when the phobic simply refuses to confront the fear.

New research and treatment, based on a possible biological cause of phobias, have focused on preventing the panic attacks, which are a hallmark of agoraphobia. The contention is that by warding off the initial panic attacks, which usually become progressively worse, full-blown agoraphobia can be prevented. Recent research claims that drugs, such as tricyclic antidepressants, stop the panic attacks in 75 percent of the cases, thus preventing agorophobia. However, when the antidepressants are withdrawn, the panic attacks often return. Drugs are sometimes also used in treating other types of phobias; for example, beta-blockers may slow down the racing hearts of people with "performance anxiety" and phobias of speaking in public. Other antianxiety drugs are being tested with some success. Some therapists now use a combination of psychological desensitization or "exposure therapy" and drugs in treating agoraphobia.

Since most phobias can now be controlled, it is essential to find the right therapist. Some phobia therapists say their patients have had an average of 200 therapy sessions, or sometimes up to 10–15 years of psychoanalysis in futile attempts to relieve the phobia before finding effective treatment.

Special phobia clinics are springing up around the country. Although these clinics do not always use precisely the same techniques, their aim is generally to expose and desensitize the person to the phobia. The treatment may include individual and group therapy, field trips to confront the phobia, and specialized drug therapy. The number of sessions required may depend on the type and seriousness of the phobia, but from 10 to 20 sessions are typical in teaching a person to successfully control phobias.

It is important to find therapy that offers broad options and is directed by, affiliated with, or supervised by a physician who can prescribe medications if necessary. Otherwise, you will not be able to get the entire range of possible treatment.

SOME LEADING PHOBIA TREATMENT CENTERS

The following phobia treatment programs are directed by physicians or affiliated with hospitals, with major medical centers, or with medical colleges.

ARIZONA
University of Arizona Health Sciences Center
Psychiatry Clinic
Tucson, AZ 85724
Stephen Shanfield, M.D., Director of
    Psychiatry Clinic
(602) 626-6254

CALIFORNIA
University of Southern California School of
    Medicine
Los Angeles Clinical Institute of Psychology
383 S. Robertson Blvd., Suite A
Beverly Hills, CA 90211
Maralyn L. Teare, M.S., M.F.C.C., Director
(213) 659-6440

TERRAP
1010 Doyle St.
Menlo Park, CA 94025
Arthur B. Hardy, M.D., Director
(415) 329-1233
Dr. Hardy is the head of TERRAP, a
    nationwide program to treat anxieties and
    phobias.

Everett A. Gladman Memorial Hospital
2633 E. 27th St.
Oakland, CA 94106
Christopher J. McCullough, Ph.D., Director
(415) 536-8111

TERRAP
900 Welch Rd., Suite 400
Palo Alto, CA 94304
Alan Ringold, M.D., Director
(415) 327-5795

San Francisco Phobia Recovery Center
85 Liberty St.
San Francisco, CA 94110
Christopher McCullough, M.D., Director
(415) 441-2583

Stanford University Medical Center
Behavioral Medicine Clinic
Stanford, CA 94305
Stewart Agras, M.D., Director
(415) 497-7107

COLORADO
Phobia Treatment
Human Performance Institute
777 S. Wadsworth
Building 4, Suite 1120
Lakewood, CO 80226
Michael Uhes, M.D., Director
(303) 988-5706

CONNECTICUT
Yale University School of Medicine
Yale Behavioral Medicine Clinic
New Haven, CT 06510
Hoyle Leight, M.D., Director of Behavioral
    Medicine Clinic
(203) 785-2112

Mid-Fairfield Child Guidance Center
74 Newton Ave.
Norwalk, CT 06851
Susan Feldman, Director (for children's
    treatment)
(203) 847-3891
Primarily treatment of children's school
    phobias.

DISTRICT OF COLUMBIA
American University
Agoraphobia & Anxiety Program
Department of Psychiatry
Washington, DC 20016
Diane Chambless, Ph.D.
(202) 885-1711

Washington Psychological Center
2139 Wisconsin Ave., N.W.
Washington, DC 20007
Allan Levanthal, M.D.
Barry McCarthy, M.D.
(202) 965-5350

FLORIDA
Seminole County Mental Health Center, Inc.
Crane's Roost Office Park, Suite 377
Altamonte Springs, FL 32701
Him Pogue, Therapist
(305) 831-2411

Agoraphobia Resource Center
2699 S. Bayshore Drive, Suite 800-E
Coconut Grove, FL 33133
Paula Levine, M.D., Director
(305) 854-0652

University of Florida Health Center
Fear and Phobias Clinic
Gainesville, FL 32610
Dr. Barbara Melamed, Director
(904) 392-4559

TERRAP
6905 W. 16th Drive
Hialeah, FL 33014
Gerald Kurtz, M.D., Director
(305) 823-8885

TERRAP
Sabal Chase Medical Center
10820 S.W. 113th Place
Miami, FL 33176
Gerald Kurtz, M.D., Director
(305) 279-4062—Medical Center
(305) 833-8885 or 822-9143—Dr. Kurtz

University of Miami School of Medicine
Phobia Clinic
Medical Arts Building
1550 N.W. 10th Ave.
Miami, FL 33136
Richard Steinbook, M.D., Director
(305) 547-6755

University of South Florida
Anxiety/Phobia Clinic
12901 N. 30th St.
Tampa, FL 33612
David V. Sheehan, M.D., Director
(813) 974-3344

GEORGIA
Atlanta Phobia Clinic
960 Johnson Ferry Rd.
Suite 215
Atlanta, GA 30342
Steven Garber, M.D., Director
(404) 256-0802

TERRAP
2531 Briarcliffe, Rd., N.E.
Atlanta, GA 30329
Rebecca Boone, M.D.
(404) 325-9602

HAWAII
Anxiety Disorder Program
Queen's Medical Center
PO Box 861
Honolulu, HI 96808
Edward Pontius, M.D., Director
(808) 547-4401

KANSAS
Anxiety Disorders Clinic
Memorial Hospital
600 Madison
Topeka, KS 66607
Connie Walters, O.T.R., Director
(913) 354-5373

LOUISIANA
Panic and Phobia Disorders Program
Tulane University Hospital
1415 Tulane Ave.
New Orleans, LA 70112
Philip T. Griffin, M.D., Director
(504) 588-5405

MAINE
Community Health and Counseling Services
43 Illinois Ave.
Bangor, ME 04401
Joseph Pickering, Executive Director
(207) 947-0366
(800) 432-7810—toll-free in Maine

MARYLAND
Jeffrey Boyd, M.D.
5654 Shields Drive
Bethesda, MD 20817
(301) 530-9395

National Institute of Mental Health
Anxiety and Affective Disorders
NIMH Building 10, Room 35239
Bethesda, MD 20892
Thomas Uhde, M.D., Director
(301) 496-6825

Center for Behavioral Medicine
Phobia Program of Washington
6191 Executive Blvd.
Rockville, MD 20852
Robert DuPont, M.D., Director
(301) 468-8980

Agoraphobia Treatment Program
6501 N. Charles St.
Towson, MD 21204
Sally Winsston, M.D., Director
(301) 823-8200

MASSACHUSETTS
Andover Phobia Center
166 N. Main St.
Andover, MA 01810
Jorge H. DeNapoli, M.D., Director
(617) 475-7249

Agoraphobia Treatment and Research of New
  England
264 Beacon
Boston, MA 02116
Stephen Fisher, M.D., Director
(617) 262-5223

Beth Israel Hospital
Outpatient Psychiatry Unit
Boston, MA 02215
Danny Silverman, M.D., Head of Outpatient
  Services
(617) 735-4735

Boston University Medical School
Biobehavioral Sciences Clinical Unit
720 Harrison Ave., Suite 911
Boston, MA 02118
Lyle Miller, M.D., Head of B.S.C. Unit
(617) 247-6138

Children's Hospital
Department of Psychology, Fagen #8
Behavioral Psychology Program
300 Longwood Ave.
Boston, MA 02115
Dennis C. Russo, Ph.D., Director
(617) 735-6720

Massachusetts General Hospital
Anxiety and Phobias Research
Boston, MA 02114
David Sheehan, M.D., Director
(617) 726-8728

Hallgarth Institute
160 MacArthur Blvd.
Bourne, MA 02532
Barbara McNamara, Director
(617) 759-2111

Lahey Clinic Medical Center
Behavioral Medicine
Burlington, MA 01805
Lyle E. Kantor, Ph.D., Director
(617) 273-8610

Cambridge Hospital
Behavioral Medicine Clinic
1493 Cambridge St.
Cambridge, MA 02139
Daniel Brown, M.D., Director
(617) 498-1148

Outpatient Psychiatric Center
Mount Auburn Hospital
Cambridge, MA 02138
Lloyd I. Sederer, M.D., Director
(617) 492-3500, x1443

Valley Clinical Associates
474 Main St.
Greenfield, MA 01301
James Shortell, M.D., Director
(413) 774-3580

Mystic Valley Health Center
186-Bedford St.
Lexington, MA 02173
Richard Weiss, M.D., Executive Director
(617) 861-0890

MICHIGAN
University of Michigan
Anxiety Disorders Program
University Hospital
APH5 Box 011
1405 E. Ann St.
Ann Arbor, MI 48109
George Curtis, M.D., Director
(313) 764-5348

TERRAP
111 S. Woodward Ave.
Birmingham, MI 48011
Lawrence A. Cantow, M.D.
(313) 642-7764 or 644-7434

Mental Health Clinic
Psychiatry Department
Providence Hospital
16001 W. 9-Mile Rd.
Southfield, MI 48037
Rhona Ahmad, M.D., Director
(313) 424-3301

MINNESOTA
Abbott-N.W. Hospital
Phobia Treatment Program
800 E. 28th St. at Chicago Ave.
Minneapolis, MN 55407
Douglas A. Hedlund, M.D., Director
(612) 874-5369

MISSOURI
County Mental Health Services
77 Westport Plaza Medical Center
St. Louis, MO 63146
John Waite, M.D., Director
(314) 434-1560

Anxiety Disorders Center
University Medical Center
1221 S. Grand Blvd.
St. Louis, MO 63104
Alec Pollard, Ph.D., Director
(314) 771-6400, x202

Washington University
Psychological Services Center
Lindell & Skinker
St. Louis, MO 63130
Amy Bertelson, Ph.D., Director
(314) 889-6555

NEBRASKA
University of Nebraska College of Medicine
42nd & Dewey Ave.
Omaha, NE 68105
Frank J. Menolascino, M.D., Chairman,
  Psychiatry
(402) 559-5100

NEW JERSEY
Mount Sinai Phobia Clinic
151 Engle St.
Englewood, NJ 07631
Barry G. Dale, D.M.D., F.A.G.D.
(201) 569-7361

NEW YORK
Phobia and Anxiety Disorders Clinic
State University of New York at Albany
1535 Western Ave.
Albany, NY 12203
David H. Parlow, Ph.D., Director
(518) 455-4127

PASS, Inc.
1042 E. 105th St.
Brooklyn, NY 11236
Seymour S. Jaffe, M.D., Director
(718) 763-0190

Long Island Jewish Hospital Medical Center
Phobia Clinic
PO Box 38
Glen Oaks, NY 11004
Charlotte M. Zitrin, M.D., Director
(718) 470-4556, 8120

Anxiety Disorders Clinic
Columbia-Presbyterian Medical Center
622 W. 168th St.
New York, NY 10032
Michael R. Liebowitz, M.D., Director
(212) 960-2367

Cornell University Medical College
151 E. 37th St.
New York, NY 10016
Herbert Fensterheim, M.D.
(212) 889-7290

Cornell University Medical College/New York
  Hospital
500 West End Ave.
New York, NY 10024
Martin N. Seif, Ph.D.
(212) 799-2549

Phobia Center
New York Psychological Center
245 E. 87th St.
New York, NY 10128
Dr. Carol Lindemann, Director
(212) 861-6841 or 860-5560

Payne Whitney Outpatient Clinic
Phobia Clinic
525 E. 68th St.
New York, NY 10021
Catherine Shear, M.D., Director
(212) 472-6277

Roosevelt Hospital Phobia Clinic
36 W. 60th St.
New York, NY 10023
Natalie Schor, Director
(212) 554-7172

Phobia Clinic
White Plains Hospital Medical Center
Davis Ave. at E. Post Rd.
White Plains, NY 10601
Manuel Zane, M.D., Director
(914) 681-1080, 1038; 949-9322
The first phobia clinic in the United States.

OHIO
Case Western Reserve University School of
  Medicine
Phobia Clinic
Cleveland, OH 44106
Barbara Fleming, Ph.D., Director
(216) 444-3557

University Hospital of Cleveland
Hanna Pavilion
2040 Abington Rd.
Cleveland, OH 44106
Alberta Tartaglia, A.C.S.W., Director
(216) 844-7840.

Riverside Hospital
Phobia Treatment Center
1600 N. Superior St.
Toledo, OH 43604
Dennis W. Kogut, Ph.D., Director
(419) 729-6323

Siva P. Kurup, M.D.
2000 E. Market St.
Warren, OH 44483
(216) 393-5566

OKLAHOMA
Oklahoma College of Osteopathic Medicine
Center for Behavioral Medicine
2345 Southwest Blvd.
Tulsa, OK 74101
Richard Wansley, Ph.D., Director
(918) 582-1980

PENNSYLVANIA
Agoraphobia and Anxiety Program
Temple University Medical School
112 Bala Ave.
Bala Cynwyd, PA 19004
Alan Goldstein, M.D., Director
Linda B. Welsh, Clinical Director
(215) 667-6490

Medical College of Pennsylvania
Temple Behavior Unit—Quarters Building
3200 Henry Ave.
Philadelphia, PA 19129
Dr. Joseph Wolpe, Director
(215) 438-9548, x33

Medical College of Pennsylvania
Phobia Clinic
3200 Henry Ave.
Philadelphia, PA 19129
Alan S. Bellack, Ph.D., Director
(215) 842-4550

Phobias and Anxieties Program
Western Psychiatric Institute and Clinic
University of Pittsburgh
School of Medicine
3811 O'Hara St.
Pittsburgh, PA 15213
Directors: Matig Mavissakalian, M.D.,
Larry Michelson, Ph.D.
(412) 624-1000

SOUTH CAROLINA
University of South Carolina
Anxiety Disorders Program
Department of Psychiatry and Behavioral
   Sciences
171 Ashley Ave. 5th Floor USB
Charleston, SC 29425
James C. Ballenger, M.D.
(803) 792-4032

TENNESSEE
Anxiety Disorders Clinic
University of Tennessee, Memphis
College of Medicine
66 N. Pauline, #633
Memphis, TN 38105
Philippe Khouri, M.D., Chairman
(901) 528-6628

TEXAS
Austin Neuropsychiatric Association
711 W. 38th St.
Suite C-35
Austin, TX 78705
Theodore Doke, Jr., M.D., Director
(512) 451-8233

University of Texas Medical Branch—
   Galveston
Psychiatry and Behavioral Sciences
   Department
Galveston, TX 77550
Rudolph Roden, M.D., Ph.D.
(409) 761-3901

San Antonio Phobia Clinic
7711 Louis Pasteur, Suite 814
San Antonio, TX 78229
Habib Nathan, M.D., Director
(512) 696-4041

UTAH
Phobias and Anxiety Disorders Clinic
University of Utah School of Medicine
50 N. Medical Drive
Salt Lake City, UT 84132
Mark E. Owens, Ph.D., Director
(801) 581-5811

VIRGINIA
Roundhouse Square Psychiatric Center
Phobia Treatment Center
1444 Duke St.
Alexandria, VA 22314
David Charney, M.D.
Jerilyn Ross, M.A.
(703) 836-7130

Henry A. Skopek, M.D.
5272 Dawes Ave.
Alexandria, VA 22301
(703) 237-0780

Anxiety Disorders Program
Medical College of Virginia
MCV Station, Box 710
Richmond, VA 23298
Prakash Ettigi, M.D., Director
(804) 786-9157

WASHINGTON
Seattle Phobia Clinic
Cabrinia Medical Tower, Suite 1910
901 Boreen Ave.
Seattle, WA 98104
Gerald Rosen, Ph.D., Director
Herbert Orenstein, M.D.
(206) 343-9474 or 623-7444

WISCONSIN
University of Wisconsin Phobia Clinic
Department of Psychiatry
Clinical Sciences Center
600 Highland Ave.
Madison, WI 53792
John H. Geist, M.D., Director
(608) 263-6056

Columbia Hospital Psychiatric Department
Phobia Clinic
2025 E. Newport Ave.
Milwaukee, WI 53211
K. Kwang Soo, M.D., Director
(414) 961-3851

Mt. Sinai Medical Center
Outpatient Psychiatry Clinic
950 N. 12th St.
Milwaukee, WI 53233
Bella Selan, M.S.W., Director Phobia
   Program
(414) 289-8150

SOURCE: *Phobia Society of America and author's survey.*

PHOBIA RESEARCH AND TREATMENT AT THE NATIONAL INSTITUTE OF MENTAL HEALTH

Researchers at the National Institute of Mental Health are conducting studies on anxiety disorders, including agoraphobia, at the Clinical Center in Bethesda, Maryland. The emphasis is on the use of drugs, namely antidepressants, to ward off panic attacks, thus preventing or treating agoraphobia. Participation is by physician referral. Your physician can contact:

National Clinical Center
National Institute of Mental Health
Bethesda, MD 20892
(301) 496-6826

ORGANIZATIONS

The Phobia Society of America
133 Rollins Ave., Suite 4-B
Rockville, MD 20852
(301) 231-5484

A national nonprofit membership organization founded by phobic people, their families and therapists. Promotes public awareness of the problems caused by panic disorder and phobias, stimulates research and development of effective treatment, and helps sufferers find appropriate treatment. The Society has a network of local chapters, sponsors conferences, develops criteria for training and certification of phobia therapists, and publishes a phobia journal. Makes referrals to phobia therapists throughout the country. Will provide more information upon request; treatment referrals if you send a self-addressed, stamped envelope.

TERRAP National Headquarters
Arthur B. Hardy, M.D., Director
1010 Doyle St.
Menlo Park, CA 94025
(415) 329-1233

TERRAP (for Territorial Apprehensiveness) is a nationwide franchise of programs to treat anxieties and phobias, especially agoraphobia. TERRAP was developed by Arthur Hardy, M.D. Will provide a list of programs in your locality.

Fear of Flying Programs

Freedom from Fear of Flying
2021 Country Club Prado
Coral Gables, FL 33134
Capt. T.W. Cummings
(305) 261-7042

SOAR Inc.
Box 747
Westport, CT 06881
(203) 259-0087
(800) 332-7359

Workshops in major U.S. cities and an audiotape program.

BOOKS

Agoraphobia, **Dr. Claire Weekes,** New York: Hawthorn Press, 1977.
Agoraphobia, Symptoms, Causes, Treatment, **Arthur B. Hardy,** Menlo Park, CA: TSC Management Corporation, 1010 Doyle St., Menlo Park, CA 94025.
The Anxiety Disease, **David V. Sheehan, M.D.,** New York: Scribner's, 1984.
Everything You Wanted to Know About Phobias But Were Afraid to Ask, **Neal Olshan,** New York: Beaufort Books, 1981.
Fearless Flying: A Passenger Guide to Modern Airline Travel, **John H. Greist** and **Georgia L. Greist,** Chicago: Nelson-Hall, 1981.
Fears and Phobias, **Tony Whitehead,** New York: Arco, 1983.
Hope and Help for Your Nerves, **Dr. Claire Weekes,** New York: Hawthorn Press, 1969.

Our Useless Fears, **Joseph Wolpe, M.D.,** and **David Wolpe,** Boston: Houghton Mifflin, 1981.
Peace from Nervous Suffering, **Dr. Claire Weekes,** New York: Hawthorn Press, 1972.
Panic: Facing Fears, Phobias and Anxiety, **Stewart Agras, M.D.,** New York: Basic Books, 1985.
Phobia: A Comprehensive Summary of Modern Treatments, **edited by Dr. Robert DuPont,** Rockville, MD: The Phobia Society of America, 1983.
Your Phobia: Understanding Your Fears Through Contextual Therapy, **Manuel Zane, M.D., and Harry Milt,** Washington: American Psychiatric Press, 1984.

MATERIALS FOR SALE

Terrap Times, bimonthly newsletter for agoraphobics.

TSC Management Corporation
1010 Doyle St.
Menlo Park, CA 94025

PM News, bimonthly newsletter on phobias.

White Plains Hospital Medical Center
Davis Ave.
White Plains, NY 10601

Audiocassette tapes

Speeches and workshop sessions from conferences sponsored by the Phobia Society of America. List and order form available from:

Caset Associates
8300 Professional Hill Drive
Fairfax, VA 22031

A Lecture by Dr. Claire Weekes, an Australian psychiatrist and international authority on phobias.
I Never Stayed in the Dark Long Enough, **Dr. Manuel Zane.**

Phobia Materials
PO Box 807
White Plains, NY 10601

Either/Or Thinking, discussion of phobias.
Relaxation Response, **Dr. Arthur Hardy.**

TSC Management Corporation
1010 Doyle St.
Menlo Park, CA 94025
(415) 329-1233

HELP BY PHONE AND MAIL

C.A.L.L. (Concerned Agoraphobics Learning to Live)
380 Tolosa Way
San Luis Obispo, CA 93401
(805) 543-3764
Daryl Woods

This self-help group has extensive telephone and mail contacts throughout the U.S.

Group By Mail
154 Chatfield Rd.
Bronxville, NY 10708
D. Jean Esterbrook
(914) 337-3220

Ms. Esterbrook, a recovered phobic, offers mutual support for phobics via correspondence at a nominal cost.

TERRAP
1010 Doyle St.
Menlo Park, CA 94025
(415) 329-1233

TERRAP offers a correspondence phobia-recovery program for those who do not have a clinic nearby or cannot leave home.

PSORIASIS

Psoriasis is a noninfectious, noncontagious, persistent skin disorder in which the body is unable to properly regulate the production of skin cells. It is characterized by scaly patches on the skin, elevated red areas, usually covered by silvery, dry scales of both living and dead skin cells. Psoriasis affects from 1–2 percent of the population, or several million Americans. It strikes men and women equally, and most frequently shows up between the ages of 15 and 35. It has also been known to strike infants as well as adults over age 50. The appearance of psoriasis in later life is generally much less severe.

The disease ranges from very mild to very severe and may even require periods of hospitalization. The disease is recurrent, going through cycles of remissions, some lasting for years, and flare-ups. It is considered a lifelong disease with no cure.

Cause: Unknown, although there is a genetic tendency toward psoriasis in at least one-third of the cases. Some scientists speculate that psoriasis might be an autoimmune deficiency, in which the body's immunological system attacks its own tissues. Psoriasis causes biochemically stimulated abnormal cell growth. Ordinarily, a normal skin cell matures in 28–30 days; in psoriasis, the cell's life cycle is only 4 days. Thus, the abnormal skin cells are produced in excess and pile up to create elevated red, scaly patches. The white scale on the red patches is composed of dead cells being sloughed off. Several events can trigger flare-ups of psoriasis, including emotional stress, some forms of infections, skin injury, pregnancy, and even cold weather.

Symptoms: Psoriasis does not follow a predictable course and is different for everyone.

Generally, mild cases are localized; affect perhaps 5 percent of the body, usually the knees, elbows, scalp, hands, and feet; and are characterized by itchy skin and red patches. More serious cases affect up to 30 percent of the body—arms, legs, torso, and head—and cause painful swelling, itching, and burning. A very severe case may affect up to 90 percent of the body, causing severe peeling of the skin, pustules, or extensive red, scaly plaques over the body. It can involve severe pain, cracking, burning sensations, and bleeding.

Common sites for psoriasis are the scalp, genital area, around the nails and on the knees and elbows. It can also show up in the ear canal, the eyelids, and in the mouth. Psoriasis does not usually appear on the face. Of course, the disease can take a severe emotional toll, ranging from embarrassment to severe depression and withdrawal.

About 5–10 percent of those with psoriasis also have psoriatic arthritis, similar to rheumatoid arthritis, with general discomfort, pain, throbbing, morning stiffness, inflammation and swelling of the joints. Why such arthritis is related to psoriasis is unknown. Psoriatic arthritis is incurable and is treated in the same general way as rheumatoid arthritis.

Diagnosis: Diagnosis is usually made by observations of the skin, family history, and finally by skin biopsy.

Treatment: Nonprescription remedies often help, especially products with coal tar and moisturizers. But in more severe cases, especially if psoriasis becomes a psychological problem, expert professional care is required. Steroids are the drugs most prescribed for psoriasis; although usually applied topically, they are in some cases injected. One of the best treatments is light—either natural or artificial. Special ultraviolet lights are often used on the entire body, sometimes in a dermatologist's office, sometimes at home. The National Psoriasis Foundation has a list of companies that sell special light-boxes to treat psoriasis. Even more effective in severe cases of psoriasis is ultraviolet light combined with coal tar (the Goeckerman regimen). In about 80 percent of the cases, psoriasis completely disappears or improves significantly. The effects usually last for a year. At one time the Goeckerman regimen was confined to hospitals, but now there are numerous "day-care" centers throughout the country where a person can get the treatment and return home at night.

The newest and most controversial treatment for psoriasis is called PUVA. The "P" stands for the drug psoralen, and the "UVA" for a type of long-wave ultraviolet light. PUVA works in about 90 percent of the cases in controlling (but not curing) psoriasis, but there are fears that the treatment may promote skin cancer. Nevertheless, the treatment, once entirely experimental, is now in fairly widespread use. PUVA is a major treatment, usually given only to people with severe cases—when psoriasis covers at least 30 percent of the body—that have not responded to other therapies. Since the PUVA treatment can be ineptly used, you should choose a physician who has had considerable experience in using the method. Dermatologists (specialists in skin disease) treat psoriasis.

SOME LEADING RESEARCH AND TREATMENT SPECIALISTS

Here are some of the universities, centers, and physicians involved in patient research with psoriasis. These are not the only centers with experience and competence in treating psoriasis, but they are among the best and in some cases may need volunteers for their studies.

CALIFORNIA
University of California, Irvine
College of Medicine
Irvine, CA 92717
Gerald D. Weinstein, M.D.
(714) 856-5515

UCLA School of Medicine
The Center for Health Sciences
Los Angeles, CA 90024
Nicholas J. Lowe, M.D.
Ronald M. Reisner, M.D.
(213) 825-2765

Psoriasis Research Institute
PO Box V
Palo Alto, CA 94305
Eugene G. Farber, M.D., Chief Director
(415) 326-1848
A non-university-affiliated, nonprofit research
   institution.

University of California, San Diego
University Hospital
225 W. Dickinson St.
San Diego, CA 92130
Irma Gigli, M.D.
(619) 294-5580

University of California Medical Center
San Francisco, CA 94143
David L. Cram, M.D.
John Epstein, M.D.
William Epstein, M.D.
Howard I. Maibach, M.D.
(415) 666-4037, 2545

Stanford University
Stanford, CA 94305
Paul Jacobs, M.D.
(415) 497-6105

CONNECTICUT
Yale University
333 Cedar St.
New Haven, CT 06510
Irwin M. Braverman, M.D.
(203) 785-4093

DISTRICT OF COLUMBIA
Washington Hospital Center
110 Irving St., N.W.
Washington, DC 20010
Thomas P. Nigra, M.D.
(202) 541-6228

FLORIDA
University of Miami
School of Medicine
1550 N.W. 10th Ave.
Miami, FL 33101
Kenneth M. Halprin, M.D.
(305) 547-6704

ILLINOIS
Northwestern University
Northwestern Medical Faculty Foundation, Inc.
Department of Dermatology
222 E. Superior St.
Chicago, IL 60611
Henry H. Roenigk, Jr., M.D.
(312) 649-8106

MARYLAND
Johns Hopkins School of Medicine
601 N. Broadway
Baltimore, MD 21205
Thomas Provost, M.D.
(301) 396-9185

MASSACHUSETTS
Harvard Medical School
Massachusetts General Hospital
Boston, MA 02114
Thomas Fitzpatrick, M.D.
(617) 726-3990, 2914

MICHIGAN
University of Michigan Medical School
1910 Taubman
Ann Arbor, MI 48109
John J. Voorhees, M.D.
(313) 936-4078

NEW YORK
Columbia University College of Physicians &
  Surgeons
630 W. 168th St.
New York, NY 10032
Alan Andrews, M.D.
(212) 694-5293

New York University Medical Center
550 First Ave.
New York, NY 10016
Irwin M. Freedberg, M.D.
(212) 340-5245

NORTH CAROLINA
Duke University Medical Center
PO Box 2907
Durham, NC 27710
Sheldon Pinnell, M.D.
(919) 684-5337

PENNSYLVANIA
Temple University
Skin and Cancer Hospital
3322 N. Broad St.
Philadelphia, PA 19140
Eugene J. Van Scott, M.D.
(215) 221-3928

University of Pennsylvania School of Medicine
229 Medical Building
36th and Hamilton Walk
Philadelphia, PA 19104
Gerald S. Lazarus, M.D.
(215) 898-3240

UTAH
University of Utah
College of Medicine
50 N. Medical Drive
Salt Lake City, UT 84132
Gerald G. Krueger, M.D.
(801) 581-7837

WASHINGTON
University of Washington Medical School
1959 N.E. Pacific St.
Seattle, WA 98195
George F. Odland, M.D.
(206) 543-5290

SOURCE: *National Psoriasis Foundation.*

PSORIASIS DAY-CARE CENTERS

Psoriasis treatment is often intensive and long term and sometimes requires hospitalization. Alternatives to hospitalization are provided by day-care programs in which the person has a full day of treatment but returns home at night. Here are some prominent day-care psoriasis treatment centers. Most offer a variety of treatment methods, including PUVA.

CALIFORNIA
Psoriasis Skin Care Medical Clinic
2801 Jefferson St.
Carlsbad, CA 92008
Richard E. Fitzpatrick, M.D.
(619) 434-7177

UCLA Psoriasis Treatment Center
11600 Wilshire Blvd.
Suite 522
Los Angeles, CA 90025
Nicholas J. Lowe, M.D.
(213) 825-6290

Psoriasis Skin Care Medical Clinic
239 Laurel St., #101
San Diego, CA 92101
Richard E. Fitzpatrick, M.D.
(619) 231-0399

University of California, San Diego
University Hospital
225 W. Dickinson St.
San Diego, CA 92130
Joseph Walter, M.D.
(619) 294-3626, 3627

San Francisco Psoriasis Treatment Center
University of California
50 Kirkham
San Francisco, CA 94143
David L. Cram, M.D.
(415) 666-4701, 5951

Stanford University Hospital and Medical
   Center
Dermatology Day Care Center and
   Phototherapy
Stanford, CA 94305
Elizabeth Able, M.D.
(415) 497-7687

FLORIDA
Psoriasis Day Care Center
Pan American Center
4530 N. Armenia Ave.
Building ''B,'' Suite 3
Tampa, FL 33603
Dr. Michael A. Scannon
(813) 877-4811

ILLINOIS
Psoriasis Treatment Center
3060 N. Arlington Heights Rd.
Arlington Heights, IL 60004
Giulio A. Leone, M.D.
(312) 394-2060

Northwestern Medical Association Clinic
222 E. Superior St.
Chicago, IL 60611
Henry H. Roenigk, Jr., M.D.
(312) 649-8106

The Soderstrom Dermatology Center, S.C.
81 Queenwood
Morton, IL 61550
C. W. Soderstrom, M.D.
(309) 263-7546

LOUISIANA
Tulane Medical Center–Psoriasis Center
1415 Tulane Ave.
New Orleans, LA 70112
Larry E. Millikan, M.D.
(504) 588-5382

MASSACHUSETTS
Massachusetts General Hospital
Dermatology Day Treatment Center
15 Parkman St.
Ambulatory Care Center, 3A-389
Boston, MA 02114
Ernesto Gonzalez, M.D.
(617) 726-8405

NEW YORK
Columbia-Presbyterian Medical Center
Vanderbilt Clinic
622 W. 168th St.
New York, NY 10032
Robert Walther, M.D.
(212) 694-2147

OHIO
University of Cincinnati College of Medicine
Department of Dermatology, Psoriasis
   Treatment Center
234 Goodman St.
Pavilion A-3, Mall Location 523
Cincinnati, OH 45267
Paul A. Lucky, M.D.
(513) 872-4644

Cleveland Clinic Foundation
Department of Dermatology
Cutaneous Care Center
9500 Euclid Ave.
Cleveland, OH 44106
Jacob Dijkstra, M.D.
(216) 444-3347

Dermatology Day Treatment Center
University Hospitals of Cleveland
2078 Abbington Rd.
Cleveland, OH 44106-5000
David Bickers, M.D.
(216) 844-7155

Psoriasis Care Center
29 W. College Ave.
Westerville, OH 43081
Frank W. Yoder, M.D.
(614) 890-1313

PENNSYLVANIA
University of Pennsylvania
Dermatology Department
Maloney 2, Hospital
3600 Spruce
Philadelphia, PA 19104
Kays Kaidbey, M.D.
Gerald Lazarus, M.D.
(215) 662-6161

Scranton Psoriasis Day Care Center
Cornell Building, Suite 822
129 N. Washington Ave.
Scranton, PA 18503
Radwan Badawi, M.D.
(717) 342-9851, 9977

TEXAS
Baylor Psoriasis Center
3600 Taston Ave.
Suite 656
Dallas, TX 75246
Alan Menter, M.D.
(214) 820-2635

UTAH
Intermountain Dermatology Foundation
Psoriasis Treatment Center
1220 E. 3900 S.
Salt Lake City, UT 84124
Billie N. Coffin
(801) 268-0435

WASHINGTON
Psoriasis Treatment Center
1105 D James St.
Seattle, WA 98104
Bernard S. Goffe, M.D.
(206) 624-3230

SOURCE: *National Psoriasis Foundation*

CLIMATOTHERAPY FOR PSORIASIS

Recently, interest has grown in "climatotherapy" for psoriasis, and some Americans are making trips to the Dead Sea for sunbathing and sea bathing. There is some evidence that a four-week treatment session is effective in controlling serious psoriasis for about six months in numerous cases, presumably because of an unusual combination of sun and sea water. Reportedly, the sun's rays in that area have a high concentration of UVA, the same kind of rays used in the PUVA treatment in the United States. The effects of this treatment are not proved, although travelers have been going to the Dead Sea for this reason for many years. New studies are being done on its effectiveness, and until they are completed experts in the United States cannot

recommend it. Nevertheless, people who want more information about it can contact:

The International Psoriasis Treatment Center at
    Ein Bokek
24 King George St.
Jerusalem 94262
Israel
Telephone: 02-231248/9
Telex: 26115

You can also get more information from tourist agencies that offer therapy trips to the Dead Sea and more medical information on the subject from the National Psoriasis Foundation.

ORGANIZATION

The National Psoriasis Foundation
Suite 210
6443 S.W. Beaverton Highway
Portland, OR 97221
(503) 297-1545

A nonprofit, membership organization. Local groups in various parts of the country. Information and self-help source for patients, physicians, and other interested persons. Provides a bimonthly bulletin and pamphlets. Acts as a clearinghouse for information on psoriasis and answers questions from the public. Offers names of physicians specializing in psoriasis treatment. Special services: The National Psoriasis Foundation has a mail-order arrangement with a pharmacy whereby you can order antipsoriasis medications at discount. For those who want to correspond with others suffering from psoriasis, the National Psoriasis Foundation has a Pen Pal Club for children, a 20-Up Club for 20 and over. The Foundation will send more information upon request.

BOOKS

Psoriasis: A Guide to One of the Commonest Skin Diseases, **Dr. Ronald A. Marks,** New York: Arco Publishing, 1981.

FREE MATERIALS

Single copies are free

Climatotherapy at the Dead Sea; psoriasis treatment at the Dead Sea.
A Guide to Understanding Psoriasis, 60 pages.
My Child Has Psoriasis; for parents, by a parent who has a child with psoriasis.
Update on Psoriasis Research; includes a discussion of experimental treatments.

National Psoriasis Foundation
6443 S.W. Beaverton Highway
Suite 210
Portland, OR 97221
(503) 297-1545

The Foundation also has materials for sale.

REHABILITATION

See also Pain, page 427, Spinal Cord Injuries, page 544, Stroke, page 268.

A number of diseases, disorders, and injuries may require care at physical rehabilitation facilities: spinal cord injury, paralysis, organic brain disease, accidental brain injury, amputation, cancer surgery, severe burns, multiple sclerosis, neuromuscular diseases, arthritis, fractures, cerebral palsy, and chronic pain.

Rehabilitation has changed significantly from the days when it consisted almost exclusively of physical therapy; much rehabilitation is now a technologically sophisticated speciality including a variety of professionals—bioengineers, physical therapists, surgeons, physiatrists (physicians who specialize in rehabilitation), orthodontists, prosthesists, rehabilitation nurses, occupational therapists, psychological counselors, speech-language pathologists, recreational therapists, audiologists, and vocational counselors. Some rehabilitation centers even specialize in certain kinds of problems, such as spinal cord injuries. Sophisticated engineering inventions, including new kinds of prostheses, now make it possible for people to recover impaired functioning. As public sensitivity to the problems of the handicapped increases, there are more services and activities, both public and private, more medical research, and more sources of information and help.

LEADING PHYSICAL REHABILITATION CENTERS

The following are comprehensive inpatient physical rehabilitation centers accredited by the Commission on Accreditation of Rehabilitation Facilities (CARF). Some of them are hospital-based. In addition, many other hospitals have inpatient and outpatient physical rehabilitation programs that you may want to check out.

It is usually suggested that you choose a rehabilitation facility near your home, if possible, because after discharge from the facility or hospital, you will probably have to continue extensive treatment and rehabilitation sessions.

Centers marked with an asterisk (*) maintain accredited spinal cord injury programs. Centers marked with # have accredited chronic pain management programs.

ALABAMA
Spain Rehabilitation Center*#
1717 Sixth Ave., S.
Birmingham, AL 35233
(205) 934-4011

ARIZONA
St. Joseph's Hospital and Health Center–
  Rehabilitation Center
PO Box 12069
Tucson, AZ 85732
(602) 296-3211

St. Mary's Hospital and Health Center–
  Regional Rehabilitation Center
PO Box 5926
Tucson, AZ 85703
(602) 622-5833

CALIFORNIA
Corona Community Hospital
Rehabilitation Unit
800 S. Main
Corona, CA 91720
(714) 737-4343

Rancho Los Amigos Medical Center*
7601 E. Imperial Highway
Downey, CA 90242
(213) 923-7022

San Joaquin General Hospital
Division of Physical Medicine and
  Rehabilitation
500 W. Hospital Rd.
French Camp, CA 95231
(209) 982-1800

Leon S. Peters Rehabilitation Center*
Fresno Community Hospital and Medical
  Center
PO Box 1232
Fresno, CA 93715
(209) 442-6000

St. Jude Hospital and Rehabilitation Center[#]
101 E. Valencia Mesa Drive
Fullerton, CA 92632
(714) 871-3280

Rehabilitation Institute[#]
Glendale Adventist Medical Center
1509 Wilson Terrace
Glendale, CA 91206
(213) 240-8000

Physical Rehabilitation Unit
Memorial Hospital of Glendale
1420 S. Central Ave.
Glendale, CA 91204
(213) 246-6711

New Directions Rehabilitation Center[#]
Centinela Hospital Medical Center
PO Box 720
Inglewood, CA 90307
(213) 673-4660

Center for Diagnostic and Rehabilitation
  Medicine*[#]
Daniel Freeman Hospital Medical Center
333 N. Prairie Ave.
Inglewood, CA 90301
(213) 674-7050

Department of Rehabilitation Medicine
La Palma Intercommunity Hospital
7901 Walker St.
La Palma, CA 90623
(714) 522-0150

Rehabilitation Center–White Memorial Medical
  Center
1720 Brooklyn Ave.
Los Angeles, CA 90033
(213) 268-5000

Paradise Valley Hospital
2400 E. Fourth St.
National City, CA 92050
(619) 470-6311

Center for Rehabilitation Medicine*[#]
Northridge Hospital Medical Center
18300 Roscoe Blvd.
Northridge, CA 91328
(213) 885-8500

Casa Colina Hospital for Rehabilitative
  Medicine*[#]
255 E. Bonita Ave.
Pomona, CA 91767
(714) 593-7521

The Robert H. Ballard Center for
  Rehabilitation
1500 W. 17th St.
San Bernadino, CA 92411
(714) 887-6333

Acute Rehabilitation Center
Mills Peninsula Hospitals
100 S. San Mateo Drive
San Mateo, CA 94401
(415) 579-2000

Center for Rehabilitation Medicine[#]
Valley Hospital Medical Center
14500 Sherman Circle
Van Nuys, CA 91405
(213) 997-0101

Valley Hospital Medical Center–Center for
  Rehabilitation Medicine[#]
14500 Sherman Circle
Van Nuys, CA 91405
(818) 908-8676

COLORADO
Rehabilitation Center#
Boulder Memorial Hospital
311 Mapleton Ave.
Boulder, CO 80302
(303) 443-0230

Capron Rehabilitation Center
Penrose Hospital
PO Box 7021
Colorado Springs, CO 80933
(303) 630-5200

Spalding Rehabilitation Hospital#
1919 Ogden St.
Denver, CO 80218
(303) 861-0504

Craig Hospital*
3425 S. Clarkson
Englewood, CO 80110
(303) 789-8242

Hilltop Rehabilitation Hospital#
1100 Patterson Rd.
Grand Junction, CO 81506
(303) 244-6007

FLORIDA
L. W. Blake Memorial Hospital
PO Box 25004
Bradenton, FL 33506
(813) 792-6611

Memorial Regional Rehabilitation Center*
3599 University Blvd., S.
Jacksonville, FL 32216
(904) 355-1761

Baptist Hospital of Miami, Inc.
Center for Rehabilitation Services
8900 N. Kendall Drive
Miami, FL 33176
(305) 596-6520

The Rehabilitation Center, University of
   Miami/Jackson Memorial Medical Center*
1611 N.W. 12th Ave.
Miami, FL 33136
(305) 325-6272

Bon Secours Hospital
1050 N.E. 125th St.
North Miami, FL 33161
(305) 891-8850

Rehabilitation Unit
Parkway Regional Medical Center
160 N.W. 170th St.
North Miami Beach, FL 33169
(305) 651-1100

Humana Hospital Lucerne*
818 S. Main Lane
Orlando, FL 32801
(305) 237-6148

Lucerne Spinal Injury Center*
Humana Hospital Lucerne
818 S. Main Lane
Orlando, FL 32801
(305) 237-6111

Rehabilitation Institute of West Florida*#
PO Box 18900
Pensacola, FL 32523-8900
(904) 474-5358

Tampa General Rehabilitation Center*
Davis Island
Tampa, FL 33606
(813) 251-7226

GEORGIA
Center for Rehabilitation Medicine#
Emory University Hospital
1441 Clifton Rd., N.E.
Atlanta, GA 30322
(404) 329-5507

The Shepherd Center for Treatment of Spinal
   Injuries, Inc.*
2020 Peachtree Rd., N.W.
Atlanta GA 30309
(404) 352-2020

Rehabilitation Services
Candler General Hospital
PO Box 9787
Savannah, GA 31412
(912) 356-6168

Roosevelt Warm Springs Institute for
   Rehabilitation
Box 1000
Warm Springs, GA 31830
(404) 655-3341

HAWAII
The Rehabilitation Hospital of the Pacific*
226 N. Kuakini St.
Honolulu, HI 96817
(808) 531-3511

IDAHO

Idaho Elks Rehabilitation Hospital, Inc.
PO Box 1100
Boise, ID 83701
(208) 343-2583

ILLINOIS

Physical Medicine and Rehabilitation
 Department
Mennonite Hospital
807 N. Main St.
Bloomington, IL 61702-2850
(309) 827-4321

Rehabilitation Unit
Holy Cross Hospital
2701 W. 68th St.
Chicago, IL 60629
(312) 434-6700

Michael Reese Hospital and Medical Center
31st at Lake Shore Drive
Chicago, IL 60616
(312) 791-2430

Rehabilitation Institute of Chicago
345 E. Superior St.
Chicago, IL 60611
(312) 908-6185

Schwab Rehabilitation Center
1401 S. California Blvd.
Chicago, IL 60608
(312) 522-2010

Alexian Brothers Medical Center
800 W. Biesterfield Rd.
Elk Grove Village, IL 60007
(312) 437-5500

Evanston Hospital Rehabilitation Unit
2650 Ridge Ave.
Evanston, IL 60201
(312) 492-6696

Rehabilitation Unit
Riverside Medical Center
350 N. Wall St.
Kankakee, IL 60901
(815) 935-7509

Rehabilitation Unit
Oak Forest Hospital
15900 S. Cicero Ave.
Oak Forest, IL 60452
(312) 928-4200

Christ Hospital of the Evangelical Hospitals
 Corporation
4440 W. 95th St.
Oak Lawn, IL 60453
(312) 425-8000

Lutheran General Hospital
Rehabilitation Medicine Unit
1775 Dempster St.
Park Ridge, IL 60068
(312) 696-2210

Institute of Physical Medicine and
 Rehabilitation
6501 N. Sheridan Rd.
Peoria, IL 61614-2932
(309) 692-8110

Methodist Medical Center Unit
Institute of Physical Medicine and
 Rehabilitation
221 N.E. Glen Oak Ave.
Peoria, IL 61636
(309) 671-2900

Franciscan Rehabilitation Center
Franciscan Medical Center
2701 17th St.
Rock Island, IL 61201
(309) 793-2011

Van Matre Rehabilitation Center
Rockford Memorial Hospital
2400 N. Rockton Ave.
Rockford, IL 61101
(815) 968-6861

Memorial Medical Center
Department of Physical Medicine and
 Rehabilitation
800 N. Rutledge St.
Springfield, IL 62781
(217) 788-3302

East Central Illinois Rehabilitation Center of
 Mercy Hospital
1400 W. Park Ave.
Urbana, IL 61801
(217) 337-2208

Marianjoy Rehabilitation Center
PO Box 795
Wheaton, IL 60189
(312) 653-7600

INDIANA
Rehabilitation Unit
Parkview Memorial Hospital
2200 Randallia Drive
Fort Wayne, IN 46805
(219) 484-6636

Rehabilitation Institute of the Methodist
  Hospital
600 Grant St.
Gary, IN 46402
(219) 886-4566

IOWA
Rehabilitation Center
St. Luke's Hospital
1026 A Ave., N.E.
Cedar Rapids, IA 52402
(319) 398-7202

Rehabilitation Medicine Program
Mercy Hospital
West Central Park at Marquette
Davenport, IA 52804
(319) 326-8503

Younker Memorial Rehabilitation Center
Iowa Methodist Medical Center
1200 Pleasant St.
Des Moines, IA 50308
(515) 283-6464

Scholtz Medical Center–Rehabilitation
  Program*
Kimball and Ridgeway Aves.
Waterloo, IA 50702
(319) 291-3336

KANSAS
Bethany Rehabilitation Center
51 N. 12th St.
Kansas City, KS 66102
(913) 281-8400

Rehabilitation Medicine Unit
St. Joseph Medical Center
3600 E. Harry St.
Wichita, KS 67218
(316) 685-1111

Cranial-Spinal Recover Unit
Wesley Medical Center
550 N. Hillside
Wichita, KS 67214
(316) 688-2060

KENTUCKY
Cardinal Hill Hospital*
2050 Versailles Rd.
Lexington, KY 40504
(606) 254-5701

Neuro-Rehabilitation Unit
Baptist Hospital Highlands
810 Barret Ave.
Louisville, KY 40204
(502) 561-3347

Amelia Brown Frazier Rehabilitation Center
DBA Frazier Rehab Center
220 Abraham Flexner Way
Louisville, KY 40202
(502) 582-2231

LOUISIANA
Rehabilitation Institute of New Orleans*
F. Edward Hebert Hospital
#1 Sanctuary Drive
New Orleans, LA 70114
(504) 363-2691

Physical Medicine and Rehabilitation Center[#]
Physicians & Surgeons Hospital
PO Box 4466
Shreveport, LA 71104
(318) 227-3950

MARYLAND
Department of Rehabilitation Medicine
Sinai Hospital of Baltimore
Belvedere Ave. at Greenspring
Baltimore, MD 21215
(301) 578-5579

Maryland Rehabilitation Center
2301 Argonne Drive
Baltimore, MD 21218
(301) 366-8800

Montebello Hospital Center
2201 Argonne Drive
Baltimore, MD 21218
(301) 554-5200

Rehabilitation Unit
The Good Samaritan Hospital of Maryland,
  Inc.
5601 Loch Raven Blvd.
Baltimore, MD 21239
(301) 323-2200

MASSACHUSETTS

Greenery Rehabilitation and Skilled Nursing
  Center
99 Chestnut Hill Ave.
Boston, MA 02135
(617) 787-3390

Rehabilitation Institute
New England Medical Center Hospitals
171 Harrison Ave.
Boston, MA 02111
(617) 956-5222

Spaulding Rehabilitation Hospital#
125 Nashua St.
Boston, MA 02114
(617) 720-6400

Braintree Hospital
250 Pond St.
Braintree, MA 02184
(617) 848-5353

Joseph P. Kennedy, Jr. Memorial Hospital
30 Warren St.
Brighton, MA 02135
(617) 254-3800

Youville Rehabilitation and Chronic Disease
  Hospital
1575 Cambridge St.
Cambridge, MA 02238
(617) 876-4344

Head Injury Center at Lewis Bay
89 Lewis Bay Rd.
Hyannis, MA 02601
(617) 775-7601

Lakeville Hospital Rehabilitation Center
Main St.
Lakeville, MA 02346
(617) 947-1231

Lenox Hill Nursing and Rehabilitative Care
  Facility
70 Granite St.
Lynn, MA 01904
(617) 581-2400

The Neurologic Center at Forest Manor
Isaac St.
Middleboro, MA 02346
(617) 947-9295

The Head Injury Center
New Pioneer Valley Nursing Home, Inc.
548 Elm St.
Northampton, MA 01060-2888
(413) 586-3150

Berkshire Rehabilitation Center, Inc.
Rehabilitation Unit, Berkshire Medical Center
741 North St.
Pittsfield, MA 01201
(413) 443-3531

Rutland Heights Hospital
Maple Ave.
Rutland, MA 01543
(617) 886-4711

Dr. J. Robert Shaughnessy Rehabilitation
  Hospital
Dove Ave.
Salem, MA 01970
(617) 745-9000

Berkshire Rehabilitation Center, Inc.
Rehabilitation Unit, Mercy Hospital
PO Box 9012
Springfield, MA 01101
(413) 781-9100

New England Sinai Hospital
PO Box 647
Stoughton, MA 02072
(617) 364-4850

New England Rehabilitation Hospital#
One Rehabilitation Way
Woburn, MA 01801
(617) 935-5050

MICHIGAN

Southwestern Michigan Rehabilitation
  Hospital, Inc.
183 West St.
Battle Creek, MI 49017
(616) 965-3206

Mary Free Bed Hospital and Rehabilitation
  Center
235 Wealthy St., S.E.
Grand Rapids, MI 49503
(616) 242-0300

Southfield Rehabilitation Center
22401 Foster Winter Drive
Southfield, MI 48075
(313) 569-1500

Wyandotte General Hospital Rehabilitation
  Center
2333 Biddle Ave.
Wyandotte, MI 48192
(313) 284-2400

MINNESOTA
Miller-Dwan Medical Center
502 E. Second St.
Duluth, MN 55805
(218) 757-8762

Knapp Rehabilitation Center
900 S. Eighth St.
Minneapolis, MN 55404
(612) 347-3780

Sister Kenny Institute*
800 E. 28th St.
Minneapolis, MN 55407
(612) 874-4463

MISSOURI
Howard A. Rusk Rehabilitation Center*
University of Missouri–Columbia Hospital and
    Clinics
One Hospital Drive
Columbia, MO 65212
(314) 882-1071

Brady Rehabilitation Services
St. John's Regional Medical Center
2727 McClelland Blvd.
Joplin, MO 64801
(417) 781-2727

The Rehabilitation Institute
3011 Baltimore Ave.
Kansas City, MO 64108
(816) 756-2250

Rehabilitation Unit
Truman Medical Center/East
7900 Lee's Summit Rd.
Kansas City, MO 64139
(816) 373-4415

MONTANA
New Hope Regional Rehabilitation Center
St. Vincent Hospital and Health Center
PO Box 35200
Billings, MT 59107
(406) 657-7724

Rehabilitation Unit
Montana Deaconess Medical Center
1101-26th St., S.
Great Falls, MT 59405
(406) 761-1200

Missoula Community Hospital Rehabilitation
    Center
2827 Fort Missoula Rd.
Missoula, MT 59801
(406) 728-4100

NEBRASKA
Madonna Professional Care Center
2200 S. 52nd St.
Lincoln, NE 68506
(402) 489-7102

Immanuel Rehabilitation Center
Immanuel Medical Center
6901 N. 72nd St.
Omaha, NE 68122
(402) 572-2121

NEW HAMPSHIRE
Northeast Rehabilitation Hospital
70 Butler St.
Salem, NH 03079
(603) 893-2900

NEW JERSEY
Lourdes Regional Rehabilitation Center
1600 Haddon Ave.
Camden, NJ 08103
(609) 757-3500

Welkind Rehabilitation Hospital
Pleasant Hill Rd.
Chester, NJ 07930
(201) 584-8145

Daughters of Miriam Center for the Aged
155 Hazel St.
Clifton, NJ 07015
(201) 772-3700

Kessler Institute for Rehabilitation
240 Central Ave.
East Orange, NJ 07018
(201) 673-1860

Robert Wood Johnson, Jr., Rehabilitation
    Institute
John F. Kennedy Medical Center
James St.
Edison, NJ 08818
(201) 321-7050

St. Lawrence Rehabilitation Center
PO Box 6367
Lawrenceville, NJ 08648
(609) 896-9500

Children's Specialized Hospital
150 New Providence Rd.
Mountainside, NJ 07091
(201) 233-3720

Rehabilitation Unit
Newton Memorial Hospital
175 High St.
Newton, NJ 07860
(201) 383-2121

Betty Bacharach Rehabilitation Hospital#
Jim Leeds Rd.
Pomona, NJ 08240
(609) 652-7000

Merwick Rehabilitation and Extended Care
   Facility
The Medical Center at Princeton
79 Bayard Lane
Princeton, NJ 08540
(609) 921-7700

Riverview Medical Center Rehabilitation Unit
35 Union St.
Red Bank, NJ 07701
(201) 741-2700

Garden State Rehabilitation Hospital
14 Hospital Drive
Toms River, NJ 08753
(201) 244-3100

Kessler Institute for Rehabilitation*
1199 Pleasant Valley Way
West Orange, NJ 07052
(201) 731-3600

Theresa Grotta Center for Rehabilitation
20 Summit St.
West Orange, NJ 07052
(201) 736-2000

NEW MEXICO
New Mexico Rehabilitation Center
"D" at E. Eyman, R.I.A.C.
Roswell, NM 88201
(505) 347-5491

NEW YORK
Kingsbrook Jewish Medical Center
585 Schenectady Ave.
Brooklyn, NY 11203
(718) 604-5000

Department of Rehabilitation Medicine
Harlem Hospital Center
506 Lenox Ave.
New York, NY 10037
(212) 491-1534

Institute of Rehabilitation Medicine
New York University Medical Center
400 E. 34th St.
New York, NY 10016
(212) 340-6200

Sunnyview Hospital and Rehabilitation Center#
1270 Belmont Ave.
Schenectady, NY 12308
(518) 382-4500

Helen Hayes Hospital
Route 9W
West Haverstraw, NY 10993
(914) 947-3000

NORTH CAROLINA
Thoms Rehabilitation Hospital, Inc.
One Rotary Drive
Asheville, NC 28803
(704) 274-2400

Charlotte Rehabilitation Hospital
1100 Blythe Blvd.
Charlotte, NC 28203
(704) 333-6634

Southeastern Regional Rehabilitation Center
Cape Fear Valley Medical Center
PO Box 2000
Fayetteville, NC 28302
(919) 323-6088

Regional Rehabilitation Center
Pitt County Memorial Hospital, Inc.
PO Box 6028
Greenville, NC 27834
(919) 757-4400

John C. Whitaker Regional Rehabilitation
   Center
3333 Silas Creek Parkway
Winston-Salem, NC 27103
(919) 773-3780

NORTH DAKOTA
Medical Center Rehabilitation Hospital
University of North Dakota
PO Box 8202, University Station
Grand Forks, ND 58202
(701) 772-8141

OHIO
Edwin Shaw Hospital
1621 Flickinger Rd.
Akron, OH 44312
(216) 784-1271

Bethesda Hospital
·Physical Rehabilitation Center
619 Oak St.
Cincinnati, OH 45206
(513) 569-6087

The Daniel Drake Memorial Hospital
151 W. Galbraith Rd.
Cincinnati, OH 45216
(513) 761-3440

Cleveland Metropolitan General Hospital/
  Highland View Hospital*
3395 Scranton Rd.
Cleveland, OH 44109
(216) 398-6000

Ohio State University Hospital*#
472 W. 8th Ave.
Columbus, OH 43210
(614) 422-5547

St. Elizabeth Rehabilitation Center
601 Edwin C. Moses Blvd., W.
Dayton, OH 45408
(513) 229-6000

Rehabilitation Unit
Euclid General Hospital
101 E. 185th St.
Euclid, OH 44119
(216) 531-9000

St. Francis Rehabilitation Hospital and Nursing
401 N. Broadway St.
Green Springs, OH 44836
(419) 639-2626

Great Lakes Rehabilitation Center of Lorain
  Community Hospital
3700 Kolbe Rd.
Lorain, OH 44053
(216) 282-9121

Comprehensive Rehabilitation Center
Medical College of Ohio Hospital
C. S. #10008
Toledo, OH 43614
(419) 381-3410

Hillside Hospital
8747 Squires Lane, N.E.
Warren, OH 44484
(216) 841-3721

Good Samaritan Medical Center and
  Rehabilitation Center*#
800 Forest Ave.
Zanesville, OH 43701
(614) 454-5469

OKLAHOMA
O'Donoghue Rehabilitation Institute
PO Box 26307
Oklahoma City, OK 73126
(405) 271-6955

Tulsa Rehabilitation Center
1120 S. Utica
Tulsa, OK 74104
(918) 584-1351

OREGON
Rehab Action Center
Sacred Heart General Hospital
Box 10905
Eugene, OR 97440
(503) 686-6862

Southern Oregon Rehabilitation Center
Providence Hospital
1111 Crater Lake Ave.
Medford, OR 97501
(503) 773-6611

Emmanuel Rehabilitation Center*#
3001 N. Gantenbein
Portland, OR 97229
(503) 280-4400

Rehabilitation Institute of Oregon
Good Samaritan Hospital and Medical Center
2010 N.W. Kearney St.
Portland, OR 97209
(503) 229-7151

PENNSYLVANIA
Good Shepherd Rehabilitation Hospital
Good Shepherd Workshop/Vocational Services
Sixth and St. John Sts.
Allentown, PA 18103
(215) 821-2121

Rehab Hospital for Special Services of Nittany
  Valley
R.D. #5, Box 451-A
Bellefonte, PA 16823
(814) 359-3421

Elizabethtown Hospital and Rehabilitation
  Center of the Pennsylvania State University*
Elizabethtown, PA 17022-0710
(717) 367-1161

Saint Vincent Rehabilitation Center
232 W. 25th St.
Erie, PA 16544
(814) 459-4000

Hiram G. Andrews Center
727 Goucher St.
Johnstown, PA 15905
(814) 255-5881

St. Joseph Hospital and Health Care Center
250 College Ave., Box 3509
Lancaster, PA 17604
(717) 291-8221

Bryn Mawr Rehabilitation Hospital
414 Paoli Pike
Malvern, PA 19355
(215) 647-3150

Rehab Hospital for Special Services
4950 Wilson Lane
Mechanicsburg, PA 17055
(717) 697-8211

Sacred Heart Hospital and Rehabilitation
  Center
1430 DeKalb St.
Norristown, PA 19401
(215) 275-4000

Department of Rehabilitation Medicine*
Thomas Jefferson University Hospital
Suite 9604, New Hospital
111 S. 11th St.
Philadelphia, PA 19107
(215) 928-6573

Magee Rehabilitation Hospital*#
Six Franklin Plaza
Philadelphia, PA 19102
(215) 864-7100

Moss Rehabilitation Hospital
12th St. & Tabor Rd.
Philadelphia, PA 19141
(215) 329-5715

Piersol Rehabilitation Center
Physical Medicine and Rehabilitation
  Department
Hospital of the University of Pennsylvania
3400 Spruce St.
Philadelphia, PA 19104
(215) 662-3242

The Rehabilitation Institute of Pittsburgh
6301 Northumberland St.
Pittsburgh, PA 15217
(412) 521-9000

St. Francis Medical Center
Department of Rehabilitation Medicine
45th St.
Pittsburgh, PA 15201
(412) 622-4212

Allied Services for the Handicapped, Inc.
PO Box 1103
Scranton, PA 18501
(717) 346-8411

D. T. Watson Rehabilitation Hospital
Camp Meeting Rd.
Sewickley, PA 15143
(412) 741-9500

Harry R. Gibson Rehabilitation Center
The Williamsport Hospital
777 Rural Ave.
Williamsport, PA 17701
(717) 321-1000

All Saints' Rehabilitation Hospital
8601 Stenton Ave.
Wyndmoor, PA 19118
(215) 248-4700

Rehab Hospital for Special Services of York
1850 Normandie Drive
York, PA 17404
(717) 767-6941

RHODE ISLAND
Vanderbilt Rehabilitation Center
Friendship St.
Newport, RI 02840
(401) 846-6400

SOUTH CAROLINA
Roger C. Peace Rehabilitation Hospital#
Greenville Hospital Center
701 Grove Rd.
Greenville, SC 29605
(803) 242-7703

TENNESSEE
Patricia Neal Rehabilitation Center*
Fort Sanders Regional Medical Center
1901 Clinch Ave., S.W.
Knoxville, TN 37916
(615) 971-1408

Baptist Memorial Hospital*#
Regional Rehabilitation Center
1025 E. H. Crump Blvd.
Memphis, TN 38104
(901) 522-6550

St. Joseph Rehabilitation Center
PO Box 178
Memphis, TN 38101-0178
(901) 529-2962

TEXAS
Baylor Institute for Rehabilitation
3504 Swiss Ave.
Dallas, TX 75204
(214) 826-7030

Dallas Rehabilitation Institute
9713 Harry Hines Blvd.
Dallas, TX 75220
(214) 358-6000

Harris Hospital–Methodist Rehabilitation Unit
1301 Pennsylvania Ave.
Fort Worth, TX 76104
(817) 334-6011

St. Joseph Hospital Rehabilitation Services
1401 S. Main St.
Fort Worth, TX 76104
(817) 336-9371

The Institute for Rehabilitation and Research*
1333 Moursund St.
Houston, TX 77030
(713) 797-1440

Medical Center Del Oro Hospital
8081 Greenbriar
Houston, TX 77054
(713) 790-8371

UTAH
Stewart Rehabilitation Center
McKay-Dee Hospital
3939 Harrison Blvd.
Ogden, UT 84409
(801) 625-2090

Rehabilitation Unit
Holy Cross Hospital
1045 E. First, S.
Salt Lake City, UT 84102
(801) 350-4111

University of Utah Health Sciences Center*
Rehabilitation Center
50 N. Medical Drive
Salt Lake City, UT 84132
(801) 581-2267

VIRGINIA
Woodrow Wilson Rehabilitation Center*
Fishersville, VA 22939
(703) 885-9600

Portsmouth General Hospital
RehabCare Unit
850 Crawford Parkway
Portsmouth, VA 23704
(804) 398-4000

WASHINGTON
Providence Hospital Center for Rehabilitation
PO Box 1067
Everett, WA 98206
(206) 258-7546

Good Samaritan Hospital and Rehabilitation
  Center
407 14th Ave., S.E.
Puyallup, WA 98371
(206) 848-6661

Physical Medicine and Rehabilitation
  Department
Sacred Heart Medical Center
W. 101-Eighth Ave. TAF-C9
Spokane, WA 99220
(509) 455-3040

Rehabilitation Department#
St. Joseph Hospital and Health Care Center
PO Box 2197
Tacoma, WA 98405
(206) 627-4101

St. Mary Medical Center
401 W. Poplar Ave.
Walla Walla, WA 99362-0312
(509) 525-3320

WEST VIRGINIA
West Virginia Rehabilitation Center
Institute, WV 25112
(304) 768-8861

Peterson Hospital
Ohio Valley Medical Center
2000 Eoff St.
Wheeling, WV 26003
(304) 234-8273

WISCONSIN
St. Elizabeth Hospital Rehabilitation Unit
1506 S. Oneida St.
Appleton, WI 54911
(414) 731-5261

L. E. Phillips Rehabilitation Unit
Sacred Heart Hospital
900 W. Clairemont Ave.
Eau Claire, WI 54701
(715) 839-4121

Neuro Rehabilitation Unit
St. Agnes Hospital
430 E. Division
Fond du Lac, WI 54935
(414) 929-1394

La Crosse Lutheran Hospital
Rehabilitation Program
1910 South Ave.
La Crosse, WI 54601
(608) 785-0530

Department of Physical Medicine and
　Rehabilitation
Madison General Hospital
202 S. Park St.
Madison, WI 53715
(608) 267-6175

Rehabilitation Center
University of Wisconsin Hospital and Clinics
600 Highland Ave.
Madison, WI 53792
(608) 263-8640

Rehabilitation Unit
St. Joseph's Hospital
611 Saint Joseph Ave.
Marshfield, WI 54449
(715) 387-1713

Department of Physical Medicine and
　Rehabilitation
St. Luke's Hospital
2900 W. Oklahoma Ave.
Milwaukee, WI 53215
(414) 649-6261

Sacred Heart Rehabilitation Hospital*
1545 S. Layton Blvd.
Milwaukee, WI 53215
(414) 383-4490

Department of Physical Rehabilitation
Theda Clark Regional Medical Center
130 Second St.
Neenah, WI 54956
(414) 729-3100

Neurological Rehabilitation Program
Mercy Medical Center
631 Hazel St.
Oshkosh, WI 54901
(414) 236-2230

SOURCE: *Commission on Accreditation of Rehabilitation Facilities.*

SOME LEADING BRAIN-INJURY CENTERS

Some centers have established programs specifically for rehabilitating people with brain injuries. The programs are generally geared toward people with brain injuries from traumas, such as automobile accidents, not from degenerative brain diseases. Here are the comprehensive brain-injury centers accredited by the Commission on Accreditation of Rehabilitation Facilities.

CALIFORNIA
Rancho Los Amigos Medical Center
7601 E. Imperial Highway
Downey, CA 90242
(213) 923-7022

COLORADO
Capron Rehabilitation Center
Penrose Hospital
PO Box 7021
Colorado Springs, CO 80933
(303) 630-5200

Hilltop Rehabilitation Hospital
1100 Patterson Rd.
Grand Junction, CO 81506
(303) 244-6007

FLORIDA
Memorial Regional Rehabilitation Center
3599 University Blvd., S.
Jacksonville, FL 32216
(904) 355-1761

Rehabilitation Institute of West Florida
PO Box 18900
Pensacola, FL 32523-8900
(904) 474-5358

KENTUCKY
Cardinal Hill Hospital
2050 Versailles Rd.
Lexington, KY 40504
(606) 254-5701

LOUISIANA
Rehabilitation Institute of New Orleans
F. Edward Hebert Hospital
#1 Sanctuary Drive
New Orleans, LA 70114
(504) 363-2691

MASSACHUSETTS
Greenery Rehabilitation and Skilled Nursing
    Center
99 Chestnut Hill Ave.
Boston, MA 02135
(617) 787-3390

Joseph P. Kennedy, Jr. Memorial Hospital
30 Warren St.
Brighton, MA 02135
(617) 254-3800

MINNESOTA
Knapp Rehabilitation Center
900 S. Eighth St.
Minneapolis, MN 55404
(612) 347-3780

NEW YORK
Sunnyview Hospital and Rehabilitation Center
1270 Belmont Ave.
Schenectady, NY 12308
(518) 382-4500

OHIO
St. Elizabeth Rehabilitation Center
601 Edwin C. Moses Blvd., W.
Dayton, OH 45408
(513) 229-6000

PENNSYLVANIA
Lake Erie Institute of Rehabilitation
137 W. Second St.
Erie, PA 16507
(814) 453-5602

Bryn Mawr Rehabilitation Hospital
414 Paoli Pike
Malvern, PA 19355
(215) 647-3150

Magee Rehabilitation Hospital
Six Franklin Plaza
Philadelphia, PA 19102
(215) 864-7100

SOURCE: *Commission on Accreditation of Rehabilitation Facilities.*

GOVERNMENT REHABILITATION RESEARCH AND TRAINING CENTERS

The federal government, through the National Institute of Handicapped Research, supports 12 centers for special research on physical rehabilitation. These centers not only help find the latest successful techniques for rehabilitation in their areas of interest but are also committed to disseminating the latest findings to the rest of the medical community and to the general public.

Such centers accept selected patients for treatment and research. The directors and staffs of the centers are considered leading authorities in their areas of rehabilitation and may be available for consultations, although, in the strictest sense, the research and training centers are not treatment centers.

ALABAMA

University of Alabama
Department of Rehabilitation Medicine
University Station
Birmingham, AL 35294
Samuel Stover, M.D.
Project Director
Special interest: Spinal cord dysfunction

CALIFORNIA

University of California Davis
Office of Research
275 Mrak Hall
Davis, CA 95616
William J. Fowler, Jr., M.D.
Project Director
(916) 752-2903
Special interest: Management of neuromuscular
  disease problems, including multiple
  sclerosis

Rancho Los Amigos Hospital
7413 Golondrinas St.
Downey, CA 90242
Bryan Kemp, Ph.D.
Project Director
(213) 922-7402
Special interest: Aging disabilities

COLORADO

University of Colorado
Health Sciences Center
4200 E. Ninth Ave.
Box C242
Denver, CO 80262
Lawrence D. Horwitz, M.D.
Project Director
(303) 394-5144
Special interest: Cardiac rehabilitation

GEORGIA

Emory University
School of Medicine
1441 Clifton Rd., N.E.
Atlanta, GA 30322
Bridgetta Rees, M.D.
Acting Project Director
(404) 329-5583
Special interest: Head injury and stroke victims

ILLINOIS

Northwestern University
Department of Rehabilitation Medicine
633 Clark St.
Evanston, IL 60201
Henry B. Betts, M.D.
Project Director
(312) 649-6017
Special interest: Brain injury and stroke

MASSACHUSETTS

Tufts—New England Medical Center, Inc.
Department of Rehabilitation Medicine
171 Harrison Ave.
Boston, MA 02111
Bruce Gans, M.D.
Project Director
(617) 955-5622
Special interest: Musculoskeletal disorders in
  children and adults, including arthritis

NEW YORK

New York University Medical Center
School of Medicine
550 First Ave.
New York, NY 10016
Leonard Diller, Ph.D.
(212) 340-6161
Special interest: Brain injury and stroke
Joseph Goodgold, M.D.
(212) 340-6105
Special interest: Management of neuromuscular
  disease, including multiple sclerosis

Yeshiva University/Einstein College of
  Medicine
Multiple Sclerosis Comprehensive Care Center
1300 Morris Park Ave.
New York, NY 10461
Labe C. Scheinberg, M.D.
(212) 430-2682
Special interest: Multiple sclerosis

TEXAS

Baylor College of Medicine
Department of Rehabilitation
1200 Moursund Ave.
Houston, TX 77030
Marcus Fuhrer, Ph.D.
Project Director
(713) 797-1440, x477
Special interest: Spinal cord dysfunction

VIRGINIA
University of Virginia Medical Center
Department of Orthopedics and Rehabilitation
Box 159, UVA Medical Center
Charlottesville, VA 22908
Robert McLaughlin, M.D.
(804) 924-5506
Special interest: Musculoskeletal arthritis and
   low back problems, including development
   of artificial joints

WASHINGTON
University of Washington
Department of Rehabilitation Medicine
BB919 Health Sciences Building
Seattle, WA 98195
Justus Lehmann, M.D.
Project Director
(206) 543-3600
Special interest: Brain trauma and stroke

SOURCE: *National Institute of Handicapped Research.*

REHABILITATION ENGINEERING CENTERS (RECs)

The federal government through the National Institute of Handicapped Research supports Rehabilitation Engineering Centers (RECs) that work with the handicapped in developing and applying technological advances.

CALIFORNIA
Rancho Los Amigos Hospital
Rehabilitation Engineering Center
7413 Golondrinas St.
Downey, CA 90242
(213) 922-7167
Donald McNeal, Ph.D.
Functional electrical stimulation

Smith-Kettelwell Institute of Visual Sciences
2200 Webster St.
San Francisco, CA 94115
(415) 563-2323
Arthur Jampolsky, M.D.
Sensory aids for blind and deaf individuals

DISTRICT OF COLUMBIA
Electronic Industries Foundation
1901 Pennsylvania Ave., N.W., Suite 700
Washington, DC 20006
(202) 955-5823
Lawrence Scadden, Ph.D.
Evaluation of technology

ILLINOIS
Northwestern University
Regional Engineering Center
633 Clark St.
Evanston, IL 60201
(312) 649-8560
Dudley Childress, Ph.D.
Prosthetics and orthotics

MASSACHUSETTS
Harvard-MIT
Children's Hospital
Medical Center
300 Longwood Ave.
Boston, MA 02115
(617) 735-6594
William Berenberg, M.D.
Quantification of human performance

Tufts-New England Medical Center
Department of Rehabilitation Medicine
171 Harrison Ave.
Boston, MA 02111
(617) 956-5031, 5625
Rick Foulds, Ph.D.
Nonvocal communication systems

MINNESOTA
University of Minnesota
Department of Physical Medicine and
   Rehabilitation
1919 University Ave.
St. Paul, MN 55455
(612) 373-8990
G. Gullickson, M.D.
Quantification of human performance

NEW YORK
The Lexington Center, Inc.
20th Ave. and 75th St.
Jackson Heights, NY 11370
(718) 899-8800
Alan Lerman, Ph.D.
New generation hearing aids

TEXAS
Dallas Rehabilitation Foundation
7850 Brookline Rd.
Dallas, TX 76235
(817) 273-2249 or (214) 637-0740
Raymond Dabney, Alfred R. Potvin
Quantification of human performance

Southwest Research Institute
Electronic Systems Division
PO Drawer 28510
6220 Culebra Rd.
San Antonio, TX 78284
(512) 684-5111
Dennis Gilstead, M.D., Ph.D.
Evaluation of technology

VERMONT
University of Vermont
Department of Orthopedics and Rehabilitation
College of Medicine
Burlington, VT 05405
(802) 656-4067
John W. Frymoyer, M.D.
Low back pain

VIRGINIA
University of Virginia Medical Center
Department of Orthopedics and Rehabilitation
PO Box 159/UVA
Charlottesville, VA 22908
(804) 977-6730
Colin McLaurin, Ph.D., Warren Stamp, M.D.
Wheelchair systems and specialized seating

WISCONSIN
University of Wisconsin
750 University Ave.
Madison, WI 53706
(608) 262-6966
Greg Vanderheiden, Ph.D.
Communication, control, and information
  processing systems

SOURCE: *National Institute of Handicapped Research.*

SPECIAL PRODUCTS FOR HANDICAPPED PERSONS

The following companies are major suppliers of a variety of devices and equipment designed especially for handicapped persons. These products include special walking, grooming, hygiene, homemaking, eating, and driving aids; for example, long-handled toothbrushes, suction eating plates, no-tip glasses, extension arms to pick up items, lifting devices, and ramps for wheelchairs. You can contact the companies listed below for more information or free catalogues.

Abbey Medical Catalogue Sales
933 E. Sandhill Ave.
Carson, CA 90746
(800) 421-5126
(800) 262-1294—California
(213) 538-5551—Los Angeles

Everest and Jennings, Inc.
1803 S. Pontius Ave.
Los Angeles, CA 90025
(800) 235-4661
(213) 479-4141

Fred Sammons, Inc.
PO Box 32
Brookfield, IL 60513
(800) 323-7305

J. A. Preston Corporation
60 Page Rd.
Clifton, NJ 07012
(800) 631-7277
(201) 777-2700—New Jersey

G. E. Miller, Inc.
484 S. Broadway
Yonkers, NY 10705
(800) 431-2924

Cleo Living Aids
3957 Mayfield Rd.
Cleveland, OH 44121
(800) 321-0595
(800) 222-2536—Ohio

Prentke Romich Company
R.D. 2, Box 191
Shreve, OH 44676
(216) 567-2001

Sears, Roebuck & Co.
Sears' Health and Convalescent Book
4640 Roosevelt Blvd.
Philadelphia, PA 19132
(215) 831-4000

Miles Kimball Co.
41 W. Eighth Ave.
Oshkosh, WI 54901
(414) 231-3800

SERVICES FOR THE HANDICAPPED

Computerized product information

ABLEDATA System
National Rehabilitation Center
4407 Eighth St., N.E.
Washington, DC 20017
(202) 635-6090

ABLEDATA System is a computerized information database, listing more than 8,000 commercially available aids and equipment for the handicapped. Will search for and print out product sources for a small fee.

Lifeline

Lifeline is the personal emergency response system, which automatically calls the local hospital when a person urgently needs help at home. Clients push a portable button they wear to summon help, or an automatic timer will notify the hospital that the individual has been inactive for a period of time and may need help. The cost of Lifeline averages $10 a month. To learn whether Lifeline is offered by a hospital near you, or for information on how to start a Lifeline program, write to:

Dr. Susan Dibner
Lifeline Systems, Inc.
400 Main St.
Waltham, MA 02254

Wheelchair exercise program

Wheelchair Workout, a 30-minute upper-body exercise program that can be done from a wheelchair or a sturdy chair, on audiocassette tape with illustrated manual. Mail order from Wheelchair Workout, 12275 Greenleaf Ave., Potomac, MD 20854. For more information call (301) 279-2994.

SPORTS ORGANIZATIONS FOR DISABLED PERSONS

CALIFORNIA
National Amputee Golf Association
5711 Yearling Court
Bonita, CA 92002
(619) 479-4578

National Foundation of Wheelchair Tennis
15441 Red Hill Ave.
Tustin, CA 92680
(714) 259-1531

Wheelchair Tennis Players Association
15441 Red Hill Ave.
Tustin, CA 92680
(714) 259-1531

Blind Sports
1939-16th Ave.
San Francisco, CA 94116
(415) 681-1939

COLORADO

Blind Outdoor Leisure Development (BOLD)
533 E. Main St.
Aspen, CO 81611
(303) 925-8922

National Archery Association
1750 E. Boulder St.
Colorado Springs, CO 80909
(303) 578-4576

National Wheelchair Athletic Association
2107 Templeton Gap Rd.
Suite C
Colorado Springs, CO 80907
(303) 632-0698

National Deaf Bowling Association
9244 E. Mansfield Ave.
Denver, CO 80237
(303) 771-9018

DISTRICT OF COLUMBIA

International Committee of Sports for the Deaf
Gallaudet College
800 Florida Ave., N.E.
Washington, DC 20002
(202) 651-5430 (voice/TDD)

National Handicapped Sports and Recreation
  Association
Farragut Station
PO Box 33141
Washington, DC 20033
(202) 429-0595

Special Olympics
1350 New York Ave., N.W.
Suite 500
Washington, DC 20005-4709
(202) 628-3630

ILLINOIS

American Blind Skiing Foundation
610 S. William St.
Mount Prospect, IL 60056
(312) 253-4292

KENTUCKY

National Wheelchair Basketball Association
110 Seaton Center
University of Kentucky
Lexington, KY 40506
(606) 257-1623

MASSACHUSETTS

Wheelchair Motorcycle Association, Inc.
101 Torrey St.
Brockton, MA 02401
(617) 583-8614

MINNESOTA

Voyageur Outward Bound School
PO Box 250
Long Lake, MN 55356
(612) 473-5476
(800) 328-2943 (outside Minnesota)

Vinland National Center
PO Box 308
3675 Ihduhapi Rd.
Loretto, MN 55357
(612) 479-3555

Ski for Light, Inc.
1455 W. Lake St.
Minneapolis, MN 55408
(612) 827-3232

MISSOURI

American Athletic Association for the Deaf
10604 E. 95th St. Terrace
Kansas City, MO 64134

NEW JERSEY

U.S. Association for Blind Athletes
55 W. California Ave.
Beach Haven Park, NJ 08008
(609) 492-1017

United States Deaf Skiers Association
159 Davis Ave.
Hackensack, NJ 07601
(201) 489-3777

NEW YORK

United States Wheelchair Sports Fund
1550 Franklin Ave.
Suite 29
Mineola, NY 11501
(516) 294-7610

Handicapped Boaters Association
PO Box 1134, Ansonia Station
New York, NY 10023
(212) 877-0310

National Association of Sports for Cerebral
  Palsied
c/o Craig Huber
66 E. 34th St.
New York, NY 10016
(212) 481-6359

OHIO
Indoor Sports Club
1145 Highland St.
Napoleon, OH 43545
(419) 592-5756

PENNSYLVANIA
National Foundation for Happy Horsemanship
  for the Handicapped, Inc.
PO Box 462
Malvern, PA 19355
(215) 644-7414

SOUTH DAKOTA
National Wheelchair Softball Association
PO Box 737
Sioux Falls, SD 57101
(605) 334-0000

VIRGINIA
American Blind Bowling Association, Inc.
3500 Terry Drive
Norfolk, VA 23518
(804) 857-7267

North American Riding for the Handicapped
  Association, Inc.
PO Box 100
Ashburn, VA 22011
(703) 471-1621

WISCONSIN
American Wheelchair Bowling Association
N54 W. 15858 Larkspur Lane
Menomonee Falls, WI 53051
(414) 781-6876

SOURCE: *Clearinghouse for the Handicapped.*

ORGANIZATIONS

Information Center for Individuals with
  Disabilities
20 Park Plaza, Room 330
Boston, MA 02116
(617) 727-5540 (voice)
(617) 727-5236 (TTV)
(800) 462-5015 (Massachusetts only)

A self-help information source for those with
disabilities and their families. Has information
on federal, state, public and private agencies
that assist the handicapped, and on such subjects
as architectural accessibility, recreation, travel
and personal care. Answers questions from the
public. Will provide more information upon request.

National Amputation Foundation
12-45 150th St.
Whitestone, NY 11357
(718) 767-0596

A national charitable, nonprofit organization
founded to assist amputee war veterans which

now serves both veteran and civilian amputees.
Services include legal counsel, vocational guidance, training in use of prosthetic devices. Has
an "Amp to Amp" program, where members
of the organization visit new amputees. Has
Prosthetic Care Center where artificial limbs are
fabricated and repaired. Active mostly in New
York area. Publishes numerous booklets, leaflets
and brochures. Will provide more information
upon request.

National Easter Seal Society, Inc.
2023 W. Ogden Ave.
Chicago, IL 60612
(312) 243-8400 (voice)
(312) 243-8880 (TDD)

A national organization with state and local societies providing services to people with disabilities from any cause, including epilepsy, cerebral
palsy, stroke, speech and hearing disorders, geriatric problems, fractures, arthritis, learning and
developmental disorders, heart disease, spina bifida, accidents, multiple sclerosis. Maintains

about 200 rehabilitation centers nationwide, with various services depending on the local unit. A major source of information and self-help. Publishes pamphlets and booklets. Referrals to services are made through local Easter Seal affiliates listed in local phone directories. Will provide more information and location of Easter Seal affiliate near you upon request.

National Institute for Rehabilitation
  Engineering
97 Decker Rd.
Butler, NJ 07405
(201) 838-2500

A nonprofit service, equipment evaluation, and training organization that will custom-design and custom-make devices and tools for handicapped persons, and train them in their use. Members include the handicapped, professionals, and other interested persons. Provides services and equipment for both major and minor disabilities. Uses a team of electronics engineers, physicists, psychologists and others to evaluate and design programs to increase a physically handicapped person's abilities and independence. Fees based on a sliding scale of ability to pay. Also gives away reconditioned equipment and clothing to certain handicapped persons who cannot pay.

National Rehabilitation Information Center
  (NARIC)
Catholic University of America
4407 Eighth St., N.E.
Washington, DC 20017
(202) 635-5826 (voice/TDD)
(800) 346-2742 (voice/TDD)

The major national source of information on disabilities from any cause, including amputation, aging, arthritis, brain damage, cardiac disorders, cerebral palsy, epilepsy, neuromuscular disorders, spinal cord injuries, deafness, blindness, mental retardation and learning disabilities. Will do computer searches for bibliographies or special devices and products. Produces ABLE-DATA system, a database of product information for the disabled and Rehabdata, a database of rehabilitation research and literature.

National Therapeutic Recreation Society
3101 Park Center Drive, 12th Floor
Alexandria, VA 22302
(703) 820-4940

A national nonprofit membership organization of therapeutic recreation specialists who work to develop recreational leisure activities for the handicapped. An information source for the public. Will help handicapped find recreational facilities, activities, resources in their area. For more information and the name of a local therapeutic recreational specialist in your area, contact the national organization.

BOOKS

Access: The Guide to a Better Life for Disabled Americans, **Lilly Bruck,** New York: Random House, 1978.

Care of the Older Adult, **Joan Carson Breitung,** New York: Tiresias Press, 1981; 116 Pinehurst Ave., New York, NY 10033.

The Disabled Homemaker, **Hoydt Anderson,** Springfield, IL: Charles C. Thomas, 1981.

Disabled? Yes. Defeated? NO: Resources for the Disabled and their Families, Friends and Therapists, **Kathleen Cruzic,** Englewood Cliffs, NJ: Prentice Hall, 1982.

Dressing with Pride: Clothing Changes for Special Needs, **Evelyn S. Kennedy,** Groton, CT: The PRIDE Foundation, 1981; 1159 Poquonnock Rd., Groton, CT 06340. Shows handicapped and elderly persons how to modify store-bought clothes for special needs.

Frommer's: A Guide for the Disabled Traveler, **Frances Barish,** New York: Simon & Schuster, 1984.

A Handbook for the Disabled: Ideas and Inventions for Easier Living, **S. Lunt,** New York: Scribner's, 1982.

Over 55: A Handbook on Health, **T. G. Duncan,** Philadelphia: Franklin Institute, 1982.

The Source Book for the Disabled, **edited by Glorya Hale,** New York: Paddington Press, 1979.

Technology for Independent Living Sourcebook, **edited by Alexandra Enders,** 1986. Association for the Advancement of Rehabilitation Technology, 1101 Connecticut Ave., Suite 700, Washington, DC 20036; (202) 857-1199.

The Wheelchair Gourmet: A Cookbook for the Disabled, **M. Blakeslee,** New York: Beautfort Books, 1981.

Stroke rehabilitation

About Stroke, **Sister Kenny Institute Staff,** Minneapolis: Sister Mary Kenny Institute, 1978; 38 pages, book-size format.

Communication Problems After a Stroke, **Lillian Kay Cohen,** Minneapolis: Sister Mary Kenny Institute, 1978; 28 pages, book-size format.

Help the Stroke Patient to Talk, **Marie C. Crickmay,** Springfield, IL: Charles C. Thomas, 1977.

Home Care for the Stroke Patient: Living in a Pattern, **Margaret Johnstone,** New York: Churchill Livingstone, 1980.

Speech After Stroke, **Stephanie Stryker,** Springfield, IL: Charles C. Thomas, 1981; a manual of drills.

Speech and Language Rehabilitation: A Workbook for the Neurologically Impaired and Language Delayed, **Robert L. Keith,** Danville, IL: Interstate Printers and Publishers, 1980; 19 N. Jackson, Danville, IL 61831.

Sourcebook for Aphasia: A Guide to Family Activities and Community Resources, Detroit: Wayne State University Press, 1982.

Stroke: A Doctor's Personal Story of Recovery, **Charles Clay Dahlberg** and **Joseph Jaffe,** New York: W. W. Norton, 1977.

Stroke: How to Prevent It/How to Survive It, **Gloria Jen Sessler,** Englewood Cliffs, NJ: Prentice-Hall, 1981.

Stroke: The New Hope and the New Help, **Arthur S. Freese,** New York: Random House, 1980.

MATERIALS, FREE AND FOR SALE

Free (single copies)

Are You Listening to What Your Child May Not Be Saying

Bicycle Safety Tips

Camps for Children With Disabilities

Points to Remember When You Meet a Person With a Disability

A Speech Pathologist Talks to the Parents of a Nonverbal Child

National Easter Seal Society
2023 W. Ogden Ave.
Chicago, IL 60612

For sale

Choosing and Using a Wheelchair, 8 pages.

First Aid for Aphasics, 19 pages.

Handy Helpful Hints for Independent Living After Stroke, 15 pages.

Organizing a Stroke Club, 16 pages.

Reflections on Managing Disability, 12 pages.

Self-Help Clothing for Children Who Have Physical Disabilities, 64 pages.

Using Everything You've Got, 12 pages.

National Easter Seal Society
2023 W. Ogden Ave.
Chicago, IL 60612

Handbook for Lower Extremity Amputees
A Manual for Below-Knee Amputees
Prosthetic Yes . . . Bionics Maybe
Things to Know About Amputation and
* Artificial Limbs*

National Amputation Foundation
12-45 150th St.
Whitestone, NY 11357

Adaptations and Techniques for the Disabled
* Homemaker*

Sister Kenny Institute
811 E. 27th St.
Minneapolis, MN 55407

SEXUAL DYSFUNCTION

Sexual dysfunction may stem from physical or emotional causes, or, especially in men, from a combination of both. The most common types of sexual problems are impotence, premature ejaculation, retarded ejaculation, anorgasmia (failure to achieve orgasm), vaginismus (a painful constriction of vaginal muscles that may prevent intercourse), and lack of desire.

If the problem is simple and straightforward, a family physician can often handle it—sometimes through elementary sex counseling and understanding. But if the problem persists or has complex psychological and physical underpinnings, it is best treated at a specialized sexual dysfunction clinic. Also, in cases of impotence, a urologist may be needed to determine if the cause is physical.

Female sexual dysfunction is usually regarded as a psychological problem and treated by behavior modification and group or individual psychotherapy. However, a woman's failure to achieve orgasm may also stem from physical problems, such as endometriosis and pelvic inflammatory disease, resulting in pain and discomfort during intercourse. In such cases, medical attention is needed to correct the underlying disease.

In the past, male sexual dysfunction also was considered to be 90–95 percent psychologically induced and amenable to psychotherapy; however, there has been a striking reversal of thinking about impotence. Although sex therapy pioneers Masters and Johnson still maintain that 80–85 percent of the cases of impotence are psychogenic, some experts now say that from 30 to 60 percent of the 10 million cases of impotence in the United States have physical causes. Recent studies link impotence to abnormalities

in the blood flow to the penis, hormonal abnormalities, such as low levels of testosterone (the male sex hormone), diseases such as diabetes, pituitary tumors, multiple sclerosis, atherosclerosis, neurological conditions, pharmaceutical drugs (notably drugs to combat high blood pressure and heart disease), and alcoholism.

Thus, many men complaining of impotence are now given a battery of diagnostic tests to determine if there is a physical cause. Such tests might include vascular measurements to determine blood flow to the penis, X-rays to reveal blockages and other abnormalities in the penis, hormone measurements (especially testosterone), and nocturnal penile tumescence tests (NPT) in sleep labs. Men usually have three to five erections a night during sleep. Laboratory monitoring during sleep can reveal whether nocturnal erections occur; if they do not this is evidence, but not proof, that the problem is physical. Such tests can identify possibly correctable organic causes before the man resorts to sex therapy. One surprising study at Boston's Beth Israel Hospital found that 35 percent of impotent men had low levels of testosterone, and nearly all of them regained potency after the deficiency was corrected. Some men with atherosclerosis regain potency after receiving drugs to increase blood flow. Men with high blood pressure may solve the problem by switching medications.

In perhaps half of the cases, emotions are at fault, and even men with clear physical problems may also need psychotherapy. According to one study, one-third of the impotent diabetic men tested regained potency after psychological therapy.

An increasingly popular way to correct impotence is with a penis implant, now used by about 30,000 men. One sophisticated device can be inflated by a tiny pump to achieve an erection. The device is entirely implanted in the body and cannot be seen; the man can inflate and deflate the penis at will by applying pressure to the scrotum. Men using the devices can often achieve ejaculation and impregnation. Many urologists now perform such surgical implants with dramatic success.

For more information on penis implants and a list of urologic surgeons who frequently perform the procedure, you can contact:

American Medical Systems
Consumer Information Department
PO Box 9
Minneapolis, MN 55440
(612) 933-4666

WHERE TO FIND HELP FOR SEXUAL DYSFUNCTION

Many of the best sexual dysfunction centers are connected with major hospitals and universities. They are not the only excellent clinics, but are among them and are sure to have personnel with excellent credentials and training. Here are some leading medical center- or hospital-based sexual dysfunction clinics. The list was compiled by *Sexual Medicine Today,* a magazine for physicians. Additionally, you can find certified therapists through the American Association of Sex Educators, Counselors, and Therapists, 11 Dupont Circle, N.W., Suite 220, Washington, DC 20036.

SOME LEADING SEXUAL DYSFUNCTION CLINICS

ALABAMA
University of Alabama at Birmingham
Marital Health Studies
Department of Psychiatry
Birmingham, AL 35294
(205) 934-2350
Director: Robert Travis, Ph.D.

ARIZONA
University of Arizona
College of Medicine
Sexual Problem Evaluation and Treatment
  Clinic
1501 N. Campbell Ave.
Tucson, AZ 85724
(602) 626-6323
Codirectors: Diane S. Fordney, M.D., M.S.,
  Peter Attarian, Ph.D.

ARKANSAS
University of Arkansas for Medical Sciences
Human Sexuality Clinic
4301 W. Markham
Slot 568
Little Rock, AR 72205
(501) 661-5900
Director: Kay Lewallen, R.N., M.S.

CALIFORNIA
The Impotency Treatment Center
3010 W. Orange, Suite 409
Anaheim, CA 92804
(714) 827-1232
and:
1211 W. La Palma Ave.
Suite 302
Anaheim, CA 92810
(714) 776-1004
Director: Daniel M. Riesenberg, M.D.

Center for Marital and Sexual Studies
5251 Los Altos Plaza
Long Beach, CA 90815
(213) 597-4425
Codirectors: William E. Hartman, Ph.D.,
  Marilyn A. Fithian, B.A.

University of California, Los Angeles School
  of Medicine
Human Sexuality Program
760 Westwood Plaza
PO Box 4
Los Angeles, CA 90024
(213) 825-0243
Codirectors: Joshua S. Golden, M.D., Lee
  Blackwell, Ph.D., Terri Price, M.A.

University of Southern California School of
  Medicine
Sex Therapy and Marital Counseling Clinic
LAC-USC Medical Center
1937 Hospital Place
Los Angeles, CA 90033
(213) 226-5329
Director: Dennis J. Munjack, M.D.

Casa Colina Hospital for Rehabilitative
  Medicine
Sexuality Clinic
255 E. Bonita Ave.
Pomona, CA 91767
(714) 593-7521
Director: Julie G. Botvin Madorsky, M.D.

University of California Medical Center, San
  Diego Department of Reproductive Medicine
Gender Dysphoria Team
225 W. Dickinson St.
San Diego, CA 92103
(619) 260-0511
Director: Joseph F. Kennedy, M.D.

University of California School of Medicine at
  San Francisco
Department of Psychiatry
Human Sexuality Program
400 Parnassus A831
San Francisco, CA 94143
(415) 476-4787, 4623
Program Director: Evalyn S. Gendel, M.D.

University of California School of Medicine at
  San Francisco
The Urology—Sexuality Clinic
400 Parnassus Ave.
San Francisco, CA 94143
(415) 476-1146 or 661-1950
Program Director: Tom Lue, M.D.

Stanford University Medical Center
Department of Psychiatry and Behavioral
  Sciences
Behavioral Medicine Clinics
Stanford Medical Center
Stanford, CA 94305
(415) 723-5868
Director: W. Stewart Agras, M.D.

CONNECTICUT
University of Connecticut Health Center
Department of Psychiatry
Sexual Education and Treatment Service
  (SETS)
263 Farmington Ave.
Farmington, CT 06032
(203) 674-2285
Director: Paul D. Reid, A.C.S.W.

Sex Therapy Program
Hartford Hospital
80 Seymour St.
Hartford, CT 06115
(203) 524-2396
Director: Alan J. Wabrek, M.D., Medical
  Sexology
Codirector of Sexual Counseling: Carolyn J.
  Wabrek, M.Ed.

Stamford Hospital Sexual Therapy Clinic
Department of Ob/Gyn
Stamford Center of Human Sexuality
Shelbourne Rd. and W. Broad St.
Stamford, CT 06904
(203) 325-7020
Codirectors: Joseph D. Waxberg, M.D., Stella
  Mostel, M.S.

GEORGIA
Emory University School of Medicine
Department of Gyn/Ob
Emory University Clinic
1365 Clifton Rd.
Atlanta, GA 30322
(404) 321-0111, x3400 or 589-4063
Director: Malcolm G. Freeman, M.D.

ILLINOIS
Cook County Hospital
Social Evaluation Clinic
1825 W. Harrison St.
Chicago, IL 60612
(312) 633-5570
Director: Wanda Sadoughi, Ph.D.

University of Chicago Hospitals and Clinics
Sexual Dysfunction/Marital Therapy Clinic
Department of Psychiatry
Box 411
5841 S. Maryland
Chicago, IL 60637
(312) 962-9703
Attn: Richard Carroll, M.D.

Loyola University of Chicago
Sexual Dysfunction Clinic
2160 S. First Ave.
Maywood, IL 60153
(312) 531-3750

Southern Illinois University
School of Medicine
Department of Ob/Gyn
PO Box 3926
Springfield, IL 62708
(217) 782-8883
Director: Robert P. Johnson, M.D.

IOWA
University of Iowa College of Medicine
The Family Stress Clinic
Department of Family Practice
2033 Steindler Building
Iowa City, IA 52242
(319) 356-4402
Director: Harold Kriesel, Ph.D.
Coordinator: Georgianna S. Hoffman, R.N.,
    M.A.

LOUISIANA
Louisiana State University Medical Center
Sex and Marital Health Clinic
Department of Urology
1542 Tulane Ave.
New Orleans, LA 70112
(504) 568-4890
Director: David M. Schnarch, Ph.D.

MARYLAND
Sexual Behaviors Consultation Unit
550 N. Broadway, Suite 114
Baltimore, MD 21205
(301) 955-6318
Director: Chester Schmidt, M.D.

The Human Behavior Foundation, Ltd.
University Professional Center
4700 Berwyn House Rd., Suite 201
College Park, MD 20740
(301) 345-2323
Director: H.L.P. Resnik, M.D.

MASSACHUSETTS
Boston University School of Medicine,
    University Hospital
New England Male Reproductive Center
720 Harrison Ave., Suite 606
Boston, MA 02118
(617) 638-8485
Director: Robert J. Krane, M.D.

Harvard Medical School, Beth Israel Hospital
Sexual Dysfunction Unit
330 Brookline Ave.
Boston, MA 02215
(617) 735-2168
Director: Joanna Perlmutter, M.D.

Tufts University School of Medicine, New
    England Medical Center Family and Couples
    Institute
171 Harrison Ave.
Boston, MA 02111
(617) 566-7508
Director: Derek Polonsky, M.D.

MICHIGAN
St. Joseph Hospital
Macomb Medical Commons
41570 Hayes
Mount Clemens, MI 48044
(313) 263-9551
Director: Donald Blain, M.D.

MINNESOTA
University of Minnesota Medical School
Department of Family Practice and Community
    Health
Program in Human Sexuality
2630 University Ave., S.E.
Minneapolis, MN 55414
(612) 376-7520
Director: Sharon B. Satterfield, M.D.

MISSOURI
University of Missouri—Columbia School of
    Medicine
Human Sexuality Clinic
Clinic 6, Outpatient
Columbia, MO 65212
(314) 882-2511
Director: Joseph Lamberti, M.D.

Masters & Johnson Institute
24 S. Kingshighway
St. Louis, MO 63108
(314) 361-2377
Chairman: William H. Masters, M.D.
Director: Virginia E. Johnson, D.Sc. (hon)

NEBRASKA
Creighton University School of Medicine
Human Sexuality Program
601 N. 30th St., Suite 5830
Omaha, NE 68131
(402) 280-4325
Director: Emmet M. Kenney, M.D.

NEW JERSEY
University of Medicine and Dentistry of New
    Jersey—Rutgers
Medical School
Sexual Counseling Service
University Heights
Piscataway, NJ 08854
(201) 463-4273, 4485
Director: Sandra Leiblum, Ph.D.

NEW YORK
Albert Einstein College of Medicine
Department of Ob/Gyn
Division of Human Sexuality
1165 Morris Park Ave.
Bronx, NY 10461
(212) 430-2655
Director: Sheila Jackman, Ph.D.

State University of New York
Downstate Medical Center
Center for Human Sexuality
450 Clarkson Ave.
Brooklyn, NY 11203
(718) 270-1750
Codirectors: Marian E. Dunn, Ph.D., Peter
    Dunn, M.D.

Long Island Jewish—Hillside Medical Center
Human Sexuality Center
PO Box 38
Glen Oaks, NY 11004
(718) 470-8208
Director: Herman Oliver, M.D.

North Shore University Hospital
Department of Ob/Gyn
Division of Human Reproduction
Sexual Dysfunction Program
300 Community Drive
Manhasset, NY 11030
(516) 562-4470
Director: Gerald M. Scholl, M.D.

Cornell University Medical College
Human Sexuality Teaching Program
Payne Whitney Clinic
New York Hospital
525 E. 68th St.
New York, NY 10021
(212) 472-6277
Director: Helen Singer Kaplan, M.D., Ph.D.

Helen S. Kaplan Institute for the Evaluation
    and Treatment of Psychosexual Disorders
30 E. 76th St.
New York, NY 10021
(212) 249-2914
Director: Helen Singer Kaplan, M.D., Ph.D.

Jewish Board of Family and Children's
    Services
Sex Therapy Clinic
120 W. 57th St.
New York, NY 10019
(212) 582-9100
Director: Clifford J. Sagar, M.D.

Lenox Hill Hospital
Psychosomatic Clinic
100 E. 77th St.
New York, NY 10021
(212) 794-4840
Program Director: Don Sloan, M.D.

Mount Sinai School of Medicine
Department of Psychiatry
Human Sexuality Program
19 E. 98th St., Room 9A
New York, NY 10019
(212) 650-6634
Director: Raul C. Schiavi, M.D.

New York Medical College
Sex and Marital Therapy Unit
215 E. 73rd St.
New York, NY 10021
(212) 772-8700
Director: Don Sloan, M.D.

New York University Medical Center
Program in Human Sexuality
550 First Ave.
New York, NY 10016
(212) 427-0885
Director: Virginia A. Sadock, M.D.

NORTH CAROLINA
Duke University Medical Center
Sex Therapy and Education Program
PO Box 3263
Durham, NC 27710
(919) 684-5322
Codirectors: John F. Steege, M.D., Anna L.
  Stout, M.D.

Section on Marital & Family Therapy
Bowman Gray School of Medicine
Marital Health Clinic
300 S. Hawthorne Rd.
Winston-Salem, NC 27103
(919) 748-4281
Director: Sallie Schumacher, Ph.D.

OHIO
University of Cincinnati Medical Center
Jewish Hospital
Department of Psychiatry
Human Sexuality Center
3216 Burnet Ave.
Cincinnati, OH 45229
(513) 872-5895
Coordinator: Kayla J. Springer, Ph.D.

Case Western Reserve University Department
  of Psychiatry
Gender Identity Clinic
Hanna Pavilion
University Hospitals
2040 Abington Rd.
Cleveland, OH 44106
(216) 844-3426 or 459-4428
Codirectors: Aaron Billowitz, M.D., Stephen
  B. Levine, M.D.

The Cleveland Clinic
Sexual Dysfunction Unit
9500 Euclid Ave., Desk 68
Cleveland, OH 44106
(216) 444-5812
Director: Suzanne Powers, Ph.D.

The Toledo Hospital
Human Sexuality Center
2142 N. Cove Blvd.
Toledo, OH 43606
(419) 471-4189
Director: Malati Multani, M.D.

PENNSYLVANIA
Sexual Behavior Center
8 N. Queen St.
Lancaster, PA 17603
(717) 397-3115
Director: Mary Kearns Condron, M.S.
Clinical supervisor: David E. Nutter, M.D.

Hahnemann Medical College and Hospital
Van Hammett Psychiatric Clinic
112 N. Broad St., 6th Floor
Philadelphia, PA 19102
(215) 448-8821
Director: Ilda V. Ficher, Ph.D.

Jefferson Medical College
Department of Psychiatry and Human Behavior
Jefferson Psychiatric Associates Sexual
  Function Center
1015 Chestnut St.
Philadelphia, PA 19107
(215) 928-6960
Acting Director: Carl Doghramji, M.D.

The Medical College of Pennsylvania
Eastern Pennsylvania Psychiatric Institute
Department of Psychiatry
Outpatient Clinics
3200 Henry Ave.
Philadelphia, PA 19129
(215) 842-4220
Treatment: Donald Cohen, Ph.D.

Temple University School of Medicine
Moss Rehabilitation Hospital
12th and Tabor Rds.
Philadelphia, PA 19141
(215) 329-5715
Director: Paul Macks, M.A.

University of Pennsylvania School of Medicine
Division of Family Study
Marriage Council of Philadelphia
4025 Chestnut St.
Philadelphia, PA 19104
(215) 382-6680
Acting Director: Martin Goldberg, M.D.

RHODE ISLAND
Kent County Memorial Hospital
Franek Clinic, Inc.
4601 Post Rd.
East Greenwich, RI 02818
(401) 884-3530
Codirectors: Bruno Franek, M.D., Marliese
    Franek, M.Ed.

SOUTH CAROLINA
Medical University of South Carolina
College of Medicine
Departments of Psychiatry and Ob/Gyn
171 Ashley Ave.
Charleston, SC 29403
(803) 792-4037

TENNESSEE
University of Tennessee
College of Medicine
Department of Psychiatry
Special Problems Unit, Sexual Dysfunction
    Clinic
66 N. Pauline, Suite 633
Memphis, TN 38105
(901) 528-5489
Codirectors: William Murphy, Ph.D., Peter
    Hoon, Ph.D.

TEXAS
University of Texas Medical Branch
Department of Ob/Gyn
Sexual Dysfunction Treatment Clinic
Galveston, TX 77550
(409) 765-1951 or 763-0016
Codirectors: L. C. Powell, Jr., M.D., Collier
    M. Cole, Ph.D.

Baylor College of Medicine
Baylor Psychiatry Clinic
1200 Moursund Ave.
Houston, TX 77030
(713) 799-4856
Director: Mariame Aviles, M.D.

University of Texas
System Cancer Center
M.D. Anderson Hospital and Tumor Institute
Department of Urology
Section of Sexual Rehabilitation
6723 Bertner Ave.
Houston, TX 77030
(713) 792-8167
Director: Andrew C. von Eschenbach, M.D.

UTAH
University of Utah Medical Center
Department of Psychiatry
50 N. Medical Drive
Salt Lake City, UT 84132
(801) 581-7951
Director: Nyla J. Cole, M.D.

VIRGINIA
The Johns Hopkins Medical Institutions
Fairfax Hospital
Department of Psychiatry
3300 Gallows Rd.
Falls Church, VA 22046
(703) 698-3626
Director: Thomas N. Wise, M.D.

WASHINGTON
University of Washington
School of Medicine
Sexual Dysfunction Clinic
4701 24th N.E., Building #1, Room 134
Seattle, WA 98105
(206) 543-3260
Codirectors: John L. Hampson, M.D., Susan
    M. Tollefson, R.N., M.A.

WISCONSIN
Good Samaritan Medical Center
Clinic of Urology
S.C. Sexual Diagnostic and Treatment Clinic
2040 W. Wisconsin Ave., Suite 401
Milwaukee, WI 53233
(414) 344-3700
Medical Director: Stuart W. Fine, M.D.

Milwaukee Psychiatric Hospital
1220 Dewey Ave.
Milwaukee, WI 53213
(414) 258-2600
Director: Phil Veenhuis, M.D.

SOURCE: *Originally compiled by* Sexual Medicine Today
and updated by the author.

ORGANIZATIONS

American Association of Sex Educators,
Counselors, and Therapists
11 Dupont Circle, N.W., Suite 220
Washington, DC 20036
(202) 462-1171

A nonprofit professional organization devoted to developing professional competency, ethical and training standards for sex educators, counselors and therapists. A source of information for the public. Answers questions, makes referrals to sex counselors and therapists in local areas. Certifies sex educators, counselors and therapists. Offers pamphlets, booklets, a journal, *Journal of Sex Education and Therapy*. Also publishes for sale a national directory listing names of about 3,000 certified sex educators,

counselors and therapists throughout the country. Will provide more information upon request.

Impotents Anonymous and Impotence Institute
of America
119 S. Ruth St.
Maryville, TN 37801
(615) 983-6064

A nonprofit national clearinghouse of information on impotence and how to overcome it. Mainly interested in establishing self-help groups for men suffering from impotence, their partners, and other interested persons. Makes medical referrals for treatment, including penis implant surgery.

BOOKS

Afterplay: A Key to Intimacy, **James Halpern** and **Mark Sherman,** New York: Stein and Day, 1979.

The Family Book About Sexuality, **Mary S. Calderone** and **Eric W. Johnson,** New York: Harper & Row, 1981.

For Yourself: The Fulfillment of Female Sexuality, **Lonnie Garfield Barbach,** New York: Doubleday, 1975.

Illustrated Manual of Sex Therapy, **Dr. Helen Singer Kaplan,** New York: New York Times Books, 1975.

Impotence, **Dr. Richard Green,** New York: Plenum Press, 1981.

Lifelong Sexual Vigor: How to Avoid and Overcome Impotence, **Marvin B. Brooks,** New York: Doubleday, 1981.

Making Love: How To Be Your Own Sex

Therapist, **Patricia E. Raley,** New York: Dial Press, 1976.

National Register of Certified Sex Educators, Counselors, and Sex Therapists, Washington, DC: American Association of Sex Educators, Counselors, and Therapists; 11 Dupont Circle, N.W., Suite 220, Washington, DC 20036. Updated annually.

The New Sex Therapy, **Dr. Helen Singer Kaplan,** New York: New York Times Books, 1974.

Sex After Sixty, **Dr. Robert Butler** and **Myrna I. Lewis,** New York: Harper & Row, 1976.

The Sex Atlas: A New Illustrated Guide, **Erwin J. Haeberle,** New York: Continuum, 1982.

SICKLE-CELL ANEMIA

See also Genetic Counseling, page 226.

Sickle-cell anemia is an inherited blood disorder, most common in populations in Africa and around the Mediterranean, including Greece, southern Italy, Spain, and among persons of African descent. About 50,000 Black Americans have the disease and about two million Afro-Americans carry the abnormal gene (sickle-cell trait) that can pass the disease on to offspring. Sickle-cell anemia is so-called because the red blood cells have an abnormal shape, resembling a sickle. Their odd shape and rigidity cause them to log-jam in the vessels, obstructing blood flow and cutting off normal oxygen supplies to the tissues and organs. Additionally, the sickled red blood cells are destroyed faster than the bone marrow can make new ones; thus, the person with sickle-cell disease is chronically anemic. An ordinary red blood cell lasts 120 days; a sickle cell lasts about 20 days.

The disease, like other genetic disorders, such as Tay-Sachs (which strikes primarily people of Middle European Jewish ancestry), is incurable. However, the life expectancy of people with sickle-cell anemia is variable and improving; some live to old age.

Cause: An abnormal gene creates a disorder of the red blood cells carrying oxygen. An individual can be born with sickle-cell anemia only if both parents carry the gene. The parents, in other words, can pass on the gene, creating the disease, even though they show no signs of illness themselves and may never know they possess the faulty gene. In such cases, there is a 25 percent chance with each pregnancy that the child will have sickle-cell anemia disease. And generally about half of their children will inherit the sickle-cell trait, enabling them to transmit the disease. It is important to point out that people with sickle-cell trait are in no danger of developing the disease, rarely show any signs of sickle cell-related illness, and have the same life expectancy as people without the trait.

Symptoms: The symptoms are quite variable, depending on the age of the individual. There may be no noticeable symptoms in the early days of life. After about six months of age, symptoms become noticeable and may include painful swelling of hands and feet, paleness, and increased susceptibility to certain infections, especially of the lungs. Characteristic of the disease are sudden bursts of pain in the extremities, back, abdomen, and chest, called "pain crisis," as the sickle cells periodically jam up.

During adolescence the infections and pain crises may subside, but other problems frequently appear: delayed puberty, impaired growth, jaundice, bone distortions, and arthritis, even stroke and other neurological complications. Adults with sickle-cell anemia are also at high risk for lung damage, chronic leg ulcers, and kidney and heart failure. Conception and pregnancy may be difficult. Some victims may be virtually free of serious symptoms; others may have only a smattering of the classic symptoms; others show most of the complications.

Diagnosis: Once suspected because of family history, the disease is fairly easy to confirm by laboratory blood tests revealing the presence of the sickled cells. Sickle-cell anemia can be detected before birth, and people carrying the sickle-cell trait can be identified by a screening test.

Treatment: Treatment is aimed at preventing or managing the complications and varies with the complication. Prevention and prompt treatment of infections are necessary. Pain relief, with drugs or other methods, is also a high priority. Some patients are treated with repeated blood transfusions. The quest for antisickling drug agents and the reversal or cure of sickle-cell has intensified in the last few years, and, with the new era of gene manipulation, a cure for sickle-cell may be in sight. There is experimental evidence that the genes of those with sickle-cell anemia can be switched on by drugs to boost the concentration of hemoglobin and the production of red blood cells temporarily.

In the interim, the ability to manage sickle-cell anemia has improved dramatically in the past few years. Because of earlier diagnoses, better comprehensive medical care by multidisciplinary teams, and better education of patients, people with sickle-cell anemia are living longer.

A screening test does detect carriers of the defective gene, and parents carrying the gene should receive genetic counseling about the risks to offspring.

COMPREHENSIVE SICKLE-CELL ANEMIA CENTERS

The federal government sponsors 10 comprehensive sickle-cell anemia centers that do basic and clinical (patient) research. These centers are considered the ultimate in knowledge about the disease and latest treatment methods, as well as about local services for patients and their families. They are also clearinghouses of educational information about sickle-cell disease. Anyone can seek help at the comprehensive centers, although most patients come through physician referrals.

CALIFORNIA
Comprehensive Sickle Cell Center
University of Southern California School of
    Medicine
2025 Zonal Ave.
Los Angeles, CA 90033
J. Julian Haywood, M.D., Director
(213) 226-7116

Comprehensive Sickle Cell Center
University of California
San Francisco General Hospital
1001 Potrero Ave.
San Francisco, CA 94110
William Mentzer, M.D., Director
(415) 821-5169

DISTRICT OF COLUMBIA
Comprehensive Sickle Cell Center
Howard University College of Medicine
2121 Georgia Ave., N.W.
Washington, DC 20059
Roland B. Scott, M.D., Director
(202) 636-7930

GEORGIA
Comprehensive Sickle Cell Center
Medical College of Georgia
1435 Laney-Walker Blvd.
Augusta, GA 39012
Titus Huisman, Ph.D., Director
(404) 838-3271

ILLINOIS
Comprehensive Sickle Cell Center
University of Illinois Medical Center
1919 W. Taylor St.
Chicago, IL 60612
Maurice Rabb, M.D., Director
(312) 996-7013

MASSACHUSETTS
Comprehensive Sickle Cell Center
Boston City Hospital
818 Harrison Ave.
Boston, MA 02118
Lillian McMahon, M.D., Director
(617) 424-5727

MICHIGAN
Comprehensive Sickle Cell Center
Wayne State University School of Medicine
Children's Hospital of Michigan
3091 Beaubien Blvd.
Detroit, MI 48201
Charles Whitten, M.D., Director
(313) 577-1546

NEW YORK
Comprehensive Sickle Cell Center
College of Physicians & Surgeons, Columbia
  University
630 W. 168th St.
New York, NY 10032
Sergio Piomelli, M.D., Director
(212) 694-5882

NORTH CAROLINA
Comprehensive Sickle Cell Center
Duke University Medical Center
Box 3934, Morris Building
Durham, NC 27710
Wendell F. Rosse, M.D., Director
(919) 684-3724

OHIO
Comprehensive Sickle Cell Center
Children's Hospital Research Foundation
Elland and Bethesda Aves.
Cincinnati, OH 45229
Bruce Cameron, M.D., Director
(513) 559-4534

SOURCE: *National Heart, Lung and Blood Institute.*

RESEARCH AND TREATMENT AT THE NATIONAL INSTITUTES OF HEALTH

Selected patients with sickle-cell anemia are being studied at the NIH Clinical Center in Bethesda, Maryland, with an emphasis on determining the effectiveness of certain therapies. Consideration for participation in research is by physician referral only. For more information your physician can contact:

Office of the Director
The Clinical Center
Building 10, Room 2C-146
National Institutes of Health
Bethesda, MD 20892
(301) 496-4891, 5093

ORGANIZATION

Sickle Cell Disease Branch
Division of Blood Diseases and Resources
National Heart, Lung, and Blood Institute
Bethesda, MD 20892
(301) 496-6931

The branch within the National Institutes of Health most concerned with sickle-cell anemia. Supports research nationwide, helps set national policy on sickle-cell, provides information to the public and to health professionals. Some publications. Will provide more information upon request.

FREE MATERIALS

*Adolescents With Sickle-Cell Anemia and
  Sickle-Cell Trait,* 6 pages.
The Family Connection, 8 pages.
Sickle-Cell Fundamentals, 15 pages.

National Sickle Cell Disease Program
National Heart, Lung, and Blood Institute
7550 Wisconsin Ave., Room 504
Bethesda, MD 20892

SLEEP DISORDERS

Since the 1970s doctors have become much more sophisticated about sleep and sleep problems. Centers and clinics where doctors diagnose, treat, and do basic research on the physiology of sleep have been established nationwide; many are connected with prestigious universities. Many people who have suffered for years with sleep problems can now get expert help. About 50 million Americans complain of sleep problems; one-third claim it is a significant problem in their lives.

TYPES OF SLEEP DISORDERS

Insomnia: The most common sleep complaint is insomnia. Almost everyone suffers from insomnia at some period of life. It can be caused by stress, major life changes, or too much caffeine. If it lasts only a day or two at a time it does not need medical attention. Some people also believe they have insomnia when in fact they are merely "short sleepers," who need only five or six hours of sleep a night. Experts say this is not abnormal unless it interferes with activity during the waking hours. Expert evaluation in a sleep laboratory will reassure "short sleepers" that they have no apparent sleeping disorder.

Chronic, real insomnia, however, is quite different. It can be debilitating, leaving the victim anxious, stressful, fatigued, depressed, and unable to function during nonsleeping hours. Doctors do not have all the answers about what controls insomnia; the scientific study of sleep is still in its infancy. Some researchers believe there are unknown physiological reasons for insomnia, but experience in sleep laboratories shows that the cause can be simple: a disturbance in the sleep cycle from irregular bedtimes, night work schedules, stimulants, mainly caffeine, sedatives, such as sleeping pills and tranquilizers.

Quite often people who cannot sleep turn to sleeping pills, but such medication has only limited use, and there is considerable evidence that it can be addicting and dangerous.

Depression is also a common cause of insomnia, especially among the elderly. One sleep expert notes that one in five insomniacs needs psychiatric help. Physical conditions, such as heart and kidney disease, asthma, pain, and angina can also cause insomnia.

After proper diagnosis, sleep specialists may try an array of methods to allay the problem. Much of the therapy is "behavioral"—changing habits. Sometimes the "biological clock" is reset by altering the sleep cycle. In other cases, doctors use drugs and psychiatric counseling.

Narcolepsy: This disorder, which affects an estimated quarter of a million Americans, is typically characterized by a susceptibility to sleepiness no matter how much sleep the person gets at night. It can afflict anyone at any age, but usually starts during the teenage years. It is thought to be a central nervous system defect, which may be inherited. There is no known cure for it, but treatment can be quite beneficial, although not always totally successful. In some people, narcolepsy is mild and does not progress;

in others, the disorder can be progressively disabling, gradually getting worse over a period of years.

The main symptom is excessive tiredness and sleepiness during the day and falling asleep at inappropriate times. Other symptoms are ''cataplexy''—a sudden loss of voluntary muscle tone usually triggered by an emotional outburst of laughter or anger; disrupted nighttime sleep; sleep paralysis; and vivid hallucinations at the beginning or end of sleep periods. Narcolepsy can be definitively diagnosed by brain-wave sleep patterns in a sleep clinic. Drugs are often prescribed to prevent the attacks of sleep.

Sleep apnea: This potentially deadly condition was virtually unrecognized before the 1970s. It is estimated that 5 percent of the population may have this problem, in which breathing suddenly ceases during sleep. One study at Stanford University's Sleep Disorders Clinic showed that the periods of apnea—not breathing—lasted from 10 to 190 seconds (more than three minutes) and sometimes occurred hundreds of times a night. Many doctors blame some sudden adult deaths during sleep on apnea, in which the cardiovascular system simply collapses.

There are two types—central and obstructive sleep apnea. In obstructive apnea, the upper airway closes when the person inhales, blocking the air passages into the lungs. Death can result. But usually the victim suddenly awakes, snorting and trying to breathe, quite unaware that he or she had stopped breathing. In some cases a ''tongue retainer'' or ''airway splint'' created by a special mask corrects the problem; in difficult cases, throat surgery is necessary. In central sleep apnea, the person stops trying to breathe. The cause of central sleep apnea is unknown. It is treated with drugs with limited success.

The signs of apnea: fitful sleep, heavy snoring, high blood pressure, and a classic sign—sleepiness during the day. Some researchers believe that people who snore are in danger of developing sleep apnea, and that heavy snoring is in fact a mild form of obstructive sleep apnea. There is also evidence that hypertension is common among snorers. Some doctors advocate simple surgery to stop severe snoring, on the theory that it may help reduce blood pressure and prevent sleep apnea. The operation widens the throat by removing some of the soft palate at the rear of the throat and part of some tissue near the tonsils. Tonsils are removed too, if they are still present.

Some other sleep disorders that may need attention are: ''nocturnal myoclonus'' (severe leg twitches every 20 to 40 seconds); sleep-related epileptic seizures; so-called ''night terrors'' (more vivid than nightmares and not remembered the next day); sleepwalking, sleep talking; bedwetting; nighttime teeth grinding, also called bruxism.

If sleep problems cannot be diagnosed or treated by a family physician and are indeed chronic (lasting for more than a month), most experts recommend evaluation at a sleep disorder clinic. If apnea is suspected, such immediate evaluation, they say, is mandatory, for the condition is life-threatening.

SOME LEADING SLEEP DISORDER CENTERS

Sleep clinics provide what family physicians cannot—overnight monitoring of sleep patterns. This is done with what is called polysomnography—the electronic tracking of heart activity, brain waves, eye movements, and movement of certain skeletal muscles. If impotence is a problem, some sleep clinics will also monitor penile erections to determine if the problem is psychological or physical. The following Sleep Disorder Clinics are accredited by the Association of Sleep Disorders Centers. Centers marked with asterisks (*) are provisional members of the Association.

ALABAMA

Sleep Disorders Center of Alabama
Affiliated with Baptist Medical Center
  Montclair
800 Montclair Rd.
Birmingham, AL 35213
Vernon Pegram, Ph.D.
(205) 592-5650

*Sleep Disorders Center
The Children's Hospital of Alabama
1600 Seventh Ave.
Birmingham, AL 35233
Drs. Virgil Wooten and Raymond Lyrene
(205) 939-9386

*Sleep/Wake Disorders Center
University of Alabama
University Station
Birmingham, AL 35294
Drs. Virgil Wooten and Edward Faught
(205) 934-7110

*North Alabama Sleep Disorders Center
Huntsville Hospital
101 Sivley Rd.
Huntsville, AL 35801
Paul Legrand, M.D.
(205) 533-8020

ARIZONA
Sleep Disorders Center
Good Samaritan Medical Center
1111 E. McDowell Rd.
Phoenix, AZ 85006
Richard M. Riedy, M.D.
(602) 239-5815

Sleep Disorders Center
University of Arizona
1501 N. Campbell Ave.
Tucson, AZ 85724
Stuart F. Quan, M.D.
(602) 626-6112

ARKANSAS
*Sleep Disorders Center
Baptist Medical Center
9601 I-630 Exit 7
Little Rock, AR 72205-7299
Drs. Robert Galbraith
(501) 227-4750

*Sleep Disorders Diagnostic and Research
Center
University of Arkansas for Medical Sciences
4301 W. Markham, Slot 555
Little Rock, AR 72205
Drs. Lawrence Scrima and Charles Hiller
(501) 661-5528

CALIFORNIA
*WMCA Sleep Disorders Center
Western Medical Center-Anaheim
1025 S. Anaheim Blvd.
Anaheim, CA 92805
Louis McNabb, M.D.
(714) 491-1159

*Sleep Disorders Center
Downey Community Hospital
11500 Brookshire Ave.
Downey, CA 90241
Mark J. Buchfuhrer, M.D.
(213) 806-5280

*Sleep Disorders Institute
St. Jude Hospital and Rehabilitation Center
101 E. Valencia Mesa Drive
Fullerton, CA 92634
Drs. Robert A. Roethe, John K. Sturman and
   Justine A. Petrie
(714) 871-3280

Sleep Disorders Center
Scripps Clinic and Research Foundation
10666 N. Torrey Pines Rd.
La Jolla, CA 92037
Richard M. Timms, M.D.
(619) 455-8087

*Sleep Disorders Center
Palma Intercommunity Hospital
7901 Walker St.
La Palma, CA 90623
Joel B. Younger, M.D.
(714) 522-0150

*Loma Linda Sleep Disorders Center
Loma Linda University Medical Center
11234 Anderson St.
Loma Linda, CA 92354
Michael Bonnet, Ph.D.
(714) 825-7084, x2703

*Sleep Disorders Center
Hollywood Presbyterian Medical Center
1300 N. Vermont St.
Los Angeles, CA 90027
Dr. Allen Rothfeld
(213) 660-3530

*Sleep Disorders Center
The Hospital of the Good Samaritan
616 S. Witmer St.
Los Angeles, CA 90017
F. Grant Buckle, M.D.
(213) 977-2206

UCLA Sleep Disorders Clinic
Department of Neurology
710 Westwood Plaza, Room 1184 RNRC
Los Angeles, CA 90024
Emery Zimmermann, M.D., Ph.D.
(213) 206-8005

Sleep Disorders Center
Holy Cross Hospital
15031 Rinaldi St.
Mission Hills, CA 91345
Elliott R. Phillips, M.D.
(818) 898-4639

Sleep Disorders Center
U.C. Irvine Medical Center
101 City Drive S.
Orange, CA 92668
Jon Sassin, M.D.
(714) 634-5777

*Sleep Disorders Center
Pomona Valley Community Hospital
1798 N. Garey Ave.
Pomona, CA 91767
Dr. Bhupat Desai
(714) 623-8715, x2135

Sleep Disorders Center
Sequoia Hospital
Whipple and Alameda
Redwood City, CA 94062
Drs. Bernhard Votteri and Robert Pavy
(415) 367-5620

*Sleep Disorders Clinic and Research Center
St. Mary's Hospital
450 Stanyan St.
San Francisco, CA 94117
Dr. Donald B. Nevins
(415) 750-5579

*Sleep Disorders Center
San Jose Hospital
675 E. Santa Clara St.
San Jose, CA 95112
Drs. Sydney Choslovsky and W. Stroud
  Connor
(408) 977-4445

*Sleep Disorders Center
S. Coast Medical Center
31872 Coast Highway
South Laguna, CA 92677
Drs. A. Tyler Pittluck and Bernard de Berry
(714) 499-1311, x2186

Sleep Disorders Program
Department of Psychiatry—TD114
Stanford University School of Medicine
Stanford, CA 94305
German Nino-Murcia, M.D.
(415) 497-6601

*Sleep Disorders Center
Torrance Memorial Hospital
3330 Lomita Blvd.
Torrance, CA 90509
Lawrence W. Kneisley, M.D.
(213) 325-9110, x2049

COLORADO
*Porter Regional Sleep Disorders Center
Porter Memorial Hospital
2525 S. Downing
Denver, CO 80210
Richard Mountain, M.D.
(303) 778-5723

Sleep Disorders Center
Presbyterian Medical Center
1719 E. 19th Ave.
Denver, CO 80218
Ian Happer, M.D.
(303) 839-6447

Sleep Disorders Center
University of Colorado Health Sciences Center
700 Delaware St.
Denver, CO 80204
Drs. Martin Reite and John Zimmerman
(303) 394-7743

CONNECTICUT
Sleep Disorders Center
The Griffin Hospital
130 Division St.
Derby, CT 06418
Deborah E. Sewitch, Ph.D., and Karl-Otto
  Liebmann, M.D.
(203) 735-7421

*New Haven Sleep Disorders Center
100 York St.
Suite 2 G
New Haven, CT 06511
Drs. Robert Watson and Alan Sholomskas
(203) 776-9578

DISTRICT OF COLUMBIA
*Sleep Disorders Center
Georgetown University Hospital
3800 Reservoir Rd., N.W.
Washington, DC 20007
Samuel J. Potolicchio, Jr., M.D.
(202) 625-2697, x2020

FLORIDA
Sleep Disorders Center
Mt. Sinai Medical Center
4300 Alton Rd.
Miami Beach, FL 33140
Martin A. Cohn, M.D.
(305) 674-2613

*Sleep Disorders Center
Sacred Heart Hospital
5151 N. Ninth Ave.
Pensacola, FL 32504
Frank V. Messina, M.D.
(904) 476-7851, x4128

GEORGIA
Sleep Disorders Center
Northside Hospital
1000 Johnson Ferry Rd.
Atlanta, GA 30342
James J. Wellman, M.D.
(404) 256-8977

HAWAII
Sleep Disorders Center
Straub Clinic and Hospital
888 S. King St.
Honolulu, HI 96813
James W. Pearce, M.D.
(808) 523-2311, x8448

IDAHO
*Idaho Sleep Disorders Center
St. Luke's Regional Medical Center
190 E. Bannock
Boise, ID 83712
Bruce T. Adornato, M.D.
(208) 386-2440

ILLINOIS
*Henrotin Sleep Disorders Center
Henrotin Hospital
111 W. Oak St.
Chicago, IL 60610
R. A. Gross, M.D.
(312) 440-7777

Sleep Disorders Center
Rush-Presbyterian-St. Luke's
1753 W. Congress Parkway
Chicago, IL 60612
Rosalind Cartwright, Ph.D.
(312) 942-5440

Sleep Disorders Center
University of Chicago
5841 S. Maryland Ave., Box 425
Chicago, IL 60637
Jean-Paul Spire, M.D.
(312) 962-1780

*Sleep Disorders Center
Neurology Service
Veterans Hospital
Hines, IL 60141
Meenal Mamdani, M.D.
(312) 343-7200, x2326

Sleep Disorders Center
Methodist Medical Center of Illinois
221 N.E. Glen Oak
Peoria, IL 61636
Drs. Duane Morgan and Richard Lee
(309) 672-4966

*Sleep Disorders Clinic and Laboratory
Carle Clinic and Hospital
611 W. Park St.
Urbana, IL 61801
Drs. Daniel L. Picchietti and Donald A.
  Greeley
(217) 337-3364

INDIANA
*Sleep Disorders Center
St. Mary's Medical Center
3700 Washington Ave.
Evansville, IN 47750
David Howard, M.D.
(812) 479-4257

*Regional Sleep Studies Laboratory
The Lutheran Hospital of Fort Wayne, Inc.
3024 Fairfield Ave.
Fort Wayne, IN 46807
Bruce J. Hopen, M.D.
(219) 458-2001

*Sleep Disorders Center
Winona Memorial Hospital
3232 N. Meridian St.
Indianapolis, IN 46208
Frederick A. Tolle, M.D.
(317) 927-2100

*Sleep Disorders Center
Lafayette Home Hospital
2400 S. St.
Lafayette, IN 47903
Fredrick Robinson, M.D.
(317) 447-6811

IOWA
*Sleep Disorders Center
Iowa Methodist Medical Center
1200 Pleasant St.
Des Moines, IA 50308
Randall R. Hanson, M.D.
(515) 283-6207

*Sleep Disorders Center
Department of Neurology
University of Iowa Hospitals and Clinics
Iowa City, IA 52242
Quentin Stokes Dickens, M.D.
(319) 356-2571

KANSAS
*Sleep Disorders Center
Wesley Medical Center
550 N. Hillside
Wichita, KS 67214
Arnold M. Barnett, M.R.C.P., F.A.C.P.
(316) 688-2660

KENTUCKY
*Sleep Disorders Center
Good Samaritan Hospital
310 S. Limestone
Lexington, KY 40508
George W. Privett, Jr., M.D.
(606) 278-0352

*Sleep Disorders Center
St. Joseph's Hospital
1 St. Joseph Drive
Lexington, KY 40504
Robert Granacher, Jr., M.D.
(606) 278-3436

Sleep Disorders Center
Humana Hospital Audubon
One Audubon Plaza Drive
Louisville, KY 40217
Carl P. Browman, Ph.D.
(502) 636-7459

LOUISIANA
*Sleep Disorders Center
Touro Infirmary
1401 Foucher
New Orleans, LA 70115
Gihan Kader, M.D.
(504) 891-7087

Tulane Sleep Disorders Center
Department of Psychiatry and Neurology
1415 Tulane Ave.
New Orleans, LA 70112
Gregory Ferriss, M.D.
(504) 588-5231

*Sleep Disorders Center
Willis-Knighton Medical Center
2600 Greenwood Rd.
Shreveport, LA 71103
Nabil A. Moufarrej, M.D.
(318) 632-4823

MARYLAND
Sleep Disorders Center
Francis Scott Key Hospital
Johns Hopkins School of Medicine
Baltimore, MD 21224
Richard Allen, Ph.D.
(301) 955-0571

National Capital Sleep Center
4520 East-West Highway
Number 406
Bethesda, MD 20814
Wallace B. Mendelson, M.D.
(301) 656-9515

MASSACHUSETTS
*Sleep Disorders Center
Boston Children's Hospital
300 Longwood Ave.
Boston, MA 02115
Richard Ferber, M.D.
(617) 735-6242

*Sleep Disorders Center
Boston University Medical Center
75 E. Newton St.
Boston, MA 02146
George F. Howard, III, M.D.
(617) 247-5206

*Sleep Disorders Unit
Harvard University School of Medicine
Beth Israel Hospital
330 Brookline Ave.
Boston, MA 02215
June Matheson, M.D.
(617) 735-3237

*Sleep-Wake Disorders Unit
University of Massachusetts
55 Lake Ave., N.
Worcester, MA 01605
Sandra Horowitz, M.D.
(617) 856-3802

MICHIGAN
*Sleep Disorders Center
University of Michigan Medical Center
1405 E. Ann St.
Ann Arbor, MI 48109
Michael S. Aldrich, M.D.
(313) 763-5118

Sleep Disorders Center
Henry Ford Hospital
2799 W. Grand Blvd.
Detroit, MI 48202
Frank Zorick, M.D.
(313) 972-1800

*Sleep Disorders Center
Ingham Medical Center
401 W. Greenlawn Ave.
Lansing, MI 48909
Samuel M. McMahon, M.D.
(517) 374-2333

MINNESOTA
*Sleep Disorders Center
Fairview Southdale Hospital
6401 France Ave., S.
Edina, MN 55435
Drs. Wilfred Corson and V. Richard Zarling
(612) 924-5058

Sleep Disorders Center
Neurology Department
Hennepin County Medical Center
Minneapolis, MN 55415
Mark Mahowald, M.D.
(612) 347-6288

Sleep Disorders Center
Methodist Hospital
6500 Excelsior Blvd.
Minneapolis, MN 55426
Mark K. Wedel, M.D.
(612) 932-6083

Sleep Disorders Center
Mayo Clinic
200 First St., S.W.
Rochester, MN 55905
Philip R. Westbrook, M.D.
(507) 285-4150

MISSISSIPPI
*Sleep Disorders Center
Division of Somnology
University of Mississippi
Jackson, MS 39216
Lawrence S. Schoen, Ph.D.
(601) 987-5552

MISSOURI
*Sleep Disorders Center
St. Mary's Hospital
101 Memorial Drive
Kansas City, MO 64108
Iftekhar Ahmed, M.D.
(816) 756-2651

*Sleep Disorders Center
Research Medical Center
2316 E. Meyer Blvd.
Kansas City, MO 64132-1199
Ronald Chisholm, Ph.D.
(816) 276-4222

Sleep Disorders Center
Deaconess Hospital
6150 Oakland Ave.
St. Louis, MO 63139
James K. Walsh, Ph.D.
(314) 768-3100

Sleep Disorders Center
St. Louis University Medical Center
1221 S. Grand Blvd.
St. Louis, MO 63104
Kristyna M. Hartse, Ph.D.
(314) 557-8704

NEBRASKA
*Sleep Disorder Center
Lutheran Medical Center
515 S. 26th St.
Omaha, NE 68103
Drs. Robert Ellingson and John Roehrs
(402) 536-6352

NEW HAMPSHIRE
*Sleep-Wake Disorders Center
Hampstead Hospital
East Rd.
Hampstead, NH 03841
J. Gila Lindsley, Ph.D.
(603) 329-5311, x240

Sleep Disorders Center
Department of Psychiatry
Dartmouth Medical School
Hanover, NH 03756
Michael Sateia, M.D.
(603) 646-7521

NEW JERSEY
*Sleep Disorders Center
Newark Beth Israel Medical Center
201 Lyons Ave.
Newark, NJ 07112
Monroe S. Karetzky, M.D.
(201) 926-7597

NEW MEXICO
*Sleep Disorders Center
Lovelace Medical Center
5400 Gibson Blvd., S.E.
Albuquerque, NM 87108
Fernando G. Miranda, M.D.
(505) 262-7250

NEW YORK
Sleep-Wake Disorders Center
Montefiore Hospital
111 E. 210th St.
Bronx, NY 10467
Michael J. Thorpy, M.D.
(212) 920-4841

*Sleep Disorders Center
Winthrop-University Hospital
259 First St.
Mineola, NY 11501
Alan M. Fein, M.D.
(516) 663-2005

Sleep Disorders Center
Columbia-Presbyterian Medical Center
161 Fort Washington Ave.
New York, NY 10032
Neil B. Kavey, M.D.
(212) 305-1860

*Institute for Sleep and Aging
Mount Sinai Medical Center
One Gustave Levy Place
New York, NY 10129
Charles Herrera, M.D.
(212) 650-5561

Sleep Disorders Center
St. Mary's Hospital
89 Genesee St.
Rochester, NY 14611
Donald W. Greenblatt, M.D.
(716) 464-3391

Sleep Disorders Center
Department of Psychiatry
SUNY at Stony Brook
Stony Brook, NY 11794
Theodore L. Baker, Ph.D.
(516) 444-2916

Sleep-Wake Disorders Center
New York Hospital–Cornell Medical Center
21 Bloomingdale Rd.
White Plains, NY 10605
Charles Pollak, M.D.
(914) 997-5751

NORTH CAROLINA
*Sleep Disorders Center
Charlotte Memorial Hospital
PO Box 32861
Charlotte, NC 28232
Dennis Hill, M.D.
(704) 331-2121

*Sleep Disorders Center
Division of Neurology
Duke University Medical Center
Durham, NC 27710
J. Scott Luther, M.D.
(919) 684-6003

NORTH DAKOTA
*TNI Sleep Disorders Center
St. Luke's Hospital
Fifth St. at Mills Ave.
Fargo, ND 58102
Philip M. Becker, M.D.
(701) 280-5673

OHIO
*Sleep Disorders Center
Bethesda Oak Hospital
619 Oak St.
Cincinnati, OH 45206
Milton Kramer, M.D.
(513) 569-6320

Sleep Disorders Center
Jewish Hospital
515 Melish Ave.
Cincinnati, OH 45229
Martin B. Scharf, Ph.D.
(513) 861-7770

Sleep Disorders Center
Department of Neurology
Cleveland Clinic
Cleveland, OH 44106
Dudley S. Dinner, M.D.
(216) 444-8732

Sleep Disorders Evaluation Center
Department of Psychiatry
Ohio State University
Columbus, OH 43210
Helmut S. Schmidt, M.D.
(614) 421-8296

*Northwest Ohio Sleep Disorders Center
The Toledo Hospital
2142 N. Cove Blvd.
Toledo, OH 43606
Frank O. Horton, III, M.D.
(419) 471-5629

OKLAHOMA
Sleep Disorders Center
Presbyterian Hospital
N.E. 13th at Lincoln Blvd.
Oklahoma City, OK 73104
William Orr, Ph.D.
(405) 271-6312

*Sleep Disorders Center
Saint Francis Hospital
6161 S. Yale
Tulsa, OK 74136
Richard M. Bregman, M.D.
(918) 494-1350

OREGON
Sleep Disorders Program
Good Samaritan Hospital
2222 N.W. Lovejoy St.
Portland, OR 97210
Gerald B. Rich, M.D.
(503) 229-8311

PENNSYLVANIA
*Sleep Disorders Center
Jefferson Medical College
1015 Walnut St., 3rd Floor
Philadelphia, PA 19107
Karl Doghramji, M.D.
(215) 928-6175

Sleep Disorders Center
The Medical College of Pennsylvania
3300 Henry Ave.
Philadelphia, PA 19129
June M. Fry, Ph.D., M.D.
(215) 842-4250

Sleep Disorders Center
Western Psychiatric Institute
3811 O'Hara St.
Pittsburgh, PA 15213
Charles F. Reynolds, III, M.D.
(412) 624-2246

Sleep Disorders Center
Department of Neurology
Crozer-Chester Medical Center
Upland-Chester, PA 19013
Calvin Stafford, M.D.
(215) 447-2689

SOUTH CAROLINA
*Sleep Disorders Center
Baptist Medical Center
Taylor at Marion Sts.
Columbia, SC 29220
Drs. Richard Bogan and Sharon Ellis
(803) 771-5557

TENNESSEE
*Sleep Disorders Center
Fort Sanders Regional Medical Center
1901 W. Clinch Ave.
Knoxville, TN 37916
Ronald W. Bryan, M.D.
(615) 971-1375

*Sleep Disorders Center
St. Mary's Medical Center
Oak Hill Ave.
Knoxville, TN 37917
Michael L. Eisenstadt, M.D.
(615) 971-6011

BMH Sleep Disorders Center
Baptist Memorial Hospital
899 Madison Ave.
Memphis, TN 38146
Helio Lemmi, M.D.
(901) 522-5704

Sleep Disorders Center
Saint Thomas Hospital
PO Box 380
Nashville, TN 37202
J. Brevard Haynes, Jr., M.D.
(615) 386-2066

TEXAS
Sleep-Wake Disorders Center
Presbyterian Hospital
8200 Walnut Hill Lane
Dallas, TX 75231
Howard P. Roffwarg, M.D.
(214) 696-8563

*Sleep Disorders Center
Sun Towers Hospital
1801 N. Oregon
El Paso, TX 79902
Gonzalo Diaz, M.D.
(915) 532-6281

Sleep Disorders Center
All Saints Episcopal Hospital
1400 Eighth Ave.
Fort Worth, TX 76101
Edgar Lucas, Ph.D.
(817) 927-6120

Sleep Disorders Center
Department of Psychiatry
Baylor College of Medicine
Houston, TX 77030
Ismet Karacan, M.D.
(713) 799-4886

*Sleep Disorders Center
Sam Houston Memorial Hospital
1624 Pech, P.O. Box 55130
Houston, TX 77055
Todd Swick, M.D.
(713) 468-4311

*Sleep Disorders Center
Pasadena Bayshore Medical Center
4000 Spencer Highway
Pasadena, TX 71504
Drs. Bernard Bradley and David Stein
(713) 944-6666

Sleep Disorders Center
Humana Hospital Metropolitan
1303 McCullough
San Antonio, TX 78212
Sabri Derman, M.D.
(512) 223-4057

Sleep Disorders Center
Scott and White Clinic
2401 S. 31st St.
Temple, TX 76508
Francisco Perez-Guerra, M.D.
(817) 774-2554

UTAH
*Sleep Disorders Center
Utah Neurological Clinic
1999 N. Columbia Lane
Provo, UT 84604
John M. Andrews, M.D.
(801) 226-2300

Intermountain Sleep Disorders Center
LDS Hospital
325 Eighth Ave.
Salt Lake City, UT 84143
Drs. James Walker and Robert J. Farney
(801) 321-1378

VIRGINIA
*Sleep Disorders Center
Norfolk General Hospital
600 Gresham Drive
Norfolk, VA 23507
Reuben H. McBrayer, M.D.
(804) 628-3322

*Sleep Disorders Center
Community Hospital of Roanoke Valley
PO Box 12946
Roanoke, VA 24029
Thomas W. DeBeck, M.D.
(703) 985-8435

WASHINGTON
*Sleep Disorders Center
Providence Medical Center
500 17th Ave. C-34008
Seattle, WA 98124
Ralph A. Pascualy, M.D.
(206) 326-5366

WISCONSIN
*Sleep Disorders Center
Gundersen Clinic, Ltd.
1836 South Ave.
La Crosse, WI 54601
Larry A. Lindesmith, M.D.
(608) 782-7300

*Sleep Disorders Center
Columbia Hospital
2025 E. Newport Ave.
Milwaukee, WI 53211
Paul A. Nausieda, M.D.
(414) 961-4650

*Sleep Disorders Center
Milwaukee Children's Hospital
1700 W. Wisconsin Ave.
Milwaukee, WI 53201
Thomas B. Rice, M.D.
(414) 931-4016

Specialty laboratories for sleep-related breathing disorders

CALIFORNIA
Sleep Apnea Center
Merritt-Peralta Medical Center
450 30th St.
Oakland, CA 94609
Drs. Jerald Kram and Richard Nusser
(415) 451-4900, x2273

Southern California Sleep Apnea Center
Lombard Medical Group
2230 Lynn Rd.
Thousand Oaks, CA 91360
Ronald A. Popper, M.D.
(805) 495-1066

PENNSYLVANIA
Sleep Disorders Center
Mercy Hospital of Johnstown
1127 Franklin St.
Johnstown, PA 15905
Drs. George Hanzel and Richard Parcinski
(814) 533-1000

SOURCE: *Association of Sleep Disorders Centers.*

SLEEP RESEARCH LABS SPONSORED BY THE NATIONAL INSTITUTE OF MENTAL HEALTH

Sleep Disorders and Research Center
Stanford University Medical Center
Stanford, CA 94305
William C. Dement, M.D.
(415) 497-7458

University of Chicago Sleep Research
  Laboratory
5741 S. Drexel Ave.
Chicago, IL 60637
(312) 753-2353

Sleep Disorders Center
Rush-Presbyterian-St. Luke's
1753 W. Congress Parkway
Chicago, IL 60612
Rosalynd Cartwright, Ph.D.
(312) 942-5440

Sleep Disorders and Research Center
Henry Ford Hospital
2799 W. Grand Blvd.
Detroit, MI 48202
(313) 876-2233

Sleep Research Laboratory
Western Psychiatric Institute
University of Pittsburgh
School of Medicine
3811 O'Hara St.
Pittsburgh, PA 15213
David J. Kupfer, M.D.
(412) 624-1000

Sleep-Wake Disorders Center
Presbyterian Hospital
8200 Walnut Hill
Dallas, TX 75231
Howard Roffwarg, M.D.
(214) 696-8563

SOURCE: *National Institute of Mental Health.*

RESEARCH AND TREATMENT AT THE NATIONAL INSTITUTES OF HEALTH

The National Institute of Mental Health conducts several research projects in its sleep laboratory in Maryland in which limited numbers of patients may participate—by physician referral only. Ongoing studies focus on insomnia and the relationship between psychiatric problems and electroencephalographic patterns of sleep. There are also studies on the role of biological rhythms in sleep disturbance and the manipulation of these rhythms as a treatment for insomnia. For further information, your physician can contact:

Gerald L. Brown, M.D.
National Institute of Mental Health
(301) 496-1337

ORGANIZATIONS

The American Narcolepsy Association
1139 Bush St., Suite D
San Carlos, CA 94070-2477

A nonprofit, membership, charitable corporation, founded by individuals afflicted with narcolepsy. Distributes information about narcolepsy and related sleep disorders; encourages sleep research in pursuit of better diagnosis, better understanding, and better treatment or cures for sleep disorders. Publishes a newsletter. Makes medical referrals to physicians throughout the country who are specialists in sleep disorders. Sponsors local mutual support groups and has some local chapters.

The Association of Sleep Disorders Centers
National Office
PO Box 2604
Del Mar, CA 92014
(619) 755-7556
Dr. Merrill Mitler

A professional association of leading experts in sleep disorders, formed to insure the highest quality services to patients seeking solutions to sleep problems. The Association sets standards and guidelines for sleep centers and acts as an accrediting body.

BOOKS

The American Medical Association Guide to Better Sleep, **Lynne Lamberg,** New York: Random House, 1984.
The Complete Book of Sleep, **Dianne R. Hales,** Reading, MA: Addison-Wesley, 1981.

Get a Better Night's Sleep, **Ian Oswald,** New York: Arco Publishers, 1983.
Get a Good Night's Sleep, **Elliot Richard Phillips,** Englewood Cliffs, NJ: Prentice Hall, 1983.

Good Night, **Norman Ford,** Rockport, MA: Para Research Inc., 1983; holistic approach to conquering insomnia.

A Good Night's Sleep, **Jerrold S. Maxmen,** New York: Norton, 1981.

The Joy of Sleep, **Shirley Motter Linde,** New York: Harper & Row, 1980.

Some Must Watch While Some Must Sleep, **William C. Dement, M.D.,** New York: Norton, 1978.

FREE MATERIALS

Keep Us Awake, 18 pages; a guide to a film about narcolepsy.

Narcolepsy: A Non-Technical Survey, fact sheet.

Sleep Apnea: A Non-Technical Presentation, fact sheet.

The American Narcolepsy Association, Inc.
1139 Bush St., Suite D
San Carlos, CA 94070-2477

SMOKING

See Cancer, page 124, Lung Diseases, page 348, Heart and Cardiovascular Diseases, page 261.

No habit inflicts such a heavy health toll as cigarette smoking. Diseases tied to smoking cause 350,000 premature deaths each year. Smoking is linked to emphysema, chronic bronchitis, colds, gastric ulcers, heart disease, and cancers of the lung, pancreas, bladder, mouth, and esophagus. Smoking is a factor in an estimated 75 percent of all lung cancers and exerts a major impact on cardiovascular diseases, including stroke. Cigarette smokers are twice as likely to have heart attacks. Smoking causes about 170,000 coronary heart disease deaths every year.

Moreover, smoking low-tar, low-nicotine cigarettes is not as protective as once thought. Some experts call the health benefits of switching to a low-tar cigarette "insignificant." In fact, smokers may increase the number of low-tar, low-nicotine cigarettes they smoke in order to maintain a certain level of nicotine in their bloodsteam. One of the most important new findings about smoking is that nicotine is an addictive drug. Smokers crave the nicotine "fix," and physical withdrawal symptoms upon quitting are quite common and real, not merely psychological as once believed. The purpose of nicotine gum, for example, is to help a person gradually withdraw, lessening the symptoms of nicotine deprivation. Such physical addiction, as well as psychological dependence, is now regarded as the prime reason so many people find it excruciatingly difficult to quit.

However, quitting is the only solution (or, of course, never starting), and millions of Americans have quit successfully with lifesaving results.

Studies show that those who do quit are always ahead in forestalling death and disease, no matter how long or how heavily they have been smoking. Overall, smokers who quit increase their chances of living by 60 percent over those who still smoke, regardless of age or smoking history, according to one large-scale study. Some experts attribute part of the falling death toll from heart disease to a general drop in the number of smokers. As far as emphysema and chronic bronchitis are concerned, the added risk of those diseases disappears about 10 years after quitting, if disability has not already developed. Even after considerable lung damage, quitting smoking slows the progression of the disability.

There are many methods and programs to help people quit smoking, and smokers respond to different techniques. Some experts say that the critical factor is the person's motivation to quit, and that if you are determined to stop, it does not matter so much which technique you choose. Studies have shown that regardless of the type of program your chances of staying off cigarettes are twice as great if you are in an organized plan than if you do it alone, although many people have successfully stopped smoking on their own.

Few studies have compared the effectiveness of stop-smoking approaches, but one major survey pinpointed five methods that "possibly work." They are hypnosis, Smokenders, Schick Clinics, self-help techniques taught by a therapist or physician, and comprehensive group counseling. Of these, the author of the survey, Dr. David Sachs, an assistant professor of medicine at Stanford University, found that nicotine gum and "aversive conditioning" to cigarette smoke seemed most effective.

SOME LEADING STOP-SMOKING PROGRAMS

Many organizations, private companies, and public health agencies sponsor smoking-cessation programs. Here are some leading ones. Some programs associated with nonprofit organizations are either free or charge a nominal to moderate fee.

Freedom From Smoking®: Behavioral change program developed by the American Lung Association (ALA) and conducted by local ALA affiliates at certain scheduled times. Contact your local ALA affiliate.

American Lung Association
National Headquarters
1740 Broadway
New York, NY 10019

Fresh Start Program: A four-session class (either twice a week for two weeks or once a week for four weeks), led by a trained ex-smoker to help you figure out your smoking patterns, set a date for quitting, learn techniques of stress management and how to keep from returning to smoking once you have quit. Conducted by local American Cancer Society units, listed in white pages of local telephone directories.

American Cancer Society
90 Park Ave.
New York, NY 10016
(212) 599-8200

Plan to Stop Smoking: Sponsored by the Seventh-day Adventist Church and organized by churches in communities. Contact the Seventh-day Adventist Church in your area.

Seventh-day Adventists
6840 Eastern Ave., N.W.
Washington, DC 20012
(800) 253-7077

Schick Centers for the Control of Smoking: Private nonmedical program, based on counter conditioning or aversive therapy techniques. Five one-hour sessions, followed by eight weeks of group sessions. For a list of Schick Centers, contact the national headquarters in Los Angeles.

Schick Centers for the Control of Smoking
1901 Ave. of the Stars
Los Angeles, CA 90067
(213) 553-9771

Smokenders: A private organization, sponsoring six-week seminars in many cities, designed to help people stop smoking. Deals with both nicotine addiction and psychological dependency. Includes weight and stress management. Claims over half a million graduates since its establishment in 1969.

Smokenders
533 Memorial Parkway
Phillipsburg, NJ 08865
(201) 454-4357

For other commercial centers, individual practitioners, and agencies, check the yellow pages under "Smoker's Information and Treatment Centers." Also check with local hospitals or medical centers. Many offer smoking-cessation programs.

OTHER SOURCES OF INFORMATION AND HELP

Action on Smoking and Health
2013 H St., N.W.
Washington, DC 20006

An advocacy organization to promote nonsmokers' rights, including regulation of cigarettes, a ban on unfair and deceptive cigarette advertising, and shifting the cost of smoking from nonsmoker to smoker. Helps secure assistance for those trying to quit smoking.

Office on Smoking and Health
U.S. Department of Health and Human
  Services
Public Health Service
5600 Fishers Lane
Bethesda, MD 20857
(301) 443-1575

The federal government agency delegated to
compile information and make health policy decisions about the dangers of smoking. Issues a
national report yearly on the latest scientific evi-

dence on hazards of cigarette smoking. Pamphlets, other publications. Will provide more
information upon request.

Antismoking helpline

(800) 4-CANCER

For more information on materials or resources
to stop smoking, you can call this toll-free line,
operated by the National Cancer Institute.

BOOKS

*The American Cancer Society's "Fresh Start:"
  21 Days to Stop Smoking,* **Dee Burton,
  Ph.D.,** New York: Pocket Books, 1986.
*How To Lose Weight and Stop Smoking
  through Self-Hypnosis,* **Robert E. Duke,**
  New York: Irvington Publishers, 1983.
The Joy of Quitting, **Dee Burton,** New York:
  Macmillan, 1979.
The Scientific Case Against Smoking, **Ruth
  Winter,** New York: Crown Publishers,
  1980.

The Stop Smoking Book for Teens, **Curtis W.
  Casewit,** New York: J. Messner, 1980.
The Stop Smoking Diet, **Jane Ogle,** New
  York: Evans, 1981.
Stop Smoking, Lose Weight, **Neil Solomon,
  M.D.,** New York: Putnam, 1981.
You Can Stop, **Jacquelyn Rogers,** New York:
  Simon & Schuster, 1977; Pocket Book
  revision, 1986.

MATERIALS, FREE AND FOR SALE

Free

*Dangers of Smoking, Benefits of Quitting and
  Relative Risks of Reduced Exposure,* 81
  pages.
The Decision is Yours, leaflet.
*Fifty Most-Often-Asked Questions About
  Smoking,* 24 pages.
*Quitter's Guide: A 7-Day Plan to Help You
  Stop Smoking Cigarettes,* 22 pages.

American Cancer Society
90 Park Ave.
New York, NY 10016

*Clearing the Air: A Guide to Quitting
  Smoking,* 32 pages.
Why Do You Smoke?
You've Kicked the Smoking Habit for Good

National Cancer Institute
9000 Rockville Pike
Building 31, 10A18
Bethesda, MD 20892
(800) 422-6239

Free or for a small donation

Freedom From Smoking® in 20 Days, self-help
  quit-smoking guide.
Help A Friend Stop Smoking, booklet.
A Lifetime of Freedom From Smoking®, a
  maintenance program.
Stop Smoking/Stay Trim, booklet.

Local American Lung Associations listed in
  the white pages of phone directories.

Audiocassettes for sale

Smokenders
533 Memorial Parkway
Phillipsburg, NJ 08865

Videocassette for sale

*In Control: A Home Video Freedom From
Smoking® Program*, local American Lung
Association affiliates.

Videocassette and audiocassette for sale

*The American Cancer Society's "Fresh Start:"
21 Days to Stop Smoking*, Simon &
Schuster, NY, 1985.

SPEECH AND LANGUAGE PROBLEMS

See also Mental Retardation and Developmental and Learning Disabilities, page 355, for more information on dyslexia; and Rehabilitation, page 460, for special resources on language rehabilitation after a stroke or other neurological disability.

Speech and language difficulties affect both children and adults; the cause of many of the problems is unknown, and unfortunately, in many cases, treatment is difficult. Included in this category are a variety of conditions, such as stuttering beginning in childhood; aphasia, the loss of the ability to understand and recall words and sentences following brain damage, often after a stroke; loss of larynx and vocal apparatus due to cancer; dyslexia (an inborn difficulty with processing language despite an average or superior intelligence); and loss of control of muscles that produce speech, as in advanced cases of Parkinson's and other neuromuscular disorders. Also, youngsters with autism and other developmental disabilities, mental retardation, cerebral palsy, and hearing impairments often have trouble with language. An estimated eight million Americans have speech and language disorders.

At least three million school-age children have speech impairments, including about a million who stutter, necessitating special education and remedial services. Approximately one-and-a-half million adults have chronic aphasia, making them unable to understand speech or form their thoughts into words. About 25,000 Americans need speech rehabilitation because they have had their larynx removed during cancer treatment.

Treatment of many of these speech disorders is varied, controversial, and constantly changing with new developments in technology or new theories. If you have tried once to correct a speech difficulty without success, you may want to try again; the chances for success may have increased.

Any child or adult with speech problems should consider help from a speech-language pathologist, also called a speech pathologist or a speech therapist. You should be sure the speech-language pathologist has professional credentials. Many states insist they be licensed. Also, the American Speech-Language-Hearing Association accredits speech-language pathologists, who meet standards of knowledge and performance set by their professional peers. The accreditation is at least a minimum guide to excellence. Many rehabilitation facilities and community associations, agencies, self-help groups, and national organizations can also refer you to speech-language pathologists.

SPEECH-LANGUAGE PATHOLOGY AND AUDIOLOGY CENTERS

Here are facilities that have been accredited by the American Speech-Language-Hearing Association for competence in speech-language pathology and/or audiology. Most of the speech-language centers are also accredited in audiology or hearing evaluation because the connection between language and hearing is so close that many practitioners are competent in both fields. A few of the centers are accredited only for audiology and are included for people with hearing problems who may want to refer to the list.

It is important to point out that these accredited facilities are often major centers of excellence in a certain location; however, they are by no means the only centers with excellent speech-language therapy services, and omission from accreditation should not be construed as a lack of competence. (The Association reports that some facilities with excellent therapists have not applied for current accreditation.) It should also be noted that these are accredited *facilities* only; the Association has a much longer list of accredited *individual* therapists who offer speech-language services. Many are on the staffs of hospitals and rehabilitation facilities. For additional speech-language therapists, you may want to consult the speech and hearing departments of leading medical centers and rehabilitation centers, as well as the American Speech-Language-Hearing Association.

ALABAMA

National Speech and Hearing Services, Inc.
2000 B S. Bridge Parkway, Suite 127
Birmingham, AL 35209
(205) 322-4477
President: Robert W. Teel
Vice President: Cecil G. Betros, Jr.
Accredited in speech-language pathology

University of Alabama at Birmingham
Speech and Hearing Clinic
Hearing Division and Speech Division
Box 187 University Station
Birmingham, AL 35294
(205) 934-4467
Director: Larry E. Adams, Ph.D.
Accredited in speech-language pathology and
  audiology

Huntsville Rehabilitation Center
Communication Services Department
316 Longwood Drive, S.W.
Huntsville, AL 35801
(205) 534-6421
Director: Barbara Zangel
Accredited in speech-language pathology and
  audiology

Speech and Hearing Center
Humanities Building, University of South
  Alabama
Mobile, AL 36688
(205) 460-6327
Director: Stephen B. Hood, Ph.D.
Accredited in speech-language pathology and
  audiology

ALASKA

State of Alaska, Department of Health and
  Social Services Communicative Disorders
  Program
1231 Gambel St.
Anchorage, AK 99501
(907) 562-2675
Director: David R. Canterbury, Ed.D.
Accredited in speech-language pathology and
  audiology

ARIZONA

Good Samaritan Medical Center
Department of Audiology
1111 E. McDowell Rd.
Phoenix, AZ 85006
(602) 247-4577
Director: Larry J. Lovering, Ph.D.
Accredited in audiology

Good Samaritan Medical Center
Institute of Rehabilitation Medicine
Department of Speech-Language Pathology
1111 E. McDowell Rd.
PO Box 2989
Phoenix, AZ 85062
(602) 239-4755
Director: Marilyn Miller Quintana, M.A.
Other language: Spanish
Accredited in speech-language pathology

St. Mary's Hospital and Health Center
Speech-Language-Hearing Clinic
1601 W. St. Mary's Rd.
Tucson, AZ 85703
(602) 622-5833, x4109
Director: Jean B. Glattke
Other language: Spanish
Accredited in speech-language pathology

ARKANSAS
Arkansas Children's Hearing and Speech
  Clinic
4815 W. Markham St.
Little Rock, AR 72201
(501) 661-2328
Director: Fred R. Beggs, M.S.
Accredited in speech-language pathology and
  audiology

CALIFORNIA
Irwin Lehrhoff and Associates, Inc.
9701 Wilshire Blvd.
One Roxbury Plaza, Suite 1200
Beverly Hills, CA 90212
(213) 273-8480
Director: Irwin Lehrhoff, Ph.D.
Other language: Spanish
Accredited in speech-language pathology

Irwin Lehrhoff and Associates, Inc.
PO Box 5658
Carmel, CA 93021
(408) 649-4564
Director: Judy Sonderman Thompson,
  Ph.D.

Los Angeles County Office of Education
Communicative Disorders Program
9300 E. Imperial Highway
Downey, CA 90242
(213) 922-6260
Director: Joan Novina
Other language: Spanish
Accredited in speech-language pathology

Rancho Los Amigos Hospital
Communication Disorders Department
7601 E. Imperial Highway
Downey, CA 90242
(213) 922-7682, 7687 (voice)
(213) 922-7684, (TTY)
Director: Frank DeRuyter, Ph.D.
Other languages: Spanish, Sign
Accredited in speech-language pathology and
  audiology

California State University–Fresno
Department of Communicative Disorders
Speech-Language-Hearing Clinic
Maple and Shaw Aves.
Fresno, CA 93740
(209) 294-2423, 2422 (voice)
(209) 294-2856, (TTY)
Director: David R. Foushee, M.A.
Other language: Sign
Accredited in speech-language pathology and
  audiology

Irwin Lehrhoff and Associates, Inc.
83 E. Shaw Ave., Suite 250
Fresno, CA 93704
(209) 229-9206
Directors: Joan Salisbury, M.S., Susan
  Lovely, M.A.

Valley Children's Hospital
Department of Speech-Language Pathology and
  Audiology
3151 N. Millbrook
Fresno, CA 93703
(209) 225-3000, x1485
Director: Carl R. Schneiderman
Other languages: Sign, Spanish, Vietnamese,
  Laosian, Hmong provided by hospital
  interpreter
Accredited in speech-language pathology and
  audiology

Veterans Administration Medical Center
Audiology and Speech Pathology Service
5901 E. Seventh St.
Long Beach, CA 90822
(213) 498-6267
Director: James L. Aten, Ph.D.
Other languages: Spanish, Sign
Accredited in speech-language pathology and
  audiology

Veterans Administration Medical Center
West Los Angeles Audiology and Speech
  Pathology Service
Wilshire and Sawtelle Blvds.
Los Angeles, CA 90073
(213) 824-3100 (voice and TTY)
Director: Douglas Noffsinger, Ph.D.
Accredited in speech-language pathology and
  audiology

Providence Speech and Hearing Center
1301 Providence Ave.
Orange, CA 92668
(714) 639-4990
Director: Margaret Anne Inman, Ph.D.
Other language: Spanish
Accredited in speech-language pathology and
 audiology

Letterman Army Medical Center
Speech Auditory Evaluation and Treatment
 Clinic
Presidio of San Francisco, CA 94129-6700
(415) 561-4950, 5267
Directors: Richard A. Dennis, Jr., Jean Nesbit,
 M.A., (speech-language pathology)
Accredited in speech-language pathology and
 audiology

Irwin Lehrhoff and Associates, Inc.
5606 El Cajon Blvd.
San Diego, CA 92115
(619) 229-6200
Director: Joan Salisbury, M.S.

San Diego State University
Communications Clinic
5300 Campanile Drive
San Diego, CA 92182
(714) 265-6477
Director: Edmund L. Thile, Ph.D.
Other languages: Sign, Spanish, Chinese
Accredited in speech-language pathology and
 audiology

Speech, Hearing, Neurosensory Center
Main Center
8001 Frost St.
San Diego, CA 92123
(714) 292-3482
Director: Chris Hagen, Ph.D.
Other language: Spanish
Accredited in speech-language pathology and
 audiology

Irwin Lehrhoff and Associates, Inc.
1850 Union St., #415
San Francisco, CA 94123
(415) 522-3771
Director: Judy Sonderman Thompson, Ph.D.

San Francisco Hearing and Speech Center
1234 Divisadero St.
San Francisco, CA 94115
(415) 921-7658
Director: Rayford C. Reddell, Ph.D.
Other languages: Spanish, Sign
Accredited in speech-language pathology and
 audiology

Saint John's Hospital and Health Center
Department of Speech and Hearing Services
1328 22nd St.
Santa Monica, CA 90404
(213) 829-6592
Director: Laurie Rauss, M.S.
Accredited in speech-language pathology and
 audiology

Stanford University Medical Center
Audiology Clinic R135
Stanford, CA 94305
(415) 497-6816 (voice)
(415) 497-7895 (TTY)
Director: Holly Hosford-Dunn, Ph.D.
Other language: Sign
Accredited in audiology

Irwin Lehrhoff and Associates, Inc.
6333 Pacific Ave., #101
Stockton, CA 95207
(209) 466-9460
Directors: Judy Sonderman Thompson, Ph.D.,
 Chris Baker, M.S.

Los Angeles County Harbor–UCLA Medical
 Center
Center for Communication Disorders
1000 W. Carson St., Building A-12
Torrance, CA 90509
(213) 533-2743
Director: Susan Kaplan, M.S.
Other language: Spanish
Accredited in speech-language pathology and
 audiology

Community Speech and Hearing Center,
 Encino-Van Nuys
7140 Balboa Blvd.
Van Nuys, CA 91406
(818) 785-2911 (voice and TTY)
Director: Howard A. Grey, Ph.D.
Other languages: Spanish, Sign
Accredited in speech-language pathology and
 audiology

UCLA Medical Center
Audiology and Speech Clinics
62-202 CHS
10833 Le Conte Ave.
West Los Angeles, CA 90024
(213) 825-5751 (audiology)
(213) 825-8551 (speech pathology)
Director: Donald E. Morgan, Ph.D.
Other languages: Most languages can be accommodated through the Translation Services Department of the Medical Center; sign language interpreters are available for audiology & speech-language services
Accredited in speech-language pathology and audiology

COLORADO
Boulder Memorial Hospital
Department of Speech Pathology and Audiology
311 Mapleton Ave.
Boulder, CO 80302
(303) 441-0437 (voice)
(303) 441-0420 (TTY)
Director: Mary Ann Keatley, Ph.D.
Accredited in speech-language pathology

The Children's Hospital
Department of Audiology and Speech Pathology
1056 E. 19th Ave.
Denver, CO 80218
(303) 861-6800 (voice)
(303) 861-6050 (TTY)
Director: Deborah Hayes, Ph.D.
Other languages: SEE, American Sign Language (ASL)
Accredited in speech-language pathology and audiology

Porter Memorial Hospital
Speech and Hearing Department
2525 S. Downing St.
Denver, CO 80210
(303) 778-5645
Director: Jerome G. Alpiner, Ph.D.
Other language: Sign
Accredited in speech-language pathology and audiology

University of Northern Colorado
Department of Communication Disorders
Greeley, CO 80639
(303) 351-2012
Director: Raymond H. Hull, Ph.D., Donna E. Bottenberg, M.A.
Accredited in speech-language pathology and audiology

Boulder Memorial Therapy Clinic
325 S. Boulder Rd.
Louisville, CO 80027
(303) 665-4484
Director: Mary Ann Keatley, Ph.D.
Other languages: French, Russian
Accredited in speech-language pathology

CONNECTICUT
East Hartford Board of Education
Language, Speech, and Hearing Services
110 Long Hill Drive
East Hartford, CT 06108
(203) 289-7411, x284, 233
Director: Linda Stachowicz
Other language: Sign
Accredited in speech-language pathology

Southern Connecticut State University
Center for Communication Disorders
501 Crescent St.
New Haven, CT 06515
(203) 397-4569
Director: Frank E. Sansone, Jr., Ph.D.
Accredited in speech-language pathology

The Southeastern Connecticut Hearing and Speech Center, Inc.
92 New London Turnpike
Norwich, CT 06360
(203) 887-1654
Director: Carmelina C. Kanzler, M.S.
Accredited in speech-language pathology and audiology

Board of Education
Language and Speech Services
195 Hillandale Ave.
Stamford, CT 06902
(203) 358-4525, x435
Director: LaWanda Green Hubbard, Sc.D.
Other language: Spanish
Accredited in speech-language pathology

Stamford School Health Program
Language, Speech, and Hearing Services
229 North St.
Stamford, CT 06901
(203) 358-4390
Director: Meryl W. Aronin, M.A.
Accredited in speech-language pathology

The University of Connecticut
Speech and Hearing Clinic
Box U-85
Storrs, CT 06268
(203) 486-2629 (voice)
(203) 486-3975 (TTY)
Director: Sandra R. Ulrich
Other language: Sign
Accredited in speech-language pathology and
   audiology

Wethersfield Board of Education
Department of Communication Development
Webb Building
51 Willow St.
Wethersfield, CT 06109
(203) 563-8181, x238
Director: Margaret D. Cafaro-Pease
Accredited in speech-language pathology

DELAWARE
Delaware Curative Workshop
Speech and Language Pathology Department
1600 Washington St.
Wilmington, DE 19802
(302) 656-2521
Director: Jan Westerhouse, M.A.
Accredited in speech-language pathology

The Medical Center of Delaware
L. L. Horne Speech and Hearing Center
501 W. 14th St.
Wilmington, DE 19899
(302) 428-2286
Director: Gary E. Fallon
Other Languages: Interpreters available through
   the Medical Center
Accredited in speech-language pathology and
   audiology

Riverside Hospital Hearing Center
700 Lea Blvd.
Wilmington, DE 19899
(302) 764-6120, x413
Director: Dr. Paul M. Imber
Accredited in audiology

DISTRICT OF COLUMBIA
Army Audiology and Speech Center
Walter Reed Army Medical Center
Washington, DC 20307-50001
(202) 576-2413
Director: Roy K. Sedge, Ph.D.
Accredited in speech-language pathology and
   audiology

Washington Hospital Center
Hearing and Speech Center
110 Irving St., N.W.
Washington, DC 20010
(202) 541-6717
Director: David M. Resnick, Ph.D.
Other languages: Spanish, Sign
Accredited in speech-language pathology and
   audiology

FLORIDA
Morton F. Plant Hospital
Department of Communicative Disorders
905 S. Fort Harrison
Clearwater, FL 33517
(813) 441-5236
Director: Beverly Payne Brown, M.S.

Morton F. Plant Hospital
323 Jeffords St.
Clearwater, FL 33517

Holiday Office Center
5800 U.S. 19 N., Suite 217
Holiday, FL 33590
(813) 937-2413
Accredited in speech-language pathology and
   audiology

Speech and Hearing Center, Inc.
1128 Laura St.
Jacksonville, FL 32206
(904) 355-3403
Director: Elaine McCray, M.A.
Other language: Spanish
Accredited in speech-language pathology and
   audiology

Central Florida Speech and Hearing Center
710 E. Bella Vista St.
Lakeland, FL 33805
(813) 686-3189 (voice or TTY)
Executive Director: L. Gay Ratcliff, M.S.
Other language: Sign
Accredited in speech-language pathology and
   audiology

Munroe Regional Medical Center
Speech Pathology Services
PO Box 6000
131 S.W. 15th St.
Ocala, FL 32678
(904) 351-7225 (voice)
(904) 351-7607 (TTY)
Director: Janet R. Thursby, M.A.
Accredited in speech-language pathology

Baptist Hospital Speech and Hearing Clinic
1000 W. Moreno
Pensacola, FL 32501
(904) 434-4957, 4958
Director: Gay Roberts
Accredited in speech-language pathology and
    audiology

The Children's Resource Center of Northwest
    Florida, Inc.
Department of Speech Pathology
6812 Lillian Highway
PO Box 3748
Pensacola, FL 32506
(904) 456-9095
Director: Deborah Henderson
Accredited in speech-language pathology

Florida State University
Department of Audiology and Speech
    Pathology
Speech and Hearing Clinic
Regional Rehabilitation Center
Tallahassee, FL 32312
(904) 644-2238
Director: William H. Haas, Ph.D.
Other language: Sign
Accredited in speech-language pathology

GEORGIA
Atlanta Speech School, Inc.
3160 Northside Parkway, N.W.
Atlanta, GA 30327
(404) 233-5332
Directors: Julia Hand, Francie Ross
Accredited in speech-language pathology and
    audiology

The Davison School
1500 N. Decatur Rd., N.E.
Atlanta, GA 30306
(404) 373-7288
Director: Lucille M. Pressnell, Ph.D.
Accredited in speech-language pathology

Easter Seal Speech and Hearing Center
2228 Starling St.
Brunswick, GA 31520
(912) 264-3141
Director: Rebecca E. Rowell, M.Ed.
Accredited in speech-language pathology

Northeast Georgia Speech Center, Inc.
621 E. Spring St.
PO Box 1482
Gainesville, GA 30503
(404) 534-5141
Director: Diane M. Brower, M.Ed.
Accredited in speech-language pathology

Gracewood State School and Hospital
Speech and Hearing Clinic
Gracewood, GA 30812
(404) 790-2101
Director: Jean F. Kernaghan, M.Ed., Ed.S.
Accredited in speech-language pathology

HAWAII
Tripler Army Medical Center
Audiology and Speech Pathology Section
Honolulu, HI 96859
(808) 433-5719, 5742
Director: Jerod L. Goldstein, Ph.D.
Accredited in speech-language pathology and
    audiology

ILLINOIS
University of Illinois
Speech and Hearing Clinic
901 S. Sixth St.
Champaign, IL 61820
(217) 333-2230
Director: Robert K. Simpson, Ph.D. (speech
    pathologist)
Other languages: Hebrew, Sign
Accredited in speech-language pathology and
    audiology

David T. Siegel Institute for Communicative
    Disorders
3031 S. Cottage Grove
Chicago, IL 60616
(312) 791-2900
Directors: Laszlo Stein, Ph.D., Frederic Curry,
    Ph.D.
Other languages: Spanish, French, Sign, ASL
Accredited in speech-language pathology and
    audiology

Institute for Juvenile Research
Henry Horner Children's Center
Illinois Department of Mental Health
Speech-Language-Hearing Service
4201 N. Oak Park Ave.
Chicago, IL 60634-1471
(312) 794-3965
Director: Joseph L. LaBelle, Ph.D.
Accredited in speech-language pathology and
    audiology

Mercy Hospital and Medical Center
Department of Speech-Language Pathology
Stevenson Expressway at King Drive
Chicago, IL 60616
(312) 567-5557
Director: Kathryn L. Adam, M.A.
Accredited in speech-language pathology

Rehabilitation Institute of Chicago
Department of Communicative Disorders
345 E. Superior St.
Chicago, IL 60611
(312) 649-6138
Director: Anita S. Halper, M.A.
Accredited in speech-language pathology and
    audiology

Rush Presbyterian-St. Luke's Medical Center
Section of Communicative Disorders
1753 W. Congress Parkway
Chicago, IL 60612
(312) 942-5332
Director: Thomas W. Jensen, Ph.D.
Accredited in speech-language pathology and
    audiology

Schwab Rehabilitation Center
Communicative Disorders Department
1401 S. California Blvd.
Chicago, IL 60608
(312) 522-2010 (voice)
(312) 522-4708 (TTY)
Director: Barbara B. Miller, M.S.
Accredited in speech-language pathology and
    audiology

Northern Illinois University
Speech and Hearing Clinic
De Kalb, IL 60115
(815) 753-1481
Director: Earl J. Seaver III, Ph.D.
Other language: Sign
Accredited in speech-language pathology and
    audiology

Dixon Developmental Center
Speech/Language, Audiology Services
2600 N. Brinton Ave.
Dixon, IL 61021
(815) 288-5561, x280 (voice)
(815) 288-5561, x501 (TDD)
Director: Jeanine M. Devlin, M.A.
Other language: Manually Coded English
    (Seeing Essential English)
Accredited in speech-language pathology and
    audiology

Jayne Shover Easter Seal Rehabilitation
    Center, Inc.
Communication Disorders Department
PO Box 883, 799 S. McLean Blvd.
Elgin, IL 60120
(312) 742-3264
Director: Gail E. Trinwith, M.S. (speech
    pathologist, Communication Disorders
    Department Head)
Accredited in speech-language pathology and
    audiology

Elaine S. Dunn, Ph.D., Ltd.
Disorders of Speech and Language
636 Church St.
Evanston, IL 60201
(312) 328-5923
Director: Elaine S. Dunn, Ph.D.
Accredited in speech-language pathology

Northwestern University, Evanston Campus
Department of Communicative Disorders
Hearing Clinic
2299 Sheridan Rd.
Evanston, IL 60201
(312) 492-3165 (voice)
(312) 492-3161 (TTY)
Director: Judith Rassi
Other languages: Spanish, Polish
Accredited in speech-language pathology and
    audiology

Northwestern University, Evanston Campus
Department of Communicative Disorders,
    Speech and Language Clinic
2299 Sheridan Rd.
Evanston, IL 60201
(312) 492-5012
Director: Margaret Aylesworth
Other languages: Spanish, Polish
Accredited in speech-language pathology and
    audiology

Loyola University Medical Center–Foster G.
  McGaw Hospital
Department of Speech Pathology and
  Audiology
2160 S. First Ave.
Maywood, IL 60153
(312) 531-3771
Director: Diane K. Traficanti, M.A.
Accredited in speech-language pathology and
  audiology

Marianjoy Rehabilitation Center
26 W. 171 Roosevelt Rd.
PO Box 795
Wheaton, IL 60189
(312) 462-4220
Director: Kathy Bollinger, M.S. (speech
  pathologist)
Accredited in speech-language pathology

INDIANA
Indiana University Speech and Hearing Center
Indiana University
Bloomington, IN 47405
(812) 335-6251
Director: Elizabeth McCrea, Ph.D. (Acting
  Director of Clinical Services)
Other language: Sign
Accredited in speech-language pathology and
  audiology

Crossroads Rehabilitation Center, Inc.
Speech Pathology and Audiology Department
3242 Sutherland Ave.
Indianapolis, IN 46205
(317) 924-3251 (voice)
(317) 924-1172 (TTY)
Director: Nancy Cole-Crawford
Accredited in speech-language pathology and
  audiology

IOWA
Mississippi Bend Area Education Agency #9
Speech and Language Services
800 23rd St.
Bettendorf, IA 52722
(319) 359-1371
Director: Robert A. Baldes
Accredited in speech-language pathology

Mississippi Bend Area Education Agency
Department of Hearing Conservation-Education
  Services
800 23rd St.
Bettendorf, IA 52722
(319) 359-1371 (voice)
(319) 324-8512 (TTY)
Director: Ronald L. Huddleston, M.A., Ed.S.
Other language: Sign
Accredited in audiology

St. Luke's Methodist Hospital
Department of Speech Pathology and
  Audiology
1026 A Ave., N.E.
Cedar Rapids, IA 52402
(319) 369-7491
Director: Ann Briggie, M.A.
Accredited in speech-language pathology and
  audiology

Des Moines Hearing and Speech Center
700 Sixth Ave.
Des Moines, IA 50309
(515) 282-5052 (voice)
(515) 282-5054 (TTY)
Director: Jaynee K. Day, B.S.W.
Accredited in speech-language pathology and
  audiology

Veterans Administration Medical Center
Audiology/Speech Pathology Service
1515 W. Pleasant St.
Knoxville, IA 50138
(515) 842-3101, x247
Director: Darrell Wheeler, M.A.
Accredited in speech-language pathology and
  audiology

KANSAS
The Capper Foundation for Crippled Children
Speech-Language Pathology Department
3500 W. 10th St.
Topeka, KS 66604
(913) 272-4060
Director: Barry R. Molineaux, M.A.
Accredited in speech-language pathology

Institute of Logopedics
2400 Jardine Drive
Wichita, KS 67219
(800) 835-1043 (toll-free)
(316) 262-8271 (in Kansas)
Directors: Frank R. Kleffner, Ph.D., David J.
   Draper, Ph.D.
Other language: Sign
Accredited in speech-language pathology and
   audiology

Irwin Lehrhoff and Associates, Inc.
PO Box 8758
Wichita, KS 67208
(316) 261-9397
Directors: Felene Boeker, M.S., Martha
   Boose, M.A.

KENTUCKY
Geiger Easter Seal Speech and Hearing Center
2201 Lexington Ave.
PO Box 151
Ashland, KY 41105-0151
(606) 324-0465
Executive Director: Mary Wells Strait
Other language: Sign
Accredited in speech-language pathology and
   audiology

Northern Kentucky Easter Seal Center
Speech and Hearing Treatment Center
212 Levassor Ave.
Covington, KY 41015
(606) 491-1171
Executive Director: Lee Z. Snyder
Director of Speech Services: Marguerite Knauf
Accredited in speech-language pathology

Albert B. Chandler Medical Center
Neurosensory and Communicative Disorders
   Program
Department of Neurology
University of Kentucky Medical Center
800 Rose St.
Lexington, KY 40536-0084
(606) 257-3390 or 233-5472
Director: William W. Green, Ph.D.
Accredited in speech-language pathology and
   audiology

Cardinal Hill Hospital
Department of Speech-Language Pathology
2050 Versailles Rd.
Lexington, KY 40504
(606) 254-5701
Director: Patricia M. Brush-Lorey, M.A.
   (speech pathologist)
Accredited in speech-language pathology

Easter Seal Hearing and Speech Center
233 E. Broadway
Louisville, KY 40202
(502) 584-9781
Director: Lois K. Hobart, M.Ed.
Accredited in speech-language pathology and
   audiology

Murray State University
Speech and Hearing Clinic
Murray, KY 42071
(502) 762-2446
Director: Leslie McColgin
Accredited in speech-language pathology and
   audiology

Eastern Kentucky University Speech-
   Language-Hearing Clinic
Department of Special Education, Eastern
   Kentucky University
Richmond, KY 40475
(606) 622-4444
Director: Mary June Moseley, Ph.D.
Accredited in speech-language pathology

LOUISIANA
Children's Hospital
Speech, Language, and Audiology Department
200 Henry Clay Ave.
New Orleans, LA 70118
(504) 899-9511, x551, 552, 553, 554
Director: Nancy T. Javier, M.A.
Other language: Spanish
Accredited in speech-language pathology and
   audiology

Louisiana State University Medical Center
Speech, Language, and Hearing Clinic
1900 Gravier St.
New Orleans, LA 70112
(504) 568-6511
Director: Dr. Donald L. Rampp
Other languages: Greek, Sign
Accredited in speech-language pathology and
   audiology

New Orleans Speech and Hearing Center
1636 Toledano St.
New Orleans, LA 70115
(504) 897-2606
Directors: John Burke, Ph.D., Jack Rosen,
  Ph.D., Emeritus
Accredited in speech-language pathology and
  audiology
Centers also in Gretna and Slidell, LA

MAINE

Pine Tree Society for Handicapped Children
  and Adults
Speech and Hearing Services
84 Front St.
PO Box 518
Bath, ME 04530
(207) 443-3341
Director: Marlene Ouellette
Other languages: Total Communication, Cued
  Speech
Accredited in speech-language pathology and
  audiology

Northeast Hearing and Speech Center, Inc.
43 Baxter Blvd.
Portland, ME 04101
(207) 775-3491
Executive Director: Deborah Parker-
  Wolfenden, M.Ed. (speech pathologist)
Other languages: Sign, Cued Speech
Accredited in speech-language pathology and
  audiology

York County Counseling Services
Speech and Hearing Program
31 Beach St.
Saco, ME 04073
(207) 282-7504
Directors: Bernard P. Henri, Ph.D.
Assistant Director: Marti Andrews, M.A.
Other language: French
Accredited in speech-language pathology and
  audiology

F. T. Hill Center for Communication Disorders
Mid Maine Medical Center, Seton Unit
Waterville, ME 04901
(207) 873-0621, Seton x383
Director: Bruce D. Olsen
Other languages: Sign, Cueing
Accredited in speech-language pathology and
  audiology

MARYLAND

Baltimore County Department of Health
Division of Speech, Language, and Hearing
Eastern Regional Health Center
9100 Franklin Square Drive
Baltimore, MD 21237
(301) 687-6500, x346
Director: Judith Silberman
Accredited in speech-language pathology and
  audiology

Baltimore County Department of Health
Division of Speech, Language, and Hearing
Hannah More Academy Center
12035 Reisterstown Rd.
Baltimore, MD 21133
(301) 833-6830
Director: Judith Silberman
Accredited in speech-language pathology and
  audiology

The Easter Seal Society of Central Maryland
Communications Disorders Program
3700 Fourth St.
Baltimore, MD 21225
(301) 355-0100
Director: Sheila Mehring
Accredited in speech-language pathology

The Kennedy Institute for Handicapped
  Children
Department of Communication Sciences and
  Disorders
707 N. Broadway
Baltimore, MD 21205
(301) 522-5450
Director: Rachel E. Stark-Seitz, Ph.D.
Other language: Sign
Accredited in speech-language pathology and
  audiology

Maryland Institute for Emergency Medical
  Services Systems "Shock Trauma Center"
University of Maryland at Baltimore
Speech-Communication Disorders Program
Satellite Speech-Communication Disorders
  Program
Montebello Center
22 S. Greene St.
Baltimore, MD 21201
(301) 528-6101
Director: Roberta Schwartz, M.Ed.
Accredited in speech-language pathology

Montebello Center
Speech and Language Rehabilitation Clinic
2201 Argonne Drive
Baltimore, MD 21218
(301) 554-5390
Director: Robin Gladstone, M.Ed.
Accredited in speech-language pathology

Kilby Easter Seal Center
6400 Laurel-Bowie Rd.
Bowie, MD 20715-4093
(301) 262-5550
Director: Warren W. Bennett, M.S.W.
Accredited in speech-language pathology

Community Hospital and Health Care Systems,
   Inc.
Department of Speech and Audiology
Hospital Rd.
Cheverly, MD 20785
(301) 341-7177 (audiology)
(301) 341-6448 (speech-language pathology)
Director: Nancy T. Harlan
Accredited in speech-language pathology and
   audiology

Prince George's County Health Department
Division of Speech and Audiology
Hospital Rd.
Cheverly, MD 20785
(301) 386-0289 (voice)
(301) 773-9788 (TTY)
Director: Nancy T. Harlan
Accredited in speech-language pathology and
   audiology

Prince George's County Health Department
Division of Speech and Audiology
D. Leonard Dyer Regional Health Center
9314 Piscataway Rd.
Clinton, MD 20735
(301) 868-8800, x185 (voice)
(301) 856-1645 (TTY)
Director: Nancy T. Harlan
Accredited in speech-language pathology and
   audiology

The Frederick Treatment Centers for Disabled
   Children and Adults
6 N. Market St.
Frederick, MD 21701
(301) 694-7241
Director: Beverly H. Whitlock, M.A.
Other language: Sign
Accredited in speech-language pathology

Leo Kanner Speech and Hearing Center
Rosewood Center
Owings Mills, MD 21117
(301) 363-0300, x2559, 2558
Director: Gretchen Tangeman, M.A.
Accredited in speech-language pathology and
   audiology

Montgomery County Public Schools
Division of Speech and Language Programs
390 Martins Lane
Rockville, MD 20850
(301) 762-0632
Director: Sally A. Veres, M.A.
Other Languages: Spanish, Portuguese,
   French, Greek, Sign
Accredited in speech-language pathology

The Treatment Centers for Disabled Children
   and Adults
1000 Twinbrook Parkway
Rockville, MD 20851
(301) 424-5200 (voice)
(301) 424-5203 (TTY)
Director: Beverly H. Whitlock, M.A.
Other languages: Sign, Spanish
Accredited in speech-language pathology and
   audiology

Baltimore County Public Schools
Special Education–Office of Communicative
   Disorders
6901 N. Charles St.
Towson, MD 21204
(301) 494-4221
Director: Margaret Shrewsbury, Ph.D.
Other language: Spanish
Accredited in speech-language pathology and
   audiology

MASSACHUSETTS
Acton Public Schools
Acton-Boxborough Regional Schools
Speech and Language Department
96 Hayward Rd.
Acton, MA 01720
(617) 264-4700, x5424
Director: Francine R. Leiboff
Accredited in speech-language pathology

Amherst-Pelham Regional Schools and
  Amherst-Pelham Schools
Language and Speech Services
Chestnut St.
Amherst, MA 01002
(413) 253-9731 (voice)
(413) 253-9734 (TTY)
Director: William R. Ensslin
Other language: Sign
Accredited in speech-language pathology

University of Massachusetts
Communication Disorders Clinic
Arnold House
Amherst, MA 01003
(413) 545-2565
Director: Charlena M. Seymour
Coordinator-Audiology: Jane Baran
Coordinator-Speech/Language Pathology:
  Patricia Mercaitis
Accredited in speech-language pathology and
  audiology

Beth Israel Hospital
Department of Audiology
330 Brookline Ave.
Boston, MA 02215
(617) 735-3171
Director: Karen H. Marcarelli, M.A.
  (audiologist)
Other language: Sign
Accredited in audiology

Boston Guild for the Hard of Hearing
283 Commonwealth Ave.
Boston, MA 02115
(617) 267-4730, (voice)
(617) 267-3496 (TTY)
Director: Nancy E. Peterson, M.Ed.
Accredited in audiology

Brigham and Women's Hospital
Speech and Hearing Division
75 Francis St.
Boston, MA 02115
(617) 732-5601
Director: Howard H. Zubick, Ph.D.
Accredited in speech-language pathology and
  audiology

Children's Hospital Medical Center, Boston
Hearing and Speech Division
300 Longwood Ave.
Boston, MA 02115
(617) 735-6460
Director: Martin C. Schultz, Ph.D.
Other language: Sign
Accredited in speech-language pathology and
  audiology

Daniels Speech and Language Clinic
Boston University Medical Center
University Hospital
75 E. Newton St.
Boston, MA 02118
(617) 247-5467
Director: Laurie Gilden Lindner, Ph.D.
Other languages: Spanish, Arabic
Accredited in speech-language pathology

Faulkner Hospital Audiology Department
1153 Centre St.
Boston, MA 02130
(617) 522-5800, x1880
Director: David Gagliardi, M.S., (audiologist)
Accredited in audiology

Massachusetts Eye and Ear Infirmary
Audiology Department
243 Charles St.
Boston, MA 02114
(617) 523-7900, x634
Director: Rhoda Kimmel Morrison
Other languages: French, Sign
Accredited in audiology

Massachusetts General Hospital
Speech-Language Pathology Department
Ambulatory Care Center, Suite 637
15 Parkman St.
Boston, MA 02114
(617) 726-2763

New England Medical Center Hospital
Speech, Hearing, and Language Center
171 Harrison Ave., Box 823
Boston, MA 02111
(617) 956-5300
Director: Hubert L. Gerstman, Ed.D.
Other languages: Hospital translator service (all
  languages), Sign
Accredited in speech-language pathology and
  audiology

Northeastern University, Hearing, Language, and Speech Clinic
133 FR
360 Huntington Ave.
Boston, MA 02115
(617) 437-2492
Directors: Robert B. Redden, Ed.D. (chair)
Helen Anis, M.A.
Other language: Spanish
Accredited in speech-language pathology and audiology

Spaulding Rehabilitation Hospital
125 Nashua St.
Boston, MA 02114
(617) 720-6726
Director: Nancy Lefkowitz, M.S.
Accredited in speech-language pathology

Braintree Hospital
Center for Communication Disorders
250 Pond St.
Braintree, MA 02184
(617) 848-5353, x192
Director: Reg L. Warren, Ph.D.
Other language: Spanish
Accredited in speech-language pathology and audiology

Joseph P. Kennedy, Jr., Memorial Hospital for Children
Audiology Department
30 Warren St.
Brighton, MA 02135
(617) 254-3800, x194
Director: Joan Salkaus, M.S.
Accredited in Audiology

Kennedy Memorial Hospital for Children
Speech-Language Pathology Department
30 Warren St.
Brighton, MA 02135
(617) 254-3800, x191
Director: Carol B. Levy, Ed.D.
Other language: Spanish
Accredited in speech-language pathology

Bunker Hill Health Center
Charlestown, MA 02129
(617) 242-5748

Chelsea Memorial Health Care Center
Chelsea, MA 02150
(617) 884-8345

Clinton Hospital Speech, Language, and Hearing Center
201 Highland St.
Clinton, MA 01510
(617) 365-4531, x85
Director: Maureen Harris, (speech pathologist)
Accredited in speech-language pathology and audiology

Dracut Public Schools
2063 Lakeview Ave.
Dracut, MA 01826
(617) 957-4633
Director: Leonard K. Smith, Ed.M.
Accredited in speech-language pathology

Burbank Hospital Speech, Language, and Hearing Center
Nichols Rd.
Fitchburg, MA 01420
(617) 343-5005
Director: Joan E. Lada, M.S.
Accredited in speech-language pathology and audiology

The Learning Center for Deaf Children
Audiology Unit
848 Central St.
Framingham, MA 01701
(617) 879-5110 (voice)
(617) 879-5423 (TTY)
Director: Linda Harrison, M.A.
Other language: Sign
Accredited in audiology

Franklin Medical Center
Communication Disorders Department
164 High St.
Greenfield, MA 01301
(413) 772-0211, x2360
Director: Mary Alice McQuade, M.S.
Accredited in speech-language pathology and audiology

Speech, Hearing, and Language Center
Lawrence General Hospital
One General St.
Lawrence, MA 01842
(617) 683-4000, x2680
Director: Francis X. Dignam
Other languages: French, Hebrew, Greek, Spanish
Accredited in speech-language pathology and audiology

MGH Revere Health Associates
Revere, MA 02151
(617) 284-0064
Director: Julie Atwood Wheelden, M.Ed.
Other languages: Spanish, French, Sign
Accredited in speech-language pathology

North Shore Children's Hospital
Department of Language, Speech and Hearing
57 Highland Ave.
Salem, MA 01970
(617) 745-2100, x266
Director: Pamela Spilatore
Other languages: Spanish, ASL, SEE
  (German, French with small children)
Accredited in speech-language pathology and
  audiology

Mercy Hospital Hearing, Speech, and
  Language Center
271 Carew St.
Springfield, MA 01106
(413) 781-9100 (voice)
(413) 788-9644 (TTY)
Director: Carole W. Tomassetti
Other languages: Spanish, Sign
Accredited in speech-language pathology and
  audiology

New England Sinai Hospital
Speech, Language, and Hearing Clinic
PO Box 647
150 York St.
Stoughton, MA 02072
(617) 364-4850
Director: Jane Mulcahy O'Hara
Accredited in speech-language pathology and
  audiology

Morton Hospital, Inc.
Speech, Hearing, and Language Center
88 Washington St.
Taunton, MA 02780
(617) 824-6911, x1329, 1336
Director: Ellen Zane, M.A.
Other language: Sign
Accredited in speech-language pathology and
  audiology

The Waltham Hospital
Center for Speech, Language, and Hearing
9 Hope Ave.
Waltham, MA 02254-9116
(617) 647-6418 (voice)
(617) 899-6831 (TTY)
Director: Patricia Hartigan Richards, M.A.
Other Language: Spanish
Accredited in speech-language pathology and
  audiology

Hahnemann Rehabilitation Center
Audiology Department
Lincoln Plaza–535 Lincoln St.
Worcester, MA 01606
(617) 792-8500 (voice)
(617) 792-8507 (TTY)
Director: Amy Tessier
Accredited in audiology

Hahnemann Rehabilitation Center
Speech-Language Pathology Department
Lincoln Plaza–535 Lincoln St.
Worcester, MA 01606
(617) 792-8500 (voice)
(617) 792-8507 (TTY)
Director: David F. Russell
Other languages: Sign, Spanish
Accredited in speech-language pathology

University of Massachusetts Medical Center
Audiology and Speech-Language Pathology
55 Lake Avenue, N.
Worcester, MA 01605
(617) 856-3996, 2398
Directors: Steven R. Fournier, M.A., Robin
  Goldberg, M.S.
Accredited in speech-language pathology and
  audiology

MICHIGAN
Sinai Hospital of Detroit
Section of Speech-Language Pathology and
  Audiology
6767 W. Outer Drive
Detroit, MI 48235
(313) 493-6315
Director: William H. Restum, Ph.D.
Accredited in speech-language pathology and
  audiology

Hurley Medical Center
Speech and Language Pathology
One Hurley Plaza
Flint, MI 48502
(313) 257-9326
Director: Vause Carlsen, M.A., (speech
 pathologist)
Accredited in speech-language pathology

McLaren General Hospital
Speech and Hearing Department
401 Ballenger Highway
Flint, MI 48502
(313) 762-2362 (voice)
(313) 762-2304 (TTY)
Director: Constance W. Novak, M.A.
Accredited in speech-language pathology and
 audiology

Mott Children's Health Center
Speech and Hearing Service
806 Tuuri Place
Flint, MI 48503
(313) 767-5750
Director: Lois Wright
Accredited in speech-language pathology and
 audiology

Comprehensive Audiologic Services
1550 E. Beltline, S.E.
Grand Rapids, MI 49506
(616) 942-1660 (voice and TTY)
Director: Cynthia L. Ellison, M.A.
Accredited in audiology

Speech and Language Services
Psychiatric Consultation Services
825 Parchment S.E.
Grand Rapids, MI 49506
(616) 957-0850
Directors: Marge Penning (speech and
 language services)
Mark W. Hinshaw, M.D. (psychiatric
 consultation services)
Other language: Sign
Accredited in speech-language pathology

Constance Brown Hearing and Speech Center
1521 Gull Rd.
Kalamazoo, MI 49001
(616) 343-2601 (voice and TTY)
Director: Alvin J. Davis
Accredited in speech-language pathology and
 audiology

Central Michigan University
Speech and Hearing Clinics
Mount Pleasant, MI 48859
(517) 774-3471 (speech pathology)
(517) 774-3904 (audiology)
(517) 774-3471 (summer resident clinic)
Director: Robert M. McLauchlin, Ph.D.
Accredited in speech-language pathology and
 audiology

Oakland Schools Speech and Hearing Clinic
2100 Pontiac Lake Rd.
Pontiac, MI 48054
(313) 858-1907 (voice)
(313) 858-1878 (TTY)
Director: Mary Lu Robertson
Other Language: Sign
Accredited in speech-language pathology and
 audiology

William Beaumont Hospital
Speech and Language Pathology Department
3601 W. Thirteen Mile Rd.
Royal Oak, MI 48072
(313) 288-8085
Director: Michael I. Rolnick, Ph.D.
Accredited in speech-language pathology

Providence Hospital
Department of Audiology and Neurological
 Evoked Potentials
16001 W. Nine Mile Rd.
PO Box 2043
Southfield, MI 48037
(313) 424-3392
Director: Bonnie Soffin
Accredited in audiology

Eastern Michigan University
Speech and Hearing Clinic
Rackham Building
Ypsilanti, MI 48197
(313) 487-4410
Director: Marjorie Chamberlain, M.A.
Accredited in speech-language pathology and
 audiology

MISSISSIPPI
Mississippi University for Women
Speech and Hearing Center
PO Box W-1340
Columbus, MS 39701
(601) 329-4750, x270; 329-4754
Director: Barbara A. Hanners, Ph.D.
  (audiologist)
Other Language: Signing Exact English
Accredited in speech-language pathology and
  audiology

University of Southern Mississippi
Speech and Hearing Clinic
PO Box 5092
Southern Station
Hattiesburg, MS 39401
(601) 266-5216
Director: Robert C. Rhodes, Ph.D.
Other language: Sign
Accredited in speech-language pathology and
  audiology

Easter Seal Speech and Language Clinic
Mississippi Easter Seal Clinic
3226 N. State St.
PO Box 4958
Jackson, MS 39216
(601) 982-7051
Director: Sandra F. Johnston, M.A.
Accredited in speech-language pathology

University of Mississippi
Speech and Hearing Center
George Hall
University, MS 38677
(601) 232-7271
Director: John T. Jacobson, Ph.D.
Other language: Sign
Accredited in speech-language pathology and
  audiology

MISSOURI
University of Missouri-Columbia Hospital and
  Clinics
Communication Disorders Unit
2R01 Rusk Rehabilitation Center
One Hospital Drive
Columbia, MO 65212
(314) 882-6988
Director: Sharon Faubel, M.A., (speech
  pathologist)
Accredited in speech-language pathology

Woodhaven Learning Center
Speech-Language Services
PO Box 1796
Columbia, MO 65205
(314) 875-6181, x234
Director: Virginia L. Reznicek, M.A., (speech
  pathologist)
Accredited in speech-language pathology

Children's Mercy Hospital
Hearing and Speech Department
24th at Gillham Rd.
Kansas City, MO 64108
(816) 234-3677
Director: Cynthia Jacobsen, Ph.D. (speech
  pathologist)
Accredited in speech-language pathology and
  audiology

Irwin Lehrhoff and Associates, Inc.
PO Box 1503
Maryland Heights, MO 63043
(314) 569-8509
Directors: Sharon Koroshec, Janet Stack, M.S.

Springfield Speech and Hearing Center
1423 N. Jefferson
Springfield, MO 65802
(417) 865-2766
Director: Susan Dye, M.A.
Accredited in speech-language pathology

Central Institute for the Deaf
Speech-Language and Hearing Clinic
818 S. Euclid
St. Louis, MO 63110
(314) 652-3200 (voice)
(314) 531-0710 (TTY)
Director: Ann E. Geers, Ph.D.
Other languages: Spanish, Sign
Accredited in speech-language pathology and
  audiology

Special School District of St. Louis County
Speech, Language, Hearing Programs
12110 Clayton Rd.
Town and Country, MO 63131
(314) 569-8222 (voice)
(314) 569-8216 (TTY)
Director: Robert L. Huskey, Ph.D.
Other language: ASL
Accredited in speech-language pathology and
  audiology

MONTANA
University of Montana
Communication Sciences and Disorders
634 Eddy Ave.
Missoula, MT 59812
(406) 243-4131
Director: Charles D. Parker
Other language: Sign
Accredited in speech-language pathology and
audiology

NEBRASKA
Educational Service Unit #9
1117 South St., Box 2047
Hastings, NE 68901
(402) 463-2847
Directors: Barb Elliot, Ed.S., Irwin Ross,
Ed.D.
Accredited in speech-language pathology

University of Nebraska
Lincoln Speech and Hearing Clinic
Department of Special Education and
Communication Disorders
202 Barkley Memorial Center
42nd and Holdrege
Lincoln, NE 68583-0738
(402) 472-2071
Director: John Bernthal, Ph.D.
Other Language: Sign
Accredited in speech-language pathology and
audiology

Boys Town National Institute for
Communication Disorders in Children
555 N. 30th St.
Omaha, NE 68131
(402) 449-6540 (voice)
(402) 449-6543 (TTY)
Director: Don W. Worthington, Ph.D.
Other languages: Spanish, Sign
Accredited in speech-language pathology and
audiology

NEW JERSEY
Robert Wood Johnson Jr. Rehabilitation
Institute
Speech and Hearing Department
James St.
Edison, NJ 08817
(201) 321-7063
Director: Patricia V. Roy
Accredited in speech-language pathology and
audiology

Hunterdon Medical Center
Speech and Hearing Department
Route 31
Flemington, NJ 08822
(201) 782-2121, x405
Director: Anne Jones, M.S.
Accredited in speech-language pathology and
audiology

Saint Barnabas Medical Center
Rehabilitation Center for Speech and Hearing
Old Short Hills Rd.
Livingston, NJ 07039
(201) 533-5786
Director: Jane Ingling Johnson, Ed.D.
Other languages: Interpreters available
Accredited in speech-language pathology and
audiology

Roosevelt Hospital
Speech Pathology and Audiology Department
PO Box 151
Metuchen, NJ 08840
(201) 321-6800, x414
Director: Carol Gruenling, M.A.
Accredited in speech-language pathology

The Matheny School
Speech and Language Department
Main St.
Peapack, NJ 07977
(201) 234-0011
Director: Janet C. Wright, M.A., (speech
pathologist)
Accredited in speech-language pathology

Department of Speech Pathology/Audiology
North Jersey Developmental Center
169 Minnisink Rd.
Totowa, NJ 07511
(201) 256-1700, x253, 254
Director: Eva Hubschman, Ph.D.
Other languages: Sign, Hungarian, German,
Hebrew
Accredited in speech-language, pathology and
audiology

William Paterson College
Speech and Hearing Clinic
300 Pompton Rd.
Wayne, NJ 07470
(201) 595-2752
Director: Gilda Walsh
Other language: Sign
Accredited in speech-language pathology

Kessler Institute for Rehabilitation
Speech and Audiology Department
West Orange Facility
1199 Pleasant Valley Way
West Orange, NJ 07052
(201) 731-3600
Director: Ruthe Udell, M.A.
East Orange Facility
Central Ave. at the Parkway
East Orange, NJ 07018
Accredited in speech-language pathology

Children's Specialized Hospital
Speech and Hearing Department
New Providence Rd.
Westfield-Mountainside, NJ 07091
(201) 233-3720
Director: Ellen B. Kandel
Accredited in speech-language pathology

NEW MEXICO
Lovelace Medical Center
Audiology Section
Department of Otorhinolaryngology
5400 Gibson Blvd., S.E.
Albuquerque, NM 87108
(505) 262-7261
Director: Catherine A.W. Mrema
Accredited in audiology

NEW YORK
The Easter Seal Society Speech and Hearing
  Center
194 Washington Ave.
Albany, NY 12210
(518) 434-4103 (voice and TTY)
Director: Jacqueline Johnson
Accredited in speech-language pathology

Hospital of the Albert Einstein College of
  Medicine
Audiology Clinic
1600 Tenbroeck Ave.
Bronx, NY 10461
(212) 904-2677
Directors: Barbara Kruger, Ph.D., Neal
  Sloane, Ph.D. (supervisor)
Other languages: Spanish, Yiddish
Accredited in audiology

Montefiore Medical Center
Speech and Hearing Center
111 E. 210th St.
Bronx, NY 10467
(212) 920-5445
Program Supervisors: Karin Sailine Riordan,
  M.A. (speech pathologist)
William Dolan, M.A. (audiologist)
Accredited in speech-language pathology and
  audiology

Mount Saint Ursula Speech Center
200th St. and Marion Ave.
Bronx, NY 10458
(212) 584-7679
Administrator: Sr. M. Winifred Danwitz,
  Ph.D.
Director: Patricia M. Sweeting, Ph.D.
Accredited in speech-language pathology

North Central Bronx Hospital
Speech-Language Pathology and Audiology
3424 Kossuth Ave.
Bronx, NY 10467
(212) 920-7581
Directors: Carl Sonn Telzak (speech)
Lisa Horowitz Zeitoun (Audiology)
Other Languages: Spanish, German
Accredited in speech-language pathology

The Brooklyn Hospital
Speech and Hearing Center
212 DeKalb Ave.
Brooklyn, NY 11201
(718) 403-8431
Director: Joyce A. Rubenstein, Ph.D.
  (coordinator)
Other language: Spanish
Accredited in speech-language pathology and
  audiology

Queens College, CUNY
Speech and Hearing Center
Augmentative Communication Center
65-30 Kissena Blvd.
Flushing, NY 11367
(718) 520-7358, 7359
Director: Joel Stark, Ph.D.
Accredited in speech-language pathology and
  audiology

Hy Weinberg Center for Communication
  Disorders
Adelphi University
Garden City, NY 11530
(516) 663-1003
Director: Ellenmorris Tiegerman, Ph.D.
Accredited in speech-language pathology and
  audiology

Hofstra University Speech and Hearing Center
Hempstead, NY 11550
(516) 560-5656
Director: Ellen Parker, Ph.D.
Accredited in speech-language pathology

Lexington Hearing and Speech Center, Inc.
74-20 25th Ave.
Jackson Heights, NY 11370
(718) 899-8800, x281; 898-5962 (both voice or
  TTY)
Directors: Denise P. O'Brien, Ph.D., Kenneth
  L. Schneider, M.D.
Other languages: Spanish, Sign
Accredited in speech-language pathology and
  audiology

North Shore University Hospital
Speech and Hearing Center
300 Community Drive
Manhasset, NY 11030
(516) 562-4600 (voice)
(516) 627-3349 (TTY)
Director: Ilene Lieberman, M.S.
Other languages: Spanish, French, Sign
Accredited in speech-language pathology and
  audiology

Long Island Jewish–Hillside Medical Center
Hearing and Speech Center
New Hyde Park, NY 11042
(718) 470-2556
Director: S. Steve Rosenbaum, Ed.D.
Accredited in speech-language pathology and
  audiology

City School District of New Rochelle
Speech-Language-Hearing Department
515 North Ave.
New Rochelle, NY 10801
(914) 632-9000, x314
Director: Ruth Aptaker (Senior speech
  pathologist)
Other languages: Gujerati, Hindi
Accredited in speech-language pathology

Beth Israel Medical Center
Department of Surgery
Division of Speech and Hearing
Nathan D. Perlman Place
New York, NY 10003
(212) 420-2760
Directors: Sylvia Balick (speech and language)
Beverly Sigal (audiology)
Other language: Sign
Accredited in speech-language pathology and
  audiology

Columbia University
Teachers College
Speech and Hearing Center
525 W. 120th St.
New York, NY 10027
(212) 678-3409
Directors: Carol N. Wilder, Ph.D., Seymour
  Rigrodsky, Ph.D.
Other languages: Spanish, French
Accredited in speech-language pathology and
  audiology

Communication and Learning Center
Marymount Manhattan College
221 E. 71st St.
New York, NY 10021
(212) 472-3800, x576, 577
Director: Joan Shapiro, Ed.D.
Other language: Sign
Accredited in speech-language pathology

Goldwater Memorial Hospital
NYU Medical Center
Speech Pathology and Audiology Service
Roosevelt Island
New York, NY 10044
(212) 750-6785, 6790
Director: Patricia Kerman-Lerner
Other languages: Spanish, Sign
Accredited in speech-language pathology and
  audiology

The Howard A. Rusk Institute of
  Rehabilitation Medicine
New York University Medical Center
440 E. 34th St.
New York, NY 10016
(212) 340-6025
Director: Martha Taylor Sarno, M.D.
Accredited in speech-language pathology

Hunter College of the City University of New
York
Center for Communication Disorders
440 E. 25th St.
New York, NY 10010
(212) 481-4464
Director: Evelyn Pollack, M.A.
Accredited in speech-language pathology and
audiology

ICD–International Center for the Disabled
340 E. 24th St.
New York, NY 10010
(212) 679-0100
Director: Dianne Slavin, M.A.
Other languages: Spanish, Italian
Accredited in speech-language pathology

Lenox Hill Hospital
Center for Communication Disorders
100 E. 77th St.
New York, NY 10021
(212) 794-4821
Directors: Carole Bloch, Maurice H. Miller
Other languages: Italian, Spanish
Accredited in speech-language pathology and
audiology

The Mount Sinai Hospital
Communication Disorders Center
One Gustave Levy Place
New York, NY 10029
(212) 650-6153 (voice and TTY)
Director: Asher Bar, Ph.D.
Other languages: Spanish, Hebrew, Yiddish,
Hungarian, Ameslan
Accredited in speech-language pathology and
audiology

New York League for the Hard of Hearing
71 W. 23rd St.
New York, NY 10010
(212) 741-7650 (voice)
(212) 255-1932 (TTY)
Directors: Ruth R. Green, M.A., Jane R.
Madell, Ph.D., Diane Brackett, Ph.D.
Other languages: Sign, Spanish
Accredited in speech-language pathology and
audiology

Donald Reed Speech Center
Phelps Memorial Hospital
North Tarrytown, NY 10591
(914) 631-5100, x3660
and:

344 Main St.
Mt. Kisco, NY 10549
(914) 666-2142
Director: Robert Schlitt
Other languages: Yiddish, French
Accredited in speech-language pathology

Hearing and Speech Center of Rochester
1000 Elmwood Ave.
Rochester, NY 14620
(716) 271-0680 (voice)
(716) 442-2985 (TTY)
Director: John N. Paris
Other language: Sign
Accredited in speech-language pathology and
audiology

Hearing and Speech Center of Rochester
Northeast Division
1245 Culver Rd.
Rochester, NY 14609
(716) 482-3372
Directors: John N. Paris, Ann Moosman,
M.A. (speech pathologist)
Accredited in speech-language pathology

Strong Memorial Hospital–University of
Rochester Medical Center
Department of Audiology and Speech
Pathology
601 Elmwood Ave.
Rochester, NY 14642
(716) 275-2501, 4803 (voice)
(716) 275-4852 (TTY)
Director: Larry E. Dalzell, Ph.D.
Accredited in speech-language pathology and
audiology

Arthur Podwall, Ph.D., and Associates
The Smithtown Commons
267 E. Main St.
Smithtown, NY 11787
(516) 360-3222
Director: Arthur Podwall, Ph.D.
Accredited in speech-language pathology and
audiology

Syosset Speech and Hearing Center
Syosset Medical Building
175 Jericho Turnpike
Syosset, NY 11791
(516) 364-1234
Director: Arthur Podwall, Ph.D.
Accredited in speech-language pathology and
audiology

State University of New York
Upstate Medical Center
Communication Disorder Unit
766 Irving Ave.
Syracuse, NY 13210
(315) 473-4806
Director: Charles T. Grimes, Ph.D.
Accredited in speech-language pathology and
   audiology

Veterans Administration Medical Center
Audiology and Speech Pathology Service
Irving Ave. and University Place
Syracuse, NY 13210
(315) 476-7461, x374
Director: Walter M. Amster, Ph.D.
Accredited in speech-language pathology and
   audiology

Blythedale Children's Hospital Department of
   Speech Pathology and Audiology
Bradhurst Ave.
Valhalla, NY 10595
(914) 592-7555, x312
Director: Eleanor Kaufman
Accredited in speech-language pathology and
   audiology

Wassaic Developmental Center
Communication Disabilities Department
Station A
Wassaic, NY 12592
(914) 877-6821
Director: Barbara Saper White, M.A.
Accredited in speech-language pathology and
   audiology

Burke Rehabilitation Center
Speech-Language and Audiology Department
785 Mamaroneck Ave.
White Plains, NY 10605
(914) 948-0050, x2308
Director: Honey K. Klein, M.S.
Accredited in speech-language pathology and
   audiology

St. Agnes Hospital Children's Rehabilitation
   Center
Speech-Language Pathology Department
305 North St.
White Plains, NY 10605
(914) 681-4660
Director: Susan Zuckerman, M.A.
Accredited in speech-language pathology

NORTH CAROLINA
Thoms Rehabilitation Hospital
Partin Speech and Hearing Center
1 Rotary Drive
Asheville, NC 28803
(704) 274-2400
Director: Dianna Hutchinson
Assistant Director: Veronica Tronolone
Accredited in speech-language pathology and
   audiology

Charlotte Speech and Hearing Center
300 S. Caldwell St.
Charlotte, NC 28202
(704) 376-1342
Director: Donald F. Bynum
Accredited in speech-language pathology and
   audiology

Charlotte Speech and Hearing Center, Inc.
Union County Speech Center
114 E. Jefferson St.
Monroe, NC 28110
(704) 283-1539
Director: Donald F. Bynum
Accredited in speech-language pathology and
   audiology

NORTH DAKOTA
University of North Dakota
Medical Center Rehabilitation Hospital
Department of Communication Disorders
1300 S. Columbia Rd.
Grand Forks, ND 58201
(701) 780-2447
Director: Jack Adien Carrol, Ph.D.
Other language: Sign
Accredited in speech-language pathology and
   audiology

OHIO
University of Akron
Speech and Hearing Center
West Hall
Akron, OH 44325
(216) 375-7884 (voice)
(216) 424-3330 (TTY)
Director: Kenneth Siloac, Ph.D.
Accredited in speech-language pathology and
   audiology

Ohio University Speech and Hearing Clinic
School of Hearing and Speech Sciences
Lindley Hall
Athens, OH 45701
(614) 594-5050
Director: Helen B. Conover
Other languages: Greek, French, Spanish
Accredited in speech-language pathology and
   audiology

Cincinnati Speech and Hearing Center
Clermont County Speech-Language-Hearing
   Services
2291 Bauer Rd.
PO Box 12
Batavia, OH 45103
(513) 732-0961 (voice and TTY)
Executive Director: Carol P. Leslie, Ph.D.
Clermont Coordinator: Patricia Zurlinden,
   M.A.
Other language: Sign

University of Cincinnati Medical Center
Division of Audiology and Speech Pathology
Mail Location #780
Cincinnati, OH 45267-0780
(513) 872-4241
Director: Robert W. Keith, Ph.D.
Accredited in speech-language pathology and
   audiology

Cleveland Clinic Foundation
Section of Communicative Disorders
Department of Otolaryngology and
   Communicative Disorders
9500 Euclid Ave.
Cleveland, OH 44106
(216) 444-6693
Director: Richard H. Nodar, Ph.D.
Other languages: The Cleveland Clinic has
   interpreters covering 38 foreign languages
Accredited in speech-language pathology and
   audiology

Cleveland Hearing and Speech Center
11206 Euclid Ave.
Cleveland, OH 44106
(216) 231-8787 (voice)
(216) 292-6333 (TTY)
Director: Harry M. Broder
Other language: Sign
Accredited in speech-language pathology and
   audiology

Cleveland State University Speech and Hearing
   Clinic
Euclid and E. 22nd St.
Cleveland, OH 44115
(216) 687-3804 (voice)
(216) 687-3808 (TTY)
Director: David A. Metz, Ph.D.
Other language: Sign
Accredited in speech-language pathology and
   audiology

Fairview General Hospital
Department of Speech Pathology and
   Audiology
18101 Lorain Ave.
Cleveland, OH 44111
(216) 476-7104 (voice)
(216) 476-7103 (TTY)
Director: Dennis A. Abahazi, Ph.D.
Other language: Sign
Accredited in speech-language pathology and
   audiology

Ohio State University
Speech and Hearing Clinic
319 Derby Hall
154 N. Oval Mall
Columbus, OH 43210
(614) 422-6251 (voice and TTY)
Director: Edward J. Hardick, Ph.D.
Other languages: Sign, major language
   interpreters available
Accredited in speech-language pathology and
   audiology

Hearing and Speech Center for Children and
   Adults of Metropolitan Dayton
730 Valley St.
Dayton, OH 45404
(513) 222-5597 (voice and TTY)
Director: Robert K. Schmidt
Accredited in speech-language pathology and
   audiology

Delaware Speech and Hearing Center
27 W. Central Ave.
Delaware, OH 43015
(614) 369-3650
Director: Guy M. Naples, M.A.
Other language: Sign
Accredited in speech-language pathology and
   audiology

Lima Memorial Hospital
Speech and Hearing Clinic
1001 Bellefontaine Ave.
Lima, OH 45804
(419) 228-3335, x2363
Director: William D. Mustain, Ph.D.
Other language: Sign
Accredited in speech-language pathology and
    audiology

Southeastern Ohio Hearing and Speech Center,
    Inc.
Doctors Hospital of Nelsonville
Nelsonville, OH 45764
(614) 753-1973
Director: Carol Kamara, Ph.D.
Other language: Sign
Accredited in speech-language pathology and
    audiology

West Central Ohio Hearing and Speech Center
2612 Elmore Drive
Springfield, OH 45505
(513) 324-2081
Director: R. Douglas Lineberger
Other language: Sign
Accredited in speech-language pathology and
    audiology

Medical College of Ohio
Speech and Hearing Service
C.S. #10008
3000 Arlington Ave.
Toledo, OH 43699
(419) 381-5040, 4012
Director: Michelle A. Ridge
Accredited in speech-language pathology and
    audiology

The Toledo Hospital Division of
    Communication Disorders
2142 N. Cove Blvd.
Toledo, OH 43606
(419) 531-5771 (speech pathology)
(419) 471-5680 (audiology)
(419) 471-5579 (TTY)
Directors: Jerry M. Higgins, Ph.D., (speech
    pathologist)
Kevin C. Webb, Ph.D., (audiologist)
Accredited in speech-language pathology and
    audiology

OKLAHOMA
University of Oklahoma Health Sciences
    Center
John W. Keys Speech and Hearing Clinic
825 N.E. 14th St.
PO Box 26901
Oklahoma City, OK 73118
(405) 271-4214
Director: Donald T. Counihan, Ph.D.
Assistant Director: Glenda J. Ochsner, Ph.D.
Accredited in speech-language pathology and
    audiology

OREGON
Clatsop County Education Service District
Speech, Language, and Hearing Program
3194 Marine Drive
Astoria, OR 97103
(503) 325-2862
Director: Donna Mary Dulcich, M.S.
Accredited in speech-language pathology

Eugene Hearing and Speech Center
1202 Almaden
PO Box 2087
Eugene, OR 97402
(503) 485-8521
Directors: Ned Risbrough, Loyal D. Ediger,
    Ph.D (audiologist), Jane McDonald, M.A.
    (speech pathologist)
Other languages: French, Spanish
Accredited in speech-language pathology and
    audiology

Irwin Lehrhoff and Associates, Inc.
840 S.E. 122nd St.
PO Box 33012
Portland, OR 97233
(503) 230-7148
Directors: Sherry Fallenstein, M.S., Kristin
    Mattson, M.S.

The Oregon Health Sciences University
Crippled Children's Division, Speech
    Pathology, Audiology
PO Box 574
Portland, OR 97207
(503) 225-8356
Director: Robert W. Blakeley, Ph.D.
Accredited in speech-language pathology and
    audiology

Portland Center for Hearing and Speech
3515 S.W. Veterans Hospital Rd.
Portland, OR 97201
(503) 228-6479
Director: Gary J. Rentschler, Ph.D.
Accredited in speech-language pathology and
  audiology

Springfield-Eugene Hearing and Speech Center
1705 Centennial, Suite #1
Springfield, OR 97477
(503) 726-1589, or 485-8521
Directors: Ned Risbrough, Loyal D. Ediger,
  Ph.D. (audiologist), Jane McDonald, M.A.
  (speech pathologist)
Other languages: French, Spanish
Accredited in speech-language pathology and
  audiology

PENNSYLVANIA

Sacred Heart Hospital Speech and Hearing
  Center
421 Chew St.
Allentown, PA 18102
(215) 776-4795
Director: John M. Page, Ph.D.
Accredited in speech-language pathology and
  audiology

Bloomsburg University
Speech, Hearing, and Language Clinic
Bloomsburg, PA 17815
(717) 389-4436
Director: Richard Angelo
Accredited in speech-language pathology and
  audiology

Capital Area Intermediate Unit
2929 Gettysburg Rd.
Camp Hill, PA 17011
(717) 737-6728 (voice)
(717) 737-6746 (TTY)
Director: Patricia H. Querry
Other languages: Sign—ASL, SEE
Accredited in speech-language pathology and
  audiology

Geisinger Medical Center, Department of
  Audiology and Speech Pathology
Danville, PA 17822
(717) 271-6379 (voice)
(717) 271-8085 (TTY)
Director: Frank Rousseau
Accredited in speech-language pathology and
  audiology

Polyclinic Medical Center
Speech and Hearing Center
2601 N. Third St.
Harrisburg, PA 17110
(717) 782-4350
Director: Richard C. Krieger, M.S.
Other language: Sign
Accredited in speech-language pathology and
  audiology

Hearing Conservation/Deaf Services Center,
  Inc.
630 Janet Ave.
Lancaster, PA 17601
(717) 397-4741 (voice)
(717) 397-7138 (TTY)
Director: Thomas W. MacConnell
Other language: Sign
Accredited in audiology

Robinson Developmental Center
Speech Pathology and Audiology Services
Clever Rd.
McKees Rocks, PA 15136
(412) 787-2350
Director: Candida G. Craven, M.A.
Other language: Sign
Accredited in speech-language pathology

Hospital of Philadelphia College of
  Osteopathic Medicine
Department of Speech and Hearing
4150 City Ave.
Philadelphia, PA 19131
(215) 581-6082 (voice)
(215) 581-6687 (TTY)
Director: Ilene Ganzman, M.S.
Accredited in speech-language pathology and
  audiology

Moss Rehabilitation Hospital
Center for Communication Disorders
12th St. and Tabor Rd.
Philadelphia, PA 19141
(215) 329-5715
Directors: Thomas A. Matsko, M.S., Janet A.
  Jamieson, M.A.
Accredited in speech-language pathology and
  audiology

Children's Hospital of Pittsburgh
Department of Communication Disorders
125 DeSoto St.
Pittsburgh, PA 15213
(412) 647-5575, 5576, 5577
Director: Lawrence A. Bloom, Ph.D.
Other languages: French, Hebrew, Sign
Accredited in speech-language pathology

The Mercy Hospital of Pittsburgh
Department of Communication Disorders
Pride and Locust St.
Pittsburgh, PA 15219
(412) 232-7773
Director: Sheila J. Winkler, Ph.D.
Accredited in speech-language pathology and
  audiology

Pittsburgh Hearing, Speech, and Deaf
  Services, Inc.
1344 Fifth Ave.
Pittsburgh, PA 15219
(412) 281-1375 (voice and TTY)
Director: Gay L. Splain, M.Ed.
Accredited in speech-language pathology and
  audiology

The Pennsylvania State University
Speech and Hearing Clinic
110 Moore Building
University Park, PA 16802
(814) 865-5414
Director: Debra R. Suffolk, M.A.
Other language: Sign
Accredited in speech-language pathology and
  audiology

RHODE ISLAND
Rhode Island Hospital
Hearing and Speech Center
593 Eddy St.
Providence, RI 02902
(401) 277-5485
Director: J. Barry Regan, Ed.D.
Other languages: Spanish, Sign
Accredited in speech-language pathology and
  audiology

SOUTH CAROLINA
University of South Carolina
Speech and Hearing Clinic/Scooter Program
1601 St. Julian Place
Columbia, SC 29204
(803) 777-2614
Director: Carol C. Coston, M.S.
Accredited in speech-language pathology and
  audiology

Pee Dee Speech and Hearing Center
153 N. Baroody St.
Florence, SC 29503
(803) 622-5601
21 Ave. N. (coastal facility)
Myrtle Beach, SC 29577
(803) 448-2913
Director: Patricia J. Vincent
Accredited in speech-language pathology and
  audiology

TENNESSEE
University of Tennessee
Department of Audiology and Speech
  Pathology
Hearing and Speech Center
Yale at Stadium Drive
Knoxville, TN 37996-2500
(615) 974-5451
Director: Harold A. Peterson, Ph.D.
Accredited in speech-language pathology and
  audiology

Memphis State University
Memphis Speech and Hearing Center
807 Jefferson Ave.
Memphis, TN 38105
(901) 525-2682
Director: Daniel S. Beasley, Ph.D.
Accredited in speech-language pathology and
  audiology

Bill Wilkerson Hearing and Speech Center
1114 19th Ave. S.
Nashville, TN 37212
(615) 320-5353
Director: Fred H. Bess, Ph.D.
Accredited in speech-language pathology and
  audiology

TEXAS

South Texas Speech Hearing and Language
   Center
PO Box 6387
3455 S. Alameda
Corpus Christi, TX 78411
(512) 852-8252
Director: Larry Higdon, M.S., (audiologist)
Other Language: Spanish
Accredited in speech-language pathology and
   audiology

Callier Center for Communication Disorders
University of Texas at Dallas
1966 Inwood Rd.
Dallas, TX 75235
(214) 783-3000
Directors: Ross J. Roeser, Ph.D (audiologist),
   Sara M. Haynes, M.S. (speech pathologist)
Other language: Spanish
Accredited in speech-language pathology and
   audiology

Irwin Lehrhoff and Associates, Inc.
PO Box 222101
Dallas, TX 75222
(814) 654-5835
Directors: Sherry Fallenstein, M.S., Janet
   Fink, M.S.
Accredited in speech-language pathology

North Texas State University
Division of Communication Disorders
Denton, TX 76203
(817) 565-2481
Director: Richard W. Stream, Ph.D.
Other language: Sign
Accredited in speech-language pathology and
   audiology

Speech and Hearing Center of El Paso, Inc.
El Paso Medical Center
1501 Arizona, Suite 1D
El Paso, TX 79902
(915) 533-2266
Director: Alice M. Lambert, M.A., SP
Other language: Spanish
Accredited in speech-language pathology and
   audiology

University of Texas Medical Branch
Center for Audiology and Speech Pathology
Bethel Hall
Texas Ave.
Galveston, TX 77550
(409) 761-2711
Directors: Lesley C. Hill, M.A., Lucinda
   Gary, M.A.
Other languages: Spanish, Sign
Accredited in speech-language pathology and
   audiology

The Battin Clinic
3931 Essex Lane
Houston, TX 77027
18100 Upper Bay Rd.
Nassau Bay, TX 77058
(713) 621-3072, 7421
Director: R. Ray Battin, Ph.D.
Assistant Director: Lynn Frankel, M.A.
Other Languages: Spanish, French, Persian,
   Armenian, American Sign Language,
   Signing Exact English
Accredited in speech-language pathology and
   audiology

Baylor College of Medicine Methodist Hospital
6501 Fannin St.
Houston, TX 77030
(713) 790-5913
Director: James F. Jerger, Ph.D.
Other language: Spanish
Accredited in speech-language pathology and
   audiology

Irwin Lehrhoff and Associates, Inc.
2539 S. Gessner, Suite 16
Houston, TX 77063
(713) 782-8145
Directors: Sherry Fallenstein, M.S., Janet
   Fink, M.S.
Accredited in speech-language pathology

University of Texas Health Science Center at
   Houston
Speech and Hearing Institute
1343 Moursund
Houston, TX 77030
(713) 792-4500
Director: Carol Lynn Waryas, Ph.D.
Other languages: Spanish, Sign
Accredited in speech-language pathology and
   audiology

Texas Tech University
Department of Speech and Hearing Sciences
Speech and Hearing Clinic
PO Box 4266
Lubbock, TX 79409
(806) 742-3907
Directors: Earlene Tash Paynter, Ph.D., Sherry
 Sancibrian, M.S.
Other languages: Spanish, Sign
Accredited in speech-language pathology and
 audiology

Richardson Independent School District
Language, Speech, and Hearing Services
400 S. Greenville Ave.
Richardson, TX 75081
(214) 238-0324
Director: Marilyn S. Duncan
Other Language: Spanish
Accredited in speech-language pathology

Brooke Army Medical Center
Auditory Treatment and Evaluation Clinic
Otolaryngology Service–Beach Pavilion
Fort Sam Houston
San Antonio, TX 78234
(512) 221-5636
Director: Lt. Col. Kenneth B. Aspinall, Ph.D.
Accredited in audiology

Harry Jersig Center
Our Lady of the Lake University
411 S.W. 24th St.
San Antonio, TX 78285
(512) 434-6711, x413
Director: Jane B. Davidson, M.A.
Other language: Spanish
Accredited in speech-language pathology and
 audiology

Irwin Lehrhoff and Associates, Inc.
PO Box 290002
San Antonio, TX 78280
(512) 299-6809
Directors: Sherry Fallenstein, M.S., Janet
 Fink, M.S.
Accredited in speech-language pathology

Southwest Texas State University
Speech, Hearing, and Language Clinic
Special Education Department
San Marcos, TX 78666
(512) 245-2157
Director: Carolyn McCall
Accredited in speech-language pathology

Vaughn Memorial Speech and Hearing Center
Medical Center Hospital
PO Drawer 6400
Tyler, TX 75711
(214) 531-8190
Director: Starr Fulcher, M.A.
Accredited in speech-language pathology and
 audiology

UTAH
Irwin Lehrhoff and Associates, Inc.
2004 S. Eighth, E.
Salt Lake City, UT 84105
(801) 584-2179
Directors: Felene Boeker, M.S., Lora Dorsey,
 M.A.

Utah Department of Health
Bureau of Communicative Disorders
44 Medical Drive
Salt Lake City, UT 84113
(801) 533-6175
Directors: Thomas Mahoney, Ph.D., Nick G.
 Cozakos, M.S.
Other languages: German, Greek
Accredited in speech-language pathology and
 audiology

VERMONT
University of Vermont
Eleanor M. Luse Center for Communication
 Disorders
Burlington, VT 05405
(802) 656-3861
Director: Mitchell B. Kramer, Ph.D.
Accredited in speech-language pathology and
 audiology

VIRGINIA
University of Virginia
Speech and Hearing Center
109 Cabell Hall
Charlottesville, VA 22903
(804) 924-7107
Director: Ralph C. Bradley, Ed.D.
Other languages: Spanish, Sign
Accredited in speech-language pathology and
 audiology

Danville Speech and Hearing Center
610 Upper St.
Danville, VA 24541
(804) 792-0650
Director: Elizabeth T. Marshall
Accredited in speech-language pathology

Woodrow Wilson Rehabilitation Center
Department of Communication Services
Fishersville, VA 22939
(703) 885-9715
Director: Linda A. Meyer, Ph.D.
Other language: Sign
Accredited in speech-language pathology and
audiology

James Madison University
Speech and Hearing Center
Harrisonburg, VA 22807
(703) 568-6491
Directors: Maynard D. Filter, Robert C.
Morris, Sr.
Accredited in speech-language pathology and
audiology

Central Virginia Speech and Hearing Center,
Inc.
Virginia Baptist Hospital
Lynchburg, VA 24503
(804) 522-4520
Director: Ernest C. Edwards, M.S.
Other language: Sign
Accredited in speech-language pathology and
audiology

Roanoke Valley Speech and Hearing Center,
Inc.
2030 Colonial Ave., S.W.
Roanoke, VA 24015
(703) 343-0165
Director: Richard R. Hawkins, M.A.
Accredited in speech-language pathology and
audiology

WASHINGTON

Hearing Speech and Deafness Center
1620 18th Ave.
Seattle, WA 98122
(206) 323-5770 (voice and TTY)
Directors: Suzanne Connors (audiologist),
Margaret Collins-Byrne (speech pathologist)
Other language: Sign
Accredited in speech-language pathology and
audiology

University of Washington Speech and Hearing
Clinic
Department of Speech and Hearing Sciences
4131 15th N.E. (JH-40)
Seattle, WA 98195
(206) 543-5440 (clinic)
(206) 543-7974 (department office)
Directors: Richard Horn, Fred D. Minifie,
Ph.D.
Accredited in speech-language pathology and
audiology

WISCONSIN

St. Elizabeth Hospital
Department of Speech Pathology
1506 S. Oneida St.
Appleton, WI 54915
(414) 738-2587
Director: Lois G. Mueller
Accredited in speech-language pathology

Sacred Heart Hospital
Speech/Language Pathology Department
900 W. Clairemont Ave.
Eau Claire, WI 54701
(715) 839-4365
Director: Lisa A. LaDew
Accredited in speech-language pathology

St. Francis Health Corporation
Department of Speech Pathology
700 West Ave. S.
La Crosse, WI 54601
(608) 785-0940
Director: Kathleen Rone
Accredited in speech-language pathology

Marshfield Clinic
Sections of Audiology and Speech-Language
Pathology
1000 N. Oak Ave.
Marshfield, WI 54449
(715) 387-5371 (audiologist)
(715) 387-5128 (speech pathologist)
(715) 387-7222 (TTY)
Directors: Richard L. Strand, M.S.
(audiologist), Marilyn Seif Workinger, M.S.
(speech pathologist)
Accredited in speech-language pathology and
audiology

SOURCE: *American Speech-Language-Hearing Association.*

SPEECH AND HEARING HOTLINE

(800) 638-TALK (8255)
(301) 897-8682—Maryland, Alaska, and
   Hawaii

The hotline operates during regular weekday business hours and answers a variety of questions, such as why your child isn't talking or has started to stutter, what to do if your spouse cannot talk normally after a stroke, where to find resources for any speech or hearing problem. Will provide literature and tell you where to find a speech-language or audiology clinic near you. Operated by the National Association for Hearing and Speech Action, which is the consumer affiliate of the American Speech-Language Hearing Association.

ORGANIZATIONS

American Speech-Language-Hearing
   Association
10801 Rockville Pike
Rockville, MD 20852
(301) 897-5700

A national professional membership organization for speech language pathologists and audiologists concerned with communication behavior and disorders. A major source of information about speech-language problems. Pamphlets, booklets, audiovisual materials, scientific journals, monographs, reports, directories. Provides the names of certified speech pathologists, audiologists and clinical centers. Will provide more information and the names of accredited speech language pathologists in your area upon request.

National Association for Hearing and Speech
   Action
10801 Rockville Pike
Rockville, MD 20852
(800) 638-8255 (voice/TDD)
(301) 897-8682 (voice/TDD)

A national organization which is the consumer affiliate of the American Speech-Language Hearing Association. Provides information about all speech, language and hearing disorders. Publishes a bimonthly newsletter, pamphlets and packets on a variety of communication disorders. Maintains a national hotline. Answers questions on all aspects of hearing and speech disorders and provides professional referrals throughout the world.

The Orton Dyslexia Society
724 York Road
Baltimore, MD 21204
(301) 296-0232
(800) ABC-D123

Nonprofit, membership organization of professionals and the public with local branches in many parts of the country. Information source for individuals, families, other interested persons on dyslexia. Booklets, pamphlets, fact sheets, audiocassette tapes, a quarterly newsletter, *Perspectives*. Answers questions from the public, maintains lists of facilities specializing in dyslexia. Will send more information and name of a local branch in your area upon request. (*See* page 372 for more information on dyslexia.)

Speech Foundation of America
PO Box 11749
Memphis, TN 38111
(901) 452-0995

A nonprofit, charitable foundation devoted to disseminating information about the prevention and treatment of stuttering. A source of information for the public. Sponsors a yearly conference on stuttering. Books and pamphlets. Can make referrals to therapists who specialize in treating stuttering in most major cities. Will provide more information upon request.

MATERIALS, FREE AND FOR SALE

Free

Answers Questions About Child Language, 2 pages.
Aphasia, 2 pages.
How Does Your Child Hear and Talk?, 8 pages.
Recognizing Communication Disorders, 8 pages.
Speech and Language Disorders and the Speech-Language Pathologist, 10 pages.

National Association for Hearing and Speech Action
10801 Rockville Pike
Bethesda, MD 20852
(301) 897-5700

First Aid for Aphasics, 19 pages; steps to take to help an aphasic.
An Open Letter to the Family of An Adult Patient with Aphasia, 4 pages.
Same Face—New Sound: Information for Laryngectomees and Their Families, 34 pages.
Understanding Stuttering: Information for Parents, 30 pages.

National Easter Seal Society
2023 W. Ogden Ave.
Chicago, IL 60612

Hearing, Speech and Language, 10 pages; NINCDS Research Program.
Stuttering: Hope Through Research, 16 pages.

National Institute of Neurological and Communicative Disorders and Stroke
9000 Rockville Pike, Building 31, Room 8A06
Bethesda, MD 20892
(301) 496-5751

For sale

If Your Child Stutters: A Guide for Parents, 48 pages.
Self-Therapy for the Stutterer, 192 pages.
To the Stutterer, 116 pages. By 24 speech pathologists who overcame stuttering.
Stuttering: Successes and Failures in Therapy, 148 pages.

Speech Foundation of America
PO Box 11749
Memphis, TN 38111

SPINA BIFIDA

See also Genetic Counseling, page 226, Rehabilitation, page 460.

Spina bifida (which literally means cleft spine) is a "neural tube" birth defect, involving damage to an embryo's developing spine and nervous system. Normally by the end of the fourth week of pregnancy, the bones of a fetus's spine close completely; in spina bifida, this does not happen, and the infant is left with an improperly formed spinal canal. The effects can be so mild as to be barely detectable, or exceedingly serious, producing various degrees of paralysis and necessitating spinal surgery soon after birth.

The number of people who have spina bifida is unknown. There are an estimated one or two cases for every 1,000 live births, and the incidence of neural tube defects is declining for an unknown reason. In the past few decades, most infants born with spina bifida died soon after birth, but because of aggressive new treatments, most spina bifida infants born today can survive.

Cause: Unknown. It is believed that the condition is at least partially genetic. Some recent studies have implicated vitamin and mineral deficiencies during pregnancy.

Symptoms: In its very slightest form, no symptoms may appear, and the condition may never be noticed. In more serious cases, a sac protrudes from the abnormal opening in the spine, sometimes exposing nerve tissue, and sometimes incorporating coverings of the spinal cord. If the neural tube fails to fuse, the spinal cord itself may protrude through the bony defect, and brain tissue may also be malformed. This is the most severe form, called anencephaly, and results in death.

The severity of symptoms depends on the type and size of the defect. Long-term effects are usually focused on the legs and may range from weak muscles to total paralysis with no feeling in the legs. Even in mild cases, bowel and bladder control are serious problems. Spina bifida is often accompanied by hydrocephalus (accumulation of fluid in the brain), which, if not relieved, can result in mental retardation.

Diagnosis: The defect, if serious, is almost always physically noticeable at birth. The defect can also be identified prior to birth by several methods, including ultrasonic scanning late in pregnancy and an alphafetoprotein test, which identifies abnormal levels of a particular biochemical early in pregnancy. Experts advise such screening, especially if the mother has given birth to one child with spina bifida. Genetic counseling is also advised.

Treatment: Treatment is controversial, focusing mainly on whether or not to perform lifesaving corrective surgery to treat the handicapped infant at the time of birth. Many argue it is a matter of medical and parental judgment. On the other hand, some groups and individuals insist immediate lifesaving surgery on spina bifida infants should always be done, regardless of the parents' wishes. Usually the surgery is done, within hours of the birth. In cases of hydrocephalus, the fluid can be drained by a permanently implanted shunt. The baby may need a daily routine of "range of motion" exercises.

In later life, children with spina bifida need special attention, and possibly orthopedic measures, to prevent stiffening of the joints and abnormalities of feet, legs and posture. An orthopedic specialist or physiatrist may prescribe corrective shoes, braces, crutches, and other devices. Some centers and specialists are also successfully using biofeedback and other behavioral techniques to train youngsters to control their fecal incontinence. Since spina bifida cannot be reversed, the main goal of treatment is manage-

ment of the condition, helping the youngster to live as normally as possible. With early and successful medical treatment, an infant born with spina bifida can expect to have a normal life span.

SOME LEADING SPECIALISTS

Here are some leading specialists in spina bifida. For a list of orthopedic surgeons and neurologists who are heads of their departments at leading medical colleges, *see* pages 621 and 630. They also may be excellent sources of treatment and/or referrals to others who are specialists in the care of spina bifida.

David McCullough, M.D.
Pediatric neurosurgeon
Children's Hospital National Medical
    Center
111 Michigan Ave., N.W.
Washington, DC 20010
(202) 745-3020

David G. McLone, M.D.
Neurologist
Children's Memorial Hospital
2300 Children's Plaza
Chicago, IL 60614
(312) 880-4373

William F. Kaplan, M.D.
Division of Urology
2300 Children's Plaza
Children's Memorial Hospital
Chicago, IL 60614
(312) 880-4428

Wilton Bunch, M.D.
Orthopedist
Loyola Medical Center
2160 S. First Ave., Building, 54, Room
    167
Maywood, IL 60153
(312) 531-3280

Richard Lindseth, M.D.
Orthopedist
702 Barnhill Drive
Indianapolis, IN 46223
(317) 264-7913

Joan Venes, M.D.
Taubman Health Center
R2128-0338
1500 E. Medical Center Drive
Ann Arbor, MI 48109
(313) 926-5016

Fred Epstein, M.D.
New York University Medical Center
550 First Ave.
New York, NY 10016
(212) 340-6419

Donald H. Reigel, M.D.
Neurolosurgeon
Suite 158, 4815 Liberty Ave.
Pittsburgh, PA 15224
(412) 682-0400

F. Brantley Scott, M.D.
Urologist
6720 Bertner, Suite B-538
Houston, TX 77030
(713) 791-4266

David Shurtleff, M.D.
Pediatrician
Children's Orthopedic Hospital and Medical
    Center
4800 Sand Point Way, N.E., PO Box C 5371
Seattle, WA 98105
(206) 526-2058

SOURCE: *Spina Bifida Association of America.*

ORGANIZATION

Spina Bifida Association of America
343 S. Dearborn St.
Chicago, IL 60604
(312) 663-1562
(800) 621-3141 (outside Illinois)

A network of more than 100 chapters nationwide, dedicated to bringing spina bifida into the public spotlight. A membership organization of adults and young people with spina bifida, their parents, and professionals offering care or services to individuals with spina bifida. Helps fund research into the cause of spina bifida and improvements in medical devices and facilities for care and treatment of the birth defect. Conducts a national conference on spina bifida, provides information, and publishes booklets and other informational materials, including a bimonthly newsletter, *The Insights*. Individuals are referred to local chapters for help.

MATERIALS, FREE AND FOR SALE

Free

Spina Bifida and Neural Tube Defects: Research Report, 6 pages

National Institute of Neurological and Communicative Disorders and Stroke
National Institutes of Health
Building 31, Room 8A06
Bethesda, MD 20892

For sale

Beyond the Family and the Institution: Residential Issues for Today

The Child With Spina Bifida.
Clinic Directory
Giant Steps for Steven
Introduction to Spina Bifida
Learning Disabilities and the Person with Spina Bifida
When Something Is Wrong With Your Baby: Looking In and Reaching Out

Spina Bifida Association of America
343 S. Dearborn St.
Chicago, IL 60604

SPINAL CORD INJURIES

See also Rehabilitation, page 460.

Spinal cord injuries are one of our most serious health problems. They happen in a second and leave a lifetime of irreversible damage. Every year about 15,000 Americans suffer paralysis and loss of sensation from spinal cord injuries. About 200,000 Americans are confined to wheelchairs because of such injuries. Almost all the paralysis comes from accidents—or war wounds—and it costs billions of dollars a year. The price tag of caring for one individual with spinal cord injury over a lifetime is put at more than $500,000. The tragedy is compounded by the fact that spinal cord injuries almost always strike the young, mostly men. About two-thirds of the victims are under age 30; the average age is 19.

Cause: Some studies show that from one-third to one-half of the spinal cord injuries are caused by motor vehicle accidents. Other common causes are gunshot wounds and athletic injuries. The spinal cord is a two-foot long bundle of nerves that fits snugly inside the 33 vertebrae that form the spinal column. The cord runs from the brain to the lower back and carries all the two-way communications between the brain and the rest of the body—the muscles, organs, and skin. The spinal cord is amply protected from minor bumps, but a severe blow can bruise or crush the spinal cord (it is rarely severed). The spinal cord then swells and begins to hemorrhage, causing death of the nerve cells and the formation of scar tissue, blocking the transmission of nerve signals below the "injury."

Symptoms: The common result of spinal cord injury is paralysis. The degree of paralysis depends on the amount of damage and its location. The loss of motor power and sensation can be total or partial. The general rule is that the higher the injury on the spinal cord, the worse the disability.

An injury to the midback may cause paralysis only of the legs and lower body; an injury to the spine at the neck may produce quadriplegia—paralysis of all limbs and the upper and lower body. Paralysis may bring complications, such as loss of bladder and bowel control, involuntary spasms, infections, and skin sores. There may be impaired sexual functioning, although most women are able to bear children. Men may or may not be able to father children through normal intercourse; some may choose artificial insemination.

Treatment: Much of the important treatment is administered in the first hours following injury; doctors do their best to minimize the tissue destruction and permanent damage. They may use drugs, surgery, and other techniques. Several drugs are in the early stages of testing in attempts to improve spinal cord functioning and lessen the permanent damage. After the patient is out of immediate danger, rehabilitation is the main concern. Rehabilitation has made giant strides. Only 10 years ago, many people paralyzed by spinal cord injuries were condemned to spend most of their lives in hospitals. Now such cases are rare; the majority of persons with spinal injuries are rehabilitated and become independent enough to leave the hospital.

The patient may need to learn to handle a number of prostheses and devices, like electronic nerve stimulators to control breathing muscles, wheelchairs, and specially equipped automobiles. New technology is constantly developing ingenious devices for people who are paralyzed. Recent research has shown that electrical stimulation of the muscles can help keep a patient's body in shape by aiding in the exercise of the muscles. A great deal of physical therapy is necessary. Patients may need to remain at rehabilitation centers for a few months, or much longer, depending on their progress. The aim of rehabilitation, of course, is to restore the individual to independence.

There is also scientific interest in the exciting possibilities of actual regeneration of the nerves, thus preventing or reversing paralysis. Researchers are experimenting with drugs and other methods to interrupt the paralysis process and possibly reverse it. There have been some successes in animals. Although nerve regeneration may be an ultimate answer in the future, scientists are far from finding such a "cure" for paralysis. Prevention, prompt initial treatment, and rehabilitation are the only current remedies for spinal cord injury.

GOVERNMENT SPINAL CORD INJURY CENTERS

The federal government, through the National Institute of Handicapped Research, sponsors a number of model spinal cord injury centers around the country that provide comprehensive, multidisciplinary care including emergency services, rehabilitation services, and long-term medical, social, psychological, and vocational services. These centers are considered among the best in the United States for the treatment and rehabilitation of spinal cord injuries.

Many patients are referred to those centers by hospitals and physicians. But patients and the families of patients can also contact the centers for admission. It is best to gain admittance to a multidisciplinary center as soon as possible after the injury. Figures for one system show that if a person paralyzed from the waist down arrives within three weeks of the injury, the average hospital stay will be about three months. If a person is referred later, the average hospital stay is at least a month longer.

These spinal cord injury centers have been compared to burn centers—the best places to be for the most comprehensive, up-to-date medical care. Although the centers prefer early referral, they will take patients at virtually any time. Some hospitals have set up spinal cord injury centers similar to the model systems supported by the federal government.

In addition, a few rehabilitation centers are now accredited especially as spinal cord injury rehabilitation centers by the Commission on Accreditation of Rehabilitation Facilities (CARF). These centers should be excellent facilities for rehabilitation. *See* Rehabilitation Centers, page 460 for those designated as spinal cord injury accredited centers.

ALABAMA
Samuel L. Stover, M.D.
Spain Rehabilitation Center
University of Alabama at Birmingham
Birmingham, AL 35294
(205) 934-3450

CALIFORNIA
Robert L. Waters, M.D.
Rancho Los Amigos Hospital
7601 E. Imperial Highway
Harriman Building 121
Downey, CA 90242
(213) 922-7167

COLORADO
Robert R. Menter, M.D.
Craig Hospital
Rocky Mountain Spinal Cord Injury Center
3425 S. Clarkson St.
Englewood, CO 80110
(303) 789-8000

GEORGIA
David F. Apple, Jr., M.D.
Shepherd Center for Treatment of Spinal
  Injuries
2020 Peachtree Rd., N.W.
Atlanta, GA 30309
(404) 352-2575

ILLINOIS
Paul R. Meyers, Jr., M.D.
Northwestern University Medical Center
Northwestern Memorial Hospital
Acute Spinal Cord Injury Service
250 E. Chicago Ave. Room 619
Chicago, IL 60611
(312) 649-3425

MASSACHUSETTS
Murray M. Freed, M.D.
Boston University
N.E. Regional Spinal Cord Injury Center
75 E. Newton St.
Boston, MA 02118
(617) 638-7300

MICHIGAN
Frederick M. Maynard, M.D.
University of Michigan
Physical Medicine & Rehabilitation
E32528 University Hospital, Box 33
Ann Arbor, MI 48109
(313) 764-9401

Leonard F. Bender, M.D.
Rehabilitation Institute of Detroit
Wayne State University
261 Mack Blvd.
Detroit, MI 48201
(313) 494-9731

NEW YORK
Kristjan T. Ragnarsson, M.D.
New York University Medical Center
Institute of Rehabilitation Medicine
400 E. 34th St.
New York, NY 10016
(212) 340-6125

Charles J. Gibson, M.D.
Strong Memorial Hospital
University of Rochester Medical Center
601 Elmwood Ave.
Rochester, NY 14642
(716) 275-3271

PENNSYLVANIA
John F. Ditunno, Jr., M.D.
Jefferson Medical College
Thomas Jefferson University
11th and Walnut St.
Philadelphia, PA 19107
(215) 928-6573

TEXAS
R. E. Carter, M.D.
The Institute for Rehabilitation & Research
Texas Medical Center
1333 Moursund Ave.
Houston, TX 77030
(713) 797-1440

VIRGINIA
Warren G. Stamp, M.D.
University of Virginia Medical Center, Box
  159
Department of Orthopedics and Rehabilitation
Charlottesville, VA 22908
(804) 924-8578

SOURCE: *National Institute of Handicapped Research.*

VETERANS ADMINISTRATION SPINAL CORD INJURY CENTERS

The Veterans Administration also maintains a group of spinal cord injury centers throughout the country. These are available to veterans only.

CALIFORNIA
VA Medical Center
5901 E. Seventh St.
Long Beach, CA 90822
Dr. Stanley Gordon
(213) 498-1313
(Affl.: University of California, Irvine)

VA Medical Center
3801 Miranda Ave.
Palo Alto, CA 94304
Dr. Inder Perkash
(415) 493-5000
(Affl.: Stanford University)

VA Medical Center
Sepulveda, CA 91343
Dr. Vasilis Nikas

FLORIDA
VA Medical Center
1201 N.W. 16th St.
Miami, FL 33125
Dr. Marilyn S. Wells
(305) 324-4455
(Affl.: University of Miami)

VA Medical Center
13000 N. 30th St.
Tampa, FL 33612
(813) 972-2000
(Affl.: Tampa Medical School)

GEORGIA
VA Medical Center
2460 Wrightsboro Rd.
Augusta, GA 30910
Dr. Janusz Markowski
(404) 321-6111
(Affl.: Medical College of Georgia)

ILLINOIS
VA Medical Center
Roosevelt Rd. & Fifth Avenue
Hines, IL 60141
Dr. Bernard A. Nemchausky
(312) 343-7200
(Affl.: Loyola University Medical School)

MASSACHUSETTS
VA Medical Center
940 Belmont St.
Brockton, MA 02401
(617) 583-4500
(Affl.: Harvard Medical School)

VA Medical Center
1400 VFW Parkway
West Roxbury, MA 02132
Dr. Bushra A. Fam
(617) 583-4500
(Affl.: Harvard University)

MISSOURI
VA Medical Center
915 N. Grand Blvd.
St. Louis, MO 63106
Dr. Robert Woolsey
(314) 487-0400
(Affl.: University of St. Louis)

NEW JERSEY
VA Medical Center
Tremont Ave. & South Center
East Orange, NJ 07019
Dr. Arthur Cytryn
(201) 676-1000
(Affl.: New Jersey State Medical School)

NEW YORK
VA Medical Center
130 W. Kingsbridge Rd.
Bronx, NY 10468
Dr. Courtney Wood
(212) 584-9000
(Affl.: Mt. Sinai Mcdical School, CUNY)

VA Medical Center
Beacon St.
Castle Point, NY 12511
Dr. Yong I. Lee
((914) 831-2000

OHIO
VA Medical Center
10701 East Blvd.
Cleveland, Oh 44016
Dr. Henry A. Bohlman
(216) 791-3800
(Affl.: Case Western Reserve University
    Medical School)

TENNESSEE
VA Medical Center
1030 Jefferson Ave.
Memphis, TN 38104
Dr. Benjamin A. Moeller, Jr.
(901) 523-8990
(Affl.: University of Tennessee)

TEXAS
VA Medical Center
2002 Holcombe Blvd.
Houston, TX 77211
Dr. Michael Krebs
(713) 795-4411
(Affl.: Baylor University Medical School)

VIRGINIA
VA Medical Center
Emancipation Drive
Hampton, VA 23667
Dr. Ralph F. Shepard
(804) 722-9961
(Affl.: Eastern Virginia Medical School)

VA Medical Center
1201 Broad Rock Rd.
Richmond, VA 23249
Dr. Robert W. Hussey
(804) 230-9001
(Affl.: Medical College of Virginia)

WASHINGTON
VA Medical Center
Seattle, WA 98208
Dr. Joel DeLisa
(206) 762-1010

WISCONSIN
VA Medical Center
5000 W. National Ave.
Wood, WI 53193
Dr. Dennis Maiman
(414) 384-2000
(Affl.: University of Wisconsin)

SOURCE: *Veterans Administration.*

GOVERNMENT-SUPPORTED RESEARCH CENTERS

The National Institute of Neurological and Communicative Disorders and Stroke supports special acute spinal cord injury research centers at the following universities. The centers are headed by the physicians listed below.

CONNECTICUT
Michael Brackew, M.D.
Associate Professor
Department of Epidemiology
Yale Medical School
60 College St.
New Haven, CT 06510
(203) 785-2808

NEW YORK
Eugene S. Flamm, M.D.
Professor and Chairman
Department of Neurosurgery
University Hospital
New York University Medical Center
New York, NY 10016
(212) 340-6414

OHIO
William E. Hunt, M.D.
Director, Division of Neurological Surgery
The University Hospitals
Ohio State University
College of Medicine
Columbus, OH 43212
(614) 421-8714

SOUTH CAROLINA
Phanor L. Perot, Jr., M.D.
Professor and Chairman
Division of Neurosurgery
The Medical University Hospital
University of South Carolina
Charleston, SC 29401
(803) 792-2421

TEXAS
Eduardo Eidelberg, M.D.
Director, Division of Neurosurgery
University of Texas
San Antonio, TX 78284
(512) 691-6136

SOURCE: *National Institute of Neurology and Communicative Disorders.*

ADDITIONAL HELP
National Center for Rehabilitation
Wright State University
Dayton, OH 45435
(513) 229-6123
Jerrold S. Petrofsky, Ph.D.
Chandler A. Phillips, M.D.

This center has been doing extensive research to help paraplegics keep in physical shape through computer-controlled electrical stimulation of muscles in paralyzed limbs. The research is aimed at rehabilitation.

ORGANIZATIONS

American Paralysis Association
PO Box 187
Short Hills, NJ 07078
(201) 379-2690
(800) 225-0292

A nonprofit organization committed to encouraging and supporting research to find a cure for paralysis caused by spinal cord or head injuries and stroke. Publishes a newsletter on central nervous system research and a medical journal, *Central Nervous System Trauma.* Has a network of local chapters. Will send research and membership information upon request.

National Spinal Cord Injury Association
149 California St.
Newton, MA 02158
(617) 964-0521

Voluntary nonprofit membership organization with 41 local chapters around the United States. Information and self-help source for patients, their families, physicians, interested persons.

Provides pamphlets, booklets, brochures. Answers questions from the public. Makes medical referrals. Sponsors conferences. Special services, counseling, makes available drugs and other medical supplies at discount. Will send more information and name of chapter in your area upon request.

Paralyzed Veterans of America
801 18th St., N.W.
Washington, DC 20006
(202) 872-1300

National nonprofit organization for spinal cord injured or diseased veterans and their families with 32 chapters around the country. Offers booklets, videotapes, a monthly magazine, *Paraplegia News,* and *Sports 'n Spokes,* a magazine of competitive sports and recreation for the wheelchair user. Special services: a national network of service offices in VA hospitals and sponsorship of wheelchair sports events. Will provide more information upon request.

BOOKS

Female Sexuality Following Spinal Cord Injury, **E. F. Becker,** Bloomington, IL: Cheever Publishing Co., 1978; PO Box 700, Bloomington, IL 61701.
Handbook for Paraplegics and Quadriplegics, Newton, MA: National Spinal Cord Injury Association, 149 California St., Newton, MA 02158.
Living with Spinal Cord Injury: Questions and Answers for Patients, Family and Friends, **Marjorie Garfunkel** and **Glen Goldfinger,** New York: New York University Medical Center. Institute for Rehabilitation Medicine, 400 E. 34th St., New York, NY 10016.
Options: Spinal Cord Injury and the Future, **Barry Corbet,** Denver, CO: A. B.

Hirschfeld Press, 1980. Available through the National Spinal Cord Injury Association, 149 California St., Newton, MA 02158.
Spinal Cord Injury: A Guide for Care, **Glenn Goldfinger** and **Marcia Hanak,** New York: New York University Medical Center, Institute for Rehabilitation Medicine, 400 E. 34th St., New York, NY 10016.
Spinal Cord Injury: A Guide for Patients and Their Families, **Lyn Phillips, et al.,** New York: Raven Press, 1986.
Who Cares? A Handbook an Sex Education and Counseling Services for Disabled People, Washington: The Sex and Disability Project, 1979; 1828 L St., N.W., Suite 704, Washington, DC 20036.

MATERIALS, FREE AND FOR SALE

Free

Spinal Cord Injury: Hope Through Research

National Institute of Neurological and
  Communicative Disorders and Stroke
9000 Rockville Pike, Building 31, Room 8A06
Bethesda, MD 20892

For sale

*National Resource Directory: An Information
  Guide for Persons with Spinal Cord Injury
  and Other Physical Disabilities*

National Spinal Cord Injury Association
149 California St.
Newton, MA 02158
(617) 964-0521

Paraplegia News, a monthly magazine that
reports on news concerning paraplegics and
wheelchair living, of interest to paraplegics,
quadriplegics, civilians and veterans: the
official organ of the Paralyzed Veterans of
America.
Spinal Cord Injury, 16 pages.

Paralyzed Veterans of America
801 18th St., N.W.
Washington, DC 20006

SUDDEN INFANT DEATH SYNDROME (SIDS)

Every year about 7,000 apparently healthy babies, most between one and six months of age, die suddenly, usually in their sleep. Sudden Infant Death Syndrome, SIDS, claims as many as two out of every 1,000 infants in the first year of life. About 90 percent of the SIDS deaths happen before six months of age, most between the second and fourth months. The peak time of death is between midnight and 8 A.M. Death is silent. SIDS, also called crib death, is a mysterious medical condition. No one really knows why it happens, what causes it, or how to prevent it. Through the years many myths and false research starts have surrounded SIDS, including theories that SIDS is hereditary, contagious or is caused by suffocation, choking or vomiting. SIDS is apparently a condition with a long history, occurring as frequently several centuries ago as it does now.

Physicians cannot identify which babies are at risk for SIDS or prevent SIDS, but research points to some risk factors in the disease. For example, a federal study of 800 babies who died of SIDS found that 70 percent of their mothers smoked during pregnancy. The study also noted that black babies were three times as likely as others to succumb to SIDS; about one-third of

SIDS infants were born to teenagers; and nearly 60 percent of the SIDS victims were male.

Furthermore, autopsies of SIDS victims show that they may not be "perfectly normal," as previously thought. They differ physically. SIDS infants often have abnormal cells around the brain stem and abnormal liver function. Low-birth-weight babies are also at special risk; the smaller the baby, the greater the risk. Additionally, at higher risk are infants from low-economic groups and the siblings of SIDS babies. The sibling of a twin who dies of SIDS, for example, is at 20 times the risk of other infants. SIDS occurs more often in the winter months.

Looking back, parents describe SIDS infants as often having had a mild respiratory tract infection in the week preceding death. Parents also observe that many SIDS infants had abnormal cries, decreased muscle tone, lack of vigor, a growth-lag, and were irritable or jittery.

Despite these patterns that offer clues, no clear causes of SIDS have emerged, and most experts believe there are multiple causes.

SIDS parents are often consumed with guilt, and support groups do exist to help them cope with the grief, anger, and anxiety surrounding SIDS.

SIDS INFORMATION AND COUNSELING PROGRAMS

If you are concerned about SIDS or suspect your infant may be at high risk, contact one of the federally supported SIDS Information and Counseling Programs listed below.

ALABAMA
SIDS Information and Counseling Program
Alabama Department of Public Health
Family Health Administration
424 Monroe St.
Montgomery, AL 36103
Beverly Boyd, M.D.
(205) 261-5673

ALASKA
Alaska SIDS Information & Counseling
  Program
Family Health Section
State Department of Health and Social Services
Pouch H-06B
Juneau, AK 99811
David Spence, M.D.
(907) 465-3100

ARKANSAS
SIDS Information and Counseling Program
Arkansas Department of Health
Maternal and Child Health Division
4815 W. Markham
Little Rock, AR 72201
Constance Morgan, R.N., M.S.N.
(501) 661-2762

CALIFORNIA
SIDS Information and Counseling Program
California Department of Health Services
Maternal and Child Health Branch
2151 Berkeley Way, Annex 4
Berkeley, CA 94704
Lyn Headley, M.D.
(415) 540-2098

COLORADO
Colorado SIDS Program
1330 Leyden St.
Suite 134
Denver, CO 80220
Sheila Marquez, R.N.
(303) 320-7771
(800) 332-1018 (in Colorado)

CONNECTICUT
SIDS Information and Counseling Program
Connecticut State Department of Health
  Services
150 Washington St.
Hartford, CT 06106
A. Verden Bolden, M.S.
(203) 566-3287

DELAWARE
SIDS Information & Counseling Program
Division of Public Health
Cooper Building
Dover, DE 19901
Richard Vehslage, A.C.S.W.
(302) 736-4744

DISTRICT OF COLUMBIA
SIDS Program
D.C. Office of Maternal & Child Health
1875 Connecticut Ave., N.W., Room 804D
Washington, DC 20009
Rose Livingston, R.N.
(202) 673-6665

FLORIDA
Florida SIDS Program
Florida State Department of Health and
  Rehabilitative Services
Children's Medical Services, HRS
1317 Winewood Blvd.
Building 5, Suite 127
Tallahassee, FL 32301
W. W. Ausbon, M.D.
(904) 488-6005

GEORGIA
Georgia SIDS Program
Child Health Programs
Division of Public Health
878 Peachtree St., N.E., Suite 212
Atlanta, GA 30306
Lillian P. Warnick, M.D.
(404) 894-6611

HAWAII
Hawaii SIDS Information and Counseling
  Program
Kapiolani Children's Medical Center
1319 Punahou St., Room 734
Honolulu, HI 96826
Dexter S. Y. Seto, M.D.
(808) 947-8587

IDAHO
SIDS Information and Counseling Program
Maternal and Child Health
Idaho Department of Health and Welfare
Child Health Bureau
Statehouse
Boise, ID 83720
Coleen Hughes, R.N., Ph.D.
(208) 334-4136

ILLINOIS
SIDS Information and Counseling Program
Illinois Department of Public Health
Division of Family Health
535 W. Jefferson St.
Springfield, IL 62761
Elsie Baukoll, M.D., M.P.H.
(217) 782-2736

INDIANA
SIDS Information and Counseling Program
Statewide SIDS Case Management System
Indiana State Board of Health
1330 W. Michigan St.
Indianapolis, IN 46206
Geraldine Wojtowicz, R.N.
(317) 633-8461

IOWA
Iowa SIDS Program
Iowa State Department of Health
Lucas State Office Building
Des Moines, IA 50319
Carolyn Adams
(515) 281-6645

KENTUCKY
SIDS Information and Counseling Program
Kentucky Department for Human
  Resources
Bureau for Health Services
Division for Maternal and Child Health
275 E. Main St.
Frankfort, KY 40621
Patricia K. Nicol, M.D.
(502) 564-4830

MAINE
Maine SIDS Program
Maine Department of Human Services
Division of Public Health Nursing
Statehouse, Station 11
Augusta, ME 04333
Helen M. Zidowecki, R.N., M.S.
(207) 289-3259

MARYLAND
Maryland SIDS Information and Counseling
  Program
University of Maryland
School of Medicine
Medical School Teaching Facility
10 S. Pine St., Suite 400
Baltimore, MD 21201
Stanford B. Friedman, M.D.
(301) 528-3542

MASSACHUSETTS
Massachusetts Center for SIDS
Boston City Hospital
Ambulatory Care Center
4th Floor, S.
818 Harrison Ave.
Boston, MA 02118
Robert Reece, M.D.
(617) 424-5742

MICHIGAN
Wayne County SIDS Center
c/o Children's Hospital of Michigan
5310 St. Antoine
Detroit, MI 48202
Herman Gray, M.D.
(313) 494-5719

SIDS Information and Counseling Program
Genessee County Health Department
310 W. Oakley
Flint, MI 48503
Bonnie Haun, R.N., M.S.
(313) 257-3585

Kent County Health Department
700 Fuller, N.E.
Grand Rapids, MI 49503
Colleen Jillson, R.N.
(616) 774-3055

Macomb County Health Department
43525 Elizabeth
Mount Clemens, MI 48043
Pamela Walsh
(313) 469-5523

Oakland County Health Department
1200 N. Telegraph Rd.
Pontiac, MI 48053
Elaine Bevan, B.S.N., M.P.H.
(313) 858-1409

MINNESOTA
Minnesota Sudden Infant Death Center
Minneapolis Children's Medical Center
2525 Chicago Ave. S.
Minneapolis, MN 55404
Ralph A. Franciosi, M.D.
(612) 874-6825

MISSISSIPPI
SIDS Information and Counseling Program
Mississippi State Department of Health
Bureau of Personal Health Services
PO Box 1700
Jackson, MS 39215
Fran Baker, M.S.W.
(601) 961-4142, 4135

MISSOURI
Sudden Infant Death Syndrome Resources,
    Inc.
1600A S. Big Bend Blvd.
St. Louis, MO 63117
Laura Hillman, M.D.
(314) 644-2056

NEBRASKA
Nebraska Department of Health
Division of Maternal and Child Health
301 Centennial Mall S.
PO Box 95007
Lincoln, NE 68509
Robert S. Grant M.D., M.P.H.
(402) 471-2907

Nebraska SIDS Program
VNA of Omaha
10840 Harvey Circle
Omaha, NE 68154
Jane Jensen, R.N., M.S.N.
(402) 571-8001

NEW HAMPSHIRE
Division of Public Health
Bureau of Maternal & Child Health
Health and Welfare Building
Hazen Drive
Concord, NH 03301
Margaret Weinberg, M.S.W.
(603) 271-4667

NEW JERSEY
SIDS New Jersey Program
New Jersey State Department of Health
CN 364
Maternal and Child Health Program
Trenton, NJ 08625
Amy Meltzer, M.D.
(609) 292-5616

NEW MEXICO
SIDS Information and Counseling Program
University of New Mexico
School of Medicine
Office of Medical Investigator
Albuquerque, NM 87131
John Smialek, M.D.
(505) 277-3053

NEW YORK
New York State SIDS Information &
    Counseling Program
Division of Children's Services
State Department of Health
Tower Building, Empire State Plaza
Room 821
Albany, NY 12237
Fr. A. Cardona, M.D., M.P.H.
(518) 474-1911

New York City Information and Counseling
    Program for Sudden Infant Death Syndrome
Office of Medical Examiner
520 First Ave., Room 506
New York, NY 10016
Olive Pitkin, M.D.
(212) 566-8170

Western New York SIDS Center
University of Rochester Medical Center
601 Elmwood Ave.
PO Box 777
Rochester, NY 14642
John Brooks, M.D.
(716) 275-2464

New York State Eastern Region Sudden Infant
    Death Syndrome Center
School of Social Welfare
Health Sciences Center
Level 2, Room 099
State University of New York
Stony Brook, NY 11794
Ruth A. Brandwein, Ph.D.
(516) 246-2582

NORTH CAROLINA

North Carolina SIDS Information and
  Counseling Program
Department of Human Resources
Division of Health Services
Maternal and Child Health Branch
PO Box 2091
Raleigh, NC 29602
Jimmie L. Rhyne, M.D.
(919) 733-7791

NORTH DAKOTA

North Dakota SIDS Management Program
North Dakota State Department of Health
Division of Maternal & Child Care
Bismarck, ND 58505
Bertie Hagberg, R.N.
(701) 224-2493
(800) 472-2286 (in North Dakota)

OHIO

Ohio SIDS Information and Counseling
  Program
Ohio Department of Health
Bureau of Maternal and Child Health
246 N. High St.
PO Box 118
Columbus, OH 43216
Ben Chukwuhmah, M.D., M.P.H.
(614) 466-4716

OKLAHOMA

SIDS Information and Counseling Program
Oklahoma State Department of Health
1000 N.E. 10th St., Room 709
PO Box 53551
Oklahoma City, OK 73152
Edd D. Rhoades, M.D.
(405) 271-5193

OREGON

Counseling Division
American SIDS Institute
1425 S.W. 20th St.
Portland, OR 97201
Janice Cram, B.A.
(503) 228-9121

SIDS Information & Counseling Program
Maternal & Child Health Program
Oregon State Health Division
PO Box 231
Portland, OR 97207
Marianne Remy, P.N.P., M.P.H.
(503) 229-5593

PENNSYLVANIA

Pennsylvania SIDS Center
Hershey Medical Center
Harrisburg, PA 17033
David Gordon
(717) 534-6509

Pennsylvania SIDS Center
One Children's Center
34th & Civic Center Blvd.
Philadelphia, PA 19104
Michael D'Antonio, Ph.D.
(215) 386-0264

RHODE ISLAND

SIDS Information and Counseling Program
Rhode Island Department of Health
Division of Family Health
Cannon Building
75 Davis St., Room 302
Providence, RI 02908
William H. Hollinshead, III, M.D.
(401) 277-2312

SOUTH CAROLINA

SIDS Information and Counseling Program
South Carolina Department of Health &
  Environmental Control
Division of Children's Health
2600 Bull St.
Columbia, SC 29201
Betty Johnson
(803) 758-5491

SOUTH DAKOTA

SIDS Information and Counseling Program
Division of Health Services
Joe Foss Building
523 E. Capitol
Pierre, SD 57501
Allen Krom, M.S.W.
(605) 773-3737

TENNESSEE
Tennessee SIDS Program
100 Ninth Ave. N., 3rd Floor
Department of Health & Environment
Division of Maternal & Child Health
Nashville, TN 37216
Millicent Stuntz, R.N., M.P.H.
(615) 741-0362

TEXAS
Texas SIDS Information & Counseling
   Program
Bureau of Maternal & Child Health
Texas Department of Health
110 W. 49th St.
Austin, TX 78756
Hilda Cover, R.N., M.S.
(512) 458-7700, x2026

North Texas SIDS Information & Counseling
   Program
P.O. Box 35728
Dallas, TX 75325
Robert J. McGovern, M.D.
(214) 668-2796

SIDS Information & Counseling Program
Harris County Health Department
2501 Dunstan
PO Box 25249
Houston, TX 77005
Francine Jensen, M.D.
(713) 526-2796

UTAH
SIDS Information and Counseling Program
Utah Department of Health
Division of Family Health Services
Bureau of Child Health
44 Medical Drive
Salt Lake City, UT 84113
Frances Frost, R.N., M.S.
(801) 533-4575

VERMONT
Vermont SIDS Health Program
Medical Services
PO Box 70
1193 North Ave.
Burlington, VT 05402
Claire LeFrancois, R.N., M.P.H.
(802) 863-7330

VIRGINIA
Virginia SIDS Program
Bureau of Maternal & Child Health
Commonwealth of Virginia
Department of Health
109 Governor St.
Richmond, VA 23219
Alice Linyear, M.D.
(804) 786-7367

WASHINGTON
SIDS Northwest Regional Center
Children's Orthopedic Hospital & Medical
   Center
4800 Sand Point Way, N.E.
Seattle, WA 98105
Nora E. Davis, M.D.
(206) 526-2100

WEST VIRGINIA
West Virginia SIDS Program
West Virginia Department of Health
Building 3, Suite 560
1800 Washington St. E.
Charleston, WV 25305
Bonnie McClung Fulcher, M.S.
(304) 348-8870

West Virginia SIDS Prevention Project
Department of Pediatrics, Room 4621
Basic Sciences Building
West Virginia University
Morgantown, WV 26506
David Myerberg, M.D.
(304) 293-7302

WISCONSIN
Wisconsin SIDS Center
PO Box 1997
Milwaukee, WI 53201
Connie Guist, R.N.
(414) 931-4049

WYOMING
Wyoming SIDS Program
Health & Medical Services
Hathaway Building, 4th Floor
Cheyenne, WY 82002
Larry Meuli, M.D.
(307) 777-6297

SOURCE: *National Sudden Infant Death Syndrome Clearinghouse.*

ORGANIZATIONS

The Guild for Infant Survival
PO Box 3841
Davenport, IA 52808
(319) 326-4653

A national voluntary membership organization for families who lose children to SIDS and for those who have high-risk SIDS youngsters. About 15 chapters in various parts of the country. Offers booklets, especially on grief and monitoring. Makes referrals to health professionals in the field. Will provide more information and the name of a local chapter near you upon request.

National Sudden Infant Death Syndrome
   Clearinghouse
8201 Greensboro Drive, Suite 600
McLean, VA 22102
(703) 821-8955 or 625-8410

An information service supported by the United States Department of Health and Human Services to provide information and educational materials to SIDS parents, the general public and health care professionals. Will answer questions from the public and send information upon request.

National Sudden Infant Death Syndrome
   Foundation
8240 Professional Place, Suite 205
Landover, MD 20785
(301) 459-3388
(800) 221-SIDS

A national voluntary mutual support organization of SIDS parents and medical professionals to support parents and further research on SIDS with about 80 chapters around the country. A source of information for the public including leaflets, audiovisual materials, a quarterly newsletter. Referrals to appropriate health professionals. Will provide more information and the name of a chapter in your locality upon request. Special services: operates a 24-hour information line on SIDS.

FREE MATERIALS

Facts About Apnea, fact sheet.
The Grief of Children, fact sheet.
Infantile Apnea and SIDS, fact sheet.
Parents and the Grieving Process, fact sheet.
Sudden Infant Death Syndrome: A Review of the Medical Literature, 1974-1979
What Is SIDS?, fact sheet.
What Parents Should Know About SIDS, fact sheet.

National SIDS Clearinghouse
8201 Greensboro Drive Suite 600
McLean, VA 22102

Facts About Sudden Infant Death Syndrome, 12-page brochure. Packet of research fact sheets.

National SIDS Foundation
8240 Professional Place, Suite 205
Landover, MD 20785

TAY-SACHS DISEASE AND RELATED DISORDERS

See also Genetic Counseling, page 226.

Tay-Sachs disease, Gaucher 's disease, Niemann-Pick disease, and Sandhoff's disease are heartbreaking disorders that begin in the womb and usually progress relentlessly after birth, leading to death at an early age—usually between two and five years. All are genetic metabolic defects of fat-storage with slightly different courses of progression. They are rare, and most commonly strike those of Eastern European (Ashkenazi) Jewish descent. However, recent studies show that other populations, notably of French-Canadian descent, are also particularly vulnerable to Tay-Sachs disease.

There is no treatment at all for Tay-Sachs, Niemann-Pick, and Sandhoff's; there is some limited experimental therapy for Gaucher's disease. The disorders, at present, can be controlled only by screening for the existence of the carrier genes, genetic counseling and, when desired, abortion.

Cause: Tay-Sachs disease results from a metabolic abnormality—in this case the absence of an enzyme—that causes fatty deposits to build up in the brain, leading to the destruction of the central nervous system. Death is inevitable by the age of five. About 85 percent of the children with Tay-Sachs are Jewish, and one in 25 American Jews is a carrier of the Tay-Sachs gene. The condition also occurs in Jews of Sephardic origin and in non-Jews, notably in some Italian Catholics.

Tay-Sachs is passed on as a recessive gene, much the same way as hair color and eye color. The gene can be carried and passed on through generations before the disease is expressed. In order to conceive a Tay-Sachs baby, both parents must be carriers. A man and a woman who are both carriers have a 25 percent chance of producing a child with Tay-Sachs with each pregnancy. There is a 50 percent chance that the child will also be a carrier. What makes the disorder so shocking is that it usually shows up in parents with no family history of the disease.

Symptoms: From birth through six months of age, the baby usually appears normal. Then subtle signs of brain damage begin to show up. By age one, the baby typically has recurring convulsions and motor control gradually deteriorates—the ability to crawl, to sit up, and to turn over are lost. As the brain destruction progresses, the stricken infant becomes blind, mentally retarded, and paralyzed, and eventually dies.

Treatment: There is no treatment; the disease is incurable. The elimination of the disorder is hoped for through prevention. This can be done by screening members of the vulnerable populations to see if they are carrying the gene and by a prenatal test, such as amniocentesis, to see if the unborn child has Tay-Sachs disease. Knowing the odds of having such a child, or that a child has been conceived with Tay-Sachs, the parents can then decide whether to consider other choices, such as adoption, artificial insemination, and abortion. If a screening test is positive, other members of the family should also be alerted so they too can be screened.

Sandhoff's disease is rarer than Tay-Sachs, but the two diseases are so similar that they can only be distinguished from each other by diagnostic laboratory tests, which show a slightly different enzyme deficiency. Other than that, the two disorders are nearly identical. Sandhoff's disease has been commonly misdiagnosed as Tay-Sachs.

Niemann-Pick disease also is a metabolic deficiency of the lipid (fat) system, leading to an enlarged liver, spleen, and lymph glands. There are several different types of the disease. The most common, the infantile form, causes general mental and physical deteriorations after the first few months of life, ending in death by age two or three. It can affect people of all ethnic origins, but the majority of infants with Niemann-Pick disease are of Ashkenazi Jewish ancestry. It is estimated that 1 Ashkenazic Jew in 100 carries the defective Niemann-Pick gene. Both Sandhoff's and Niemann-Pick diseases are rarer than Tay-Sachs.

Another similar though more common genetic metabolic disorder is Gaucher's disease. It can be found in all racial and ethnic groups, but once again is concentrated in the Ashkenazi Jewish population. As many as 1 in 12 persons in that ethnic group may carry the gene, and as many as 10,000 Americans may have Gaucher's. There are three distinct types of the disorder. The most common, which can appear at any age, generally causes an enlarged spleen and liver, bone pain, and orthopedic complications. The infantile type, just as in Tay-Sachs, shows up several months after birth, strikes the central nervous system, and results in death before age two. The third type also involves the nervous system, with symptoms of seizures, mental retardation, and erratic movements. It generally appears between the ages of 10 and 20, and although it is not fatal, it does shorten the life span.

Gaucher's is also incurable, but several therapies are being tried, including enzyme replacement and bone marrow transplantation. A test that was recently developed at the National Institutes of Health can predict whether a youngster with Gaucher's has the type that will eventually attack the central nervous system.

The presence of Gaucher's, Niemann-Pick and Sandhoff's can be detected by testing the fetus. There is no reliable mass screening test to determine who is carrying the defective gene for these three disorders. But once a person has had a child with these disorders, enzyme level tests can determine whether others in the family are carrying the gene. As with Tay-Sachs, both parents must carry the gene before there is a possibility of the appearance of the disorder in their offspring; then, the chances are one in four.

TAY-SACHS SCREENING

The screening test for carriers of the Tay-Sachs gene in vulnerable populations is common but is occasionally subject to misinterpretation. Therefore, authorities say it is critical that the blood analysis, or assay, is done by experienced physicians, preferably in a hospital lab that processes a large number of such tests, to keep mistakes at a minimum. Especially in borderline cases, an uncritical reading of the results by an inexperienced technician could result in a mistaken finding.

The National Tay-Sachs and Allied Diseases Association has a nationwide directory of experienced hospital laboratories that do blood screening for carriers of the Tay-Sachs gene and the allied genetic diseases. You, your physician, or your genetic counselor can contact the Association for the name of such a laboratory in your area, or of a medical center that uses one of the experienced laboratories. (Often the blood is collected in one hospital lab for analysis.)

In addition, you can refer to the list of genetic counseling centers on page 227. Most of them have screening services, as well as prenatal detection for a variety of disorders, including Tay-Sachs disease.

SOME LEADING SPECIALISTS AND CENTERS

The following centers and specialists have a special interest and experience in diagnosing, managing, preventing, and screening for Tay-Sachs and the related disorders.

California Tay-Sachs Disease Prevention
  Program
Harbor UCLA Medical Center
Division of Medical Genetics
1124 W. Carson
Torrance, CA 90502
Dr. Michael Kaback
(213) 775-7333

University of Colorado Medical Center
Department of Pediatrics
Box C-233
4200 E. Ninth Ave.
Denver, CO 80262
Dr. Stephen Goodman
(303) 394-7301

University of Miami School of Medicine
Division of Genetics
Mailman Center
1641 N.W. 12th Ave.
Miami, FL 33131
Paul M. Tocci, Ph.D.
(305) 547-6446

Emory University School of Medicine
2040 Ridgewood Drive
Atlanta, GA 30322
Dr. Louis J. Elsas II
Director Division of Medical Genetics
(404) 329-5731

Michael Reese Hospital
Division of Medical Genetics
2959 S. Cottage Grove
Chicago, IL 60616
Dr. Eugene Pergament
(312) 791-3848

Johns Hopkins Hospital
John F. Kennedy Institute
Tay-Sachs Screening Program
707 Broadway
Baltimore, MD 21205
Dr. Haig H. Kazazian, Jr.
(301) 955-3075

National Institutes of Health
Clinical Center, Building 10, Room 3D04
9000 Rockville Pike
Bethesda, MD 20892
Dr. Roscoe O. Brady
(301) 496-3285

Development Evaluation Clinic
Children's Hospital
300 Longwood Ave.
Boston, MA 02115
Dr. Allen C. Crocker
(617) 735-6509

Eunice Kennedy Shriver Center
Tay-Sachs Prevention Program
200 Trapelo Rd.
Waltham, MA 02154
Dr. Edwin H. Kolodny
(617) 893-0600

Center for Jewish Genetic Diseases
Mount Sinai School of Medicine
Division of Medical Genetics
Annenberg Building 17-76
100th St. and Fifth Ave.
New York, NY 10029
Dr. R. J. Desnick
(212) 650-6944

Thomas Jefferson University School of
  Medicine
Tay-Sachs Prevention Program
1015 Walnut St., Room 107
Philadelphia, PA 19107
Dr. Eugene E. Grebner
Dr. Laird G. Jackson
(215) 928-6955

The Hospital for Sick Children
Tay-Sachs Screening Program
555 University Ave.
Toronto, Ontario M5G 1X8
Canada
Dr. J. Alexander Lowden
(416) 597-1500

SOURCE: *National Tay-Sachs & Allied Diseases Association; for a more extensive directory, contact the Association.*

RESEARCH AND TREATMENT AT THE NATIONAL INSTITUTES OF HEALTH

Extensive studies on Gaucher's, Tay-Sachs, and Niemann-Pick diseases are being carried out at the National Institutes of Health's Clinical Center in Bethesda, Maryland, under the supervision of Dr. John A. Barranger, one of the acknowledged experts in the world on Gaucher's disease. Services include diagnosis of the disease and genetic counseling. Selected patients may participate in research that includes experimental enzyme replacement therapy. Acceptance is by physician referral only. For more information your physician can contact:

Office of Director
The Clinical Center
Building 10, Room 2C-146
National Institutes of Health
Bethesda, MD 20892
(301) 496-4891

or:

Roscoe O. Brady, M.D.
(301) 496-3285

or:

John A. Barranger, M.D.
(301) 496-1465

ORGANIZATIONS

Gaucher's Disease Research Foundation
9319 Meadow Hill Rd.
Ellicott City, MD 21043

A nationwide nonprofit organization dedicated to research on Gaucher's and support of individuals and families affected by Gaucher's. Keeps a "Gaucher's Disease Registry" that documents cases of Gaucher's mostly for physicians and scientists. (Address: Gaucher's Disease Registry, 4418 E. Chapman, Orange, CA 92669.) Also operates a Family Support Network, which will place a person who has had experience with Gaucher's in contact with others in need of support. Contact the main organization at above address. Publishes a newsletter. Will answer questions from the public and provide more information upon request.

The National Tay-Sachs & Allied Diseases Association
92 Washington Ave.
Cedarhurst, NY 11516
(516) 569-4300

A national support and information organization for those affected by Tay-Sachs and allied diseases. Local parent groups in several parts of the country. Has a Parent Peer Group in which parents who have been through experiences with Tay-Sachs children offer emotional support and practical guidance to parents with children newly diagnosed with the diseases. Has a directory of test centers and laboratories. Makes referrals to screening centers. Will provide more information upon request.

FREE MATERIALS

Gaucher's Disease: Facts for Patients and their Families

Gaucher's Disease Research Foundation
9319 Meadow Hill Rd.
Ellicott City, MD 21043

What Every Family Should Know About Tay Sachs and Allied Diseases

National Tay-Sachs & Allied Diseases Association
92 Washington Ave.
Cedarhurst, NY 11516
(516) 569-4300

ADDITIONAL SPECIALISTS AND SOURCES

Some leading specialists and referral sources for:

Allergies and Asthma (Allergists)

Arthritis and Rheumatology (Rheumatologists)

Digestive Diseases: Colon, Stomach, Liver (Gastroenterologists)

Ear, Nose, and Throat (Otolaryngologists)

Endocrinology and Diabetes (Endocrinologists)

Eye Diseases and Vision Problems (Ophthalmologists)

Heart and Cardiovascular Diseases (Cardiologists)

Neurology—Diseases and Disorders of the Nervous System (Neurologists)

Orthopedic (Bone and Musculoskeletal) Problems (Orthopedic Surgeons)

Pulmonary (Lung) Diseases (Pulmonary Specialists)

Skin Disorders (Dermatologists)

If you need help in finding a specialist for any problems noted above, in addition to those listed in the body of *Health Care U.S.A.*, you or your primary physician may find the following names a useful reference source. The physicians listed here are all leaders in their fields as shown by the fact that they have been chosen to head departments or divisions in their specialties at medical schools accredited by the Association of American Medical Colleges.

Many of these physicians have been chosen by their peers as the "finest specialists" in the nation, according to the book, *The Best Doctors in the U.S.*, by John Pekkanen (Seaview Books). They are listed here to help health consumers gain access to the latest, most effective, safe therapies.

Contrary to public belief, many physicians at medical schools are surprisingly accessible for patient treatment, consultations, and referrals. Most of them see private patients, if sometimes on a restricted schedule. But even if you do not end up being treated by such physicians, you may benefit from their suggestions on who else to consult. The office staff of such a specialist can often direct you to outstanding persons and places for care in your locality.

Although there are other medical specialties, these 11 we.e selected because they are most applicable to the diseases and disorders discussed in earlier sections of this book. In some cases, the lists of specialists offer an additional, geographically broader source of help than those noted in the body of the book.

The addresses and phone numbers may be for the physician's private office, but usually they are the general numbers and addresses of the medical college with which the physician is affiliated.

562

ALLERGIES AND ASTHMA (ALLERGISTS)

The physicians listed below are some of the leading specialists in allergies and immunology. They may be available for treatment and consultations or may be able to refer you to someone else. All are heads of allergy departments at medical colleges accredited by the Association of American Medical Colleges.

ALABAMA
William J. Koopman, M.D.
Director, Division of Clinical Immunology and
   Rheumatology
Director of Multipurpose Arthritis Center
Department of Medicine
University of Alabama at Birmingham
THT 429A
University Station
Birmingham, AL 35294
(205) 934-5306

ARIZONA
Eric P. Gall, M.D.
Chief, Immunology
University of Arizona College of Medicine
Arizona Health Sciences Center
1501 N. Campbell Ave.
Tucson, AZ 85724
(602) 626-0111

CALIFORNIA
M. Eric Gershwin, M.D.
Chief, Rheumatology-Allergy
School of Medicine TB 192
University of California, Davis
Davis, CA 95616
(916) 453-3096

Sudhir Gupta, M.D.
Chief, Basic and Clinical Immunology
   (includes allergy)
University of California, Irvine
California College of Medicine
Irvine, CA 92717
(714) 856-7108

Andrew Saxon, M.D.
Chief, Department of Allergy/Immunology
UCLA Center for the Health Sciences
Los Angeles, CA 90024
(213) 825-9111

Stephen Wasserman, M.D.
Chief, Division of Allergy
University of California, San Diego
Medical Center
225 Dickinson St.
San Diego, CA 92103
(619) 294-6911

Oscar L. Frick, M.D.
Chief, Department of Pediatrics
University of California, San Francisco
San Francisco, CA 94143
(415) 666-1401

Abba Terr, M.D.
Clinic Chief
Samuel Strober, M.D.
Division Chief
Allergy Clinic
Division of Immunology
Stanford University Medical Center
Stanford, CA 94305
(415) 723-6001

COLORADO
Henry N. Claman, M.D.
Charles Kirkpatrick, M.D.
Chairmen, Clinical Immunology
University of Colorado School of Medicine
4200 E. Ninth Ave.
Denver, CO 80262
(303) 399-1211

CONNECTICUT
Philip W. Askenase, M.D.
Head, Section of Clinical Immunology
Carleton R. Palm, M.D.
Head, Pediatric Allergy
Yale University School of Medicine
333 Cedar St.
New Haven, CT 06510
(203) 785-4142, 4081

DISTRICT OF COLUMBIA
S. V. Spagnolo, M.D.
Chief, Pulmonary Diseases and Allergy
George Washington University Medical Center
2150 Pennsylvania Ave., N.W.
Washington, DC 20037
(202) 676-3633

Joseph A. Bellanti, M.D.
Director, Immunology Center
Georgetown University Hospital
3800 Reservoir Rd., N.W.
Washington, DC 20007
(202) 625-0100

Floyd J. Malveaux, M.D.
Chief, Allergies
Howard University Hospital
2041 Georgia Ave., N.W.
Washington, DC 20060
(202) 745-6741

FLORIDA
Richard S. Panush, M.D.
Chief, Allergy and Rheumatology
University of Florida College of Medicine
Box J-215, J. Hillis Miller Health Center
Chief, Allergy and Rheumatology
Gainesville, FL 32610
(904) 392-4681

Richard E. Lockey, M.D.
Chief, Division of Allergy and Immunology
University of South Florida College of
  Medicine
James A. Haley Veterans Hospital
13000 N. 30th St., VAR 111-D
Tampa, FL 33612
(813) 972-7631

GEORGIA
Betty B. Wray, M.D.
Chief, Allergy and Immunology
Medical College of Georgia Hospital
Augusta, GA 30912
(404) 828-3531

ILLINOIS
Roy Patterson, M.D.
Northwestern University Medical School
Chief, Allergy/Immunology
303 E. Chicago Ave.
Chicago, IL 60611
(312) 908-2000

Henry Gewurz, M.D.
Chairman, Immunology/Microbiology
Rush-Presbyterian-St. Luke's Medical Center
1753 W. Congress Parkway
Chicago, IL 60612
(312) 942-6554

Truman O. Anderson, M.D.
Chief, Allergy
University of Illinois College of Medicine at
  Chicago
1853 W. Polk St.
Chicago, IL 60612
(312) 996-3500

INDIANA
Angenieta A. Biegel, M.D.
Chief, Allergy-Immunology
Indiana University School of Medicine
Riley Hospital for Children, SO9
702 Barnhill Drive
Indianapolis, IN 46223
(317) 264-8971

IOWA
Hal Richerson, M.D.
University of Iowa Hospitals and Clinics
Chief, Allergy and Immunology
Iowa City, IA 52242
(319) 353-4843

KANSAS
Daniel J. Stechschulte, M.D.
Director, Division of Allergy, Clinical
  Immunology, & Rheumatology
University of Kansas Medical Center
39th & Rainbow Blvd.
Kansas City, KS 66103
(913) 588-6008

KENTUCKY
Hobert L. Pence, M.D.
Chief, Allergy/Immunology
University of Louisville School of Medicine
Department of Medicine
Louisville, KY 40292
(502) 583-1427

LOUISIANA
Stephen H. Leech, M.C., C.B., Ph.D.
Chief, Allergy and Clinical Immunology
LSU School of Medicine
New Orleans, LA 70112
(504) 568-4580

John E. Salvaggio, M.D.
Chairman, Department of Medicine
Tulane University School of Medicine
Section of Allergy & Immunology
1430 Tulane Ave.
New Orleans, LA 70112
(504) 588-5176

Bettina C. Hilman, M.D.
Chief, Pulmonary and Allergy
Department of Pediatrics
Louisiana State University School of Medicine
  in Shreveport
PO Box 33932
Shreveport, LA 71130
(318) 674-5000

MARYLAND
Philip S. Norman, M.D.
Chief, Clinical Immunology
Johns Hopkins University School of Medicine
720 Rutland Ave.
Baltimore, MD 21205
(301) 955-5000

John Kastor, M.D.
Chief, Department of Medicine
University of Maryland School of Medicine
655 W. Baltimore St.
Baltimore, MD 21201
(301) 528-6352

MASSACHUSETTS
Peter Pochi, M.D.
Chief, Allergies
Boston University School of Medicine
80 E. Concord St.
Boston, MA 02118
(617) 247-5000

Albert L. Sheffer, M.D.
Chief, Allergies
Brigham and Women's Hospital
Harvard Medical School
110 Francis St.
Boston, MA 02115
(617) 732-5500

Raif S. Geha, M.D.
Chief, Allergies
Children's Hospital
Harvard Medical School
300 Longwood Ave.
Boston, MA 02115
(617) 735-6000

Ross E. Rocklin, M.D.
Chief, Allergy Division
Tufts University School of Medicine
New England Medical Center
171 Harrison Ave.
Boston, MA 02111
(617) 956-5333

MICHIGAN
William R. Solomon, M.D.
Chief, Allergy
Allergy Clinic
University of Michigan Medical Center
3214 A. Alfred Taubman Health Care Center
Ann Arbor, MI 48109
(313) 936-5634

MINNESOTA
Malcolm N. Blumenthal, M.D.
Head, Allergy
Department of Medicine
University of Minnesota Medical School
Box 434 UMHC
Minneapolis, MN 55455
(612) 624-5456

Charles E. Reed, M.D.
Chief, Allergic Diseases
Gerald J. Gleich, M.D.
Chief, Immunology
Mayo Graduate School of Medicine
200 First St., S.W.
Rochester, MN 55905
(507) 284-2511

MISSOURI
Lynn I. De Marco, M.D.
Chief, Allergy/Immunology/Rheumatology
University of Missouri
Kansas City School of Medicine
2411 Holmes St.
Kansas City, MO 64108
(816) 276-1910

Raymond G. Slavin, M.D.
Director, Allergy/Immunology
St. Louis University School of Medicine
1402 S. Grand Blvd.
St. Louis, MO 63104
(314) 577-8456

Charles W. Parker, M.D.
Chief, Allergy and Immunology
Washington University School of Medicine
660 S. Euclid Ave.
St. Louis, MO 63110
(314) 362-9000

NEBRASKA
Robert G. Townley, M.D.
Creighton University School of Medicine
Chief, Allergy
California at 24th St.
Omaha, NE 68178
(402) 280-2940

NEW HAMPSHIRE
Harold M. Friedman, M.D.
Chief, Allergy
Dartmouth Medical School
Hanover, NH 03756
(603) 646-7505

NEW JERSEY
David Gocke, M.D.
Chief, Infectious Disease and Immunology
Lawrence D. Frenkel, M.D.
Director, Pediatric Allergy, Immunology, and
  Infectious Diseases
UMDNJ–Robert Wood Johnson Medical
  School
(formerly Rutgers)
UMDNJ Medical Education Building
Academic Health Science Building, CN19
New Brunswick, NJ 08903
(201) 937-7710, 7894

James M. Oleske, M.D.
Chief, Pediatric Allergy, Immunology, and
  Infectious Diseases
University of Medicine and Dentistry of New
  Jersey
Children's Hospital of Newark
15 S. Ninth St.
Newark, NJ 07107
(201) 268-8000

NEW YORK
Robert W. Raymond, M.D.
Chief, Allergy
Albany Medical College of Union University
47 New Scotland Ave.
Albany, NY 12208
(518) 445-5582

Elliott Middleton, Jr., M.D.
Chief, Allergy Division
SUNY at Buffalo School of Medicine
Buffalo General Hospital
100 High St.
Buffalo, NY 14203
(716) 845-2985

William J. Davis, M.D.
Columbia-Presbyterian Medical Center
630 W. 168th St.
New York, NY 10021
(212) 649-2500

Gregory W. Siskind, M.D.
Chief, Allergy and Immunology
Cornell University Medical College
1300 York Ave.
New York, NY 10021
(212) 472-6794

H. Sherwood Lawrence, M.D.
Chief, Immunology and Infectious Diseases
New York University School of Medicine
550 First Ave.
New York, NY 10016
(212) 340-7300

John P. Leddy, M.D.
Chief, Immunology/Rheumatology
University of Rochester Medical Center
601 Elmwood Ave.
Rochester, NY 14642
(716) 275-2891

Angelo Taranta, M.D.
Chief, Rheumatology and Immunology
New York Medical College
Elmwood Hall
Valhalla, NY 10595
(914) 347-5000

NORTH CAROLINA
Rebecca Buckley, M.D.
Chief, Pediatric Immunology/Allergy/
  Pulmonary
Duke University Medical Center
Department of Allergy/Immunology
Durham, NC 27710
(919) 684-2922

James D. Crapo, M.D.
Chief, Allergy
Duke University Medical Center
Box 3005
Durham, NC 27710
(919) 684-2498

W. James Metzger, M.D.
Chief, Allergy
East Carolina University School of Medicine
Greenville, NC 27834
(919) 757-2570

OHIO

Evelyn V. Hess, M.D.
Chief, Immunology (Rheumatic Diseases)
University of Cincinnati Medical Center
231 Bethesda Ave.
Cincinnati, OH 45267-0563
(513) 872-4701

E. Regis McFadden, M.D.
Director, Asthma and Allergic Disease Center
Case Western Reserve University School of
  Medicine
University Hospitals of Cleveland
2119 Abington Rd.
Cleveland, OH 44106
(216) 844-8668

James Tennenbaum, M.D.
Chief, Division of Allergy
Ohio State University Hospitals
3018-3A University Hospitals Clinic
456 Clinic Drive
Columbus, OH 43210
(614) 421-8061

J. Harlan Dix, M.D.
Chief, Allergy
Northeastern Ohio Universities College of
  Medicine
4209 State Route 44
PO Box 95
Rootstown, OH 44272
(216) 325-2511

OKLAHOMA

Morris Reichlin, M.D.
Chief, Section of Immunology
University of Oklahoma Health Sciences
  Center
825 N.E. 13th St.
Oklahoma City, OK 73104
(405) 271-7766

OREGON

Bernard Pirofsky, M.D.
Chief, Immunology, Allergy, and
  Rheumatology
Oregon Health Sciences University School of
  Medicine
3181 Sam Jackson Park Rd.
Portland, OR 97201
(503) 225-8311

PENNSYLVANIA

Herbert C. Mansmann, Jr., M.D.
Chief, Allergy
Jefferson Medical College of Thomas Jefferson
  University
11th and Walnut St.
Philadelphia, PA 19107
(215) 928-8912

Eliot Dunsky, M.D.
Director, Allergy
Hahnemann University School of Medicine
Broad & Vine Sts.
Philadelphia, PA 19102
(205) 448-7754

Leonard Girsh, M.D.
Chief, Allergy
Medical College of Pennsylvania
3300 Henry Ave.
Philadelphia, PA 19129
(215) 842-6000

Burton Zweiman, M.D.
Chief, Allergy and Immunology
Hospital of the University of Pennsylvania
3400 Spruce St.
Philadelphia, PA 19104
(215) 662-2425

Philip Fireman, M.D.
Director, Allergy and Immunology
University of Pittsburgh School of Medicine
Children's Hospital of Pittsburgh
One Children's Place
Fifth Ave. at DeSoto St.
Pittsburgh, PA 15213
(412) 647-5080

SOUTH CAROLINA
Stephen A. Sahn, M.D.
Director, Pulmonary and Critical Care
E. Carvile LeRoy, M.D.
Director, Rheumatology and Immunology
Medical University of South Carolina
171 Ashley Ave.
Charleston, SC 29425
(803) 792-3161, 2000

Robert A. Vande Stouwe, M.D., Ph.D.
Chief, Allergy, Immunology, and
    Rheumatology
University of South Carolina School of
    Medicine
Columbia, SC 29208
(803) 765-6563

SOUTH DAKOTA
D. W. Humphreys, M.D.
Chief, Division of Allergy
Department of Medicine
University of South Dakota School of
    Medicine
2501 W. 22nd St.
Sioux Falls, SD 57105
(605) 339-6790

TENNESSEE
J. Kelly Smith, M.D.
Chief, Allergy-Immunology
East Tennessee State University
Quillen-Dishner College of Medicine
PO Box 21, 106A
Johnson City, TN 37614
(615) 928-6426

Tai June Yoo, M.D., Ph.D.
Chief, Division of Allergy/Immunology
Henry Herrod, M.D.
Chief, Section of Pediatric Allergy/
    Immunology
University of Tennessee, Memphis
College of Medicine
956 Court Ave.
Memphis, TN 38163
(901) 528-6663, 5930

Lawrence Prograis, M.D.
Head, Division of Allergy and Immunology
Meharry Medical College School of Medicine
1005 D. B. Todd Blvd.
Nashville, TN 37207
(615) 327-6111

Samuel R. Marney, M.D.
Director, Allergy Division
Vanderbilt University Medical Center
1161 21st Ave., S.
Nashville, TN 37232
(615) 322-7424

TEXAS
Timothy Sullivan, M.D.
Chief, Allergy
University of Texas Health Science Center at
    Dallas
5323 Harry Hines Blvd.
Dallas, TX 75235
(214) 688-3111

David Huston, M.D.
Chief, Allergy Section
Baylor College of Medicine
6565 Fannin
Mail Station F501
Houston, TX 77030
(713) 799-4951

William T. Shearer, M.D., Ph.D.
Chief, Section of Allergy and Immunology
Department of Pediatrics
Baylor College of Medicine
1200 Moursund Ave.
Houston, TX 77030
(713) 799-4951

William T. Kniker, M.D.
Chief, Clinical Immunology, Department of
    Pediatrics
University of Texas at San Antonio
7703 Floyd Curl Drive
San Antonio, TX 78284
(512) 691-6257

G. W. Brasher, M.D.
Chair, Allergy/Immunology
Texas A&M University College of Medicine
Scott and White Clinic
Temple, TX 76508
(817) 745-2516

UTAH
Robert Griffiths, M.D.
Director, Allergy Clinic
University of Utah School of Medicine
50 N. Medical Drive
Salt Lake City, UT 84132
(801) 581-2676

VIRGINIA
Thomas A. E. Platts-Mills, M.D.
Head, Allergy Division
Department of Internal Medicine
University of Virginia School of Medicine
Charlottesville, VA 22908
(804) 924-2098

Lawrence B. Schwartz, M.D., Ph.D.
Chief, Allergy & Immunology
Medical College of Virginia
MCV Station, Box 263
Richmond, VA 23298
(804) 786-9685

WASHINGTON
Seymour J. Klebanoff, M.D.
Head, Allergy Division
University of Washington School of Medicine,
 RM-13
Seattle, WA 98195
(206) 543-3780

WEST VIRGINIA
Eric P. Brestel, M.D.
Chief, Allergy and Clinical Immunology
West Virginia University School of Medicine
Morgantown, WV 26506
(304) 293-4121

WISCONSIN
William W. Busse, M.D.
Chief, Allergy
University of Wisconsin Medical School
University Hospital and Clinics
600 Highland Ave., Room H6/360
Madison, WI 53792
(608) 263-6400

Jordan N. Fink, M.D.
Chief, Allergy
Medical College of Wisconsin
8700 W. Wisconsin Ave.
Milwaukee, WI 53226
(414) 257-6095

ARTHRITIS AND RHEUMATOLOGY (RHEUMATOLOGISTS)

The physicians listed below are some of the leading specialists in rheumatology (the study of a variety of disorders characterized by inflammation and degeneration of metabolic derangement of the connective tissue structures, especially the joints; rheumatism confined to the joints is called arthritis). These doctors may be available for consultations and treatment or may be able to refer you to someone else. All are heads of rheumatology at medical colleges accredited by the Association of American Medical Colleges.

ALABAMA
William J. Koopman, M.D.
Director, Division of Clinical Immunology and
 Rheumatology
University of Alabama School of Medicine
University of Alabama at Birmingham
THT 429A
University Station
Birmingham, AL 35294
(205) 934-5306

Joe Hardin, M.D.
Chief, Rheumatology
University of South Alabama College of
 Medicine
307 University Blvd.
Mobile, AL 36688
(205) 460-7174

ARKANSAS
Eleanor A. Lipsmeyer, M.D.
Chief, Rheumatology
University of Arkansas College of Medicine
4301 W. Markham St., Slot 640
Little Rock, AR 72205
(501) 661-5586

CALIFORNIA
M. Eric Gershwin, M.D.
Chief, Rheumatology/Allergy
University of California, Davis
School of Medicine
Davis, CA 95616
(916) 752-0331

George Friou, M.D.
Chief, Rheumatology
University of California, Irvine
California College of Medicine
Irvine, CA 92717
(714) 856-5907

Steen Mortesen, M.D.
Chief, Rheumatology
Loma Linda University School of Medicine
Loma Linda, CA 92350
(714) 824-4909

Bevra Hahn, M.D.
Chief, Rheumatology
University of California at Los Angeles
UCLA School of Medicine
Los Angeles, CA 90024
(213) 825-6439

David Horwitz, M.D.
Chief, Rheumatology
University of Southern California School of
   Medicine
2025 Zonal Ave.
Los Angeles, CA 90033
(213) 224-7880

Nathan J. Zvaifler, M.D.
Chief, Rheumatic Diseases Division
University of California, San Diego
Medical Center
225 Dickinson St.
San Diego, CA 92103
(619) 294-5982

Walter Epstein, M.D.
Acting Chairman
Department of Rheumatology
University of California, San Francisco
School of Medicine
513 Parnassus Ave.
San Francisco, CA 94143
(415) 476-1001

James Fries, M.D.
Clinic Chief
Samuel Strober, M.D.
Division Chief
Rheumatology and Arthritis/Immunology
   Clinic
Division of Immunology
Stanford University Medical Center
Stanford, CA 94305
(415) 723-6001

COLORADO
William Arend, M.D.
Chief, Rheumatic Diseases
University of Colorado School of Medicine
4200 E. Ninth Ave.
Denver, CO 80262
(303) 399-1211

CONNECTICUT
Naomi Rothfield, M.D.
Chief, Rheumatology
University of Connecticut Health Center
Farmington, CT 06032
(203) 674-2160

Stephen E. Malawista, M.D.
Head, Section of Rheumatology
Yale University School of Medicine
333 Cedar St.
New Haven, CT 06510
(203) 785-2454

DISTRICT OF COLUMBIA
Patience White, M.D.
Director, Rheumatology Division
George Washington University
Medical Center
2150 Pennsylvania Ave., N.W.
Washington, DC 20037
(202) 676-3203

Paul Katz, M.D.
Director, Rheumatology
Georgetown University School of Medicine
3900 Reservoir Rd., N.W.
Washington, DC 20007
(202) 625-7201

FLORIDA
Richard S. Panush, M.D.
Chief, Rheumatology and Allergy
University of Florida College of Medicine
Box J-215, J. Hillis Miller Health Center
Gainesville, FL 32610
(904) 392-4681

David S. Howell, M.D.
Chief, Rheumatology and Arthritis
University of Miami School of Medicine
PO Box 016099 (R-699)
Miami, FL 33101
(305) 547-6467

Bernard F. Germain, M.D.
Professor and Director, Division of
  Rheumatology
University of South Florida
College of Medicine
12901 N. 30th St., Box 19
Tampa, FL 33612
(813) 974-2681

GEORGIA
Colon H. Wilson, Jr., M.D.
Chief, Rheumatology
Emory University School of Medicine
Atlanta, GA 30322
(404) 329-6123

Joseph P. Bailey, Jr., M.D.
Chief, Rheumatology
Medical College of Georgia Hospital
Augusta, GA 30912
(404) 828-2981

ILLINOIS
Thomas J. Schnitzer, M.D.
Chief, Section of Rheumatology
Rush-Presbyterian-St. Luke's Medical Center
1753 W. Congress Parkway
Chicago, IL 60612
(312) 942-8268

Michael A. Becker, M.D.
Chief, Section of Rheumatology
University of Chicago Medical Center
5841 S. Maryland Ave.
Chicago, IL 60637
(312) 947-1000

John Skosey, M.D.
Chief, Rheumatology
University of Illinois College of Medicine
1853 W. Polk St.
Chicago, IL 60612
(312) 996-3500

John A. Robinson, M.D.
Chief, Immunology/Rheumatology and Allergy
Loyola University of Chicago Stritch School of
  Medicine
2160 S. First Ave.
Maywood, IL 60153
(312) 531-3000

Nicholas Joyce-Clark, M.D.
Chief, Rheumatology
University of Health Sciences
Chicago Medical School
3333 Green Bay Rd.
North Chicago, IL 60064
(312) 578-3000

Roger B. Traycoff, M.D.
Chief, Rheumatology
Southern Illinois University School of
  Medicine
800 N. Rutledge
PO Box 3926
Springfield, IL 62708
(217) 782-3318

INDIANA
Kenneth Brandt, M.D.
Chief, Rheumatology Section
Department of Medicine
Indiana University Medical Center
Clinical Building 492
541 Clinical Drive
Indianapolis, IN 46223
(317) 264-4225

Murray Passo, M.D.
Chief, Rheumatology Section
Department of Pediatrics
Indiana University Medical Center
Riley Hospital for Children, A562
702 Barnhill Drive
Indianapolis, IN 46223
(317) 264-2172

IOWA
Robert Ashman, M.D.
Chief, Rheumatology
University of Iowa College of Medicine
100 College of Medicine Administration
  Building
Iowa City, IA 52242
(319) 353-4843

KENTUCKY
Ronald Saykaly, M.D.
Chief, Rheumatology
University of Kentucky College of Medicine
800 Rose St.
Lexington, KY 40536
(606) 233-5000

Peter Hasselbacher, M.D.
Chief, Rheumatology
University of Louisville School of Medicine
Louisville, KY 40292
(502) 588-5233

LOUISIANA
Joseph J. Biundo, Jr., M.D.
Chief, Rheumatology and Rehabilitation
  Medicine
Louisiana State University School of Medicine
1542 Tulane Ave.
New Orleans, LA 70112
(504) 568-4643

Oren Gum, M.D.
Chief, Arthritis and Rheumatology
Tulane University School of Medicine
1430 Tulane Ave.
New Orleans, LA 70112
(504) 588-5437

Robert E. Wolf, M.D., Ph.D.
Chief, Rheumatology
Louisiana State University School of Medicine
PO Box 33932
Shreveport, LA 71130
(318) 674-5000

MARYLAND
Mary Betty Stevens, M.D.
Chief, Rheumatology
Johns Hopkins University School of Medicine
720 Rutland Ave.
Baltimore, MD 21205
(301) 955-5000

Barry Handwerger, M.D.
Chief, Rheumatology
University of Maryland School of Medicine
Baltimore, MD 21201
(301) 528-5888

MASSACHUSETTS
K. Frank Austin, M.D.
Chief, Rheumatology
Harvard Medical School
25 Shattuck St.
Boston, MA 02115
(617) 732-1000

Juan J. Canoso, M.D.
Acting Division Chief, Rheumatology
Tufts University School of Medicine
New England Medical Center
171 Harrison Ave.
Boston, MA 02111
(617) 956-5789

David Giansiracusa, M.D.
Chief, Rheumatology
University of Massachusetts Medical School
55 Lake Ave. N.
Worcester, MA 01605
(617) 856-2146

MICHIGAN
Giles G. Bole, M.D.
Chief, Rheumatology
University of Michigan Medical Center
3918 A. Alfred Taubman Health Care Center
Ann Arbor, MI 48109
(313) 936-5560

Felix Fernandez-Madrid, M.D.
Chief, Rheumatology
Wayne State University
School of Medicine
University Health Center
4201 St. Antoine
Detroit, MI 48201
(313) 577-1133

MINNESOTA
Ronald Messner, M.D.
Head, Rheumatology
University of Minnesota Medical School
Box 108 UMHC
Minneapolis, MN 55455
(612) 625-1155

Doyt L. Conn, M.D.
Chief, Rheumatology
Mayo Medical School
200 First St., S.W.
Rochester, MN 55905
(507) 284-3671

MISSISSIPPI
Valee Harisdangkul, M.D.
Chief, Rheumatology
University of Mississippi School of Medicine
2500 N. State St.
Jackson, MS 39216
(601) 984-5540

MISSOURI
Gordon Sharp, M.D.
Chief, Rheumatology
University of Missouri
Columbia School of Medicine
One Hospital Drive
Columbia, MO 65212
(314) 882-1566

Terry L. Moore, M.D.
Director, Rheumatology
St. Louis University School of Medicine
1402 S. Grand Blvd.
St. Louis, MO 63104
(314) 577-8467

John P. Atkinson, M.D.
Chief, Rheumatology
Washington University School of Medicine
660 S. Euclid Ave.
St. Louis, MO 63110
(314) 362-9000

NEBRASKA
Jay G. Kenik, M.D.
John A. Hurley, M.D.
Co-Chiefs, Rheumatology
Creighton University School of Medicine
California at 24th St.
Omaha, NE 68178
(402) 280-4180

Lynell W. Klassen, M.D.
Chief, Rheumatology
University of Nebraska College of Medicine
42nd St. and Dewey Ave.
Omaha, NE 68105
(402) 559-7288

NEW HAMPSHIRE
G. James Morgan, Jr., M.D.
Department of Rheumatology
Dartmouth Medical School
Hanover, NH 03756
(603) 646-7505

NEW JERSEY
James R. Seibold, M.D.
Chief, Rheumatology
University of Medicine and Dentistry of New
   Jersey
Robert Wood Johnson Medical School
(formerly Rutgers)
UMDNJ Medical Education Building
Academic Health Science Building CN 19
New Brunswick, NJ 08903
(201) 937-7704

Phoebe Krey, M.D.
Chief, Rheumatology
University of Medicine and Dentistry of New
   Jersey
New Jersey Medical School
100 Bergen St.
Newark, NJ 07103
(201) 456-4300

NEW MEXICO
Arthur D. Bankhurst, M.D.
Chief, Rheumatology
Department of Medicine
University of New Mexico School of Medicine
Albuquerque, NM 87131
(505) 277-4761

NEW YORK
Lee E. Bartholomew, M.D.
Chief, Rheumatology
Albany Medical College of Union University
47 New Scotland Ave.
Albany, NY 12208
(518) 445-5582

Harold Keiser, M.D.
Division Head, Rheumatology
Albert Einstein College of Medicine
Bronx, NY 10461
(212) 430-2078

Charles Steinman, M.D.
Chief, Rheumatology
SUNY Health Science Center at Brooklyn
450 Clarkson Ave.
Brooklyn, NY 11203
(718) 270-1978

Robert Kaprove, M.D.
Erie County Medical Center
Buffalo, NY 14215
(716) 898-4800
Affiliated with SUNY at Buffalo School of
  Medicine

Floyd Green, M.D.
Chief, Rheumatology & Arthritis Division
SUNY at Buffalo School of Medicine
Veterans Administration Medical Center
3495 Bailey Ave.
Buffalo, NY 14215
(716) 834-9200

Leonard Chess
Chief, Rheumatology
Columbia-Presbyterian Medical Center
630 W. 168th St.
New York, NY 10032
(212) 694-3645

Charles L. Christian, M.D.
Chief, Rheumatology
Cornell University Medical College
1300 York Ave.
New York, NY 10021
(212) 606-1328

Harry Spiera, M.D.
Chief, Rheumatology
The Mount Sinai Medical Center
1 Gustave L. Levy Place
New York, NY 10029
(212) 650-6792

Gerald Weissmann, M.D.
Chief, Rheumatology
New York University School of Medicine
550 First Ave.
New York, NY 10016
(212) 340-7300

Allen Kaplan, M.D.
Division Head, Allergy, Rheumatology, and
  Immunization Clinic
SUNY at Stony Brook Health Sciences Center
Stony Brook, NY 11794
(516) 444-2272

Paul E. Phillips, M.D.
Chief, Division of Clinical Immunology
Chief, Rheumatology Section
SUNY Health Science Center at Syracuse
Syracuse, NY 13210
(315) 473-5663

Angelo Taranta, M.D.
Chief, Rheumatology
New York Medical College
Elmwood Hall
Valhalla, NY 10595
(914) 347-5000

NORTH CAROLINA
John P. Winfield, M.D.
Chief, Rheumatology
University of North Carolina
Chapel Hill School of Medicine
Chapel Hill, NC 27514
(919) 966-4191

Ralph Snyderman, M.D.
Chief, Rheumatology
Duke University Medical Center
Box 3005
Durham, NC 27710
(919) 684-2498

Edward L. Treadwell, M.D.
Chief, Rheumatology
East Carolina University School of Medicine
Greenville, NC 27834
(919) 757-2570

Robert A. Turner, M.D.
Chief, Rheumatology
Bowman Gray School of Medicine
300 S. Hawthorne Rd.
Winston-Salem, NC 27103
(919) 748-4209

OHIO
Evelyn B. Hess, M.D.
Chief, Immunology (Rheumatic Diseases)
University of Cincinnati Medical Center
231 Bethesda Ave.
Cincinnati, OH 45267-0563
(513) 872-4701

Roland W. Moskowitz, M.D.
Director, Division of Rheumatic Diseases
University Hospitals of Cleveland
2074 Abington Rd.
Cleveland, OH 44106
(216) 844-3168

Ronald L. Whisler, M.D.
Director, Rheumatology
Ohio State University Hospitals
4813 University Hospitals Clinic
456 Clinic Drive
Columbus, OH 43210
(614) 421-8093

Andrew C. Raynor, M.D.
Chief, Rheumatology
Northeastern Ohio Universities College of
   Medicine
4209 State Route 44
Rootstown, OH 44272
(216) 325-2511

Thomas C. Namey, M.D.
Chief, Rheumatology
Medical College of Ohio at Toledo
Caller Service No. 10008
Toledo, OH 43699
(419) 381-4172

OREGON
Bernard Pirofsky, M.D.
Chief, Rheumatology
Oregon Health Sciences University School of
   Medicine
3181 S.W. Sam Jackson Park Rd.
Portland, OR 97201
(503) 225-8311

PENNSYLVANIA
Rafael DeHoratius, M.D.
Director, Rheumatology
Hahnemann University School of Medicine
Broad and Vine Sts.
Philadelphia, PA 19102
(215) 448-3482

John L. Abruzzo, M.D.
Chief, Rheumatology
Jefferson Medical College of Thomas Jefferson
   University
11th & Walnut Sts.
Philadelphia, PA 19107
(215) 928-6942

Bruce I. Hoffman, M.D.
Chief, Rheumatology
Medical College of Pennsylvania
3300 Henry Ave.
Philadelphia, PA 19129
(215) 842-6000

Charles D. Tourtellotte, M.D.
Chief, Rheumatology
Temple University School of Medicine
3400 N. Broad St.
Philadelphia, PA 19140
(215) 221-4046

Robert B. Zurier, M.D.
Chief, Rheumatology
Hospital of the University of Pennsylvania
3400 Spruce St.
Philadelphia, PA 19104
(215) 662-3681

Thomas A. Medsger, Jr., M.D.
Chief, Division of Rheumatology and Clinical
   Immunology
985 Scaife Hall
Department of Medicine
University of Pittsburgh School of Medicine
Pittsburgh, PA 15261
(412) 624-2722

PUERTO RICO
Esther González, M.D.
Chief, Rheumatology
University of Puerto Rico School of Medicine
Medical Sciences Campus
GPO Box 5067
San Juan, PR 00936
(809) 758-2525, x1825

SOUTH CAROLINA
E. Carwile LeRoy, M.D.
Director, Rheumatology and Immunology
Medical University of South Carolina
171 Ashley Ave.
Charleston, SC 29425
(803) 792-2000

Robert A. Vande Stouwe, M.D., Ph.D.
Chief, Allergy, Immunology, and
   Rheumatology
University of South Carolina School of
   Medicine
Columbia, SC 29208
(803) 765-6563

SOUTH DAKOTA
Alan D. Morris, M.D.
Chief, Rheumatology
University of South Dakota School of
   Medicine
2501 W. 22nd St.
Sioux Falls, SD 57105
(605) 339-6790

TENNESSEE
David P. Lurie, M.D.
Chief, Rheumatology
East Tennessee State University
Quillen-Dishner College of Medicine
PO Box 21,106A
Johnson City, TN 37614
(615) 928-6426

Arnold E. Postlethwaite, M.D.
Director, Division of Connective Tissue
  Diseases
University of Tennessee, Memphis
College of Medicine
956 Court Ave., Box 3A
Memphis, TN 38163
(901) 528-5774

Theodore P. Pincus, M.D.
Director, Rheumatology
Vanderbilt University Medical Center
1161 21st Ave., S.
Nashville, TN 37232
(615) 322-4746

TEXAS
Peter Lipsky, M.D.
Chief, Rheumatology and Arthritis
University of Texas Health Science Center at
  Dallas
5323 Harry Hines Blvd.
Dallas, TX 75235
(214) 688-3111

Donald Marcus, M.D.
Chief, Rheumatology
Baylor College of Medicine
One Baylor Plaza
Houston, TX 77030
(713) 799-6015

Frank C. Arnett, M.D.
Director, Rheumatology
University of Texas Health Science Center at
  Houston
PO Box 20708
Houston, TX 77225
(713) 792-5900

Bruce A. Bartholomew, M.D.
Chief, Rheumatology
Texas Tech University Health Sciences Center
  School of Medicine
4th St. and Indiana Ave.
Lubbock, TX 79430
(806) 743-3155

Norman Talal, M.D.
Chief, Clinical Immunology (rheumatoid
  arthritis, etc.)
University of Texas Health Science Center at
  San Antonio
7703 Floyd Curl Drive
San Antonio, TX 78284
(512) 691-6341

A. Dean Steele, M.D.
Chief, Rheumatology
Texas A&M University College of Medicine
Scott & White Clinic
Temple, TX 76508
(817) 774-4060

UTAH
John R. Ward, M.D.
Chief, Rheumatology
University of Utah School of Medicine
50 N. Medical Drive
Salt Lake City, UT 84132
(801) 581-7724

VIRGINIA
John Davis, IV, M.D.
Division Head, Rheumatology
University of Virginia School of Medicine
Box 395, Medical Center
Charlottesville, VA 22908
(804) 924-5213

Shaun Ruddy, M.D.
Chairman, Immunology & Connective Tissue
  Diseases
Medical College of Virginia
MCV Station, Box 263
Richmond, VA 23298
(804) 786-9685

WASHINGTON
P. J. Fialkow, M.D.
Chief, Medicine
University of Washington School of Medicine,
  RG-2D
Seattle, WA 98195
(206) 543-3293

WEST VIRGINIA
John C. Huntwork, M.D.
Acting Chief, Rheumatology
Marshall University School of Medicine
Huntington, WV 25701
(304) 526-6113

Anthony G. DiBartolomeo, M.D.
Chief, Rheumatology
West Virginia University School of Medicine
Morgantown, WV 26506
(304) 293-4121

WISCONSIN
Walter S. Sundstrom, M.D.
Chief, Rheumatology
University of Wisconsin Medical School
1300 University Ave.
Madison, WI 53706
(608) 263-4900

Robert W. Lightfoot, Jr., M.D.
Chief, Rheumatology
Medical College of Wisconsin
8700 W. Wisconsin Ave.
Milwaukee, WI 53226
(414) 257-6356

DIGESTIVE DISEASES: COLON, STOMACH, AND LIVER (GASTROENTEROLOGISTS)

The physicians listed below are some of the leading specialists in gastroenterology (bowel, stomach, and liver diseases). They may be available for consultations and treatment or can refer you to other specialists. All are the heads of divisions or departments of gastroenterology at medical colleges accredited by the Association of American Medical Colleges.

ALABAMA
Basil I. Hirschowitz, M.D.
Director, Gastroenterology Division
University of Alabama at Birmingham
LHR 404
University Station
Birmingham, AL 35294
(205) 934-6060

ARIZONA
David L. Earnest, M.D.
Chief, Gastroenterology
University of Arizona College of Medicine
Arizona Health Sciences Center
1501 N. Campbell Ave.
Tucson, AZ 85724
(602) 626-0111

ARKANSAS
Chao Chan, M.D.
Acting Chief, Gastroenterology
University of Arkansas College of Medicine
4301 W. Markham St., Slot 567
Little Rock, AR 72205
(501) 661-5177

CALIFORNIA
Daniel Hollander, M.D.
Chief, Gastroenterology
University of California, Irvine
California College of Medicine
Irvine, CA 92717
(714) 856-7455

Helen Ranney, M.D.
Chief, Department of Medicine
University of California, San Diego
School of Medicine
La Jolla, CA 92093
(619) 543-3542

Raymond Herber, M.D.
Chief, Gastroenterology
Loma Linda University School of Medicine
Loma Linda, CA 92350
(714) 824-4905

Arthur Schwabe, M.D.
Chief, Division of Gastroenterology
University of California at Los Angeles
School of Medicine
Department of Medicine
Division of Gastroenterology
Los Angeles, CA 90024
(213) 825-6373

Jorge E. Valenzuela, M.D.
Chief, Gastroenterology
Telfer B. Reynolds, M.D. (liver specialist)
Allan G. Redeker, M.D. (liver specialist)
University of Southern California School of
  Medicine
Department of Medicine
2025 Zonal Ave.
Los Angeles, CA 90033
(213) 226-7994, 7622

Neville R. Pimstone, M.D.
Chief, Gastroenterology
University of California, Davis Medical Center
4301 X St.
Sacramento, CA 95817
(916) 453-3751

Jon I. Isenberg, M.D.
Chief, Division of Gastroenterology
University of California, San Diego
Medical Center
225 Dickinson St.
San Diego, CA 92103
(619) 294-6248

Robert K. Ockner, M.D.
Chief, Gastroenterology
University of California
San Francisco, CA 94143
(415) 666-9000

Gary M. Gray, M.D.
Division Chief
Keith Taylor, M.D.
Clinic Chief
Gastroenterology Clinic
Division of Gastroenterology
Stanford University Medical Center
Stanford, CA 94305
(415) 723-5488

COLORADO
Francis R. Simon, M.D.
Chief, Gastroenterology Section
University of Colorado Health Sciences
111 E, VA Medical Center
Denver, CO 80220
(303) 399-1211

CONNECTICUT
Joel Levin, M.D.
Chief, Gastroenterology
University of Connecticut Health Center
Farmington, CT 06032
(203) 674-3238

James L. Boyer, M.D.
Head, Division of Digestive Diseases
Department of Internal Medicine
Joyce Gryboski, M.D.
Head, Section of Pediatric Gastroenterology
Yale University School of Medicine
333 Cedar St.
New Haven, CT 06510
(203) 785-4130, 4081

DISTRICT OF COLUMBIA
Hans Fromm, M.D.
Director, Gastroenterology Division
George Washington University
Medical Center
2150 Pennsylvania Ave., N.W.
Washington, DC 20037
(202) 676-4418

Stanley B. Benjamin, M.D.
Chief, Gastroenterology
Georgetown University Hospital
3800 Reservoir Rd., N.W.
Washington, DC 20007
(202) 625-8783

Victor Scott, M.D.
Chief, Gastroenterology
Howard University Hospital
2041 Georgia Ave., N.W.
Washington, DC 20060
(202) 636-6270

FLORIDA
Philip P. Toskes, M.D.
Chief, Gastroenterology
University of Florida College of Medicine
PO Box J-214
Gainesville, FL 32610
(904) 392-3331

Martin Kalser, M.D.
Chief, Gastroenterology
University of Miami School of Medicine
1201 N.W. 16th St. (111B)
Miami, FL 33125
(305) 549-6132

H. Worth Boyce, M.D.
Director, Digestive Diseases
University of South Florida College of
  Medicine
12901 N. 30th St., Box 19
Tampa, FL 33612
(813) 974-2034

GEORGIA
John T. Galambos, M.D.
Chief, Gastroenterology
Emory University School of Medicine
69 Butler St.
Atlanta, GA 30303
(404) 329-6123

Francis J. Tedesco, M.D.
Chief, Gastroenterology
Medical College of Georgia Hospital
Augusta, GA 30912
(404) 828-2238

ILLINOIS
J. Donald Ostrow, M.D.
Chief, Gastroenterology
Northwestern University Medical School
Northwestern Memorial Hospital
1420 Wesley Pavilion
251 Chicago Ave.
Chicago, IL 60611
(312) 908-8649

Seymour Sabesin, M.D.
Director, Section of Digestive Diseases
Rush-Presbyterian-St. Luke's Medical Center
1725 W. Harrison St.
Chicago, IL 60612
(312) 942-5861

Thomas Brasitus, M.D.
Chief, Joint Section of Gastroenterology
Alfred Baker, M.D.
Director, Liver Disease Unit
University of Chicago Medical Center
Michael Reese Hospital and Medical Center
5841 S. Maryland Ave.
Chicago, IL 60637
(312) 947-1000

Thomas J. Layden, M.D.
Chief, Section of Gastroenterology
University of Illinois at Chicago
840 S. Wood St.
Chicago, IL 60612
(312) 996-7000

Martin G. Durkin, M.D.
Chief, Gastroenterology
Loyola University Medical Center
2160 S. First Ave.
Maywood, IL 60153
(312) 531-3000

James B. Hammond, M.D.
Chief, Gastroenterology
University of Health Sciences
Chicago Medical School
3333 Green Bay Rd.
North Chicago, IL 60064
(312) 578-3000

Stephen Holt, M.D.
Chief, Gastroenterology
Southern Illinois School of Medicine
800 N. Rutledge
Springfield, IL 62708
(217) 782-3318

INDIANA
Joseph F. Fitzgerald, M.D.
Chief, Gastroenterology Section
Department of Pediatrics
Indiana University Medical Center
Riley Hospital for Children, P122
702 Barnhill Drive
Indianapolis, IN 46223
(317) 264-3774

Lawrence Lumeng, M.D.
Chief, Gastroenterology Section
Department of Medicine
Indiana University Medical Center
University Hospital N541
926 W. Michigan St.
Indianapolis, IN 46223
(317) 274-4377

IOWA
James Christensen, M.D.
Chief, Gastroenterology—Hepatology
University of Iowa Hospitals & Clinics
Iowa City, IA 52242
(319) 356-2456

KANSAS
Norton J. Greenberger, M.D.
Chairman, Department of Medicine
University of Kansas College of Health
    Sciences
39th & Rainbow Blvd.
Kansas City, KS 66103
(913) 588-6001

KENTUCKY
Craig J. McClain, M.D.
Chief, Gastroenterology
University of Kentucky Medical Center
Department of Medicine, GI Division
Room MN 654
Lexington, KY 45036
(606) 233-5000

Richard N. Redinger, M.D.
Chief, Gastroenterology/Hepatology
Department of Medicine
University of Louisville School of Medicine
Louisville, KY 40292
(502) 588-7963

LOUISIANA
Fred M. Hunter, M.D.
Chief, Gastroenterology
Louisiana State University
School of Medicine
1542 Tulane Ave.
New Orleans, LA 70112
(504) 568-8841

Kemal Akdamar, M.D.
Chairman, Gastroenterology
Tulane University School of Medicine
1430 Tulane Ave.
New Orleans, LA 70112
(504) 588-5329

MARYLAND
Thomas R. Hendrix, M.D.
Chief, Gastroenterology
Johns Hopkins Hospital
Baltimore, MD 21205
(301) 955-5000

Sudbirk K. Dutta, M.D.
Acting Chief, Gastroenterology
University of Maryland School of Medicine
655 W. Baltimore St.
Baltimore, MD 21201
(301) 528-5780

MASSACHUSETTS
Kurt J. Isselbacher, M.D.
Executive Committee Chairman, Department
    of Medicine
Harvard Medical School
Massachusetts General Hospital
Boston, MA 02114
(617) 726-2000

Marshall M. Kaplan, M.D.
Chief, Gastroenterology Division
Department of Medicine
Tufts University School of Medicine
New England Medical Center
171 Harrison Ave.
Boston, MA 02111
(617) 956-5877

Gregory L. Eastwood, M.D.
Chief, Gastroenterology
University of Massachusetts Medical Center
55 Lake Ave.
North Worcester, MA 01605
(617) 856-3068

MICHIGAN
Tadataka Yamada, M.D.
Chief, Gastroenterology
University of Michigan Medical Center
3912 A. Alfred Taubman Health Care Center
Ann Arbor, MI 48109
(313) 936-4770

David Bull, M.D.
Chief, Gastroenterology
Wayne State University
School of Medicine
Harper Hospital
3990 John R
Detroit, MI 48201
(313) 494-8601

MINNESOTA
Joseph Bloomer, M.D.
Head, Gastroenterology and Hepatology
Department of Medicine
University of Minnesota Medical School
Box 36 UMHC
Minneapolis, MN 55455
(612) 625-8999

Harvey I. Sharp, M.D.
Head, Gastroenterology
Department of Pediatrics
University of Minnesota Medical School
Box 279 UMHC
Minneapolis, MN 55455
(612) 624-0685

Albert D. Newcomer, M.D.
Chief, Gastroenterology
Mayo Clinic–Mayo Medical School
200 First St., S.W.
Rochester, MN 55905
(507) 284-2511

MISSISSIPPI
James L. Achord, M.D.
Chief, Digestive Diseases
University of Mississippi Medical Center
2500 N. State St.
Jackson, MS 39216
(601) 984-4540

MISSOURI
E. Lee Forker, M.D.
Chief, Division of GI & Liver
Department of Medicine, M463
University of Missouri
School of Medicine
One Hospital Drive
Columbia, MO 65212
(314) 882-3984

Timothy T. Schubert, M.D.
Chief, Gastroenterology
Department of Medicine
University of Missouri–Kansas City School of
  Medicine
2411 Holmes St.
Kansas City, MO 64108
(816) 276-1950

John S. Farrell, M.D.
Director, Gastroenterology
St. Louis University School of Medicine
1325 S. Grand Blvd.
St. Louis, MO 63104
(314) 577-8765

David H. Alpers, M.D.
Chief, Gastroenterology
Washington University School of Medicine
660 S. Euclid
St. Louis, MO 63110
(314) 454-2000

NEBRASKA
Harry J. Jenkins, Jr., M.D.
Chief, Gastroenterology
Creighton University School of Medicine
California at 24th St.
Omaha, NE 68178
(402) 449-4692

Rowena K. Zetterman, M.D.
Chief, Division of Digestive Disease &
  Nutrition
University of Nebraska College of Medicine
42nd St. & Dewey Ave.
Omaha, NE 68105
(402) 559-6209

NEW HAMPSHIRE
Maurice L. Kelley, Jr., M.D.
Chief, Gastroenterology
Dartmouth Medical School
Hitchcock Clinic
2 Maynard St.
Hanover, NH 03755
(603) 646-5000

NEW JERSEY
Shelly Ludwig, M.D.
Chief, Gastroenterology
UMDNJ–Robert Wood Johnson Medical
  School (Formerly Rutgers)
UMDNJ Medical Education Building
Academic Health Science Building CN19
New Brunswick, NJ 08903
(201) 937-7788

Carroll M. Leevy, M.D.
Chief, Liver Diseases
George Hamilton, M.D.
Chief, Gastroenterology
Department of Medicine
University of Medicine & Dentistry of New
  Jersey
New Jersey Medical School
100 Bergen St.
Newark, NJ 07103
(201) 456-4300

NEW MEXICO
Robert G. Strickland, M.D.
Chief, Division of Gastroenterology
Department of Medicine
University of New Mexico School of Medicine
Albuquerque, NM 87131
(505) 277-4755

NEW YORK
John B. Rodgers, M.D.
Chief, Gastroenterology
Department of Medicine
Albany Medical College
Albany, NY 12208
(518) 445-3125

Louis Sherwood, M.D.
Chief, Medicine
Albert Einstein College of Medicine
1300 Morris Park Ave.
Bronx, NY 10461
(212) 430-2000

Eugene W. Strauss, M.D.
Chief, Gastroenterology
SUNY Health Science Center at Brooklyn
450 Clarkson Ave.
Brooklyn, NY 11203
(718) 270-1112

Milton M. Weiser, M.D.
Chief, GI and Liver Disease
SUNY at Buffalo School of Medicine
Buffalo General Hospital
100 High Street
Buffalo, NY 14203
(716) 845-5600

Emanuel Lebenthal, M.D.
Chief, Gastroenterology
Children's Hospital
SUNY at Buffalo School of Medicine
Buffalo, NY 14203
(716) 878-7793

Robert M. Glickman, M.D.
Chief, Department of Medicine
Columbia-Presbyterian Medical Center
630 W. 168th St.
New York, NY 10032
(212) 694-2500

David Zakim, M.D.
Chief, Digestive Diseases
Cornell University Medical College
New York, NY 10021
(212) 472-4570

Henry D. Janowitz, M.D.
Chief, Gastroenterology
Fenton Schaffner, M.D.
Chief, Hepatology
The Mt. Sinai Medical Center
1 Gustave L. Levy Place
New York, NY 10029
(212) 650-6749, 7369

Norman B. Javitt, M.D.
Director, Division of Hepatic Disease
Arthur E. Lindner, M.D.
Chief, Gastroenterology
New York University Medical Center
550 First Ave.
New York, NY 10016
(212) 340-5111

Laurence S. Jacobs, M.D.
Chief, Gastroenterology
University of Rochester Medical Center
601 Elmwood Ave.
Rochester, NY 14642
(716) 275-4711

Douglas Brand, M.D.
Division Head, Gastroenterology-Hepatology
SUNY at Stony Brook
T-17, R060
Stony Brook, NY 11794
(516) 444-2122

Robert A. Levine, M.D.
Chief, Section of Gastroenterology
SUNY Health Science Center at Syracuse
750 E. Adams St.
Syracuse, NY 13210
(315) 473-5540

William S. Rosenthal, M.D.
Chairman, Gastroenterology
New York Medical College
Munger Pavilion, Room 206
Valhalla, NY 10595
(914) 347-5000

NORTH CAROLINA
Don W. Powell, M.D.
Chief, Division of Digestive Disease &
   Nutrition
326 Burnett—Womack Building
University of North Carolina
Chapel Hill, NC 27514
(919) 962-2211

Malcolm P. Tyor, M.D.
Chief, Gastroenterology
Duke University Medical Center
Box 3902
Durham, NC 27710
(919) 684-5587

Thomas F. O'Brien
Chief, Gastroenterology
East Carolina University School of Medicine
Greenville, NC 27834
(919) 757-4652

Donald O. Castell, M.D.
Chief, Gastroenterology
Bowman Gray School of Medicine
300 S. Hawthorne Rd.
Winston-Salem, NC 27103
(919) 748-4621

OHIO
Ralph A. Giannella, M.D.
Chief, Digestive Diseases
University of Cincinnati Medical Center
231 Bethesda Ave.
Cincinnati, OH 45267-0595
(513) 872-5244

Anthony S. Tavill, M.D.
Director, Division of Gastroenterology
Case Western Reserve University School of
  Medicine
Cleveland Metropolitan General Hospital
2119 Abington Rd.
Cleveland, OH 44106
(216) 459-5681

Fred B. Thomas, M.D.
Director, Division of Gastroenterology
Ohio State University Hospitals
N-214 Doan Hall
410 W. 10th Ave.
Columbus, OH 43210
(614) 421-8462

James F. King, M.D.
Chief, Gastroenterology
Northeastern Ohio Universities College of
  Medicine
4209 State Route 44
Rootstown, OH 44272
(216) 325-2511

Frank S. McCullough, M.D.
Chief, Gastroenterology
Medical College of Ohio at Toledo
Toledo, OH 43699
(419) 381-4172

OKLAHOMA
Jack D. Welsh, M.D.
Chief, Digestive Diseases and Nutrition
Oklahoma Memorial Hospital
PO Box 26307
Oklahoma City, OK 73126
(405) 271-5428

OREGON
Clifford S. Melnyk, M.D.
Chief, Gastroenterology
Oregon Health Sciences University School of
  Medicine
3181 S.W. Sam Jackson Park Rd.
Portland, OR 97201
(503) 225-8311

PENNSYLVANIA
Frederick A. Wilson, M.D.
Chief, Gastroenterology Division
Pennsylvania State University College of
  Medicine
Milton S. Hershey Medical Center
PO Box 850
Hershey, PA 17033
(717) 531-8521

Harris R. Clearfield, M.D.
Director, Gastroenterology
Hahnemann University School of Medicine
Broad and Vine Sts.
Philadelphia, PA 19102
(215) 448-8101

Steven R. Peiken, M.D.
Acting Chief, Gastroenterology
Jefferson Medical College of Thomas Jefferson
  University
11th and Walnut St.
Philadelphia, PA 19107
(215) 928-6944

Walter Rubin, M.D.
Chief, Gastroenterology
The Medical College of Pennsylvania
3300 Henry Ave.
Philadelphia, PA 19129
(215) 842-6000

Stanley H. Lorber, M.D.
Chief, Gastroenterology
Temple University Hospital
3401 N. Broad St.
Philadelphia, PA 19140
(215) 221-2000

Sidney Cohen, M.D.
Chief, Gastroenterology Section
Hospital of the University of Pennsylvania
3400 Spruce St.
Philadelphia, PA 19104
(215) 662-2168

David H. Van Thiel, M.D.
Chief, Gastroenterology
University of Pittsburgh School of Medicine
1000 J Scaife Hall
Pittsburgh, PA 15261
(412) 624-2550

PUERTO RICO
Esther Torres, M.D.
Chief, Gastroenterology
University of Puerto Rico
Medical Sciences Campus
School of Medicine
GPO Box 5067
San Juan, PR 00936
(809) 754-3649

SOUTH CAROLINA
Clarence W. Legerton, M.D.
Director, Gastroenterology
Medical University of South Carolina
171 Ashley Ave.
Charleston, SC 29425
(803) 792-2302

John L. Orchard, M.D.
Chief, Gastroenterology and Metabolism
University of South Carolina
School of Medicine
Columbia, SC 29208
(803) 733-3112

SOUTH DAKOTA
Robert R. Raszkowski, M.D.
Chief, Division of Gastroenterology
Department of Medicine
University of South Dakota
School of Medicine
2501 W. 22nd St.
Sioux Falls, SD 57105
(605) 339-6790

TENNESSEE
Eapen Thomas, M.D.
Chief, Gastroenterology
East Tennessee State University
Quillen-Dishner College of Medicine
PO Box 21,106A
Johnson City, TN 37614
(615) 928-6426

Charles Mansbach, M.D.
Chief, Division of Gastroenterology
University of Tennessee, Memphis
College of Medicine
951 Court Ave., 555D
Memphis, TN 38163
(901) 528-5813

L. O. P. Perry, M.D.
Head, Division of Gastroenterology
Meharry Medical College School of Medicine
1005 D. B. Todd Blvd.
Nashville, TN 37207
(615) 327-6111

G. Dewey Dunn, M.D.
Director, Gastroenterology
Vanderbilt University Medical Center
1161 21st Ave., S.
Nashville, TN 37232
(615) 322-4856

TEXAS
John Dietschy, M.D.
Chief, Gastroenterology
University of Texas Health Science Center at
  Dallas
5323 Harry Hines Blvd.
Dallas, TX 75235
(214) 688-3111

William P. Deiss, Jr., M.D.
Chief, Internal Medicine
Division of Gastroenterology
(ME4 1180JSH)
Department of Internal Medicine
University of Texas Medical Branch
Galveston, TX 77550
(409) 671-2441

Eliot Alpert, M.D.
Chief, Gastroenterology
Baylor College of Medicine
The Methodist Hospital
6565 Fannin, B-503
Houston, TX 77030
(713) 790-3311

Larry Scott, M.D.
Interim Division Director, Division of
  Gastroenterology
University of Texas Health Science Center at
  Houston
PO Box 20708
Houston, TX 77225
(713) 792-5422

Robert R. Secrest, M.D.
Chief, Gastroenterology-Hepatology
Texas Tech University Health Science Center
  School of Medicine
Fourth St. and Indiana Ave.
Lubbock, TX 79430
(806) 743-3000

Steven Schenker, M.D.
Chief, Division of Gastroenterology &
  Nutrition
University of Texas Health Science Center at
  San Antonio
7703 Floyd Curl Drive
San Antonio, TX 78284
(512) 691-6514

Walter P. Dyck, M.D.
Chief, Gastroenterology
Texas A&M University College of Medicine
Scott & White Clinic
Temple, TX 76502
(817) 939-1844

UTAH
Keith G. Tolman, M.D.
Chief, Gastroenterology, Hepatology, and
  Nutrition
University of Utah School of Medicine
50 N. Medical Drive
Salt Lake City, UT 84132
(801) 581-7802

VERMONT
Edward L. Krawitt, M.D.
Chief, Gastroenterology
Department of Medicine
University of Vermont
Given Building Room C-317
Burlington, VT 05405
(802) 656-2554

VIRGINIA
Edward C. Wilson, M.D.
Head, Division of Gastroenterology
University of Virginia Hospital
Jefferson Park Ave.
Charlottesville, VA 22908
(804) 924-0211

Z. Reno Vlahcevic, M.D.
Chairman, Gastroenterology
Medical College of Virginia
MCV Station, Box 711
Richmond, VA 23298
(804) 786-9598

WASHINGTON
David R. Saunders, M.D.
Head, Division of Gastroenterology
University of Washington School of Medicine,
  RG 24
Seattle, WA 98195
(206) 543-3183

WEST VIRGINIA
James Moore, M.D.
Chief, Gastroenterology
Marshall University School of Medicine
Huntington, WV 25701
(304) 526-0561

Ronald D. Gaskins, M.D.
Chief, Gastroenterology
West Virginia University School of Medicine
Morgantown, WV 26506
(304) 293-4121

WISCONSIN
John F. Morrissey, M.D.
Chief, Gastroenterology
University of Wisconsin Medical School
Department of Medicine
600 Highland Ave., J5/235
Madison, WI 53792
(608) 263-6400

Konrad H. Soergel, M.D.
Chief, Gastroenterology
Medical College of Wisconsin
Froedtert Memorial Lutheran Hospital
9200 W. Wisconsin Ave.
Milwaukee, WI 53226
(414) 259-3028

EAR, NOSE, AND THROAT (OTOLARYNGOLOGISTS)

The physicians listed below are some of the leading specialists in otolaryngology, the medical and surgical treatment of the head and neck, including ear, nose, and throat. They may be available for consultations and treatment or may be able to refer you to someone else. All are heads of departments or divisions of otolaryngology at medical colleges accredited by the Association of American Medical Colleges.

ALABAMA
Julius N. Hicks, M.D.
Director, Division of Otorhinolaryngology
Department of Surgery
University of Alabama at Birmingham
OHB 345
University Station
Birmingham, AL 35294
(205) 934-9765

Milton Leigh, M.D.
Chief, Otolaryngology Surgery
University of South Alabama College of
  Medicine
307 University Blvd.
Mobile, AL 36688
(205) 460-7174

ARIZONA
Stanley W. Coulthard, M.D.
Chief, Otorhinolaryngology Surgery
University of Arizona Health Sciences Center
1501 N. Campbell Ave.
Tucson, AZ 85724
(602) 626-0111

ARKANSAS
James Y. Suen, M.D.
Chief, Otolaryngology and Maxillofacial
  Surgery
University of Arkansas for Medical Sciences
University of Arkansas College of Medicine
University Hospital
4301 W. Markham, Slot 543
Little Rock, AR 72205
(501) 661-5140

CALIFORNIA
Irving Rappaport, M.D.
Chief, Otolaryngologic Surgery
University of California, Irvine
California College of Medicine
Irvine, CA 92717
(714) 634-6928

Robert P. Rowe, M.D.
Chief, Otolaryngology
Loma Linda University
Barton & Anderson Sts.
Loma Linda, CA 92354
(714) 796-7311

Paul H. Ward, M.D.
Chief, Head and Neck Surgery
University of California
Los Angeles School of Medicine
Department of Otolaryngology
Los Angeles, CA 90024
(213) 825-9111

Dale Rice, M.D.
Chief, Otolaryngology
University of Southern California School of
  Medicine
1200 N. State St.–Room 4136
Los Angeles, CA 90033
(213) 226-7315

Victor Passy, M.D.
Chief, Otolaryngology
University of California, Irvine Medical Center
101 City Drive S.
Orange, CA 92668
(714) 634-5753

Richard A. Chole, M.D., Ph.D.
Acting Chair, Otorhinolaryngology
School of Medicine
University of California, Davis
4301 X St.
Sacramento, CA 95817
(916) 453-2831, 2801

Alan M. Nahum, M.D.
Chief, Head and Neck Surgery Division
University of California, San Diego Medical
  Center
225 Dickinson St.
San Diego, CA 92103
(619) 294-6322

Roger Boles, M.D.
University of California, San Francisco
Chief, Department of Otolaryngology, A-717
400 Parnassus Ave.
San Francisco, CA 94143
(415) 666-9000

Willard E. Fee, Jr., M.D.
Clinic and Division Chief
Division of Otolaryngology
Stanford University Medical Center
Stanford, CA 94305
(415) 723-5281

COLORADO
Bruce W. Jafek, M.D.
Chief, Otolaryngology
University of Colorado Health Sciences Center
4200 E. Ninth Ave. (B-210)
Denver, CO 80262
(303) 399-1211

CONNECTICUT
Gerald Leonard, M.D.
Chief, Otolaryngology
University of Connecticut Health Center
Department of Otolaryngology
Farmington, CT 06032
(203) 674-3372

Clarence T. Sasaki, M.D.
Head, Section of Otolaryngology
Yale University School of Medicine
333 Cedar St.
New Haven, CT 06510
(203) 785-2593

DISTRICT OF COLUMBIA
William Wilson, M.D.
Director, Otolaryngology Division
George Washington University
Medical Center
2150 Pennsylvania Ave., N.W.
Washington, DC 20037
(202) 676-5550

Hugh O. DeFries, M.D.
Chief, Otolaryngology Surgery
Georgetown University Hospital
3800 Reservoir Rd., N.W.
Washington, DC 20007
(202) 625-0100

Ernest M. Myers, M.D.
Chief, Rhinotolaryngology
Howard University College of Medicine
520 W. St., N.W.
Washington, DC 20059
(202) 745-1432

FLORIDA
Nicholas J. Cassissi, M.D., D.D.S.
Chief, Otolaryngology Surgery
University of Florida College of Medicine
J. Hillis Miller Health Center
Box J 264
Gainesville, FL 32610
(904) 392-5000

James R. Chandler, M.D.
University of Miami School of Medicine
Chief, Department of Otolaryngology, D-48
PO Box 16960
Miami, FL 33101
(305) 547-6418

James N. Endicott, M.D.
Chief, Division of Otolaryngology
University of South Florida
College of Medicine
James A. Haley Veterans Hospital
13000 N. 30th St., Room 112-A
Tampa, FL 33612
(813) 972-7585

GEORGIA
John S. Turner, Jr., M.D.
Chief, Otolaryngology Surgery
The Emory Clinic
1365 Clifton Rd., N.E.
Atlanta, GA 30322
(404) 321-0111

Edward S. Porubsky, M.D.
Chief, Otolaryngology
Medical College of Georgia Hospital
Augusta, GA 30912
(404) 828-2047

ILLINOIS
George A. Sisson, M.D.
Chairman, Otolaryngology and Head and Neck
  Surgery
Northwestern University Medical School
303 E. Chicago Ave.
Chicago, IL 60611
(312) 908-8649

David D. Caldarelli, M.D.
Chairman, Otolaryngology and
  Bronchoescophagology
Rush-Presbyterian-St. Luke's Medical Center
1753 W. Congress Parkway
Chicago, IL 60612
(312) 942-5000

William Panje, M.D.
Chief, Section of Otolaryngology/Head and
  Neck Surgery
University of Chicago Medical Center
5841 S. Maryland Ave.
Chicago, IL 60637
(312) 947-1000

Edward L. Applebaum, M.D.
Chief, Otolaryngology
University of Illinois Hospital
1855 W. Taylor St.
Chicago, IL 60612
(312) 996-7000

Gregory J. Matz, M.D.
Chief, Otolaryngology
Loyola University of Chicago
Stritch School of Medicine
2160 S. First Ave.
Maywood, IL 60153
(312) 531-3000

Horst R. Konrad, M.D.
Chief, Otolaryngology Surgery
Southern Illinois University School of
  Medicine
800 N. Rutledge St.
PO Box 3926
Springfield, IL 62708
(217) 782-3318

INDIANA
Raleigh E. Lingeman, M.D.
Chairman, Department of Otolaryngology–
  Head and Neck Surgery
Indiana University Medical Center
Riley Hospital for Children, A56
702 Barnhill Drive
Indianapolis, IN 46223
(317) 630-8954

IOWA
Brian F. McCabe, M.D.
Chief, Otolaryngology
University of Iowa Hospitals
Department of Otolaryngology
Iowa City, IA 52242
(319) 356-1616

KANSAS
C. W. Norris, M.D.
Chairman, Otorhinolaryngology
University of Kansas Medical Center
39th and Rainbow Blvd.
Kansas City, KS 66103
(913) 588-6720

KENTUCKY
Serge A. Martinez, M.D.
Chief, Otolaryngology
Department of Surgery
University of Louisville School of Medicine
Louisville, KY 40292
(502) 588-6994

LOUISIANA

George D. Lyons, M.D.
Head, Otorhinolaryngology and
   Biocommunication
Louisiana State University School of Medicine
1542 Tulane Ave.
New Orleans, LA 70112
(504) 568-4785

Harold G. Tabb, M.D.
Chief, Otolaryngology
Tulane University School of Medicine
1430 Tulane Ave., Suite 2000
New Orleans, LA 70112
(504) 588-5451

Frederick J. Stucker, Jr., M.D.
Chairman, Otolaryngology/Head and Neck
   Surgery
Louisiana State University School of Medicine
   in Shreveport
PO Box 33932
Shreveport, LA 71130
(318) 674-6180

MARYLAND

George T. Nager, M.D.
Chief, Otolaryngology
Johns Hopkins University School of Medicine
720 Rutland Ave.
Baltimore, MD 21205
(301) 955-5000

Cyrus L. Blanchard, M.D.
Chief, Otolaryngology Surgery
University of Maryland Hospital
22 S. Greene St.
Room 4-1181
Baltimore, MD 21201
(301) 528-2121

MASSACHUSETTS

M. Stuart Strong, M.D.
Chief, Otolaryngology Surgery
Boston University Hospital
75 E. Newton St.
Boston, MA 02118
(617) 247-5000

Joseph Nadol, M.D.
Chief, Otolaryngology
Harvard Medical School
Massachusetts Eye and Ear Infirmary
243 Charles St.
Boston, MA 02114
(617) 523-7900

Werner D. Chasin, M.D.
Otolaryngologist-in-Chief
Tufts University School of Medicine
New England Medical Center
171 Harrison Ave.
Boston, MA 02111
(617) 956-5494

James P. Hughes, M.D.
Chief, Otolaryngology
University of Massachusetts Medical School
55 Lake Ave., N.
Worcester, MA 01605
(617) 856-4161

MICHIGAN

Charles J. Krause, M.D.
Chairman, Department of Otolaryngology
University of Michigan Medical Center
1904N A. Alfred Taubman Health Care Center
Ann Arbor, MI 48109
(313) 936-7483

Robert H. Mathog, M.D.
Chief, Otolaryngology
Wayne State University
School of Medicine
540 E. Canfield Ave.
Detroit, MI 48201
(313) 577-0804

Richard Dean, M.D.
Chief, Surgery
Michigan State University
College of Human Medicine
East Lansing, MI 48824
(517) 353-6625

MINNESOTA

Arndt J. Duvall, M.D.
Chief, Otolaryngology
University of Minnesota Medical School
Box 396 UMHC
Minneapolis, MN 55455
(612) 625-3200

H. Bryan Neel, III, M.D.
Chief, Otorhinolaryngology
Mayo Medical School
200 First St., S.W.
Rochester, MN 55905
(507) 284-3671

MISSISSIPPI
Winsor V. Morrison, M.D.
Chief, Otolaryngology Surgery
University of Mississippi Medical Center
Jackson, MS 39216
(601) 984-5160

MISSOURI
William E. Davis, M.D.
Chief, Otolaryngology Surgery
University of Missouri Medical Center
807 Stadium Rd.
Columbia, MO 65212
(312) 882-4141

William H. Friedman, M.D.
Chief, Otolaryngology
St. Louis University School of Medicine
1325 S. Grand Blvd.
St. Louis, MO 63104
(314) 577-8887

John M. Fredrickson, M.D.
Head, Otolaryngology
Washington University School of Medicine
660 S. Euclid, Box 8115
St. Louis, MO 63110
(314) 362-7552

NEBRASKA
Patrick E. Brookhouser, M.D.
Chief, Otolaryngology
Creighton University School of Medicine
California at 24th St.
Omaha, NE 68178
(402) 449-6501

Anthony J. Yonkers, M.D.
Chairman, Otolaryngology and Maxillofacial
  Surgery
University of Nebraska College of Medicine
42nd and Dewey Ave.
Omaha, NE 68105
(402) 559-4433

NEW HAMPSHIRE
Nathan A. Geurkink, M.D.
Chief, Otolaryngology/Audiology
Dartmouth Medical School
Hanover, NH 03756
(603) 646-7505

NEW JERSEY
Barry Skobel, M.D.
Chief, Otolaryngology
University of Medicine and Dentistry of New
  Jersey
Robert Wood Johnson Medical School
(formerly Rutgers)
1150 Amboy Ave.
Edison, NJ 08837
(201) 548-3200

Anthony F. Jahn, M.D.
Chief, Otolaryngology
University of Medicine and Dentistry of New
  Jersey
New Jersey Medical School
100 Bergen St., H-586
Newark, NJ 07107
(201) 456-4300

NEW MEXICO
Fred S. Herzon, M.D.
Chief, Otorhinolaryngology Surgery
Department of Surgery
University of New Mexico School of Medicine
Albuquerque, NM 87131
(505) 843-2336

NEW YORK
Jerome C. Goldstein, M.D.
Chief, Otolaryngology Surgery
Albany Medical College
47 New Scotland Ave.
Albany, NY 12208
(518) 445-3125

Robert J. Ruben, M.D.
Chief, Otolaryngology
Albert Einstein College of Medicine
1300 Morris Park Ave.
Bronx, NY 10461
(212) 920-4141

Abraham Shulman, M.D.
Chief, Otolaryngology
SUNY Health Science Center at Brooklyn
450 Clarkson Ave.
Brooklyn, NY 11203
(718) 270-1638

John M. Lore, Jr., M.D.
Chairman, Otolaryngology
SUNY at Buffalo
Seton Professional Building, Suite 208
2121 Main St.
Buffalo, NY 14214
(714) 831-2000

Maxwell Abramson, M.D.
Chief, Otolaryngology
Columbia-Presbyterian Medical Center
Presbyterian Hospital
622 W. 168th St.
New York, NY 10032
(212) 694-2500

Robert W. Selfe, M.D.
Chief, Otorhinolaryngology
Cornell University Medical College
New York Hospital
525 E. 68th St.
New York, NY 10021
(212) 472-8386

Hugh F. Biller, M.D.
Chief, Otolaryngology
The Mount Sinai Medical Center
1 Gustave L. Levy Place
New York, NY 10029
(212) 650-6141

Frank E. Lucente, M.D.
Chairman, Otolaryngology
New York Medical College
New York Eye & Ear Infirmary
310 E. 14th St.
New York, NY 10003
(212) 598-1420

Noel L. Cohen, M.D.
Chief, Otorhinolaryngology
New York University Medical Center
550 First Ave.
New York, NY 10016
(212) 340-7300

Arthur S. Hengerer, M.D.
Chief, Otolaryngology Surgery
University of Rochester Medical Center
601 Elmwood Ave.
Rochester, NY 14642
(716) 275-2754

Richard R. Gacek, M.D.
Chief, Otolaryngology
SUNY Health Science Center at Syracuse
750 E. Adams St.
Syracuse, NY 13210
(315) 473-5540

NORTH CAROLINA
Newton D. Fischer, M.D.
Chief, Otolaryngology Surgery
University of North Carolina
610 Burnet-Womack Building 229 H
Chapel Hill, NC 27514
(919) 962-2211

William R. Hudson, M.D.
Chief, Otolaryngology Surgery
Duke University Medical Center
Box 3805
Durham, NC 27710
(919) 684-8111

William A. Bost, M.D.
Chief, Otorhinolaryngology
East Carolina University School of Medicine
Greenville, NC 27834
(919) 752-5227

Robert I. Kohut, M.D.
Chief, Otolaryngology
Bowman Gray School of Medicine
300 S. Hawthorne Rd.
Winston-Salem, NC 27103
(919) 748-4161

NORTH DAKOTA
John N. Youngs, M.D.
Chief, Otolaryngology Surgery
University of North Dakota School of
  Medicine
Grand Forks, ND 58202
(701) 780-6301

OHIO
Donald A. Shumrick, M.D.
Chief, Otolaryngology and Maxillofacial
    Surgery
University of Cincinnati Medical Center
231 Bethesda Ave.
Cincinnati, OH 45267-0528
(513) 872-4155

Anthony J. Maniglia, M.D.
Chairman, Department of Otolaryngology
Case Western Reserve University School of
    Medicine
University Hospitals of Cleveland
2074 Abington Rd.
Cleveland, OH 44106
(216) 844-3001

David E. Schuller, M.D.
Chairman, Otolaryngology
Ohio State University Hospitals
4102 University Hospitals Clinic
456 Clinic Drive
Columbus, Ohio 43210
(614) 421-8074

Robert A. Goldenberg, M.D.
Chair, Otolaryngology
Wright State University School of Medicine
PO Box 927
Dayton, OH 45401
(513) 275-1646

Joseph P. Yut, M.D.
Chief, Otolaryngology
Northeastern Ohio Universities College of
    Medicine
4209 Star Route 44
Rootstown, OH 44272
(216) 325-2511

OKLAHOMA
J. Gail Neely, M.D.
Chief, Otorhinolaryngology
University of Oklahoma Health Sciences,
    South Pavilion
PO Box 26307
Oklahoma City, OK 73126
(405) 271-5504

OREGON
Alexander J. Schleuning, M.D.
Chief, Otolaryngology
Oregon Health Sciences University Hospital
3181 S.W. Sam Jackson Park Rd.
Portland, OR 97201
(503) 225-8311

PENNSYLVANIA
George H. Conner, M.D.
Chief, Otolaryngology
Pennsylvania State University College of
    Medicine
Milton S. Hershey Medical Center
Department of Otolaryngology
Hershey, PA 17033
(717) 531-8521

Robert Wolfson, M.D.
Chairman, Otorhinolaryngology
Hahnemann University School of Medicine
Broad and Vine Sts.
Philadelphia, PA 19102
(215) 448-7703

Louis D. Lowry, M.D.
Chief, Otolaryngology
Jefferson Medical College of Thomas Jefferson
    University Hospital
11th & Walnut Sts.
Philadelphia, PA 19107
(215) 928-6784

Frank I. Marlowe, M.D.
Chief, Otolaryngology
Medical College of Pennsylvania
3300 Henry Ave.
Philadelphia, PA 19129
(215) 842-6000

Max L. Ronis, M.D.
Chief, Otorhinology
Temple University Hospital
3400 N. Broad St.
Philadelphia, PA 19140
(215) 221-2000

James B. Snow, Jr., M.D.
Chief, Otorhinolaryngology and Human
    Communication
Hospital of the University of Pennsylvania
3400 Spruce St.
Philadelphia, PA 19104
(215) 662-2653

Eugene N. Myers, M.D.
Chairman, Otolaryngology
University of Pittsburgh School of Medicine
Eye and Ear Hospital
230 Lothrop St., Suite 1115
Pittsburgh, PA 15213
(412) 647-2110

PUERTO RICO
Juan Trinidad, M.D.
Chief, Otolaryngology
University of Puerto Rico
Medical Sciences Campus
School of Medicine
GPO Box 5067
San Juan, PR 00936
(809) 758-2525, x1910

SOUTH CAROLINA
Warren Y. Adkins, M.D.
Chairman, Otolaryngology and Communicative
  Sciences
Medical University of South Carolina
171 Ashley Ave.
Charleston, SC 29425
(803) 792-3531

Alan H. Brill, M.D.
Chief, Otolaryngology Surgery
University of South Carolina School of
  Medicine
Columbia, SC 29208
(803) 254-4158

SOUTH DAKOTA
Vernon Stensland, M.D.
Chief, Otorhinolaryngology Surgery
University of South Dakota School of
  Medicine
2501 W. 22nd St.
Sioux Falls, SD 57105
(605) 331-3225

TENNESSEE
Floyd B. Goffin, M.D.
Chief, Otolaryngology Surgery
East Tennessee State University
Quillen-Dishner College of Medicine
PO Box 19,750A
Johnson City, TN 37614
(615) 928-6426

Richard W. Babin, M.D.
Chairman, Otolaryngology and Maxillofacial
  Surgery
University of Tennessee, Memphis
College of Medicine
956 Court Ave., B226
Memphis, TN 38163
(901) 528-5885

Joseph L. B. Forrester, M.D.
Chief, Otolaryngology Surgery
Meharry Medical College School of Medicine
1005 D. B. Todd Blvd.
Nashville, TN 37207
(615) 327-6342

TEXAS
William L. Meyerhoff, M.D., Ph.D.
Chief, Otorhinolaryngology
University of Texas Health Sciences Center
5323 Harry Hines Blvd.
Dallas, TX 75235
(214) 688-3111

Byron J. Bailey, M.D.
Chief, Otolaryngology
University of Texas Medical Branch Hospitals
John Sealy Hospital
Galveston, TX 77550
(409) 761-1011

Bobby R. Alfrod, M.D.
Chief, Otorhinolaryngology and
  Communicative Sciences
Baylor College of Medicine
One Baylor Plaza
Houston, TX 77030
(713) 799-4951

Robert A. Jahrsdoerfer, M.D.
Chairman, Otolaryngology-Head and Neck
  Surgery
University of Texas Health Science Center at
  Houston
6431 Fannin, Suite 6132
Houston, TX 77030
(713) 792-5866

George A. Gates, M.D.
Chief, Otorhinolaryngology Surgery
University of Texas Health Science Center at
  San Antonio
7703 Floyd Curl Drive
San Antonio, TX 78284
(512) 691-6563

Tibor Ruff, M.D.
Chief, Otolaryngology
Texas A&M University College of Medicine
Scott & White Clinic
Temple, TX 76508
(817) 774-2581

UTAH
James L. Parkin, M.D.
Chief, Otolaryngology Surgery
University of Utah School of Medicine
50 N. Medical Drive
Salt Lake City, UT 84132
(801) 581-7514

VERMONT
Robert A. Sofferman, M.D.
Chief, Otolaryngology Surgery
Medical Center Hospital of Vermont
1 S. Prospect St.
Burlington, VT 05401
(802) 656-4535

VIRGINIA
Robert C. Cantrell, M.D.
Chief, Otolaryngology
University of Virginia Medical Center
Department of Otolaryngology
PO Box 430
Charlottesville, VA 22908
(804) 924-0211

Gary Schechter, M.D.
Chief, Otolaryngology Surgery
Eastern Virginia Medical School
Department of Otolaryngology
901 Hampton Blvd.
Norfolk, VA 23507
(804) 628-3481

George H. Williams, M.D.
Chairman, Otolaryngology
Medical College of Virginia
MCV Station, Box 146
Richmond, VA 23298
(804) 786-9336

WASHINGTON
Charles W. Cummings, M.D.
Chief, Otolaryngology
University of Washington School of Medicine,
  R L-30
Seattle, WA 98195
(206) 543-5230

WEST VIRGINIA
Joseph B. Touma, M.D.
Acting Chief, Otolaryngology
Marshall University School of Medicine
Huntington, WV 25701
(304) 529-2407

Philip M. Sprinkle, M.D.
Chief, Otolaryngology
West Virginia University Medical Center
Department of Otolaryngology
Morgantown, WV 26506
(304) 293-0111

WISCONSIN
James H. Brandenburg, M.D.
Chief, Otolaryngology Surgery
University of Wisconsin Hospital and Clinics
800 Highland Avenue, F 4/2
Madison, WI 53792
(608) 263-6400

Roger H. Lehman, M.D.
Chief, Otolaryngology Surgery
Medical College of Wisconsin
Clement J. Zablocki VA Medical Center
Department of Otolaryngology
5000 W. National Ave.
Milwaukee, WI 53295
(414) 384-2000

ENDOCRINOLOGY AND DIABETES (ENDOCRINOLOGISTS)

The physicians listed below are some of the leading specialists in endocrinology, the treatment of diseases related to hormone-secreting glands, such as diabetes. These physicians may be available for consultations and treatment or may be able to refer you to someone else. All are heads of endocrinology or diabetes departments or divisions at medical colleges accredited by the Association of American Medical Colleges.

ALABAMA

Rex S. Clements, M.D.
Director, Division of Endocrinology and
    Metabolism
Department of Medicine
University of Alabama at Birmingham
DB 414
University Station
Birmingham, AL 35294
(205) 934-3410

J. Claude Bennett, M.D.
Acting Director, Diabetes Research and
    Training Center
University of Alabama at Birmingham
MEF 621
University Station
Birmingham, AL 35294
(205) 934-5304

Alan M. Siegel, M.D.
Chief, Endocrinology
University of South Alabama College of
    Medicine
307 University Blvd.
Mobile, AL 36688
(205) 460-7174

ARIZONA

David G. Johnson, M.D.
Chief, Endocrinology
University of Arizona College of
    Medicine
Arizona Health Sciences Center
1501 N. Campbell Ave.
Tucson, AZ 85724
(602) 626-0111

ARKANSAS

Robert W. Harrison, M.D.
Chief, Endocrinology
University of Arkansas College of
    Medicine
4301 W. Markham St., Slot 587
Little Rock, AR 72205
(501) 661-5130

CALIFORNIA

Grant Gwinup, M.D.
Chief, Endocrinology
University of California, Irvine
California College of Medicine
Irvine, CA 92717
(714) 856-7374

Jerrold Olefsky, M.D.
Chief, Endocrinology/Metabolism Division
University of California, San Diego
School of Medicine
La Jolla, CA 92093
(619) 452-4310

J. Lamont Murdoch, M.D.
Chief, Endocrinology
Loma Linda University School of Medicine
Loma Linda, CA 92350
(714) 824-4911

Andre J. Van Herle, M.D.
Acting Chief, Division of Endocrinology
University of California, Los Angeles
UCLA School of Medicine
Los Angeles, CA 90024
(213) 825-5366

Richard Horton, M.D.
Chief, Endocrinology
George Bray, M.D.
Chief, Diabetes
University of Southern California School of
    Medicine
2025 Zonal Ave.
Los Angeles, CA 90033
(213) 226-4635, 4719

Thomas T. Aoki, M.D.
Chief, Endocrinology and Metabolism
University of California, Davis Medical Center
4301 X St., FOLB II, Building C
Sacramento, CA 95817
(916) 453-3739

Lloyd H. Smith, Jr., M.D.
Chief, Department of Medicine
University of California, San Francisco
School of Medicine
513 Parnassus Ave.
San Francisco, CA 94143
(415) 666-9000

David Feldman, M.D.
Division Chief
Carlos Camargo, M.D.
Clinic Chief
Endocrinology Clinic
Division of Endocrinology
David Feldman, M.D.
Division Chief
Fredric Kraemer, M.D.
Clinic Chief
Diabetes and Metabolism Clinic
Stanford University Medical Center
Stanford, CA 94305
(415) 723-6054

COLORADO
Jerrold M. Olefsky, M.D.
Chief, Endocrinology
University of Colorado School of Medicine
4200 E. Ninth Ave.
Denver, CO 80262
(303) 399-1211

CONNECTICUT
Lawrence G. Raisz, M.D.
Chief, Endocrinology and Metabolism
University of Connecticut Health Center
Farmington, CT 06032
(203) 674-2129

Howard Rasmussen, M.D.
Head, Section of Endocrinology
William Tamborlane, M.D.
Head, Section of Pediatric Endocrinology
Yale University School of Medicine
333 Cedar St.
New Haven, CT 06510
(203) 785-4181, 4648

DISTRICT OF COLUMBIA
Kenneth L. Becker, M.D.
Director, Endocrinology Division
George Washington University
Medical Center
2150 Pennsylvania Ave., N.W.
Washington, DC 20037
(202) 676-3695

Richard C. Eastman, M.D.
Chief, Endocrinology
Georgetown University School of Medicine
3900 Reservoir Rd., N.W.
Washington, DC 20007
(202) 625-8728

FLORIDA
Thomas J. Merimee, M.D.
Chief, Endocrinology
University of Florida College of Medicine
Box J-215, J. Hillis Miller Health Center
Gainesville, FL 32610
(904) 392-2616

J. Maxwell McKenzie, M.D.
Chief, Endocrinology
University of Miami School of Medicine
PO Box 016099 (R-699)
Miami, FL 33101
(305) 549-7023

Robert V. Farese, M.D.
Professor of Medicine
Director, Division of Endocrinology and
   Metabolism
Associate Chief of Staff for Research and
   Development
James A. Haley Veterans Hospital
13000 N. 30th St., VA Research Building
   #208
Tampa, FL 33612
(813) 972-7662

GEORGIA
Lawrence S. Phillips, M.D.
Chief, Endocrinology
Emory University School of Medicine
Atlanta, GA 30322
(404) 588-3645

Virendra B. Mahesh, M.D.
Chief, Endocrinology
Medical College of Georgia Hospital
Augusta, GA 30912
(404) 828-2781

ILLINOIS
Norbert Freinkel, M.D.
Director, Center for Endocrinology,
   Metabolism, & Nutrition
Northwestern University Medical School
303 E. Chicago Ave.
Chicago, IL 60611
(312) 908-8023

John G. Bagdade, M.D.
Director, Section of Endocrinology
Rush-Presbyterian-St. Luke's Medical
  Center
1753 W. Congress Parkway
Chicago, IL 60612
(312) 942-6163

Leslie DeGroot, M.D.
Chief, Section of Endocrinology
Director, Thyroid Study Unit
University of Chicago Medical Center
5841 S. Maryland Ave.
Chicago, IL 60637
(312) 947-1000

Gerald A. Williams, M.D.
Chief, Endocrinology and Metabolism
University of Illinois College of Medicine
1853 W. Polk St.
Chicago, IL 60612
(312) 996-3500

Marion H. Brooks, M.D.
Chief, Endocrinology
Loyola University of Chicago
Stritch School of Medicine
2160 S. First Ave.
Maywood, IL 60153
(312) 531-3000

Kenneth A. Fisher, M.D.
Chief, Endocrinology
University of Health Sciences
Chicago Medical School
3333 Green Bay Rd.
North Chicago, IL 60064
(312) 578-3000

Norman Soler, M.D.
Chief, Endocrinology
Southern Illinois University School of
  Medicine
800 N. Rutledge
PO Box 3926
Springfield, IL 62708
(217) 782-3318

INDIANA
C. Conrad Johnston, M.D.
Chief, Endocrinology & Metabolism Section
Department of Medicine
Indiana University Medical Center
Emerson Hall 421
545 Barnhill Drive
Indianapolis, IN 46223
(317) 264-8554

James Wright, M.D.
Chief, Endocrinology Section
Department of Pediatrics
Indiana University Medical Center
Riley Hospital for Children A586
702 Barnhill Drive
Indianapolis, IN 46223
(317) 264-3973

IOWA
Daryl K. Granner, M.D.
Chief, Endocrinology
University of Iowa College of Medicine
100 College of Medicine Administration
  Building
Iowa City, IA 52242
(319) 353-4843

KANSAS
R. Neil Schimke, M.D.
Director, Division of Metabolism,
  Endocrinology, & Genetics
University of Kansas Medical Center
39th & Rainbow Blvd.
Kansas City, KS 66103
(913) 588-6043

KENTUCKY
Theodore A. Kotchen, M.D.
Chief, Endocrinology
University of Kentucky College of Medicine
800 Rose St.
Lexington, KY 40536
(606) 233-5000

Ellis Samols, M.D.
Chief, Endocrinology/Metabolism
Department of Medicine
University of Louisville School of Medicine
Veterans Administration Medical Center
800 Zorn Ave.
Louisville, KY 40206
(502) 895-3401

LOUISIANA
John F. Wilber, M.D.
Chief, Endocrinology
Louisiana State University School of Medicine
1542 Tulane Ave.
New Orleans, LA 70112
(504) 568-6446

Cyril Y. Bowers, M.D.
Chief, Endocrinology
Tulane University School of Medicine
1430 Tulane Ave.
New Orleans, LA 70112
(504) 588-5441

Steven Levine
Chief, Endocrinology
Louisiana State University
School of Medicine in Shreveport
PO Box 33932
Shreveport, LA 71130
(318) 674-5000

MARYLAND
Robert L. Ney, M.D.
Chief, Endocrinology
Johns Hopkins University School of Medicine
720 Rutland Ave.
Baltimore, MD 21205
(301) 955-5000

Thomas B. Connor, M.D.
Chief, Endocrinology
University of Maryland School of Medicine
655 W. Baltimore St.
Baltimore, MD 21201
(301) 528-6219

MASSACHUSETTS
Sidney Ingbar, M.D.
Chief, Endocrinology
Beth Israel Hospital
Harvard Medical School
330 Brookline Ave.
Boston, MA 02215
(617) 735-2029

Gordon Williams, M.D.
Chief, Endocrinology
Brigham & Women's Hospital
Harvard Medical School
75 Francis St.
Boston, MA 02115
(617) 732-5661

Michael Rosenblatt, M.D.
Chief, Endocrinology
Massachusetts General Hospital
Harvard Medical School
32 Fruit St.
Boston, MA 02114
(617) 726-3966

Seymour Reichlin, M.D.
Division Chief, Endocrinology
Tufts University School of Medicine
New England Medical Center
171 Harrison Ave.
Boston, MA 02111
(617) 956-5692

Lewis E. Braverman, M.D.
Chief, Endocrinology
Aldo A. Rossini, M.D.
Chief, Diabetes
University of Massachusetts Medical School
55 Lake Ave. N.
Worcester, MA 01605
(617) 856-3115, 3206

MICHIGAN
John Marshall, M.D.
Chief, Endocrinology and Metabolism
University of Michigan Medical Center
3920 A. Alfred Taubman Health Care Center
Ann Arbor, MI 48109
(313) 936-5505

James R. Sowers, M.D.
Chief, Endocrinology
Wayne State University
School of Medicine
540 E. Canfield
Detroit, MI 48201
(313) 577-5036

MINNESOTA
Jack Oppenheimer, M.D.
Head, Endocrinology
Department of Medicine
University of Minnesota Medical School
Box 91 UMHC
Minneapolis, MN 55455
(612) 624-5150

B. Lawrence Riggs, M.D.
Chief, Endocrinology
Mayo Medical School
200 First St., S.W.
Rochester, MN 55905
(507) 284-3671

MISSISSIPPI
Herbert G. Langford, M.D.
Chief, Endocrinology and Hypertension
University of Mississippi Medical Center
2500 N. State St.
Jackson, MS 39216
(601) 984-5525

MISSOURI
Thomas Burns, M.D.
Chief, Endocrinology
University of Missouri
Columbia School of Medicine
One Hospital Drive
Columbia, MO 65212
(314) 882-1566

Nathaniel Winer, M.D.
Chief, Endocrinology
University of Missouri
Kansas City School of Medicine
2411 Holmes St.
Kansas City, MO 64108
(816) 296-1910

Stewart Albert, M.D.
Acting Division Director, Endocrinology
St. Louis University School of Medicine
1402 S. Grand Blvd.
St. Louis, MO 63104
(314) 577-8458

Philip E. Cryer, M.D.
Chief, Endocrinology
Washington University School of Medicine
660 S. Euclid Ave.
St. Louis, MO 63110
(314) 362-7617

NEBRASKA
Robert R. Recker, M.D.
Chief, Endocrinology
Creighton University School of Medicine
California at 24th St.
Omaha, NE 68178
(402) 280-4470

Joseph C. Shipp, M.D.
Chief, Diabetes, Endocrinology, and
  Metabolism
University of Nebraska College of Medicine
42nd St. and Dewey Ave.
Omaha, NE 68105
(402) 559-7229

NEW HAMPSHIRE
Lee A. Witters, M.D.
Chief, Endocrinology
Dartmouth Medical School
Hanover, NH 03756
(603) 646-7505

NEW JERSEY
Avedis K. Khachadurian, M.D.
Chief, Endocrinology
University of Medicine and Dentistry of New
  Jersey
Robert Wood Johnson Medical School
(formerly Rutgers)
UMDNJ Medical Education Building
Academic Health Science Building CN19
New Brunswick, NJ 08903
(201) 937-7749

Margo P. Cohen, M.D.
Chief, Endocrinology
University of Medicine and Dentistry of New
  Jersey
New Jersey Medical School
100 Bergen St.
Newark, NJ 07103
(201) 456-4300

NEW MEXICO
R. Phillip Eaton, M.D.
Chief, Endocrinology
Department of Medicine
University of New Mexico School of Medicine
Albuquerque, NM 87131
(505) 277-4656

NEW YORK
A. David Goodman, M.D.
Chief, Endocrinology
Albany Medical College of Union University
47 New Scotland Ave.
Albany, NY 12208
(518) 445-5582

Norman Fleisher, M.D.
Division Head, Endocrinology
Albert Einstein College of Medicine
Bronx, NY 10461
(212) 430-2908

Harold Lebovitz, M.D.
Chief, Endocrinology and Diabetes
SUNY Health Science Center at Brooklyn
450 Clarkson Ave.
Brooklyn, NY 11203
(718) 270-1333

Paul Davis, M.D.
Chief, Endocrinology
Erie County Medical Center
SUNY Buffalo School of Medicine
Buffalo, NY 14215
(716) 898-3850

Andrew Frantz, M.D.
Chief, Division of Endocrinology
Columbia-Presbyterian Medical Center
630 W. 168th St.
New York, NY 10032
(212) 694-4006

Marvin Gershengorn, M.D.
Chief, Endocrinology
Cornell University Medical College
1300 York Ave.
New York, NY 10021
(212) 472-4896

Terry Davies, M.D.
Chief, Endocrinology
The Mount Sinai Medical Center
1 Gustave L. Levy Place
New York, NY 10029
(212) 650-6627

Charles S. Hollander, M.D.
Chief, Endocrinology
New York University School of Medicine
550 First Ave.
New York, NY 10016
(212) 340-7300

Dean H. Lockwood, M.D.
Chief, Endocrinology
University of Rochester Medical Center
601 Elmwood Ave.
Rochester, NY 14642
(716) 275-2896

David H. P. Streetan, M.D.
Chief, Endocrinology
SUNY Health Science Center at Syracuse
College of Medicine
Syracuse, NY 13210
(315) 473-5726

A. Louis Southren, M.D.
Gary G. Gordon, M.D.
Chairmen, Endocrinology
New York Medical College
Elmwood Hall
Valhalla, NY 10595
(914) 347-5000

NORTH CAROLINA
T. Kenney Gray, M.D.
Chief, Endocrinology
University of North Carolina at Chapel Hill
School of Medicine
Chapel Hill, NC 27514
(919) 966-3336

Francis A. Neelon, M.D.
Chief, Endocrinology
Duke University Medical Center
Box 3005
Durham, NC 27710
(919) 684-2498

Jose F. Caro, M.D.
Chief, Endocrinology
East Carolina University School of Medicine
Greenville, NC 27834
(919) 757-2570

Emery C. Miller, Jr., M.D.
Chief, Endocrinology
Bowman Gray School of Medicine
300 S. Hawthorne Rd.
Winston-Salem, NC 27103
(919) 748-2076

NORTH DAKOTA
William Newman, M.D.
Chief, Endocrinology
University of North Dakota
School of Medicine
UND Medical Education Center
Fargo, ND 58102
(701) 293-4133

OHIO

Lawrence Frohman, M.D.
Chief, Endocrinology
University of Cincinnati Medical Center
231 Bethesda Ave.
Cincinnati, OH 45267-0547
(513) 872-4444

Janice Douglas, M.D.
Acting Director, Endocrinology
University Hospitals of Cleveland
2074 Abington Rd.
Cleveland, OH 44106
(216) 844-3194

Jack M. George, M.D.
Director, Endocrinology and Metabolism
Ohio State University Hospitals
N-1111 Doan Hall
410 W. 10th Ave.
Columbus, OH 43210
(614) 421-8730

Everett Burgess, Jr., M.D.
Chief, Endocrinology
Northeastern Ohio Universities College of
    Medicine
4209 State Route 44
PO Box 95
Rootstown, OH 44272
(216) 325-2511

Roberto Franco-Szenz, M.D.
Chief, Endocrinology
Medical College of Ohio at Toledo
Caller Service No. 10008
Toledo, OH 43699
(419) 381-4172

OKLAHOMA

David C. Kem, M.D.
Chief, Section of Endocrinology, Metabolism,
    Hypertension
Oklahoma Memorial Hospital
PO Box 26307
Oklahoma City, OK 73190
(405) 271-5896

OREGON

Monte A. Greer, M.D.
Chief, Endocrinology
Oregon Health Sciences University School of
    Medicine
3181 S.W. Sam Jackson Park Rd.
Portland, OR 97201
(503) 225-8311

PENNSYLVANIA

Richard J. Santen, M.D.
Chief, Endocrinology
Pennsylvania State University College of
    Medicine
500 University Drive
PO Box 850
Hershey, PA 17033
(717) 531-8521

Leslie Rose, M.D.
Director, Endocrinology
Hahnemann University School of Medicine
Broad and Vine Sts.
Philadelphia, PA 19102
(215) 448-8114

Joseph A. Glennon, M.D.
Chief, Endocrinology
Jefferson Medical College of Thomas Jefferson
    University
11th and Walnut Sts.
Philadelphia, PA 19107
(215) 928-8663

Doris Bartuska, M.D.
Chief, Endocrinology
Medical College of Pennsylvania
3300 Henry Ave.
Philadelphia, PA 19129
(215) 842-6000

Bertram J. Channick, M.D.
Chief, Endocrinology
Temple University School of Medicine
3400 N. Broad St.
Philadelphia, PA 19140
(215) 221-4046

John G. Haddad, Jr., M.D.
Chief, Endocrinology
Albert J. Winegrad, M.D.
Chief, Diabetes
Hospital of the University of Pennsylvania
3400 Spruce St.
Philadelphia, PA 19104
(215) 662-3790

Alan G. Robinson, M.D.
Chief, Endocrinology and Metabolism
University of Pittsburgh School of Medicine
930 Scaife Hall
Pittsburgh, PA 15261
(412) 648-9770

PUERTO RICO

Francisco Aguiló, M.D.
Chief, Endocrinology
University of Puerto Rico School of Medicine
Medical Sciences Campus
GPO Box 5067
San Juan, PR 00936
(809) 754-3633

SOUTH CAROLINA

John A. Colwell, M.D., Ph.D.
Chief, Endocrinology
Medical University of South Carolina
171 Ashley Ave.
Charleston, SC 29425
(803) 792-2528

Howard R. Nankin, M.D.
Chief, Endocrinology
University of South Carolina School of
  Medicine
Columbia, SC 29208
(803) 733-3112

SOUTH DAKOTA

J. M. McMillin, M.D.
Chief, Endocrinology
University of South Dakota School of
  Medicine
2501 W. 22nd St.
Sioux Falls, SD 57105
(605) 339-6790

TENNESSEE

Abbas E. Kitabchi, Ph.D., M.D.
Director, Endocrinology and Metabolism and
  Clinical Research Center
University of Tennessee, Memphis
College of Medicine
951 Court Ave., 335M
Memphis, TN 38163
(901) 528-5802

Elizabeth Schriock, M.D.
Assistant Professor, Section on Pediatric
  Endocrinology and Diabetes
University of Tennessee, Memphis
College of Medicine
956 Court Ave., B318
Memphis, TN 38163
(901) 528-5930

L. W. McNeil, M.D.
Chief, Endocrinology
Meharry Medical College School of Medicine
1005 D. B. Todd Blvd.
Nashville, TN 37207
(615) 327-6518

David N. Orth, M.D.
Director, Endocrinology
Oscar B. Crofford, Jr., M.D.
Director, Diabetes and Metabolism
Vanderbilt University Medical Center
1161 21st Ave., S.
Nashville, TN 37232
(615) 322-4871, 2197

TEXAS

Jean Wilson, M.D.
Chief, Endocrinology
University of Texas Health Science Center at
  Dallas
5323 Harry Hines Blvd.
Dallas, TX 75235
(214) 688-3111

James Field, M.D.
Chief, Endocrinology
Baylor College of Medicine
One Baylor Plaza
Houston, TX 77030
(713) 791-4200

Alton L. Steiner, M.D.
Chief, Endocrinology
University of Texas Health Science Center at
  Houston
PO Box 20708
Houston, TX 77225
(713) 792-5508

Gregory R. Mundy, M.D.
Chief, Endocrinology
University of Texas Health Science Center at
    San Antonio
7703 Floyd Curl Drive
San Antonio, TX 78284
(512) 691-6524

P. F. Gilliland, M.D.
Chief, Endocrinology
Texas A&M University College of Medicine
Scott & White Clinic
Temple, TX 76508
(817) 774-2461

UTAH
Don H. Nelson, M.D.
Chief, Endocrinology and Metabolism
University of Utah School of Medicine
50 N. Medical Drive
Salt Lake City, UT 84132
(801) 581-7761

VERMONT
Edward S. Horton, M.D.
Chief, Endocrinology
University of Vermont College of Medicine
E109 Given Building
Burlington, VT 05405
(802) 656-2530

VIRGINIA
Michael O. Thorner, M.D.
Division Head, Endocrinology
University of Virginia School of Medicine
Box 395, Medical Center
Charlottesville, VA 22908
(804) 924-2656

Hershel Estep, M.D.
Chief, Endocrinology
Eastern Virginia Medical School
700 Olney Rd., P.O. Box 1980
Norfolk, VA 23501
(804) 628-3584

William G. Blackard, M.D.
Chairman, Endocrinology
Medical College of Virginia
MCV Station, Box 155
Richmond, VA 23298
(804) 786-9228

WASHINGTON
Philip J. Fialkow, M.D.
Chief, Medicine
University of Washington School of Medicine,
    RG-20
Seattle, WA 98195
(206) 543-3293

WEST VIRGINIA
Bruce S. Chertow, M.D.
Chief, Endocrinology
Marshall University School of Medicine
Huntington, WV 25701
(304) 526-0561

Stanley R. Shane, M.D.
Chief, Metabolism—Endocrinology
West Virginia University School of Medicine
Morgantown, WV 26506
(304) 293-4121

WISCONSIN
Donald S. Schalch, M.D.
Chief, Endocrinology
University of Wisconsin Medical School
1300 University Ave.
Madison, WI 53706
(608) 263-4900

Ronald K. Kalkhoff, M.D.
Chief, Endocrine/Metabolic Medicine
Medical College of Wisconsin
9200 W. Wisconsin Ave.
Milwaukee, WI 53226
(414) 259-2934

EYE DISEASES AND VISION PROBLEMS (OPHTHALMOLOGISTS)

The physicians listed below are some of the leading specialists in ophthalmology, the treatment of eye diseases and disorders. These physi-cians may be available for consultations and treatment or may be able to refer you to someone else. All are heads of divisions or departments of ophthalmology at medical colleges accredited by the Association of American Medical Colleges.

ALABAMA
Harold W. Skalka, M.D.
Chairman, Ophthalmology
University of Alabama at Birmingham
EFH-1
University Station
Birmingham, AL 35294
(205) 934-2014

Leonard S. Rich, M.D.
Chief, Ophthalmology Surgery
University of South Alabama College of
  Medicine
307 University Blvd.
Mobile, AL 36688
(205) 460-7174

ARIZONA
Barton C. Hodes, M.D.
Chief, Ophthalmology
University of Arizona College of Medicine
Arizona Health Sciences Center
1501 N. Campbell Ave.
Tucson, AZ 85724
(602) 626-0111

ARKANSAS
John P. Schock, M.D.
Chief, Ophthalmology
University of Arkansas College of Medicine
4301 W. Markham St., Slot 523
Little Rock, AR 72205
(501) 661-5150

CALIFORNIA
John L. Keltner, M.D.
Chief, Ophthalmology
University of California, Davis
School of Medicine
Davis, CA 95616
(916) 453-2608

Edward K. Wong, M.D.
Acting Chief, Ophthalmology
University of California, Irvine
California College of Medicine
Irvine, CA 92717
(714) 856-6255

Stuart J. Brown, M.D.
Chief, Ophthalmology
University of California, San Diego
School of Medicine
La Jolla, CA 92093
(619) 452-3713

James J. McNeill, M.D.
Chief, Ophthalmology
Loma Linda University School of Medicine
Loma Linda, CA 92350
(714) 796-4818

Bradley R. Straatsma, M.D.
Chief, Ophthalmology
University of California, Los Angeles
UCLA School of Medicine
Jules Stein Eye Institute
800 Westwood Plaza
Los Angeles, CA 90024
(213) 825-6373

Steven J. Ryan, Jr., M.D.
Chief, Ophthalmology
University of Southern California School of
  Medicine
2025 Zonal Ave.
Los Angeles, CA 90033
(213) 224-7167

Stuart I. Brown, M.D.
Chairman, Department of Ophthalmology
University of California, San Diego
Medical Center
225 Dickinson St.
San Diego, CA 92103
(619) 294-6244

Stephen G. Kramer, M.D.
Chief, Ophthalmology
University of California, San Francisco
School of Medicine
513 Parnassus Ave.
San Francisco, CA 94143
(415) 666-9000

Michael Marmor, M.D.
Clinic and Division Chief
Ophthalmology Clinic
Division of Ophthalmology
Stanford University Medical Center
Stanford, CA 94305
(415) 723-5517

COLORADO
Phillip E. Ellis, M.D.
Chief, Ophthalmology
University of Colorado School of Medicine
4200 E. Ninth Ave.
Denver, CO 80262
(303) 399-1211

CONNECTICUT
Peter Donshik, M.D.
Co-Chief (Clinical), Ophthalmology
Daniel Taylor, M.D.
Co-Chief (Research), Ophthalmology
University of Connecticut Health Center
Farmington, CT 06032
(203) 674-2804

Marvin L. Sears, M.D.
Chairman, Department of Ophthalmology and
  Visual Science
Head, Yale Eye Center
Yale University School of Medicine
333 Cedar St.
New Haven, CT 06510
(203) 785-2731

DISTRICT OF COLUMBIA
Mansour F. Armaly, M.D.
Chairman, Ophthalmology Department
George Washington University
Medical Center
2150 Pennsylvania Ave., N.W.
Washington, DC 20037
(202) 676-4048

Michael A. Lemp, M.D.
Chairman, Ophthalmology
Georgetown University School of Medicine
3900 Reservoir Rd., N.W.
Washington, DC 20007
(202) 625-7121

Claude L. Cowan, M.D.
Chief, Ophthalmology
Howard University College of Medicine
520 W St., N.W.
Washington, DC 20059
(202) 745-1257

FLORIDA
Melvin L. Rubin, M.D.
Chairman, Ophthalmology
University of Florida College of Medicine
Box J-215, J. Hillis Miller Health Center
Gainesville, FL 32610
(904) 392-3451

Edward W. D. Norton, M.D.
Chief, Ophthalmology
University of Miami School of Medicine
PO Box 016099 (R-699)
Miami, FL 33101
(305) 326-6032

William E. Layden, M.D.
Chairman, Ophthalmology Department
University of South Florida College of
  Medicine
12901 N. 30th St., Box 21
Tampa, FL 33612
(813) 974-3170

GEORGIA
Louis Wilson, M.D.
Acting Director, Emory Eye Center
Emory University School of Medicine
Atlanta, GA 30322
(404) 321-0111, x3424

Malcolm N. Luxenberg, M.D.
Chief, Ophthalmology
Medical College of Georgia Hospital
Augusta, GA 30912
(404) 828-2791

ILLINOIS
Lee Jampol, M.D.
Chairman, Ophthalmology
Northwestern University Medical School
303 E. Chicago Ave.
Chicago, IL 60611
(312) 908-8649

William Deutsch, M.D.
Chairman, Ophthalmology
Rush-Presbyterian-St. Luke's Medical Center
1725 W. Harrison St.
Chicago, IL 60612
(312) 942-5370

J. Terry Ernest, M.D.
Chairman, Joint Department of Ophthalmology
University of Chicago Medical Center
Michael Reese Hospital and Medical Center
5841 S. Maryland Ave.
Chicago, IL 60637
(312) 947-1000

Morton F. Goldberg, M.D.
Chief, Ophthalmology
University of Illinois College of Medicine
1853 W. Polk St.
Chicago, IL 60612
(312) 996-3500

James E. McDonald, M.D.
Chief, Ophthalmology
Loyola University of Chicago
Stritch School of Medicine
2160 S. First Ave.
Maywood, IL 60153
(312) 531-3000

Walter I. Fried, M.D.
Chief, Ophthalmology
University of Health Sciences
Chicago Medical School
3333 Green Bay Rd.
North Chicago, IL 60064
(312) 578-3000

Stephen A. Kwedar, M.D.
Chief, Ophthalmology Surgery
Southern Illinois University School of
   Medicine
1027 S. Seventh
Springfield, IL 62704
(217) 528-7541

INDIANA
Merrill Grayson, M.D.
Acting Chairman, Department of
   Ophthalmology
Indiana University Medical Center
702 Rotary Circle
Indianapolis, IN 46223
(317) 264-8129

IOWA
Charles D. Phelps, M.D.
Chief, Ophthalmology
University of Iowa College of Medicine
100 College of Medicine Administration
   Building
Iowa City, IA 52242
(319) 353-4843

KANSAS
Theodore Lawwill, M.D.
Chairman, Ophthalmology
University of Kansas Medical Center
School of Medicine
39th and Rainbow Blvd.
Kansas City, KS 66103
(913) 588-6600

KENTUCKY
Donald R. Bergsma, M.D.
Chief, Ophthalmology
University of Kentucky College of Medicine
800 Rose St.
Lexington, KY 40536
(606) 233-5000

Thom Zimmerman, M.D.
Chairman, Department of Ophthalmology
University of Louisville School of Medicine
Louisville, KY 40292
(502) 588-5477

LOUISIANA
Herbert E. Kaufman, M.D.
Head, Ophthalmology
Louisiana State University School of Medicine
136 S. Roman St.
New Orleans, LA 70112
(504) 568-6700

Delmar Caldwell, M.D.
Chief, Ophthalmology
Tulane University School of Medicine
1430 Tulane Ave.
New Orleans, LA 70112
(504) 588-5312

James Ganley, M.D., Dr.P.H.
Chairman, Ophthalmology
Louisiana State University
School of Medicine in Shreveport
PO Box 33932
Shreveport, LA 71130
(318) 674-5000

MARYLAND
Arnall Patz, M.D.
Chief, Ophthalmology
Johns Hopkins University School of Medicine
720 Rutland Ave.
Baltimore, MD 21205
(301) 955-5000

Richard D. Richards, M.D.
Chief, Ophthalmology
University of Maryland School of Medicine
655 W. Baltimore St.
Baltimore, MD 21201
(301) 528-5918

MASSACHUSETTS
Howard M. Leibowitz, M.D.
Chief, Ophthalmology
Boston University School of Medicine
80 E. Concord St.
Boston, MA 02118
(617) 247-5000

Claes H. Dohlman, M.D.
Chief, Ophthalmology
Harvard Medical School
25 Shattuck St.
Boston, MA 02115
(617) 732-1000

Bernard Schwartz, M.D.
Ophthalmologist-in-Chief
Tufts University School of Medicine
New England Medical Center
171 Harrison Ave.
Boston, MA 02111
(617) 956-5485

John W. Gittinger, Jr., M.D.
Chief, Ophthalmology Surgery
University of Massachusetts Medical School
55 Lake Ave., N.
Worcester, MA 01605
(617) 856-2289

MICHIGAN
Paul R. Lichter, M.D.
Chairman, Department of Ophthalmology
University of Michigan Medical Center
W. K. Kellogg Eye Center
1000 Wall St.
Ann Arbor, MI 48105
(313) 763-5874

Robert S. Jampel, M.D.
Chief, Ophthalmology
Wayne State University School of Medicine
540 E. Canfield Ave.
Detroit, MI 48201
(313) 577-1320

MINNESOTA
Donald J. Doughman, M.D.
Chief, Ophthalmology
University of Minnesota Medical School
Box 293 UMHC
Minneapolis, MN 55455
(612) 625-4400

Robert R. Waller, M.D.
Chief, Ophthalmology
Mayo Medical School
200 First St., S.W.
Rochester, MN 55905
(507) 284-3671

MISSISSIPPI
Samuel B. Johnson, M.D.
Chief, Ophthalmology
University of Mississippi Medical Center
2500 N. State St.
Jackson, MS 39216
(601) 984-5020

MISSOURI
Robert Burns, M.D.
Chief, Ophthalmology
University of Missouri
Columbia School of Medicine
One Hospital Drive
Columbia, MO 65212
(314) 882-1566

Felix N. Sabates, M.D.
Chief, Ophthalmology
University of Missouri
Kansas City School of Medicine
2411 Holmes St.
Kansas City, MO 64108
(816) 556-3501

Lawrence Hirst, M.D.
Chairman, Ophthalmology
St. Louis University School of Medicine
3655 Vista Ave.
St. Louis, MO 63110
(314) 772-9200, x2398

Bernard Becker, M.D.
Head, Ophthalmology
Washington University School of Medicine
660 S. Euclid Ave.
St. Louis, MO 63110
(314) 362-7156

NEBRASKA
Ira A. Priluck, M.D.
Chief, Ophthalmology
Creighton University School of Medicine
California at 24th St.
Omaha, NE 68178
(402) 280-4531

Raymond E. Records, M.D.
Chairman, Ophthalmology
University of Nebraska College of Medicine
42nd St. and Dewey Ave.
Omaha, NE 68105
(402) 559-4276

NEW HAMPSHIRE
Gault M. Farrell, M.D.
Chief, Ophthalmology
Dartmouth Medical School
Hanover, NH 03756
(603) 646-7505

NEW JERSEY
Alphonse Cinotti, M.D.
Chief, Ophthalmology
University of Medicine and Dentistry of New
   Jersey
New Jersey Medical School
100 Bergen St.
Newark, NJ 07103
(201) 456-4300

NEW MEXICO
Robert W. Reidy, M.D.
Chief, Ophthalmology
Department of Surgery
University of New Mexico School of Medicine
Albuquerque, NM 87131
(505) 277-4151

NEW YORK
Richard S. Smith, M.D.
Chief, Ophthalmology
Albany Medical College of Union University
47 New Scotland Ave.
Albany, NY 12208
(518) 445-5582

Paul Henkind, M.D., Ph.D.
Chief, Ophthalmology
Albert Einstein College of Medicine of
   Yeshiva University
1300 Morris Park Ave.
Bronx, NY 10461
(212) 430-2000

Joseph Monte, M.D.
Chief, Ophthalmology
State University of New York at Buffalo
School of Medicine
Buffalo General Hospital
100 High St.
Buffalo, NY 14203
(716) 845-2534

Charles J. Campbell, M.D.
Chief, Ophthalmology
Columbia-Presbyterian Medical Center
630 W. 168th St.
New York, NY 10032
(212) 694-2725

D. Jackson Coleman, M.D.
Chief, Ophthalmology
Cornell University Medical College
1300 York Ave.
New York, NY 10021
(212) 472-5293

Steven M. Podos, M.D.
Chief, Ophthalmology
The Mount Sinai Medical Center
1 Gustave L. Levy Place
New York, NY 10029
(212) 650-7321

Goodwin M. Breinin, M.D.
Chief, Ophthalmology
New York University School of Medicine
550 First Ave.
New York, NY 10016
(212) 340-7300

Henry S. Metz, M.D.
Chief, Ophthalmology
University of Rochester Medical Center
601 Elmwood Ave.
Rochester, NY 14642
(716) 275-3256

John A. Hoepner, M.D.
Chairman, Ophthalmology
State University of New York Health Science
  Center at Syracuse
750 E. Adams St.
Syracuse, NY 13210
(315) 473-7115

Michael W. Dunn, M.D.
Chief, Ophthalmology
New York Medical College
Elmwood Hall
Valhalla, NY 10595
(914) 347-5000

NORTH CAROLINA

David E. Eifring, M.D.
Chief, Ophthalmology
University of North Carolina at Chapel Hill
School of Medicine
Chapel Hill, NC 27514
(919) 966-5296

Robert E. Machemer, M.D.
Chairman, Ophthalmology
Duke University Medical Center
Box 3005
Durham, NC 27710
(919) 684-2498

Steven M. White, M.D.
Chief, Ophthalmology
East Carolina University School of Medicine
Greenville, NC 27834
(919) 758-5800

M. Madison Slusher, M.D.
Chief, Ophthalmology
Bowman Gray School of Medicine
300 S. Hawthorne Rd.
Winston-Salem, NC 27103
(919) 748-4091

NORTH DAKOTA

James R. Olson, M.D.
Chief, Ophthalmology
University of North Dakota School of
  Medicine
Grand Forks, ND 58202
(701) 780-6000

OHIO

Joel G. Sacks, M.D.
Chief, Ophthalmology
University of Cincinnati Medical Center
231 Bethesda Ave.
Cincinnati, OH 45267-0527
(513) 872-5151

William H. Havener, M.D.
Chairman, Ophthalmology
Ohio State University Hospitals
5100 University Hospitals Clinic
456 Clinic Drive
Columbus, OH 43210
(614) 421-8160

John D. Bullock, M.D.
Chair, Ophthalmology
Wright State University School of Medicine
PO Box 927
Dayton, OH 45401
(513) 226-0524

Daniel Mathias, M.D.
Chief, Ophthalmology Surgery
Northeastern Ohio Universities College of
  Medicine
4209 State Route 44
FPO Box 95
Rootstown, OH 44272
(216) 325-2511

Norman C. Johnson, M.D.
Acting Chief, Ophthalmology
Medical College of Ohio at Toledo
Caller Service No. 10008
Toledo, OH 43699
(419) 381-4172

OKLAHOMA

Thomas E. Acers, M.D.
Chief, Ophthalmology
University of Oklahoma Health Sciences
  Center
PO Box 26901
Oklahoma City, OK 73190
(405) 271-4066

OREGON

Frederick T. Fraunfelder, M.D.
Chief, Ophthalmology
Oregon Health Sciences University School of
  Medicine
3181 S.W. Sam Jackson Park Rd.
Portland, OR 97201
(503) 225-8311

PENNSYLVANIA
Joseph W. Sassani, M.D.
Acting Chief, Ophthalmology
The Milton S. Hershey Medical Center
The Pennsylvania State University
Hershey, PA 17033
(717) 531-8521

David B. Soll, M.D.
Chairman, Ophthalmology
Hahnemann University School of Medicine
Broad and Vine Sts.
Philadelphia, PA 19102
(215) 448-7880

William S. Tasman, M.D.
Chief, Ophthalmology
Jefferson Medical College of Thomas Jefferson
   University
1025 Walnut St.
Philadelphia, PA 19107
(215) 928-3149

Herbert J. Nevyas, M.D.
Chief, Ophthalmology
Medical College of Pennsylvania
3300 Henry Ave.
Philadelphia, PA 19129
(215) 842-6000

Guy H. Chan, M.D.
Chief, Ophthalmology
Temple University
School of Medicine
3400 N. Broad St.
Philadelphia, PA 19140
(215) 221-4046

Theodore Krupin, M.D.
Chief, Ophthalmology
Hospital of the University of Pennsylvania
Scheie Eye Institute
51 N. 39th St.
Philadelphia, PA 19104
(215) 662-8100

Charles Nichols, M.D.
Director, Department of Ophthalmology
Hospital of the University of Pennsylvania
3400 Spruce St.
Philadelphia, PA 19104
(215) 662-2762

Richard Thoft, M.D.
Chairman, Ophthalmology
University of Pittsburgh
School of Medicine
Eye and Ear Hospital
230 Lothrop St.
Pittsburgh, PA 15213
(412) 647-2205

PUERTO RICO
Victor Díaz-Bonnet, M.D.
Acting Chief, Ophthalmology
University of Puerto Rico
School of Medicine
Medical Sciences Campus
GPO Box 5067
San Juan, PR 00936
(809) 758-2525, x1927

SOUTH CAROLINA
William W. Vallotton, M.D.
Chairman, Ophthalmology
Medical University of South Carolina
171 Ashley Ave.
Charleston, SC 29425
(803) 792-2492

James G. Ferguson, M.D.
Chief, Ophthalmology
University of South Carolina
School of Medicine
Columbia, SC 29208
(803) 254-4398

SOUTH DAKOTA
Thomas H. Willcockson, M.D.
Chief, Ophthalmology
University of South Dakota School of
   Medicine
2501 W. 22nd St.
Sioux Falls, SD 57105
(605) 665-9638

TENNESSEE
Barbara O. Kimbrough, M.D.
Chief, Ophthalmology
East Tennessee State University
Quillen-Dishner College of Medicine
PO Box 19, 750A
Johnson City, TN 37614
(615) 928-6426

Roger L. Hiatt, M.D.
Chairman, Department of Ophthalmology
University of Tennessee, Memphis
College of Medicine
956 Court Ave., D228
Memphis, TN 38163
(901) 528-5883

J. H. Logan, M.D.
Acting Chairman, Division of Ophthalmology
Meharry Medical College School of Medicine
1005 D. B. Todd Blvd.
Nashville, TN 37207
(615) 327-6111

Axel C. Hansen, M.D.
Chief, Ophthalmology
Meharry Medical College School of Medicine
1005 D. B. Todd Blvd.
Nashville, TN 37207
(615) 327-6636

James H. Elliott, M.D.
Chairman, Ophthalmology
Vanderbilt University Medical Center
1161 21st Ave., S.
Nashville, TN 37232
(615) 322-2031

TEXAS
James P. McCulley, M.D.
Chief, Ophthalmology
University of Texas Southwestern Medical
  School at Dallas
5323 Harry Hines Blvd.
Dallas, TX 75235
(214) 688-3111

John C. Barber, M.D.
Chief, Ophthalmology
University of Texas Medical School at
  Galveston
Galveston, TX 77550
(409) 761-2671

Dan B. Jones, M.D.
Chief, Ophthalmology
Baylor College of Medicine
One Baylor Plaza
Houston, TX 77030
(713) 799-4951

Richard S. Ruiz, M.D.
Chief, Ophthalmology
University of Texas Health Science Center at
  Houston
PO Box 20708
Houston, TX 77225
(713) 792-5920

James Price, M.D., Ph.D.
Chief, Ophthalmology
Texas Tech University Health Sciences Center
  School of Medicine
Fourth St. and Indiana Ave.
Lubbock, TX 79430
(806) 743-2412

Wichard A. J. van Heuven, M.D.
Chief, Ophthalmology
University of Texas Health Science Center at
  San Antonio
7703 Floyd Curl Drive
San Antonio, TX 78284
(512) 567-5100

Richard D. Cunningham, M.D.
Chief, Ophthalmology
Texas A&M University College of Medicine
Scott & White Clinic & Hospital
Temple, TX 76508
(817) 774-2294

UTAH
Randall J. Olson, M.D.
Chief, Ophthalmology
University of Utah School of Medicine
50 N. Medical Drive
Salt Lake City, UT 84132
(801) 581-6384

VERMONT
Phil A. Aitken, M.D.
Chief, Ophthalmology Surgery
University of Vermont College of Medicine
Burlington, VT 05405
(802) 656-4516

VIRGINIA
Brian P. Conway, M.D.
Chief, Ophthalmology
University of Virginia School of Medicine
Box 395, Medical Center
Charlottesville, VA 22908
(804) 924-0211

Earl Crouch, M.D.
Chief, Ophthalmology Surgery
Eastern Virginia Medical School
700 Olney Rd.
Norfolk, VA 23501
(804) 446-5600

Andrew P. Ferry, M.D.
Chairman, Ophthalmology
Medical College of Virginia
MCV Station, Box 262
Richmond, VA 23298
(804) 786-9680

WASHINGTON
Robert E. Kalina, M.D.
Chief, Ophthalmology
University of Washington School of Medicine,
   RJ-10
Seattle, WA 98195
(206) 543-3883

WEST VIRGINIA
Albert C. Esposito, M.D.
Chief, Ophthalmology
Marshall University School of Medicine
Huntington, WV 25701
(304) 526-0530

George W. Weinstein, M.D.
Chief, Ophthalmology
West Virginia University School of Medicine
Morgantown, WV 26506
(304) 293-3757

WISCONSIN
Matthew D. David, M.D.
Chief, Ophthalmology
University of Wisconsin Medical School
1300 University Ave.
Madison, WI 53706
(608) 263-4900

Richard O. Schultz, M.D.
Chief, Ophthalmology
Medical College of Wisconsin
8700 W. Wisconsin Ave.
Milwaukee, WI 53226
(414) 257-5541

HEART AND CARDIOVASCULAR DISEASES (CARDIOLOGISTS)

The physicians listed below are some of the leading specialists in heart and cardiovascular diseases. These physicians may be available for consultations and treatment or may be able to refer you to someone else. All are heads of cardiology departments or divisions at medical colleges accredited by the Association of American Medical Colleges.

ALABAMA
Gerald M. Pohost, M.D.
Director, Cardiovascular Disease
University of Alabama at Birmingham
University Station
Birmingham, AL 35294
(205) 934-3642

Loren F. Parmley, Jr., M.D.
Chief, Cardiology
University of South Alabama
College of Medicine
307 University Blvd.
Mobile, AL 36688
(205) 460-7174

ARIZONA
Gordon A. Ewy, M.D.
Chief, Cardiology
University of Arizona College of Medicine
Arizona Health Sciences Center
1501 N. Campbell Ave.
Tucson, AZ 85724
(602) 626-0111

ARKANSAS
Joseph A. Franciosa, M.D.
Chief, Cardiology
University of Arkansas
College of Medicine
4301 W. Markham St., Slot 532
Little Rock, AR 72205
(501), 661-5880

CALIFORNIA
Zakauddin Vera, M.D.
Chief, Cardiovascular Medicine
University of California, Davis
School of Medicine
Davis, CA 95616
(916) 453-3764

Walter L. Henry, M.D.
Chief, Cardiology
University of California, Irvine
California College of Medicine
Irvine, CA 92717
(714) 634-6752

John Ross, Jr., M.D.
Chief, Cardiology Division
University of California, San Diego
School of Medicine
La Jolla, CA 92093
(619) 452-3347

Roy V. Jutzy, M.D.
Chief, Cardiology
Loma Linda University School of Medicine
Loma Linda, CA 92350
(714) 824-2413, 0800

Alan M. Fogelman, M.D.
Professor of Medicine and Chief, Cardiology
University of California, Los Angeles
UCLA School of Medicine
Los Angeles, CA 90024
(213) 825-5280

Shahbudin Rahimtoola, M.D.
Chief, Cardiology
University of Southern California
School of Medicine
2025 Zonal Ave.
Los Angeles, CA 90033
(213) 226-7264

Lloyd H. Smith, Jr., M.D.
Chief, Department of Medicine
University of California, San Francisco
School of Medicine
513 Parnassus Ave.
San Francisco, CA 94143
(415) 666-9000

Donald C. Harrison, M.D.
Division Chief
William Hancock, M.D.
Clinic Chief
Cardiology Clinic
Division of Cardiology
Stanford University Medical Center
Stanford, CA 94305
(415) 723-7491

COLORADO
Lawrence Horwitz, M.D.
Chief, Cardiology
University of Colorado School of Medicine
4200 E. Ninth Ave.
Denver, CO 80262
(303) 399-1211

CONNECTICUT
Arnold M. Katz, M.D.
Chief, Cardiology
University of Connecticut Health Center
Farmington, CT 06032
(203) 674-2770

Barry L. Zaret, M.D.
Head, Section of Cardiology
Yale University School of Medicine
333 Cedar St.
New Haven, CT 06510
(203) 785-4144

DISTRICT OF COLUMBIA
Allan M. Ross, M.D.
Director, Cardiology Division
George Washington University
Medical Center
2150 Pennsylvania Ave., N.W.
Washington, DC 20037
(202) 676-3777

Charles Rackley, M.D.
Chairman, Medicine
Georgetown University School of Medicine
3900 Reservoir Rd., N.W.
Washington, DC 20007
(202) 625-7225

Charles L. Curry, M.D.
Chief, Cardiology
Howard University College of Medicine
520 W St., N.W.
Washington, DC 20059
(202) 745-6100

FLORIDA
C. Richard Conti, M.D.
Chief, Cardiology
University of Florida College of Medicine
Box J-215, J. Hillis Miller Health Center
Gainesville, FL 32610
(904) 392-3481

Robert J. Myerburg, M.D.
Chief, Cardiology
University of Miami School of Medicine
PO Box 016099 (R-699)
Miami, FL 33101
(305) 547-6881

Stephen P. Glasser, M.D.
Director, Division of Cardiology
University of South Florida College of
    Medicine
12901 N. 30th St., Box 19
Tampa, FL 33612
(813) 974-2880

GEORGIA
Robert C. Schlant, M.D.
Chief, Cardiology
Emory University School of Medicine
Woodruff Medical Center Administration
    Building
Atlanta, GA 30322
(404) 588-4440

Leo G. Horan, M.D.
Acting Chief, Cardiology
Medical College of Georgia Hospital
Augusta, GA 30912
(404) 828-2426

ILLINOIS
Michael Lesch, M.D.
Chief, Cardiology
Northwestern University Medical School
303 E. Chicago Ave.
Chicago, IL 60611
(312) 908-8649

Joseph W. Messer, M.D.
Director, Section of Cardiology
Rush-Presbyterian-St. Luke's Medical Center
1753 W. Congress Parkway
Chicago IL 60612
(312) 942-6014

Morton Arnsdorf, M.D.
Chief, Section of Cardiology
University of Chicago Medical Center
5841 S. Maryland Ave.
Chicago, IL 60637
(312) 947-1000

Raymond J. Pietras, M.D.
Chief, Cardiology
University of Illinois
College of Medicine
1853 W. Polk St.
Chicago, IL 60612
(312) 996-3500

Patrick J. Scanlon, M.D.
Chief, Cardiology
Loyola University of Chicago
Stritch School of Medicine
2160 S. First Ave.
Maywood, IL 60153
(312) 531-3000

Max H. Weil, M.D., Ph.D.
Chief, Cardiology
University of Health Sciences
Chicago Medical School
3333 Green Bay Rd.
North Chicago, IL 60064
(312) 578-3000

Stuart Frank, M.D.
Chief, Cardiology
Southern Illinois University
School of Medicine
800 N. Rutledge
PO Box 3926
Springfield, IL 62708
(217) 782-0185

INDIANA

Charles Fisch, M.D.
Chief, Cardiology Section
Department of Medicine
Indiana University Medical Center
Krannert Institute of Cardiology
960 Locke St.
Indianapolis, IN 46223
(317) 630-6238

Donald Girod, M.D.
Chief, Cardiology Section
Department of Pediatrics
Indiana University Medical Center
Riley Research 126
702 Barnhill Drive
Indianapolis, IN 46223
(317) 264-8906

IOWA

Allyn L. Mark, M.D.
Chief, Cardiovascular Diseases
University of Iowa College of Medicine
100 College of Medicine Administration
  Building
Iowa City, IA 52242
(319) 353-4843

KANSAS

Marvin I. Dunn, M.D.
Director, Division of Cardiovascular Disease
University of Kansas Medical Center
39th & Rainbow Blvd.
Kansas City, KS 66103
(913) 588-6015

KENTUCKY

Anthony DeMaria, M.D.
Chief, Cardiology
University of Kentucky College of Medicine
800 Rose St.
Lexington, KY 40536
(606) 233-5000

Gurbachan S. Sohi, M.D.
Chief, Cardiology
Department of Medicine
University of Louisville School of Medicine
Louisville, KY 40292
(502) 588-7959

LOUISIANA

Gerald S. Berenson, M.D.
Chief, Cardiology
Louisiana State University School of Medicine
1542 Tulane Ave.
New Orleans, LA 70112
(504) 568-4605

John H. Phillips, Jr., M.D.
Chief, Cardiology
Tulane University School of Medicine
1430 Tulane Ave.
New Orleans, LA 70112
(504) 588-5152

Henry G. Hanley, M.D.
Chief, Cardiology
Louisiana State University
School of Medicine in Shreveport
PO Box 33932
Shreveport, LA 71130
(318) 674-5000

MARYLAND

Myron L. Weisfeldt, M.D.
Chief, Cardiology
Johns Hopkins University
School of Medicine
720 Rutland Ave.
Baltimore, MD 21205
(301) 955-5000

Leonard Scherlis, M.D.
Chief, Cardiology
University of Maryland
School of Medicine
655 W. Baltimore St.
Baltimore, MD 21201
(301) 528-6522

MASSACHUSETTS

William Grossman, M.D.
Chief, Cardiology
Beth Israel Hospital
Harvard Medical School
330 Brookline Ave.
Boston, MA 02215
(617) 735-2191

Thomas Smith, M.D.
Chief, Cardiology
Brigham & Women's Hospital
Harvard Medical School
75 Francis St.
Boston, MA 02115
(617) 732-5500

Edgar Haber, M.D.
Chief, Cardiology
Massachusetts General Hospital
Harvard Medical School
32 Fruit St.
Boston, MA 02114
(617) 726-2887

Herbert Levine, M.D.
Division Chief, Cardiology
Tufts University School of Medicine
New England Medical Center
171 Harrison Ave.
Boston, MA 02111
(617) 956-5911

Joseph S. Alpert, M.D.
Chief, Cardiovascular Medicine
University of Massachusetts Medical School
55 Lake Ave., N.
Worcester, MA 01605
(617) 856-3191

MICHIGAN
Bertram Pitt, M.D.
Chief, Cardiology
University of Michigan Medical Center
3910 A. Alfred Taubman Health Care Center
Ann Arbor, MI 48109
(313) 936-5255

Joshua Wynne, M.D.
Chief, Cardiology
Wayne State University
School of Medicine
Harper Hospital
3990 John R
Detroit, MI 48201
(313) 745-2636

MINNESOTA
Jay Cohn, M.D.
Head, Cardiovascular Medicine
Department of Medicine
University of Minnesota Medical School
Box 488 UMHC
Minneapolis, MN 55455
(612) 625-9100

Robert L. Frye, M.D.
Chief, Cardiovascular Diseases
Mayo Medical School
200 First St., S.W.
Rochester, MN 55905
(507) 284-3671

MISSISSIPPI
Thomas M. Blake, M.D.
Chief, Cardiology
University of Mississippi Medical Center
2500 N. State St.
Jackson, MS 39216
(601) 984-2250

MISSOURI
Richard Martin, M.D.
Chief, Cardiology
University of Missouri
Columbia School of Medicine
One Hospital Drive
Columbia, MO 65212
(314) 882-1566

Harry R. Gibbs, M.D.
Chief, Cardiology
University of Missouri
Kansas City School of Medicine
2411 Holmes St.
Kansas City, MO 64108
(816) 276-1970

Harold L. Kennedy, M.D.
Chief, Cardiology
St. Louis University School of Medicine
1325 S. Grand Blvd.
St. Louis, MO 63104
(314) 577-8890

Burton E. Sobel, M.D.
Chief, Cardiology
Washington University School of Medicine
660 S. Euclid Ave.
St. Louis, MO 63110
(314) 362-8900

NEBRASKA
Michael H. Sketch, M.D.
Chief, Cardiology
Creighton University School of Medicine
California at 24th St.
Omaha, NE 68178
(402) 280-4566

Toby R. Engel, M.D.
Chief, Cardiology
University of Nebraska College of Medicine
42nd St. and Dewey Ave.
Omaha, NE 68105
(402) 559-5151

NEW HAMPSHIRE
Ellis L. Rolett, M.D.
Chief, Cardiology
Dartmouth Medical School
Hanover, NH 03756
(603) 646-7505

NEW JERSEY
John B. Kostis, M.D.
Chief, Cardiology
University of Medicine and Dentistry of New
  Jersey
Robert Wood Johnson Medical School
(formerly Rutgers)
UMDNJ Medical Education Building
Academic Health Science Building CN19
New Brunswick, NJ 08903
(201) 937-7855

Timothy J. Regan, M.D.
Chief, Cardiology
University of Medicine and Dentistry of New
  Jersey
New Jersey Medical School
100 Bergen St.
Newark, NJ 07103
(201) 456-4300

NEW MEXICO
Jonathan Abrams, M.D.
Chief, Cardiology
Department of Medicine
University of New Mexico School of Medicine
Albuquerque, NM 87131
(505) 277-4253

NEW YORK
Joseph T. Doyle, M.D.
Chief, Cardiology
Albany Medical College of Union University
47 New Scotland Ave.
Albany, NY 12208
(518) 445-5582

Edmund Sonneblick, M.D.
Division Head, Cardiology
Albert Einstein College of Medicine
1300 Morris Park Ave.
Bronx, NY 10461
(212) 430-2461

Richard Stein, M.D.
Director and Chief, Cardiology
SUNY Health Science Center at Brooklyn
450 Clarkson Ave.
Brooklyn, NY 11203
(718) 270-2606

Francis Klocke, M.D.
Chief, Cardiology
Erie County Medical Center
SUNY at Buffalo School of Medicine
Buffalo, NY 14215
(716) 896-1568

Djavad Arani, M.D.
Chief, Angiology
Buffalo General Hospital
Buffalo, NY 14203
(716) 845-6465
Affiliated with SUNY at Buffalo School of
  Medicine

David Dean, M.D.
Chief, Cardiology
Veterans Administration Hospital
Buffalo, NY 14215
(716) 834-9200
Affiliated with SUNY at Buffalo School of
  Medicine

Jay Thomas Bigger, Jr., M.D.
Chief, Cardiology
Columbia-Presbyterian Medical Center
630 W. 168th St.
New York, NY 10032
(212) 694-4093

John H. Laragh, M.D.
Chief, Cardiology
Cornell University Medical College
1300 York Ave.
New York, NY 10021
(212) 472-5464

Valentin Fuster, M.D.
Chief, Cardiology
The Mount Sinai Medical Center
1 Gustave L. Levy Place
New York, NY 10029
(212) 650-7911

Arthur C. Fox, M.D.
Chief, Cardiology
New York University School of Medicine
550 First Ave.
New York, NY 10016
(212) 340-7300

William B. Hood, Jr., M.D.
Chief, Cardiology
University of Rochester Medical Center
601 Elmwood Ave.
Rochester, NY 14642
(716) 275-7736

Peter Cohn, M.D.
Division Head, Cardiology
SUNY at Stony Brook
Health Sciences Center
Stony Brook, NY 11794
(516) 444-1060

Harold Smulyan, M.D.
Chief, Section of Cardiology
Veterans Administration Hospital
SUNY Health Science Center at Syracuse
766 Irving Ave.
Syracuse, NY 13210
(315) 476-7461

Michael V. Herman, M.D.
Chief, Cardiology
New York Medical College
Elmwood Hall
Valhalla, NY 10595
(914) 347-5000

NORTH CAROLINA
Leonard S. Gettes, M.D.
Chief, Cardiology
University of North Carolina at Chapel Hill
School of Medicine
Chapel Hill, NC 27514
(919) 966-5203

Joseph C. Greenfield, Jr., M.D.
Chief, Cardiology
Duke University Medical Center
Box 3005
Durham, NC 27710
(919) 684-2498

Allen F. Bowyer, M.D.
Chief, Cardiology
East Carolina University School of Medicine
Greenville, NC 27834
(919) 757-4651

Henry S. Miller, Jr., M.D.
Chief, Cardiology
Bowman Gray School of Medicine
300 S. Hawthorne Rd.
Winston-Salem, NC 27103
(919) 748-4208

NORTH DAKOTA
Gopal Das, M.D.
Chief, Cardiology
University of North Dakota
School of Medicine
UND Medical Education Center
Fargo, ND 58102
(701) 293-4133

OHIO
Noble O. Fowler, M.D.
Chief, Cardiology
University of Cincinnati Medical Center
231 Bethesda Ave.
Cincinnati, OH 45267-0542
(513) 872-4721

Robert E. Botti, M.D.
Director, Division of Cardiology
Case Western Reserve University School of
    Medicine
University Hospitals of Cleveland
2074 Abington Rd.
Cleveland, OH 44106
(216) 844-3153

Richard P. Lewis, M.D.
Director, Cardiology
The Ohio State University Hospitals
669 Means Hall
1654 Upham Drive
Columbus, OH 43210
(614) 421-4967

George I. Litman, M.D.
Chief, Cardiology
Northeastern Ohio University College of
  Medicine
4209 State Route 44
PO Box 95
Rootstown, OH 44272
(216) 325-2511

Richard F. Leighton, M.D.
Chief, Cardiology
Medical College of Ohio at Toledo
Caller Service No. 10008
Toledo, OH 43699
(419) 381-4172

OKLAHOMA
Ralph Lazzara, M.D.
Chief, Cardiovascular Section
University of Oklahoma Health Sciences
  Center
PO Box 26901
Oklahoma City, OK 73190
(405) 271-4742

OREGON
Frank E. Kloster, M.D.
Chief, Cardiology
Oregon Health Sciences University School of
  Medicine
3181 S.W. Sam Jackson Park Rd.
Portland, OR 97201
(503) 225-8311

PENNSYLVANIA
David M. Leaman, M.D.
Chief, Cardiology
The Milton S. Hershey Medical Center
The Pennsylvania State University
Hershey, PA 17033
(717) 531-8521

Bernard Segal, M.D.
Director, Likoff Cardiovascular Institute
Hahnemann University School of Medicine
Broad and Vine Sts.
Philadelphia, PA 19102
(215) 448-8063

Albert N. Brest, M.D.
Chief, Cardiology
Jefferson Medical College of Thomas Jefferson
  University
11th and Walnut Sts.
Philadelphia, PA 19107
(215) 928-6051

Steven Meister, M.D.
Chief, Cardiology
Medical College of Pennsylvania
3300 Henry Ave.
Philadelphia, PA 19129
(215) 842-6000

James Spann, M.D.
Chief, Cardiology
Temple University School of Medicine
3400 N. Broad St.
Philadelphia, PA 19140
(215) 221-4046

Mark E. Josephson, M.D.
Chief, Cardiovascular
Hospital of the University of Pennsylvania
3400 Spruce St.
Philadelphia, PA 19104
(215) 662-2185

James A. Shaver, M.D.
Director, Division of Cardiology
University of Pittsburgh School of Medicine
Presbyterian-University Hospital
Pittsburgh, PA 15261
(412) 647-3429

PUERTO RICO
Mario R. García-Palmieri, M.D.
Chief, Cardiology
University of Puetro Rico School of Medicine
Medical Sciences Campus
GPO Box 5067
San Juan, PR 00936
(809) 758-2525, x1821

SOUTH CAROLINA
James F. Spann, Jr., M.D.
Director, Cardiology and Gazes Cardiac
  Research Institute
Medical University of South Carolina
171 Ashley Ave.
Charleston, SC 29425
(803) 792-3355

Donald E. Saunders, Jr., M.D.
Chief, Cardiology
University of South Carolina
School of Medicine
Columbia, SC 29208
(803) 765-7438

SOUTH DAKOTA
Robert Talley, M.D.
Professor and Chief, Cardiology
University of South Dakota School of
    Medicine
2501 W. 22nd St.
Sioux Falls, SD 57105
(605) 339-6790

TENNESSEE
John Douglas, M.D.
Chief, Cardiology
East Tennessee State University
Quillen-Dishner College of Medicine
PO Box 21, 160A
Johnson City, TN 37614
(615) 928-6426

Jay M. Sullivan, M.D.
Chief, Division of Cardiovascular Diseases
University of Tennessee, Memphis
College of Medicine
951 Court Ave., 353D
Memphis, TN 38163
(901) 528-5750

Bruce Alpert, M.D.
Chief, Pediatric Cardiology Section
University of Tennessee, Memphis
College of Medicine
848 Adams Ave., 4th Floor
Le Bonheur Children's Medical Center
Memphis, TN 38103
(901) 522-3380

J. E. Hinds, M.D.
Head, Division of Cardiology
Meharry Medical College School of Medicine
1005 D. B. Todd Blvd.
Nashville, TN 37207
(615) 327-6111

John Thomas, M.D.
Chief, Cardiology
Meharry Medical College School of Medicine
1005 D. B. Todd, Jr. Blvd.
Nashville, TN 37208
(615) 327-6277

Gottlieb C. Friesinger, III, M.D.
Director, Cardiology
Vanderbilt University Medical Center
1161 21st Ave., S.
Nashville, TN 37232
(615) 322-2318

TEXAS
Michael E. DeBakey, M.D.
Chief, Surgery
Robert Roberts, M.D.
Chief, Cardiology
Baylor College of Medicine
One Baylor Plaza
Houston, TX 77030
(713) 799-4951, 3064

Gerald V. Naccarelli, M.D.
Acting Division Director, Cardiology
University of Texas Health Science Center at
    Houston
PO Box 20708
Houston, TX 77225
(713) 792-5178

M. Wayne Cooper, M.D.
Chief, Cardiology
Texas Tech University
Health Sciences Center School of Medicine
Fourth St. and Indiana Ave.
Lubbock, TX 79430
(806) 743-3156

Robert A. O'Rourke, M.D.
Chief, Cardiology
University of Texas Health Science Center at
    San Antonio
7703 Floyd Curl Drive
San Antonio, TX 78284
(512) 691-6011

L. E. Watson, M.D.
Chief, Cardiology
Texas A&M University College of Medicine
Scott & White Clinic
Temple, TX 76508
(817) 774-2491

UTAH
Jay W. Mason, M.D.
Chief, Cardiology
University of Utah School of Medicine
50 N. Medical Drive
Salt Lake City, UT 84132
(801) 581-7715

VERMONT
Martin M. Le Winter, M.D.
Chief, Cardiology
University of Vermont College of Medicine
Medical Center Hospital of Vermont
Burlington, VT 05405
(802) 656-3734

VIRGINIA
George Beller, M.D.
Division Head, Cardiology
University of Virginia School of Medicine
Box 395, Medical Center
Charlottesville, VA 22908
(804) 924-2134

Douglas Moore, M.D.
Chief, Cardiology
E. Virginia Medical School
700 Olney Rd.
PO Box 1980
Norfolk, VA 23501
(804) 628-3584

David W. Richardson, M.D.
Chairman, Cardiology
Medical College of Virginia
MCV Station, Box 15
Richmond, VA 23298
(804) 786-9704

WASHINGTON
P.J. Fialow, M.D.
Chief, Department of Medicine
University of Washington School of Medicine
Seattle, WA 98195
(206) 543-3293

WEST VIRGINIA
Robert C. Touchon, M.D.
Chief, Cardiology
Marshall University School of Medicine
Huntington, WV 25701
(304) 429-4775

Abnash C. Jain, M.D.
Chief, Cardiology
West Virginia University School of Medicine
Morgantown, WV 26506
(304) 293-4121

WISCONSIN
A. James Liedtke, M.D.
Chief, Cardiology
University of Wisconsin Medical School
1300 University Ave.
Madison, WI 53706
(608) 263-4900

Harold L. Brooks, M.D.
Chief, Cardiology
Medical College of Wisconsin
8700 W. Wisconsin Ave.
Milwaukee, WI 53226
(414) 257-6070

NEUROLOGY: DISEASES AND DISORDERS OF THE NERVOUS SYSTEM (NEUROLOGISTS)

The physicians listed below are some of the leading specialists in neurology, the treatment of disorders of the nervous system. They may be available for consultations and treatment or may be able to refer you to someone else. All are heads of departments of neurology at medical colleges accredited by the Association of American Medical Colleges.

ALABAMA
John N. Whitaker, M.D.
Chairman, Neurology
University of Alabama at Birmingham
OHB 358
University Station
Birmingham, AL 35294
(205) 934-2402

Paul R. Dyken, M.D.
Chairman, Neurology
University of South Alabama College of
  Medicine
2451 Fillingim St.
Mobile, AL 36617
(205) 471-7841

ARIZONA
Colin Bamford, M.D.
Acting Chief, Department of Neurology
University of Arizona College of Medicine
University of Arizona Health Sciences Center
Tucson, AZ 85724
(602) 626-0111

ARKANSAS
Dennis D. Lucy, Jr., M.D.
Chief, Neurology
University of Arkansas for Medical Sciences
4301 W. Markham, Slot 500
Little Rock, AR 72205
(501) 661-5135

CALIFORNIA
Arnold Starr, M.D.
Chief, Neurology
University of California, Irvine
California College of Medicine
Irvine, CA 92717
(714) 856-6088

Donald Miller, M.D.
Chief, Neurology
Loma Linda University Medical Center
Department of Neurology
Loma Linda, CA 92350
(714) 824-4907

Leslie P. Weiner, M.D.
Chief, Neurology
University of Southern California School of
  Medicine
1200 N. State St.
Los Angeles, CA 90033
(213) 226-7381

Robert Baloh, M.D.
Acting Chair, Neurology
University of California, Los Angeles
School of Medicine
Reed Neurological Research Center
710 Westwood Plaza
Los Angeles, CA 90024
(213) 825-6373

Andrew Gabor, M.D.
Chief, Neurology
University of California, Davis Medical Center
4301 X St., Professional Building, Room 210
Sacramento, CA 95817
(916) 453-3520

Robert Katzman, M.D.
Chairman, Department of Neurosciences
University of California, San Diego
Medical Center
225 Dickinson St.
San Diego, CA 92103
(619) 294-6720

Robert A. Fishman, M.D.
Chief, Neurology
University of California, San Francisco
School of Medicine
Room 794-M, 505 Parnassus Ave.
San Francisco, CA 94143
(415) 666-9000

David A. Prince, M.D.
Department Chairman
Bruce Ransom, M.D.
Chief, Neurology Clinic
Department of Neurology
Stanford University Medical Center
Stanford, CA 94305
(415) 723-6469

COLORADO
James H. Austin, M.D.
Chief, Neurology
University of Colorado Medical Center
4200 E. Ninth Ave.
Denver, CO 80262
(303) 399-1211

CONNECTICUT
James O. Donaldson, M.D.
Acting Head, Neurology
University of Connecticut Health Center
Farmington, CT 06032
(203) 674-3186

Gilbert H. Glaser, M.D.
Chairman, Department of Neurology
Yale University School of Medicine
333 Cedar St.
New Haven, CT 06510
(203) 436-4771

DISTRICT OF COLUMBIA
Gaetano Molinari, M.D.
Chairman, Neurology Department
George Washington University
Medical Center
2150 Pennsylvania Ave., N.W.
Washington, DC 20037
(202) 676-4061

Desmond S. O'Doherty, M.D.
Director, Neurology
Georgetown University School of Medicine
3800 Reservoir Rd., N.W.
Washington, DC 20007
(202) 625-7125

Don H. Wood, M.D.
Chief, Neurology
Howard University Hospital
2041 Georgia Ave., N.W.
Washington, DC 20060
(202) 636-6270

FLORIDA
Melvin Greer, M.D.
Chairman, Neurology
University of Florida College of Medicine
Department of Neurology, Box J236
Gainesville, FL 32610
(904) 392-3491

Peritz Scheinberg, M.D.
Chief, Neurology
University of Miami
Department of Neurology D4-5
PO Box 016960
Miami, FL 33101
(305) 547-6731

Leon D. Prockop, M.D.
Chairman, Department of Neurology
University of South Florida College of
    Medicine
12901 N. 30th St., Box 55
Tampa, FL 33612
(813) 974-2794

GEORGIA
Robert F. Kibler, M.D.
Chief, Neurology
Emory University
Department of Neurology
69 Butler St., S.E.
Atlanta, GA 30303
(404) 329-6123

Thomas R. Swift, M.D.
Chief, Neurology
Medical College of Georgia Hospital
Augusta, GA 30912
(404) 828-4583

ILLINOIS
Donald H. Harter, M.D.
Chairman, Neurology
Northwestern University Medical School
Northwestern Memorial Hospital
Superior St. & Fairbanks Court
Chicago, IL 60611
(312) 908-8649

Harold W. Klawans, M.D.
Acting Chairman, Neurological Sciences
Rush-Presbyterian-St. Luke's Medical Center
1725 W. Harrison St.
Chicago, IL 60612
(312) 942-8010

Barry G.W. Arnason, M.D.
Chairman, Department of Neurology
Director, Brain Research Institute
University of Chicago Medical Center
5841 S. Maryland Ave.
Chicago, IL 60637
(312) 947-1000

John S. Garvin, M.D.
Chief, Neurology
University of Illinois
College of Medicine
University of Illinois Hospital
912 S. Wood St.
Chicago, IL 60612
(312) 996-3500

Gastone G. Celesia, M.D.
Chief, Neurology
Loyola University
Stritch School of Medicine
2160 S. First Ave.
Maywood, IL 60153
(312) 531-3000

Charles E. Morris, M.D.
Chairman, Department of Neurology
Chicago Medical School
VA Center, Building 50
North Chicago, IL 60064
(312) 578-3000

Krishna Kalyan-Raman, M.D.
Chief, Neurology
University of Illinois
College of Medicine at Peoria
One Illini Drive
Peoria, IL 61656
(309) 671-3000

James B. Couch, M.D., Ph.D.
Chief, Neurology
Southern Illinois University School of
  Medicine
800 N. Rutledge
Springfield, IL 62708
(217) 782-3318

INDIANA
Mark L. Dyken, M.D.
Chairman, Neurology
Indiana University Medical Center
Emerson Hall 125
545 Barnhill Drive
Indianapolis, IN 46223
(317) 264-4455

David Dunn, M.D.
Chief, Pediatric Neurology Section
Department of Neurology
Indiana University Medical Center
Riley Hospital for Children, N102
702 Barnhill Drive
Indianapolis, IN 46223
(317) 264-8747

IOWA
Maurice W. Van Allen, M.D.
Chief, Neurology
University of Iowa College of Medicine
2151 Carver Pavilion
Iowa City, IA 52242
(319) 353-4843

KANSAS
Arthur R. Dick, M.D.
Acting Chief, Neurology
University of Kansas Medical Center
39th & Rainbow Blvd.
Kansas City, KS 66103
(913) 588-6975

KENTUCKY
Norman H. Bass, M.D.
Chief, Neurology
University of Kentucky Medical Center
800 Rose St.
Lexington, KY 40506
(606) 233-5000

William H. Olson, M.D.
Chairman, Department of Neurology
University of Louisville School of Medicine
Louisville, KY 40292
(502) 588-7981

LOUISIANA
Earl R. Hackett, M.D.
Head, Neurology
Louisiana State University School of Medicine
Department of Neurology
1542 Tulane Ave.
New Orleans, LA 70112
(504) 568-4080

Joseph B. Green, M.D.
Chairman, Psychiatry and Neurology
Tulane University School of Medicine
1415 Tulane Ave.
New Orleans, LA 70112
(504) 588-5246

Larry J. Embree, M.D.
Chairman, Neurology
Louisiana State University School of Medicine
  in Shreveport
PO Box 33932
Shreveport, LA 71130
(318) 674-5000

MARYLAND
Guy M. McKhann, M.D.
Chief, Neurology
Johns Hopkins Hospital
600 N. Wolfe St.
Baltimore, MD 21205
(301) 955-3282

Kenneth P. Johnson, M.D.
Chief, Neurology
University of Maryland Hospital
Redwood & Green Sts.
Baltimore, MD 21201
(301) 528-6438

MASSACHUSETTS

Robert G. Feldman, M.D.
Chief, Neurology
Boston University School of Medicine
80 E. Concord St.
Boston, MA 02118
(617) 247-5000

Alfred Pope, M.D.
Chief, Executive Committee, Neurology-
  Neuropathology
Harvard Medical School
25 Shattuck St.
Boston, MA 02115
(617) 732-1000

Joseph B. Martin, M.D.
Harvard Department of Neurology
Chief, Neurology, Massachusetts General
  Hospital
Neurology Service
Boston, MA 02114
(617) 726-2000

Charles F. Barlow, M.D.
Chief, Neurology
Harvard Medical School
Children's Hospital Medical Center
300 Longwood Ave.
Boston, MA 02115
(617) 735-6000

Louis R. Caplan, M.D.
Neurologist-in-Chief
Tufts University School of Medicine
New England Medical Center
171 Harrison Ave.
Boston, MA 02111
(617) 956-5450

David A. Drachman, M.D.
Chief, Neurology
University of Massachusetts Medical School
55 Lake Ave., N.
Worcester, MA 01605
(617) 856-3081

MICHIGAN

Sid Gilman, M.D.
Chairman, Department of Neurology
University of Michigan Medical Center
1914 A. Alfred Taubman Health Care Center
Ann Arbor, MI 48109
(313) 936-9070

John C. McHenry, M.D.
Acting Chairman, Neurology
Wayne State University School of Medicine
University Health Center
Department of Neurology
4201 St. Antoine
Detroit, MI 48201
(313) 577-1242

Raymond Murray, M.D.
Chief, Medicine
Michigan State University
College of Human Medicine
East Lansing, MI 48824
(517) 353-6625

MINNESOTA

Arthur C. Klassen, M.D.
Chief, Neurology
University of Minnesota Medical School
Box 295 UMHC
Minneapolis, MN 55455
(612) 625-9900

Burton A. Sandok, M.D.
Chief, Neurology
Mayo Graduate School of Medicine
200 First St., S.W.
Rochester, MN 55905
(507) 284-3671

MISSISSIPPI

Robert D. Currier, M.D.
Chairman, Neurology
University of Mississippi Medical Center
2500 N. State St.
Jackson, MS 39216
(601) 984-5500

MISSOURI

James D. Dexter, M.D.
Chief, Neurology
University of Missouri
Columbia School of Medicine
University of Missouri Hospital and Clinics
Columbia, MO 65212
(314) 882-3133

Violet Matovich, M.D.
Chief, Neurology
University of Missouri–Kansas City School of
  Medicine
Truman Medical Center
2301 Holmes
Kansas City, MO 64108
(816) 556-3534

John B. Selhorst, M.D.
Chairman, Neurology
St. Louis University School of Medicine
3660 Vista Ave.
St. Louis, MO 63110
(314) 577-6082

William M. Landau, M.D.
Head, Neurology
Washington University School of Medicine
660 S. Euclid
St. Louis, MO 63110
(314) 362-7177

NEBRASKA
Donald R. Bennett, M.D.
Chief, Neurology
Creighton University School of Medicine
California at 24th St.
Omaha, NE 68178
(402) 280-4686

Donald R. Bennett, M.D.
Chairman, Neurology
University of Nebraska College of Medicine
42nd & Dewey Ave.
Omaha, NE 68105
(402) 559-4496

NEW HAMPSHIRE
Alexander G. Reeves, M.D.
Chief, Neurology
Dartmouth-Hitchcock Medical Center
Hanover, NH 03755
(603) 646-7505

NEW JERSEY
Robert C. Duvoisin, M.D.
Chairman, Neurology
UMDNJ–Robert Wood Johnson Medical
  School (formerly Rutgers)
UMDNJ Medical Education Building
Academic Health Science Building CN19
New Brunswick, NJ 08903
(201) 937-7732

Stuart D. Cook, M.D.
Chief, Neurology
University of Medicine and Dentistry
New Jersey Medical School
100 Bergen St.
Newark, NJ 07103
(201) 456-4300

NEW MEXICO
Gary Rosenburg, M.D.
Chairman, Neurology
University of New Mexico School of Medicine
2211 Lomas Blvd.
Albuquerque, NM 87131
(505) 277-3342

NEW YORK
Kevin D. Barron, M.D.
Chief, Neurology
Albany Medical Center
47 New Scotland Ave.
Albany, NY 12208
(518) 445-5582

Herbert Schaumberg, M.D.
Acting Chief, Neurology
Albert Einstein College of Medicine
1300 Morris Park Ave.
Bronx, NY 10461
(212) 430-2833

Roger Q. Cracco, M.D.
Chairman and Chief, Neurology
SUNY Health Science Center at Brooklyn
450 Clarkson Ave.
PO Box 1213
Brooklyn, NY 11203
(718) 270-2051

Michael Cohen, M.D.
Chairman, Neurology
State University of New York at Buffalo
School of Medicine
Children's Hospital
219 Bryant St.
Buffalo, NY 14222
(716) 878-7325

Lewis P. Rowland, M.D.
Chief, Neurology
Columbia-Presbyterian Medical Center
710 W. 168th St.
New York, NY 10032
(212) 694-5852

Fred Plum, M.D.
Chief, Neurology
Cornell University Medical Center
New York Hospital
525 E. 68th St.
New York, NY 10021
(212) 472-5744

Clark T. Randt, M.D.
Chief, Neurology
New York University Medical Center
550 First Ave.
New York, NY 10016
(212) 340-7300

Melvin D. Yahr, M.D.
Chief, Neurology
The Mount Sinai Medical Center
1 Gustave L. Levy Place
New York, NY 10029
(212) 650-7301

Richard Satran, M.D.
Acting Chief, Neurology
University of Rochester Medical Center
6011 Imwood Ave.
Rochester, NY 14642
(716) 275-2776

Robert Y. Moore, M.D.
Chief, Neurology
SUNY at Stony Brook Health Sciences Center
L 12, Room 020
Department of Neurology
Stony Brook, NY 11794
(516) 444-1451

Carl J. Crosley, M.D.
Acting Chairman, Neurology
State University of New York Health Science
  Center at Syracuse
750 E. Adams St.
Syracuse, NY 13210
(315) 473-4627

Robert J. Strobos, M.D.
Chief, Neurology
New York Medical College
Munger Pavilion
Valhalla, NY 10595
(914) 347-5000

NORTH CAROLINA
James N. Hayward, M.D.
Chief, Neurology
University of North Carolina School of
  Medicine
North Carolina Memorial Hospital
751 Burnett-Womack Building 229H
Chapel Hill, NC 27514
(919) 966-2526

Allen D. Roses, M.D.
Chief, Neurology
Duke University Medical Center
Box M2900
Durham, NC 27710
(919) 684-2498

B. Todd Troost, M.D.
Chief, Neurology
William T. McLean, Jr., M.D.
Chief, Pediatric Neurology
Bowman Gray School of Medicine
North Carolina Baptist Hospital
300 S. Hawthorne Rd.
Winston-Salem, NC 27103
(919) 748-4101

NORTH DAKOTA
Generoso G. Gascon, M.D.
Chief, Neurology
University of North Dakota School of
  Medicine
UND Medical Education Center
Fargo, ND 58102
(701) 293-4101

OHIO
Frederick J. Samaha, M.D.
Chief, Neurology
University of Cincinnati Medical Center
231 Bethesda Ave.
Cincinnati, OH 45267-0525
(513) 872-5431

Robert B. Daroff, M.D.
Chairman, Neurology
Case Western Reserve University
School of Medicine
University Hospitals of Cleveland
2074 Abington Rd.
Cleveland, OH 44106
(216) 844-3193

George W. Paulson, M.D.
Chairman, Neurology
Ohio State University Hospitals
447 Means Hall
1654 Upham Drive
Columbus, OH 43210
(614) 421-4963

Samuel E. Pitner, M.D.
Chair, Neurology
Wright State University School of Medicine
PO Box 927
Dayton, OH 45401
(513) 223-9948

Gerald Dean Timmons, M.D.
Chief, Neurology
Northeastern Ohio Universities College of
  Medicine
4209 State Route 44
PO Box 95
Rootstown, OH 44272
(216) 325-2511

Peter White, M.D.
Acting Chairman, Neurology
Mark Rayport, M.D.C.M., Ph.D.
Chairman, Neurological Surgery
Medical College of Ohio
C.S. 10,008
Toledo, OH 43699
(419) 381-4172

OKLAHOMA
John W. Nelson, M.D.
Chief, Neurology
University of Oklahoma Health Sciences
  Center
PO Box 26901
Oklahoma City, OK 73190
(405) 271-4113

OREGON
John P. Hammerstad, M.D.
Chief, Neurology
Oregon Health Sciences University
School of Medicine
3181 S.W. Sam Jackson Park Rd.
Portland, OR 97201
(503) 225-8311

PENNSYLVANIA
Richard B. Tenser, M.D.
Acting Chief, Neurology
The Milton S. Hershey Medical Center
The Pennsylvania State University
Hershey, PA 17033
(717) 531-8521

Elliott L. Mancall, M.D.
Chairman, Neurology
Hahnemann University School of Medicine
Broad and Vine Sts.
Philadelphia, PA 19102
(215) 448-8092

Robert Jay Schwartzman, M.D.
Chief, Neurology
Jefferson Medical College of Thomas Jefferson
  University Hospital
11th and Walnut Sts.
Philadelphia, PA 19107
(215) 928-7310

Rosalie A. Burns, M.D.
Chairman, Neurology
Medical College of Pennsylvania
3300 Henry Ave.
Philadelphia, PA 19129
(215) 842-6000

Milton Alter, M.D.
Chief, Neurology
Temple University School of Medicine
Temple University Hospital
3401 N. Broad St.
Philadelphia, PA 19140
(215) 221-4046

Donald H. Silberberg, M.D.
Chief, Neurology
Hospital of the University of Pennsylvania
3400 Spruce St.
Philadelphia, PA 19104
(215) 662-3386

Oscar M. Reinmuth, M.D.
Chairman, Neurology
University of Pittsburgh
School of Medicine
322 Scaife Hall
Pittsburgh, PA 15261
(412) 624-2596

PUERTO RICO
Luis P. Sánchez-Longo, M.D.
Chief, Neurology
University of Puerto Rico
Medical Sciences Campus
School of Medicine
GPO Box 5067
San Juan, PR 00936
(809) 754-3784

SOUTH CAROLINA
Edward L. Hogan, M.D.
Chairman, Neurology
Medical University of South Carolina
171 Ashley Ave.
Charleston, SC 29425
(803) 792-3224

William L. Brannon, M.D.
Chief, Neurology
University of South Carolina
School of Medicine
Columbia, SC 29208
(803) 733-2300

SOUTH DAKOTA
George C. Flora, M.D.
Chief, Neurology
University of South Dakota School of
   Medicine
2501 W. 22nd St.
Sioux Falls, SD 57105
(605) 339-6648

TENNESSEE
John A. Churchill, M.D.
Chief, Neurology
East Tennessee State University
Quillen-Dishner College of Medicine
PO Box 21,160A
Johnson City, TN 37614
(615) 928-6426

Gerald Golden, M.D.
Acting Chairman, Department of Neurology
University of Tennessee, Memphis
College of Medicine
956 Court Ave., B212
Memphis, TN 38163
(901) 528-5876

Calvin L. Calhoun, M.D.
Chief, Neurology
Meharry Medical College School of Medicine
1005 D. B. Todd Blvd.
Nashville, TN 37207
(615) 233-6204

Gerald M. Fenichel, M.D.
Chairman, Neurology
Vanderbilt University Medical Center
1161 21st Ave., S.
Nashville, TN 37232
(615) 322-3461

TEXAS
Roger N. Rosenberg, M.D.
Chief, Neurology
University of Texas Health Science Center
Southwestern Medical School
Dallas, TX 75235
(214) 688-3111

John R. Calverley, M.D.
Chief, Neurology
University of Texas Medical Branch Hospitals
Galveston, TX 77550
(409) 761-2646

Stanley H. Appel, M.D.
Chief, Neurology
Baylor College of Medicine
Department of Neurology
Houston, TX 77030
(713) 799-4951

Frank M. Yatsu, M.D.
Chairman, Neurology
University of Texas Health Science Center at
   Houston
PO Box 20708
Houston, TX 77225
(713) 792-5777

J. Donald Easton, M.D.
Chief, Neurology
University of Texas Health Science Center at
   San Antonio
7703 Floyd Curl Drive
San Antonio, TX 78284
(512) 696-9660, x408

Allen B. Follender, M.D.
Chief, Neurology
Texas A&M University College of Medicine
Scott and White Clinic
Temple, TX 76508
(817) 774-2465

UTAH
J. Richard Baringer, M.D.
Chief, Neurology
University of Utah School of Medicine
50 N. Medical Drive
Salt Lake City, UT 84132
(801) 581-4283

VERMONT
Walter G. Bradley, M.D.
Chief, Neurology
University of Vermont College of Medicine
Burlington, VT 05405
(802) 656-4588

VIRGINIA
Thomas R. Johns, M.D.
Chief, Neurology
University of Virginia School of Medicine
PO Box 304
Charlottesville, VA 22908
(804) 924-0211

James E. Etheridge, Jr., M.D.
Chief, Neurology
Eastern Virginia Medical School
Medical Center Hospitals
855 W. Brambleton Ave.
Norfolk, VA 23510
(804) 446-5600

Robert J. De Lorenzo, M.D., Ph.D., M.P.H.
Chairman, Neurology
Medical College of Virginia
MCV Station, Box 599
Richmond, VA 23298
(804) 786-9721

WASHINGTON
Philip D. Swanson, M.D., Ph.D.
Chief, Neurology
University of Washington School of Medicine,
  RG-27
Seattle, WA 98195
(206) 543-2340

WEST VIRGINIA
Carl McComas, M.D.
Chief, Neurology
Marshall University School of Medicine
Huntington, WV 25701
(304) 526-0561

Ludwig Gutmann, M.D.
Chief, Neurology
West Virginia University Medical Center
Morgantown, WV 26505
(304) 293-3527

WISCONSIN
Henry S. Schutta, M.D.
Chief, Neurology
University of Wisconsin Hospital and Clinics
600 Highland Ave.
Room H 6-570
Madison, WI 53792
(608) 263-4900

Michael P. McQuillen, M.D.
Chief, Neurology
Medical College of Wisconsin
9200 W. Wisconsin Ave.
Milwaukee, WI 53226
(414) 257-2881

ORTHOPEDIC (BONE AND MUSCULOSKELETAL) PROBLEMS (ORTHOPEDIC SURGEONS)

The physicians listed below are some of the leading specialists in orthopedic surgery. They may be available for consultations and treatment or may be able to refer you to someone else.

All are heads of departments or divisions of orthopedic surgery at medical colleges accredited by the Association of American Medical Colleges.

ALABAMA
Kurt M. Niemann, M.D.
Chief, Division of Orthopedics
University of Alabama at Birmingham
MEF 508
University Station
Birmingham, AL 35294
(205) 934-4667

Lewis D. Anderson, M.D.
Chief, Orthopedic Surgery
University of South Alabama Medical Center
2451 Fillingim St.
Mobile, AL 36617
(205) 471-7937

ARIZONA
Robert G. Volz, M.D.
Chief, Orthopedic Surgery
University of Arizona College of Medicine
Arizona Health Sciences Center
Tucson, AZ 85724
(602) 626-0111

ARKANSAS
Carl L. Nelson, M.D.
Chief, Orthopedic Surgery
University of Arkansas College of Medicine
4301 W. Markham St., Slot 531
Little Rock, AR 72205
(501) 661-5251

CALIFORNIA
Michael W. Chapman, M.D.
Chief, Orthopedic Surgery
University of California, Davis
School of Medicine
Davis, CA 95616
(916) 453-2709

Mark M. Hoffer, M.D.
Chief, Orthopedic Surgery
University of California, Irvine
California College of Medicine
Irvine, CA 92717
(714) 634-5754

George J. Wiesseman, M.D.
Chief, Orthopedic Surgery
Loma Linda University Medical Center
Loma Linda, CA 92350
(714) 796-4808

Harlan C. Amstutz, M.D.
Chief, Division of Orthopedic Surgery
UCLA School of Medicine
Room 76-125 CHS
Los Angeles, CA 90024
(213) 825-0628

Augusto Sarmiento, M.D.
Chief, Orthopedics
University of Southern California
School of Medicine
Los Angeles—USC Medical Center
1200 N. State St.
Los Angeles, CA 90033
(213) 226-2622

Wayne H. Akeson, M.D.
Chief, Orthopedic Surgery Division
University of California, San Diego
Medical Center
225 Dickinson St.
San Diego, CA 92103
(619) 294-5944

William R. Murray, M.D.
Chief, Orthopedic Surgery
University of California—San Francisco
School of Medicine
414-U
Parnassus Ave.
San Francisco, CA 94143
(415) 666-9000

Eugene E. Bleck, M.D.
Division Chief
Donald Nagel, M.D.
Clinic Chief
Orthopedics Clinic
Division of Orthopedic Surgery
Stanford University Medical Center
Stanford, CA 94305
(415) 723-6518

COLORADO
James S. Miles, M.D.
Chief, Orthopedic Surgery
4200 E. Ninth Ave.
Denver, CO 80262
(303) 399-1211

CONNECTICUT
Harry R. Gossling, M.D.
Head, Orthopedic Surgery
University of Connecticut Health Center
Farmington, CT 06032
(203) 674-3367

Gary L. Friedlaender, M.D.
Head, Section of Orthopedic Surgery
Yale University School of Medicine
333 Cedar St.
New Haven, CT 06510
(203) 785-2579

DISTRICT OF COLUMBIA
John P. Adams, M.D.
Chairman, Orthopedic Surgery Department
George Washington University
Medical Center
2150 Pennsylvania Ave., N.W.
Washington, DC 20037
(202) 676-4380

Peter I. Kenmore, M.D.
Director, Orthopedic Surgery
Georgetown University School of Medicine
Georgetown University Hospital
3800 Reservoir Rd., N.W.
Washington, DC 20007
(202) 625-0100

Charles H. Epps, Jr., M.D.
Chief, Orthopedic Surgery
Howard University Hospital
2041 Georgia Ave., N.W.
Washington, DC 20060
(202) 745-1182

FLORIDA
R. William Petty, M.D.
Chairman, Orthopedic Surgery
University of Florida College of Medicine
J. H. Miller Health Center
PO Box J-246
Gainesville, FL 32610
(904) 392-5000

John Bowker, M.D.
Acting Chief, Orthopedics and Rehabilitation
University of Miami School of Medicine
PO Box 016960, D-27
Miami, FL 33101
(305) 549-6108

Phillip G. Spiegel, M.D.
Chairman, Department of Orthopedic Surgery
University of South Florida
College of Medicine
12901 N. 30th St., Box 36
Tampa, FL 33612
(813) 974-3322

GEORGIA
Richard S. Riggins, M.D.
Chief, Orthopedics
Emory University School of Medicine
Grady Memorial Hospital
80 Butler St., S.E.
Atlanta, GA 30303
(404) 588-4473

Monroe I. Levine, M.D.
Chief, Orthopedics
Medical College of Georgia Hospital
Augusta, GA 30912
(404) 828-2742

ILLINOIS
Michael F. Schafer, M.D.
Chairman, Orthopedic Surgery
Northwestern University Medical School
#9-037
303 E. Chicago Ave.
Chicago, IL 60611
(312) 908-8649

Jorge O. Galante, M.D.
Chairman, Orthopedic Surgery
Rush-Presbyterian-St. Luke's Medical Center
1753 W. Congress Parkway
Chicago, IL 60612
(312) 942-5850

Lawrence A. Pottenger, M.D.
Chief, Section of Orthopedic Surgery
University of Chicago Medical Center
5841 S. Maryland Ave.
Chicago, IL 60637
(312) 947-1000

Robert D. Ray, M.D., Ph.D.
Chief, Orthopedic Surgery
University of Illinois Hospital
840 S. Wood St.
Chicago, IL 60612
(312) 996-7000

Sidney J. Blair, M.D.
Chief, Orthopedic Surgery
Loyola University Medical Center
2160 S. First St.
Maywood, IL 60153
(312) 531-3000

E. Shannon Stauffer, M.D.
Chief, Orthopedic Surgery
Southern Illinois University
School of Medicine
800 N. Rutledge
Springfield, Il. 62708
(217) 782-8864

INDIANA
Richard E. Lindseth, M.D.
Acting Chairman, Department of Orthopedic
    Surgery
Indiana University Medical Center
Riley Hospital for Children 1182
702 Barnhill Drive
Indianapolis, IN 46223
(317) 264-7913

IOWA
Reginald R. Cooper, M.D.
Chief, Orthopedic Surgery
University of Iowa Hospitals
Iowa City, IA 52242
(319) 356-3470

KANSAS
Frederick W. Reckling, M.D.
Director, Section of Orthopedic Surgery
University of Kansas Medical Center
39th & Rainbow Blvd.
Kansas City, KS 66103
(913) 588-6129

KENTUCKY
Thomas D. Brower, M.D.
Chief, Orthopedic Surgery
University of Kentucky College of Medicine
800 Rose St.
Lexington, KY 40536
(606) 233-5000

Kenton Leatherman, M.D.
Acting Chairman, Department of Orthopedic
    Surgery
University of Louisville School of Medicine
Louisville, KY 40292
(502) 588-5319

LOUISIANA
Robert D. D'Ambrosia, M.D.
Head, Orthopedics
Louisiana State University School of Medicine
1542 Tulane Ave.
New Orleans, LA 70112
(504) 568-4680

Ray J. Haddad, Jr., M.D.
Chairman, Orthopedic Surgery
Tulane University School of Medicine
1430 Tulane Ave.
New Orleans, LA 70112
(504) 588-5192

James A. Albright, M.D.
Chairman, Orthopedic Surgery
Louisiana State University School of Medicine
    in Shreveport
PO Box 33932
Shreveport, LA 71130
(318) 674-6180

MARYLAND
Lee H. Riley, Jr., M.D.
Chief, Orthopedic Surgery
Johns Hopkins Hospital
Johns Hopkins University School of Medicine
600 N. Wolfe St.
Baltimore, MD 21205
(301) 955-6096

John E. Kenzora, M.D.
Chief, Orthopedic Surgery
University of Maryland Hospital
NGW 58
Baltimore, MD 21201
(301) 528-2121

MASSACHUSETTS
Robert E. Leach, M.D.
Chief, Orthopedic Surgery
Boston University School of Medicine
75 E. Newton St.
Boston, MA 02118
(617) 247-5000, 5430

Clement B. Sledge, M.D.
Chief, Orthopedic Surgery
Harvard Medical School
Brigham & Women's Hospital
25 Shattuck St.
Boston, MA 02115
(617) 732-1000

Seymour Zimbler, M.D.
Orthopedic Surgeon-in-Chief
Tufts University School of Medicine
New England Medical Center
171 Harrison Ave.
Boston, MA 02111
(617) 956-5169

Arthur M. Papas, M.D.
Chief, Orthopedic Surgery
University of Massachusetts Medical School
55 Lake Ave., N.
Worcester, MA 01605
(617) 856-2171

MICHIGAN
Larry S. Matthews, M.D.
Section Head, Orthopedic Surgery
University of Michigan Medical Center
2912D A. Alfred Taubman Health Care Center
Ann Arbor, MI 48109
(313) 936-5710

Richard L. LaMont, M.D.
Chairman, Orthopedic Surgery
Wayne State University School of Medicine
University Health Center
4201 St. Antoine St.
Detroit, MI 48201
(313) 577-0804

Richard Dean, M.D.
Chief, Surgery
Michigan State University College of Human
  Medicine
East Lansing, MI 48824
(517) 353-8730

MINNESOTA
Roby C. Thompson, Jr., M.D.
Chief, Orthopedic Surgery
University of Minnesota Medical School
Box 189 UMHC
Minneapolis, MN 55455
(612) 625-1177

Anthony J. Bianco, Jr., M.D.
Chief, Orthopedic Surgery
Mayo Medical School
200 First St., S.W.
Rochester, MN 55905
(507) 284-3671

MISSISSIPPI
James L. Hughes, M.D.
Chief, Orthopedic Surgery
University of Mississippi Medical Center
2500 N. State St.
Jackson, MS 39216
(601) 984-5135

MISSOURI
William C. Allen, M.D.
Chief, Orthopedic Surgery
University of Missouri Medical Center
807 Stadium Rd.
Columbia, MO 65212
(314) 882-4141

James Hamilton, M.D.
Chief, Orthopedic Surgery
University of Missouri–Kansas City School of
  Medicine
2411 Holmes St.
Kansas City, MO 64108
(816) 556-3561

Robert E. Burdge, M.D.
Chairman, Orthopedic Surgery
St. Louis University School of Medicine
1325 S. Grand Blvd.
St. Louis, MO 63104
(314) 557-8850

Paul Manske, M.D.
Chief, Orthopedic Surgery
Washington University School of Medicine
660 S. Euclid Ave.
St. Louis, MO 63110
(314) 362-4080

NEBRASKA
John F. Connolly, M.D.
Chief, Orthopedic Surgery
Creighton University School of Medicine
California at 24th St.
Omaha, NE 68178
(402) 280-4342

John F. Connolly, M.D.
Chairman, Orthopedic Surgery and
  Rehabilitation
University of Nebraska College of Medicine
42nd & Dewey Ave.
Omaha, NE 68105
(402) 559-4287

NEW HAMPSHIRE
Leland W. Hall, M.D.
Chief, Orthopedic Surgery
Dartmouth-Hitchcock Medical Center
2 Maynard St.
Hanover, NH 03755
(603) 646-5133

NEW JERSEY
Joseph P. Zawadsky, M.D.
Chief, Orthopedic Surgery
University of Medicine and Dentistry of New
  Jersey—Robert Wood Johnson Medical
  School (formerly Rutgers)
St. Peter's Medical Center
254 Easton Ave., Room 32F
New Brunswick, NJ 08903
(201) 645-0691

Andrew B. Weiss, M.D.
Chief, Orthopedic Surgery
University of Medicine and Dentistry of New
  Jersey
New Jersey Medical School
100 Bergen St.
Newark, NJ 07103
(201) 456-4300

NEW MEXICO
George E. Omer, M.D.
Chairman, Department of Orthopedics
University of New Mexico Medical Center
Albuquerque, NM 87131
(505) 843-4107

NEW YORK
Richard L. Jacobs, M.D.
Chief, Orthopedic Surgery
Albany Medical College of Union University
Albany Medical Center
New Scotland Ave.
Albany, NY 12208
(518) 445-3125

Edward T. Habermann, M.D.
Chief, Orthopedic Surgery
Montefiore Hospital and Medical Center
Albert Einstein College of Medicine
111 E. 210th St.
Bronx, NY 10467
(212) 920-4141

Stanley L. Gordon, M.D.
Chief, Orthopedic Surgery
State University of New York Health Science
  Center at Brooklyn
PO Box 40, 450 Clarkson Ave.
Brooklyn, NY 11203
(718) 270-1716

Eugene R. Mindell, M.D.
Chief, Orthopedic Surgery
State University of New York at Buffalo
Erie County Medical Center
462 Grider St.
Buffalo, NY 14215
(716) 898-3000

Philip D. Wilson, Jr., M.D.
Chief, Orthopedic Surgery
Cornell University Medical College
Hospital for Special Surgery
535 E. 70th St.
New York, NY 10021
(212) 535-6888

Robert S. Siffert, M.D.
Chief, Orthopedic Surgery
The Mount Sinai Medical Center
1 Gustave L. Levy Place
New York, NY 10029
(212) 650-6144

Theodore R. Waugh, M.D.
Chief, Orthopedic Surgery
New York University School of Medicine
New York University Medical Center
550 First Ave.
New York, NY 10016
(212) 340-7300

C. McCollister Evarts, M.D.
Chief, Orthopedic Surgery
University of Rochester Medical Center
PO Box 665, 601 Elmwood Ave.
Rochester, NY 14642
(716) 275-5167

Roger Dee, M.D.
Chief, Orthopedic Surgery
State University of New York at Stony Brook
Health Science Center
T-18, R020
Stony Brook, NY 11794
(516) 444-1484

David G. Murray, M.D.
Chief, Orthopedic Surgery
State University of New York Health Science
   Center at Syracuse
750 E. Adams St.
Syracuse, NY 13210
(315) 473-4472

Robert J. Schultz, M.D.
Chief, Orthopedic Surgery
New York Medical College
Department of Orthopedic Surgery
Valhalla, NY 10595
(914) 347-5000

NORTH CAROLINA
Frank C. Wilson, M.D.
Chief, Orthopedic Surgery
University of North Carolina School of
   Medicine
236 Burnett-Womack Building 229h
Chapel Hill, NC 27514
(919) 962-2211

J. Leonard Goldner, M.D.
Chief, Division of Orthopedic Surgery
Duke University Medical Center
Box 3706
Durham, NC 27710
(919) 684-8111

John L. Wooten, M.D.
Chief, Orthopedic Surgery
East Carolina University School of Medicine
Greenville, NC 27834
(919) 752-4613

Anthony G. Gristina, M.D.
Chief, Orthopedic Surgery
Bowman Gray School of Medicine
Winston-Salem, NC 27103
(919) 748-4340

NORTH DAKOTA
J. Donald Opgrande, M.D.
Chief, Orthopedic Surgery
University of North Dakota School of
   Medicine
Fargo, ND 58102
(701) 232-0054

OHIO
Buel S. Smith, M.D.
Chief, Orthopedic Surgery
Northeastern Ohio Universities College of
   Medicine
Akron General Medical Center
400 Wabash Ave.
Akron, OH 44307
(216) 384-6000

Clark N. Hopson, M.D.
Chief, Orthopedic Surgery
University of Cincinnati Medical Center
231 Bethesda Ave.
Cincinnati, OH 45267-0212
(513) 872-4592

Kingsbury G. Heiple, M.D.
Chairman, Orthopedics
Case Western Reserve University School of
   Medicine
University Hospitals of Cleveland
2074 Abington Rd.
Cleveland, OH 44106
(216) 844-3046

Sheldon R. Simon, M.D.
Director, Division of Orthopedic Surgery
Ohio State University Hospitals
N-843 Doan Hall
410 W. 10th Ave.
Columbus, OH 43210
(614) 421-8710

W. Thomas Jackson, M.D.
Chief, Orthopedic Surgery
Medical College of Ohio
C.S. 10,008
Toledo, OH 43699
(419) 381-4172

OKLAHOMA
Joseph A. Kopta, M.D.
Chief, Orthopedic Surgery and Rehabilitation
University of Oklahoma Health Sciences
   Center
PO Box 26901
Oklahoma City, OK 73190
(405) 271-4426

OREGON
Rodney K. Beals, M.D.
Chief, Orthopedic Surgery
Oregon Health Sciences University Hospital
3181 S.W. Sam Jackson Park Rd.
Portland, OR 97201
(503) 225-8311

PENNSYLVANIA
Robert B. Greer, III, M.D.
Chief, Orthopedic Surgery
Milton S. Hershey Medical Center
Pennsylvania State University
Hershey, PA 17033
(717) 531-8521

Arnold T. Berman, M.D.
Chairman, Orthopedic Surgery and
  Rehabilitation
Hahnemann University School of Medicine
Broad and Vine St.
Philadelphia, PA 19102
(215) 448-8168

Richard H. Rothman, M.D., Ph.D.
Chief, Orthopedic Surgery
Jefferson Medical College of Thomas Jefferson
  University
1015 Walnut St.
Philadelphia, PA 19107
(215) 928-6212

Henry H. Sherk, M.D.
Chief, Orthopedic Surgery
Hospital of the Medical College of
  Pennsylvania
3300 Henry Ave.
Philadelphia, PA 19129
(215) 842-6000

John W. Lachman, M.D.
Chief, Orthopedic Surgery
Temple University Hospital
3401 N. Broad St.
Philadelphia, PA 19140
(215) 221-2000

Carl T. Brighton, M.D.
Chairman, Orthopedic Surgery
Hospital of the University of Pennsylvania
3400 Spruce St.
Philadelphia, PA 19104
(215) 662-3350

Albert B. Ferguson, Jr., M.D.
Chairman, Department of Orthopedic Surgery
University of Pittsburgh School of Medicine
Falk Building, 4th Floor
3601 Fifth Ave.
Pittsburgh, PA 15213
(412) 648-3290

PUERTO RICO
Rafael Fernández-Feliberty, M.D.
Chief, Orthopedics
University of Puerto Rico
Medical Sciences Campus
School of Medicine
GPO Box 5067
San Juan, PR 00936
(809) 758-2525, x1907

RHODE ISLAND
James H. Herndon, M.D.
Chief, Orthopedic Surgery
Brown University Program in Medicine
Rhode Island Hospital
593 Eddy St.
Providence, RI 02902
(401) 227-4000

SOUTH CAROLINA
John B. McGinty, M.D.
Chairman, Orthopedic Surgery
Medical University of South Carolina
171 Ashley Ave.
Charleston, SC 29425
(803) 792-3856

Edward E. Kimbrough, M.D.
Chief, Orthopedics
University of South Carolina School of
  Medicine
Columbia, SC 29208
(803) 765-6812

SOUTH DAKOTA
Robert E. VanDemark, M.D.
Chief, Orthopedic Surgery
University of South Dakota School of
  Medicine
2501 W. 22nd St.
Sioux Falls, SD 57105
(605) 335-3707

TENNESSEE
Joseph K. Maloy, M.D.
Chief, Orthopedic Surgery
East Tennessee State University
Quillen-Dishner College of Medicine
PO Box 19,750A
Johnson City, TN 37614
(615) 928-6426

Rocco A. Calandruccio, M.D.
Chairman, Department of Orthopedic Surgery
University of Tennessee, Memphis
College of Medicine
956 Court Ave., A302, Box 13
Memphis, TN 38163
(901) 528-5880

Wallace P. Dooley, M.D.
Head, Division of Orthopedic Surgery
Meharry Medical College School of Medicine
1005 D. B. Todd Blvd.
Nashville, TN 37207
(615) 327-6111

Dan M. Spengler, M.D.
Chairman, Orthopedics and Rehabilitation
Vanderbilt University Medical Center
1161 21st Ave., S.
Nashville, TN 37232
(615) 322-7156

TEXAS
Donald E. Pisar, M.D.
Chief, Orthopedic Surgery
Texas A&M University College of Medicine
Medical Sciences Building
College Station, TX 77843
(817) 774-2706

Vert Mooney, M.D.
University of Texas Southwestern Medical
   School
Chief, Orthopedics Division
5323 Harry Hines Blvd.
Dallas, TX 75235
(214) 688-3111

William W. Robertson, M.D.
Acting Chief, Orthopedic Surgery
(Lubbock Branch)
Texas Tech University
Health Sciences Center
4800 Alberta
El Paso, TX 79905
(915) 534-5900

E. Burke Evans, M.D.
Chief, Orthopedic Surgery
207 Clinical Sciences Building
University of Texas Medical Branch
Galveston, TX 77550
(409) 761-1011

Hugh S. Tullos, M.D.
Chief, Orthopedic Surgery
Baylor College of Medicine
6560 Fannin, Suite 2100
Houston, TX 77030
(713) 799-4951

Bruce Browner, M.D.
Chief, Orthopedic Surgery
University of Texas Health Science Center at
   Houston
6431 Fannin, Room 6154 MSMB
Houston, TX 77030
(713) 792-5636

W. W. Robertson, M.D.
Chief, Texas Tech University Health Sciences
   Center
Department of Orthopedic Surgery
Lubbock, TX 79430
(806) 743-3111

Charles A. Rockwood, M.D.
Chief, Orthopedics
University of Texas Health Science Center at
   San Antonio
7703 Floyd Curl Drive
San Antonio, TX 78284
(512) 691-6140

UTAH
Harold K. Dunn, M.D.
Chief, Orthopedic Surgery
University of Utah School of Medicine
50 N. Medical Drive
Salt Lake City, UT 84132
(801) 581-7601

VERMONT
John W. Frymoyer, M.D.
Chairman, Department of Orthopedic and
   Rehabilitative Medicine
James Howe, M.D.
Head of Residency Program
University of Vermont College of Medicine
Given Building
Burlington, VT 05405
(802) 656-2250

VIRGINIA

Warren G. Stamp, M.D.
Chief, Orthopedic Surgery
University of Virginia Medical Center
PO Box 159
Charlottesville, VA 22908
(804) 924-0211

Curtis V. Spear, M.D.
Chief, Orthopedic Surgery
Eastern Virginia Medical School
Medical Center Hospitals
30 Medical Tower
Norfolk, VA 23507
(804) 461-1688

John A. Cardea, M.D.
Chairman, Orthopedic Surgery
Medical College of Virginia
MCV Station, Box 153
Richmond, VA 23298
(804) 786-9295

WASHINGTON

Frederick A. Matsen III, M.D.
Chief, Orthopedics
University of Washington School of Medicine,
  RK-10
Seattle, WA 98195
(206) 543-3690

WEST VIRGINIA

Thomas F. Scott, M.D.
Acting Chief, Orthopedic Surgery
Marshall University School of Medicine
Huntington, WV 25701
(304) 526-6905

Eric L. Radin, M.D.
Chief, Department of Orthopedic Surgery
West Virginia University Medical School
Morgantown, WV 26506
(304) 293-0111

WISCONSIN

Andrew A. McBeath, M.D.
Chief, Orthopedic Surgery
University of Wisconsin Hospital and Clinics
600 Highland Ave., Room G5/327
Madison, WI 53792
(608) 263-1344

Bruce J. Brewer, M.D.
Chief, Orthopedic Surgery
Medical College of Wisconsin
Milwaukee County Medical Complex
8700 W. Wisconsin Ave.
Milwaukee, WI 53226
(414) 257-5432

PULMONARY (LUNG) DISEASES (PULMONARY SPECIALISTS)

The physicians listed below are some of the leading physicians who specialize in lung diseases. You or your primary physician can contact them for consultations or treatment. If they are not available, they can refer you to someone else on their staffs. All are heads of pulmonary-disease departments at medical colleges accredited by the Association of American Medical Colleges.

ALABAMA

Dick D. Briggs, Jr., M.D.
Director, Division of Pulmonary and Critical
  Care Medicine
Department of Medicine
University of Alabama at Birmingham
THT 215
University Station
Birmingham, AL 35294
(205) 934-5400

John B. Bass, Jr., M.D.
Chief, Pulmonary Diseases
University of South Alabama
College of Medicine
Mobile, AL 36617
(205) 471 7887

ARIZONA

Benjamin Burrows, M.D.
Chief, Pulmonary Diseases
University of Arizona College of Medicine
Tucson, AZ 85724
(602) 626-6114

ARKANSAS

Charles Hiller, M.D.
Chief, Pulmonary
University of Arkansas College of Medicine
4301 W. Markham St., Slot 555
Little Rock, AR 72205
(501) 661-5525

CALIFORNIA
John B. West, M.D.
Chief, Pulmonary Physiology
University of California, San Diego
La Jolla, CA 92093
(619) 452-4190

Philip Gold, M.D.
Chief, Pulmonary Diseases
Loma Linda University Medical Center
Loma Linda, CA 92354
(714) 796-7311, x3232

Kaye H. Kilburn, M.D.
Chief, Pulmonary Diseases
Los Angeles County–University of Southern
  California Medical Center
Los Angeles, CA 90033
(213) 224-7514

Donald F. Tierney, M.D.
Chief, Pulmonary
University of California, Los Angeles
School of Medicine
Los Angeles, CA 90024
(213) 825-5316

Archie F. Wilson, M.D., Ph.D.
Chief, Pulmonary Diseases
University of California (Irvine) Medical
  Center
Orange, CA 92668
(714) 634-5150

Glen A. Lillington, M.D.
Chief, Pulmonary Medicine
University of California, Davis Medical Center
Sacramento, CA 95817
(916) 453-3564

Kenneth M. Moser, M.D.
Chief, Pulmonary and Critical Care Divisions
University of California, San Diego
Medical Center
225 Dickinson St.
San Diego, CA 92103
(619) 294-5970

H. B. Kaltreider, M.D.
University of California, San Francisco
San Francisco General Hospital
San Francisco, CA 94100
(415) 648-5010

James Theodore, M.D.
Thomas Raffin, M.D.
Clinic Co-Chiefs
Edward Rubenstein, M.D.
Acting Division Chief
Chest Clinic
Division of Respiratory Medicine
Stanford University Medical Center
Stanford, CA 94305
(415) 723-5841

COLORADO
Thomas L. Petty, M.D.
Chief, Pulmonary Diseases
University of Colorado Health Sciences Center
Denver, CO 80262
(303) 394-7767

CONNECTICUT
Stephen B. Sulavik, M.D.
Chief, Pulmonary Medicine
University of Connecticut Health Center
Farmington, CT 06032
(203) 674-3585

Herbert Y. Reynolds, M.D.
Head, Pulmonary Section
Yale University School of Medicine
333 Cedar St.
New Haven, CT 06510
(203) 785-4163

DISTRICT OF COLUMBIA
Sam V. Spagnolo, M.D.
Director, Pulmonary Diseases & Allergy
George Washington University
Medical Center
2150 Pennsylvania Ave., N.W.
Washington, DC 20037
(202) 676-3633

Hall G. Canter, M.D.
Chief, Pulmonary Diseases
Georgetown University Medical Center
Washington, DC 20007
(202) 625-7211

Earl M. Armstrong, M.D.
Chief, Pulmonary Diseases
Howard University Hospital
Washington, DC 20060
(202) 745-6796

FLORIDA

A. Jay Block, M.D.
Chief, Pulmonary Diseases
University of Florida College of Medicine
PO Box J-225
Gainesville, FL 32610
(904) 374-6063

Adam Wanner, M.D.
Chief, Pulmonary Diseases
University of Miami
Pulmonary Division R-120
Miami, FL 33101
(305) 674-2610

Allan L. Goldman, M.D.
Professor and Director, Division of Pulmonary
    and Critical Care Medicine
University of South Florida
College of Medicine
James A. Haley Veterans Hospital
13000 N. 30th St., 111-C
Tampa, FL 33612
(813) 972-7543

GEORGIA

G. Michael Duffell, M.D.
Chief, Pulmonary Diseases
Emory University School of Medicine
Atlanta, GA 30322
(404) 321-0111, x3368

William A. Speir, Jr., M.D.
Chief, Pulmonary Diseases
Medical College of Georgia Hospital
Augusta, GA 30912
(404) 828-2566

ILLINOIS

Lewis J. Smith, M.D.
Chief, Pulmonary Diseases
Northwestern University
McGaw Medical Center
Chicago, IL 60611
(312) 908-8163

Roger Bone, M.D.
Chairman, Internal Medicine
Rush-Presbyterian-St. Luke's Medical Center
1753 W. Congress Parkway
Chicago, IL 60612
(312) 942-5269

Lawrence D. H. Wood, M.D.
Chief, Section of Pulmonary Medicine
University of Chicago Medical Center
5841 S. Maryland Ave.
Chicago, IL 60637
(312) 947-1000

Melvin Lopata, M.D.
Chief, Respiratory Medicine
University of Illinois College of Medicine
Chicago, IL 60680
(312) 996-8039

J. T. Sharp, M.D.
Chief, Pulmonary Diseases
Loyola University of Chicago
Stritch School of Medicine
Maywood, IL 60153
(312) 343-7200

Eric C. Rackow, M.D.
Chief, Pulmonary Diseases
University of Health Sciences
Chicago Medical School
3333 Green Bay Rd.
North Chicago, IL 60064
(312) 578-3000

Lanie E. Eagleton, M.D.
Chief, Pulmonary Medicine
Southern Illinois University School of
    Medicine
801 N. Rutledge
Springfield, IL 62708
(217) 782-0187

INDIANA

Richard E. Brashear, M.D.
Chief, Pulmonary Diseases Section
Department of Medicine
Indiana University Medical Center
University Hospital N559
926 W. Michigan St.
Indianapolis, IN 46223
(317) 264-2136

Howard Eigen, M.D.
Chief, Pulmonology Section
Department of Pediatrics
Indiana University Medical Center
Riley Hospital for Children 293
702 Barnhill Drive
Indianapolis, IN 46223
(317) 264-7208

IOWA
Gary M. Hunninghake, M.D.
Chief, Pulmonary Diseases
University of Iowa College of Medicine
Iowa City, IA 52242
(319) 353-6690

KANSAS
William E. Ruth, M.D.
Chief, Pulmonary Diseases
University of Kansas Medical Center
39th and Rainbow Blvd.
Kansas City, KS 66103
(913) 588-6044

KENTUCKY
N. K. Burki, M.D.
Chief, Pulmonary Diseases
University of Kentucky Medical Center
Lexington, KY 40536
(606) 233-5045

William H. Anderson, M.D.
Chief, Respiratory and Environmental
   Medicine
Department of Medicine
University of Louisville School of Medicine
Louisville, KY 40242
(502) 588-5841

LOUISIANA
Warren Summer, M.D.
Chief, Pulmonary Critical Care Medicine
Louisiana State University Medical Center
New Orleans, LA 70112
(504) 568-4634

Hans Weill, M.D.
Chief, Pulmonary Diseases
Tulane University School of Medicine
1430 Tulane Ave.
New Orleans, LA 70112
(504) 588-2250

Ronald George, M.D.
Chief, Pulmonary Diseases Section
Department of Medicine
Louisiana State University
School of Medicine in Shreveport
PO Box 33932
Shreveport, LA 71130
(318) 674-5920

MARYLAND
Gareth M. Green, M.D.
Chief, Respiratory Medicine
The Johns Hopkins Medical Institutions
Baltimore, MD 21205
(301) 955-3900

Lewis Rubin, M.D.
Chief, Pulmonary Diseases
University of Maryland School of Medicine
Baltimore, MD 21205
(301) 528-6251

MASSACHUSETTS
Gordon L. Snider, M.D.
Chief, Pulmonary
Boston University Medical Center
Boston, MA 02118
(617) 247-5277

Barry L. Fanburg, M.D.
Division Chief, Pulmonary
Tufts University School of Medicine
New England Medical Center
171 Harrison Ave.
Boston, MA 02111
(617) 956-5871

Richard S. Irwin, M.D.
Chief, Pulmonary Medicine
University of Massachusetts
Worcester, MA 01605
(617) 856-3121

MICHIGAN
Joseph P. Lynch, III, M.D.
Acting Chief, Pulmonary and Critical Care
   Medicine
University of Michigan Medical Center
3916 A. Alfred Taubman Health Care Center
Ann Arbor, MI 48109
(313) 936-5040

Richard Carlson, M.D., Ph.D.
Chief, Pulmonary Medicine
Wayne State University
School of Medicine
540 E. Canfield
Detroit, MI 48201
(313) 577-1460

MINNESOTA

Peter Bitterman, M.D.
Head, Pulmonary Diseases
Department of Medicine
University of Minnesota Medical School
Box 132 UMHC
Minneapolis, MN 55455
(612) 624-0999

David R. Sanderson, M.D.
Chief, Thoracic Diseases
Mayo Graduate School of Medicine
Mayo Medical School
Rochester, MN 55905
(507) 284-2511

MISSISSIPPI

Joe R. Norman, M.D.
Chief, Pulmonary Diseases
University of Mississippi Medical Center
Jackson, MS 39216
(601) 984-5650

MISSOURI

E. V. Sunderrajan, M.D.
Chief, Pulmonary Diseases
University of Missouri
Columbia School of Medicine
Columbia, MO 65212
(314) 443-2511

George Reisz, M.D.
Chief, Pulmonary Diseases
University of Missouri–Kansas City School of
    Medicine
Kansas City, MO 64108
(816) 276-1940

Thomas Hyers, M.D.
Director, Pulmonary Medicine
St. Louis University School of Medicine
1325 S. Grand Blvd.
St. Louis, MO 63104
(314) 577-8856

John A. McDonald, M.D.
Chief, Pulmonary Diseases
Washington University School of Medicine
St. Louis, MO 63110
(314) 362-8980

NEBRASKA

Walter J. O'Donohue, Jr., M.D.
Chief, Pulmonary
Creighton University School of Medicine
California at 24th St.
Omaha, NE 68131
(402) 449-4486

Stephen I. Rennard, M.D.
Chief, Pulmonary Diseases
University of Nebraska College of Medicine
42nd St. and Dewey Ave.
Omaha, NE 68105
(402) 559-4087

NEW HAMPSHIRE

Peter B. Barlow, M.D.
Chief, Pulmonary Medicine
Dartmouth Hitchcock Medical Center
Hanover, NH 03577
(603) 646-5261

NEW JERSEY

Norman H. Edelman, M.D.
Chief, Pulmonary Diseases
UMDNJ–Robert Wood Johnson Medical
    School (formerly Rutgers)
New Brunswick, NJ 08903
(201) 937-7840

Lee B. Reichman, M.D.
Chief, Pulmonary Diseases
University of Medicine & Dentistry of New
    Jersey University Hospital
100 Bergen St.
Newark, NJ 07103
(201) 456-6110, 6111

NEW MEXICO

Andre W. Van As, M.D.
Chief, Pulmonary Medicine
University of New Mexico School of Medicine
Albuquerque, NM 87108
(505) 265-1711, x2375

NEW YORK

Brendan Keogh, M.D.
Chief, Pulmonary Diseases
Albany Medical Center
Albany, NY 12208
(518) 439-9158

Louis Sherwood, M.D.
Chief, Department of Medicine
Albert Einstein College of Medicine
Bronx Municipal Hospital Center
Bronx, NY 10461
(212) 430-2182

Robert Klocke, M.D.
Chief, Pulmonary & Respiratory Division
SUNY at Buffalo School of Medicine
Erie County Medical Center
Buffalo, NY 14215
(716) 894-1212

Alvin S. Teirstein, M.D.
Chief, Pulmonary Diseases
The Mount Sinai Medical Center
1 Gustave L. Levy Place
New York, NY 10029
(212) 650-5901

Edward Crandall, M.D.
Chief, Pulmonary Medicine
New York Hospital—Cornell Medical Center
New York, NY 10029
(212) 472-5621

John H. McClement, M.D.
Chief, Pulmonary Diseases
New York University Medical Center
Bellevue Hospital Medical Center
N.Y. VA Hospital
New York, NY 10016
(212) 561-3704

Matthew G. Marin, M.D.
Mark J. Utell, M.D.
Chairmen, Pulmonary Diseases
University of Rochester Medical Center
Rochester, NY 14642
(716) 275-4861

Edward Bergofsky, M.D.
Division Head, Pulmonary Disease
SUNY at Stony Brook Health Sciences Center
T-17, R040
Stony Brook, NY 11794
(516) 444-1776

J. H. Auchincloss, M.D.
Chief, Pulmonary Section
State University of New York Health Science
    Center of Syracuse
750 E. Adams St.
Syracuse, NY 13210
(315) 473-5663

Daniel J. Stone, M.D.
Chief, Pulmonary Diseases
New York Medical College
Valhalla, NY 10595
(914) 347-7517

NORTH CAROLINA
Philip A. S. Bromberg, M.D.
Chief, Pulmonary Diseases
University of North Carolina at Chapel Hill
Chapel Hill, NC 27514
(919) 966-2531

James D. Crapo, M.D.
Chief, Pulmonary Diseases
Duke University Medical Center
Durham, NC 27710
(919) 684-6266

Yash P. Kataria, M.D.
Chief, Pulmonary Diseases
East Carolina University School of Medicine
Greenville, NC 27834
(919) 757-4653

Byron D. McLees, M.D.
Chief, Pulmonary Diseases
Bowman Gray School of Medicine
Winston-Salem, NC 27103
(919) 748-4325

NORTH DAKOTA
Jerry Greene, M.D.
Chief, Pulmonary Medicine
University of North Dakota School of
    Medicine
UND Medical Education Center
Fargo, ND 58102
(701) 232-3241, x430

OHIO
Robert G. Loudon, M.D.
Chief, Pulmonary Diseases
University of Cincinnati Medical Center
231 Bethesda Ave.
Cincinnati, OH 45267-0564
(513) 872-4831

Neil S. Cherniack, M.D.
Director, Division of Pulmonary Medicine
Department of Medicine
Case Western Reserve University
University Hospitals of Cleveland
2074 Abington Rd.
Cleveland, OH 44106
(216) 844-3120

James E. Gadek, M.D.
Director, Division of Pulmonary Diseases
Ohio State University Hospitals
N-325 Means Hall
1654 Upham Drive
Columbus, OH 43210
(614) 421-4925

Stephen L. Demeter, M.D.
Chief, Pulmonary
Northeastern Ohio Universities College of
  Medicine
4209 State Route 44
Rootstown, OH 44272
(216) 325-2511

Abdul Memon, M.D.
Chief, Pulmonary Medicine
Medical College of Ohio
C.S. 10,008
Toledo, OH 43699
(419) 381-4267

OKLAHOMA
Sami I. Said, M.D.
Section Head, Pulmonary
University of Oklahoma Health Sciences
  Center
PO Box 26901
Oklahoma City, OK 73126
(405) 271-6173

OREGON
M. J. Edwards, M.D.
Chief, Chest Diseases
Oregon Health Sciences University
Portland, OR 97201
(503) 225-7680

PENNSYLVANIA
Clifford W. Zwillich, M.D.
Chief, Pulmonary Diseases
Pennsylvania State University
College of Medicine
Hershey, PA 17033
(717) 531-8521

Robert A. Promisloff, D.O.
Acting Director, Pulmonary Diseases
Hahnemann University School of Medicine
Philadelphia, PA 19102
(215) 448-8013

James E. Fish, M.D.
Chief, Pulmonary Diseases
Jefferson Medical College of Thomas Jefferson
  University
11th and Walnut Sts.
Philadelphia, PA 19107
(215) 928-6590

Lee W. Greenspan, M.D.
Chief, Pulmonary Medicine
Medical College of Pennsylvania
Philadelphia, PA 19129
(215) 842-6000

A. B. Cohen, M.D.
Chief, Pulmonary Diseases
Temple University Health Sciences Center
Philadelphia, PA 19140
(215) 456-6950

A. P. Fishman, M.D.
Director, Cardiovascular Pulmonary
Hospital of the University of Pennsylvania
3400 Spruce St.
Philadelphia, PA 19104
(215) 662-3194

Robert M. Rogers, M.D.
Chief, Pulmonary Medicine
University of Pittsburgh School of Medicine
440 Scaife Hall
Pittsburgh, PA 15261
(412) 624-1929

PUERTO RICO
Rafael Rodríguez Servera, M.D.
Chief, Pulmonary
University of Puerto Rico
Medical Sciences Campus
School of Medicine
GPO Box 5067
San Juan, PR 00936
(809) 758-2525, x1827

SOUTH CAROLINA
Stephen A. Sahn, M.D.
Director, Pulmonary and Critical Care
Medical University of South Carolina
171 Ashley Ave.
Charleston, SC 29425
(803) 792-3161

Gerald Olsen, M.D.
Chief, Pulmonary Diseases
University of South Carolina School of
   Medicine
Columbia, SC 29208
(803) 776-6575

SOUTH DAKOTA
Rodney R. Parry, M.D.
Chief, Division of Pulmonary Medicine
University of South Dakota School of
   Medicine
2501 W. 22nd St.
Sioux Falls, SD 57105
(605) 339-6790

TENNESSEE
William Dralle, M.D.
Chief, Pulmonary
East Tennessee State University
Quillen-Dishner College of Medicine
PO Box 21,160A
Johnson City, TN 37614
(615) 928-6426

John R. Hoidal, M.D.
Chief, Division of Pulmonary Medicine
University of Tennessee, Memphis
College of Medicine
956 Court Ave., H314
Memphis, TN 38163
(901) 528-5757

J. M. Stinson, M.D.
Head, Division of Pulmonary Diseases
Meharry Medical College School of Medicine
1005 D. B. Todd Blvd.
Nashville, TN 37207
(615) 327-6111

Kenneth L. Brigham, M.D.
Director, Pulmonary Medicine
Vanderbilt University Medical Center
Nashville, TN 37232
(615) 322-3412

TEXAS
Alan Pierce, M.D.
Chief, Pulmonary
University of Texas Health Science Center at
   Dallas
5323 Harry Hines Blvd.
Dallas, TX 75235
(214) 688-3111

Keith Wilson
Chief, Pulmonary Diseases
Baylor College of Medicine
One Baylor Plaza
Houston, TX 77030
(713) 790-2076

David R. Dantzker, M.D.
Chief, Pulmonary Medicine
University of Texas Health Science Center at
   Houston
Houston, TX 77025
(713) 792-5110

Kenneth Nugent, M.D.
Chief, Pulmonary
Texas Tech University Health Science Center
Fourth St. at Indiana Ave.
Lubbock, TX 79430
(806) 743-3155

Stephen Jenkinson, M.D.
Acting Chief, Pulmonary Diseases
University of Texas Health Science Center at
   San Antonio
7703 Floyd Curl Drive
San Antonio, TX 78284
(512) 696-9660, x6492

Ronald E. Walsh, M.D.
Chief, Pulmonary Medicine
Texas A&M
University College of Medicine
Scott and White Memorial Hospital
Temple, TX 76508
(817) 774-2478

W. G. Avery, M.D.
Chief, Pulmonary Diseases
The University of Texas Health Center at Tyler
Tyler, TX 75710
(214) 877-3451, x5059

UTAH
Attilio D. Renzetti, Jr., M.D.
Chief, Respiratory and Occupational Medicine
University of Utah School of Medicine
50 N. Medical Drive
Salt Lake City, UT 84132
(801) 581-7806

VERMONT
Gerald S. Davis, M.D.
Chief, Pulmonary Diseases
University of Vermont College of Medicine
Burlington, VT 05405
(802) 656-2182

VIRGINIA

Frederick L. Glauser, M.D.
Chief, Pulmonary and Critical Care Medicine
Medical College of Virginia
MCV Station, Box 50
Richmond, VA 23298
(804) 786-9071

WASHINGTON

John Butler, M.D.
Head, Respiratory Diseases Division
University of Washington School of Medicine,
  RM-12
Seattle, WA 98195
(206) 543-3166

WEST VIRGINIA

Nancy Munn, M.D.
Chief, Pulmonary Diseases
Marshall University School of Medicine
Huntington, WV 25701
(304) 429-4615

N. Leroy Lapp, M.D.
Chief, Pulmonary Medicine
West Virginia University Medical Center
Morgantown, WV 26506
(304) 293-4661

WISCONSIN

Guillermo A. Do Pico, M.D.
Chief, Pulmonary Medicine
University of Wisconsin Hospital and Clinics
Center for Health Sciences
Madison, WI 53792
(608) 263-3035

Donald P. Schlueter, M.D.
Chief, Pulmonary Medicine
Medical College of Wisconsin
Milwaukee, WI 53226
(414) 257-6355

SKIN DISORDERS (DERMATOLOGISTS)

The physicians listed below are some of the leading specialists in skin disorders and diseases. They may be available for treatment and consultations or may be able to refer you to someone else. All are heads of dermatology departments at medical colleges accredited by the Association of American Medical Colleges.

ALABAMA

W. Mitchell Sams, Jr., M.D.
Chairman, Department of Dermatology
University of Alabama at Birmingham
NHB 225
University Station
Birmingham, AL 35294
(205) 934-4141

CALIFORNIA

Gerald D. Weinstein, M.D.
Chairman, Dermatology
University of California, Irvine
California College of Medicine
Irvine, CA 92717
(714) 856-5925

Edwin T. Wright, M.D.
Chief, Dermatology
J. L. Pettis Memorial Veterans Hospital
Loma Linda, CA 92357
(714) 825-7084
Affiliated with Loma Linda University School
  of Medicine

Ronald Reisner, M.D.
Head, Division of Dermatology
University of California, Los Angeles School
  of Medicine
Los Angeles, CA 90024
(213) 825-0631

Thomas Rea, M.D.
Chief, Dermatology
University of Southern California School of
  Medicine
1200 N. State St.—Room 8841
Los Angeles, CA 90033
(213) 226-3373

Irma Gigli, M.D.
Chief, Dermatology Division
University of California, San Diego
Medical Center
225 Dickinson St.
San Diego, CA 92103
(619) 294-6863

Paul Jacobs, M.D.
Department Chairman and Clinic Chief
Dermatology Clinic
Department of Dermatology
Stanford University Medical Center
Stanford, CA 94305
(415) 723-6316

CONNECTICUT
Jane Grant-Kels, M.D.
Chief, Dermatology
University of Connecticut Health Center
Farmington, CT 06032
(203) 674-3474

Richard L. Edelson, M.D.
Chairman, Department of Dermatology
Yale University School of Medicine
333 Cedar St.
New Haven, CT 06510
(203) 785-4632

DISTRICT OF COLUMBIA
Mervyn Elgart, M.D.
Chairman, Dermatology Department
George Washington University
Medical Center
2150 Pennsylvania Ave., N.W.
Washington, DC 20037
(202) 676-4058

Virginia Sulica, M.D.
Head, Division of Dermatology
Georgetown University School of Medicine
3900 Reservoir Rd., N.W.
Washington, DC 20007
(202) 625-7259

Harold Minus, M.D.
Head, Division of Dermatology
Howard University College of Medicine
520 W St., N.W.
Washington, DC 20059
(202) 636-6270

FLORIDA
Franklin P. Flowers
Chief, Division of Dermatology
University of Florida College of Medicine
PO Box J-277
Gainesville, FL 32610
(904) 392-4984

William H. Eaglestein, M.D.
Chief, Dermatology and Cutaneous Surgery
University of Miami School of Medicine
PO Box 016099 (R-250)
Miami, FL 33101
(305) 547-6734

Neil A. Fenske, M.D.
Director of the Division of Dermatology
University of South Florida College of
  Medicine
12901 N. 30th St., Box 19
Tampa, FL 33612
(813) 974-2854

GEORGIA
Marilynne McKay, M.D.
Acting Chairman, Department of Dermatology
Emory University School of Medicine
Atlanta, GA 30322
(404) 727-5872

J. Graham Smith, Jr., M.D.
Chief, Dermatology
Medical College of Georgia Hospital
Augusta, GA 30912
(404) 828-3291

ILLINOIS
Henry H. Roenigk, Jr., M.D.
Chairman, Dermatology
Northwestern University Medical School
303 E. Chicago Ave.
Chicago, IL 60611
(312) 908-8173

Frederick Malkinson, M.D.
Chairman, Dermatology
Rush-Presbyterian-St. Luke's Medical Center
1725 W. Harrison St.
Chicago, IL 60612
(312) 942-6096

Allan L. Lorincz, M.D.
Chief, Section of Dermatology
University of Chicago Medical Center
5841 S. Maryland Ave.
Chicago, IL 60637
(312) 947-1000

INDIANA
Arthur L. Norins, M.D.
Chairman, Department of Dermatology
Indiana University Medical Center
Regenstrief Health Center 524
1100 W. Michigan St.
Indianapolis, IN 46223
(317) 630-6691

KANSAS
James T. Kalivas, M.D.
Director, Division of Dermatology
University of Kansas Medical Center
Kansas City, KS 66103
(913) 588-6028

KENTUCKY
Lafayette G. Owen, M.D.
Chief, Dermatology
Department of Medicine
University of Louisville
School of Medicine
Louisville, KY 40292
(502) 588-7287

LOUISIANA
Ricardo G. Mora, M.D.
Acting Head, Dermatology
LSU School of Medicine
1542 Tulane Ave.
New Orleans, LA 70112
(504) 568-4885

Larry E. Millikan, M.D.
Chairman, Dermatology
Tulane University School of Medicine
1430 Tulane Ave.
New Orleans, LA 70112
(504) 588-5114

MARYLAND
Thomas Provost, M.D.
Head, Division of Dermatology
Johns Hopkins University School of Medicine
720 Rutland Ave.
Baltimore, MD 21205
(301) 955-3345

Joseph Burnett, M.D.
Chief, Dermatology
University of Maryland School of Medicine
655 W. Baltimore St.
Baltimore, MD 21201
(301) 528-5766

MASSACHUSETTS
Thomas Fitzpatrick, M.D.
Head, Division of Dermatology
Harvard Medical School
Massachusetts General Hospital
Boston, MA 02114
(617) 726-2914

David S. Feingold, M.D.
Dermatologist-in-Chief
Tufts University School of Medicine
New England Medical Center
171 Harrison Ave.
Boston, MA 02111
(617) 956-5235

Rita Berman, M.D.
Chief, Department of Dermatology
University of Massachusetts Medical School
Worcester, MA 01605
(617) 856-2209

MICHIGAN
John J. Voorhees, M.D.
Chairman, Dermatology
University of Michigan Medical Center
1910F A. Alfred Taubman Health Care Center
Ann Arbor, MI 48109
(313) 936-4080

Ken Hashimoto, M.D.
Chief, Dermatology
Wayne State University
School of Medicine
540 E. Canfield
Detroit, MI 48201
(313) 577-5057

MINNESOTA
Peter Lynch, M.D.
Chief, Dermatology
University of Minnesota Medical School
Box 98 UMHC
Minneapolis, MN 55455
(612) 625-8625

MISSOURI
Joseph Duvall, M.D.
Acting Director, Dermatology
St. Louis University School of Medicine
1325 S. Grand Blvd.
St. Louis, MO 63104
(314) 577-6070

Arthur Z. Eisen, M.D.
Chief, Dermatology
Washington University School of Medicine
660 S. Euclid
St. Louis, MO 63110
(314) 362-9000

NEBRASKA
Ramon M. Fusaro, M.D.
Chief, Dermatology
Creighton University School of Medicine
California at 24th St.
Omaha, NE 68178
(402) 280-4507

NEW JERSEY
Richard S. Berger, M.D.
Acting Chief, Dermatology
UMDNJ–Robert Wood Johnson Medical
  School (formerly Rutgers)
UMDNJ Medical Education Building
Academic Health Science Building CN19
New Brunswick, NJ 08903
(201) 937-7688

Robert Schwartz, M.D.
Chief, Dermatology
University of Medicine and Dentistry of New
  Jersey
New Jersey Medical School
100 Bergen St.
Newark, NJ 07103
(201) 456-4300

NEW MEXICO
Walter Burgdorf, M.D.
Chairman, Department of Dermatology
University of New Mexico School of Medicine
Albuquerque, NM 87131
(505) 277-4757

NEW YORK
Alan R. Shalita, M.D.
Chairman and Chief, Dermatology
SUNY Health Science Center at Brooklyn
450 Clarkson Ave.
Brooklyn, NY 11203
(718) 270-1229

Frederick Helm, M.D.
Chairman of Dermatology
SUNY at Buffalo School of Medicine
50 High St., Suite 609
Buffalo, NY 14203
(716) 885-0707

Leonard Harber, M.D.
Chairman, Department of Dermatology
Columbia Presbyterian Medical Center
630 W. 168th St.
New York, NY 10032
(212) 305-3497

Raul Fleischmajer, M.D.
Chief, Dermatology
The Mount Sinai Medical Center
1 Gustave L. Levy Place
New York, NY 10029
(212) 650-8151

George Hambrick, M.D.
D. Martin Carter, M.D.
Co-Chiefs, Dermatology
New York Hospital–Cornell Medical Center
525 E. 68th St.
New York, NY 10021
(212) 472-8025

Fuad Farah, M.D.
Chief, Section of Dermatology
SUNY Health Science Center at Syracuse
750 E. Adams St.
Syracuse, NY 13210
(315) 473-5540

NORTH CAROLINA
Billy E. Jones, M.D.
Chief, Dermatology
East Carolina University School of Medicine
Greenville, NC 27834
(919) 757-2570

Joseph L. Jorizzo, M.D.
Chief, Dermatology
Bowman Gray School of Medicine
Winston-Salem, NC 27103
(919) 748-3926

OHIO

James J. Nordlund, M.D.
Director, Department of Dermatology
University of Cincinnati Medical Center
231 Bethesda Ave.
Cincinnati, OH 45267-0592
(513) 872-6242

David Bickers, M.D.
Chairman, Department of Dermatology
Case Western Reserve University School of
  Medicine
Veterans Administration Medical Center
10701 East Blvd.
Cleveland, OH 44106
(216) 791-3800

Charles Camisa, M.D.
Director, Division of Dermatology
Ohio State University Hospitals
4731 University Hospitals Clinic
456 Clinic Drive
Columbus, OH 43210
(614) 421-8111

Arnold Schroeter
Chair, Dermatology
Wright State University School of Medicine
PO Box 927
Dayton, OH 45401
(513) 268-3465

Linda Alston, M.D.
Chief, Dermatology
Northeastern Ohio Universities College of
  Medicine
4209 State Route 44
Rootstown, OH 44272
(216) 325-2511

E. Dorinda Shelley, M.D.
Chief, Dermatology
Medical College of Ohio
C.S. 10,008
Toledo, OH 43699
(419) 381-4267

OKLAHOMA

Mark Allen Everett, M.D.
Head, Dermatology
University of Oklahoma Health Sciences
  Center
619 N.E. 13th
Oklahoma City, OK 73104
(405) 271-6111

PENNSYLVANIA

Donald P. Lookingbill, M.D.
Chief, Dermatology
The Milton S. Hershey Medical Center
The Pennsylvania State University
Hershey, PA 17033
(717) 531-8521

Henry Maguire, M.D.
Professor & Director, Dermatology
Hahnemann University School of Medicine
Broad & Vine Sts.
Philadelphia, PA 19102
(215) 448-8252

Herbert A. Luscombe, M.D.
Chief, Dermatology
Jefferson Medical College of Thomas Jefferson
  University
11th and Walnut Sts.
Philadelphia, PA 19107
(215) 928-6680

Bernard Kirshbaum, M.D.
Chief, Dermatology
Medical College of Pennsylvania
3300 Henry Ave.
Philadelphia, PA 19129
(215) 842-6000

Gerald Lazarus, M.D.
Chairman, Dermatology
Hospital of the University of Pennsylvania
3400 Spruce St.
Philadelphia, PA 19104
(215) 662-2536

SOUTH CAROLINA

John C. Maize, M.D.
Acting Chairman, Dermatology
Medical University of South Carolina
171 Ashley Ave.
Charleston, SC 29425
(803) 792-5858

J. Richard Allison, M.D.
Chief, Dermatology
University of South Carolina School of
  Medicine
Columbia, SC 29208
(803) 765-6563

SOUTH DAKOTA
Helen Jane Hare, M.D.
Section Head, Dermatology
University of South Dakota School of
   Medicine
Rapid City Regional Hospital
Box 6020
Rapid City, SD 57701
(605) 342-3280, 3716

TENNESSEE
Stuart S. Leicht, M.D.
Chief, Dermatology
East Tennessee State University
Quillen-Dishner College of Medicine
PO Box 21,160A
Johnson City, TN 37614
(615) 928-6426

E. William Rosenberg, M.D.
Chief, Division of Dermatology
University of Tennessee, Memphis
College of Medicine
956 Court Ave., E332
Memphis, TN 38163
(901) 528-5795

T. W. Johnson, M.D.
Head, Division of Dermatology
Meharry Medical College School of Medicine
1005 D. B. Todd Blvd.
Nashville, TN 37207
(615) 327-6111

Lloyd E. King, Jr., M.D., Ph.D.
Director, Dermatology
Vanderbilt University Medical Center
1161 21st Ave., S.
Nashville, TN 37232
(615) 322-6485

TEXAS
Paul Bergstresser, M.D.
Chief, Dermatology
University of Texas Health Science Center at
   Dallas
5323 Harry Hines Blvd.
Dallas, TX 75235
(214) 688-3111

Robert E. Jordon, M.D.
Chairman, Department of Dermatology
University of Texas Health Science Center at
   Houston
PO Box 20708
Houston, TX 77225
(713) 792-2121

Darl Vander Ploeg, M.D.
Chief, Dermatology
University of Texas Health Science Center at
   San Antonio
7703 Floyd Curl Drive
San Antonio, TX 78284
(512) 691-6351

D. P. Posey, M.D.
Chief, Dermatology
Texas A&M University College of Medicine
Scott & White Clinic
Temple, TX 76508
(817) 774-4060

UTAH
Gerald G. Krueger, M.D.
Chief, Dermatology
University of Utah School of Medicine
50 N. Medical Drive
Salt Lake City, UT 84132
(801) 581-7837

VERMONT
Paul A. Krusinski, M.D.
Chief, Dermatology
University of Vermont College of Medicine
Burlington, VT 05405
(802) 656-4570

VIRGINIA
Peyton E. Weary, M.D.
Chairman, Department of Dermatology
University of Virginia Medical Center
Box 134
Charlottesville, VA 22908
(804) 924-0211

W. Kenneth Blaylock, M.D.
Chairman, Dermatology
Medical College of Virginia
MCV Station, Box 565
Richmond, VA 23298
(804) 786-9361

WEST VIRGINIA
Charles L. Yarbrough, M.D.
Chief, Dermatology
Marshall University School of Medicine
Huntington, WV 25701
(304) 529-0900

WISCONSIN
Derek J. Crupps, M.D.
Chief, Dermatology
University of Wisconsin Medical School
University Hospital and Clinics
600 Highland Ave.
Room F4/225
Madison, WI 53706
(608) 263-6230

Thomas J. Russell, M.D.
Chief, Dermatology
Medical College of Wisconsin
9200 W. Wisconsin Ave.
Milwaukee, WI 53226
(414) 259-3855

SOURCE: *Author's survey of medical colleges.*

NOTE TO OUR READERS

We have tried to make sure the names, addresses, and phone numbers of sources in this directory are correct. But we realize changes do occur and that errors in such a vast enterprise have a way of creeping in. We invite readers to note any items that need alteration by writing to Jean Carper, *Health Care U.S.A.*, Prentice Hall Press, Gulf+Western Building, One Gulf+Western Plaza, New York, NY 10023.

ABOUT THE AUTHOR

JEAN CARPER is the author of ten other books on consumer and health subjects and a contributor to numerous national publications, including the *Washington Post* and *Reader's Digest*. She was formerly the Washington medical correspondent for Cable News Network.

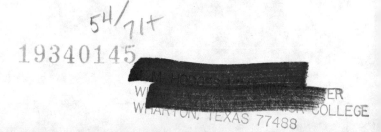